PATIENT CARE IN PLASTIC SURGERY

Bernard M. Barrett, Jr., M.D., F.A.C.S.
Associate Clinical Professor of Plastic Surgery,
Baylor College of Medicine;
Associate Chief of Plastic Surgery,
St. Luke's Episcopal Hospital,
Texas Medical Center,
Houston, Texas

SECOND EDITION

with 102 illustrations

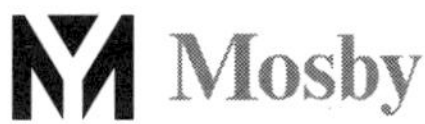

St. Louis Baltimore Boston Carlsbad Chicago Naples New York Philadelphia Portland
London Madrid Mexico City Singapore Sydney Tokyo Toronto Wiesbaden

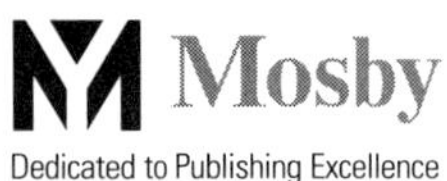

A Times Mirror Company

Publisher: Anne Patterson
Editor: Robert Hurley
Developmental Editor: Christine Pluta
Project Manager: Dana Peick
Production Editor: Dottie Martin
Copy Editors: Dottie Martin, Albert G. Zusman
Designer: Amy Buxton
Manufacturing Manager: J. A. McAllister
Cover art: Cindi Harwood Rose

SECOND EDITION

Printed in the United States of America
Composition by Carlisle Communications, Ltd.
Printing/binding by Maple-Vail Book MFG Group

Mosby-Year Book, Inc.
11830 Westline Industrial Drive
St. Louis, Missouri 63146

Library of Congress Cataloging-in-Publication Data
Patient care in plastic surgery / (edited by) Bernard M. Barrett, Jr.
—2nd ed.
p. cm.
Rev. ed. of: Manual of patient care in plastic surgery. 1982.
Includes bibliographic references and index.
ISBN 0-8151-0563-0 (pbk.)
1. Surgery, Plastic—Handbooks, manuals, etc. 2. Therapeutics, Surgical—Handbooks, manuals, etc. I. Barrett, Bernard M. II. Manual of patient care in plastic surgery.
[DNLM: 1. Surgery, Plastic—handbooks. 2. Preoperative Care—handbooks. 3. Postoperative Care—handbooks. WO 39 P298 1995]
RD118.M375 1995
617.9′5—dc20
DNLM/DLC
for Library of Congress 95-44090
CIP

95 96 97 98 99 / 9 8 7 6 5 4 3 2 1

Contributors

Jerome E. Adamson, M.D.
Professor, Retired,
Department of Plastic and Reconstructive Surgery,
Eastern Virginia Medical School,
Norfolk, Virginia
Chapter 8 **Prevention of Complications**

Joseph Agris, M.D., D.D.S., F.A.C.S.
Clinical Assistant Professor,
Baylor College of Medicine;
The Methodist Hospital;
St. Luke's Episcopal Hospital;
Texas Children's Hospital;
Texas Medical Center,
Houston, Texas
Chapter 39 **Cutaneous Laser Surgery**
Chapter 41 **Pressure Ulcers**

Louis C. Argenta, M.D.
Professor and Chairman,
Bowman Gray School of Medicine;
Professor and Chairman,
Wake Forest University Physicians;
North Carolina Baptist Hospital,
Winston-Salem, North Carolina
Chapter 30 **Tissue Expansion**

Daniel C. Baker, M.D.
Associate Professor of Surgery (Plastic),
New York University;
Attending Surgeon,
Manhattan Eye, Ear & Throat Hospital;
Tisch Hospital,
New York, New York
Chapter 14 **Eyelid Surgery**

James L. Baker, Jr., M.D., F.A.C.S.
Clinical Professor of Plastic Surgery,
University of South Florida;
Adjunct Clinical Professor of Surgery,
University of Central Florida;
Winter Park Hospital;
Florida Hospital;
Orlando Regional Medical Center,
Winter Park, Florida
Chapter 25 **Breast Augmentation and Capsular Contractures**

Thomas J. Baker, M.D., F.A.C.S.
Associate Clinical Professor of Surgery (Plastic),
University of Miami;
Senior Attending Physician,
Mercy Hospital,
Miami, Florida
Chapter 18 **Chemical Peeling and Dermabrasion**

Bernard M. Barrett, Jr., M.D., F.A.C.S.
Associate Clinical Professor of Plastic Surgery,
Baylor College of Medicine;
Associate Chief of Plastic Surgery,
St. Luke's Episcopal Hospital,
Texas Medical Center,
Houston, Texas
Editor
Chapter 1 **Patient Selection**
Chapter 2 **Preoperative Evaluation and Preparation**
Chapter 4 **Postoperative Management**
Chapter 15 **Face- and Neck-Lift**
Chapter 22 **Cleft Lip and Palate**

Craig B. Bass, M.D., F.A.C.S.
Plastic Surgery Centre,
Ketchum, Idaho
Chapter 34 **Burns**

Martin L. Bell, M.D., J.D.
Plastic Surgery Center of Baton Rouge,
Baton Rouge, Louisiana
Chapter 20 **Surgical Hair Restoration**

John Bostwick III, M.D.
Professor of Surgery,
Chairman, Division of Plastic Surgery,
Emory University,
Atlanta, Georgia
Chapter 27 **Breast Reconstruction After Mastecotomy**

Burt D. Brent, M.D.
Associate Clinical Professor,
Stanford University;
El Camino Hospital,
Mountain View, California
Chapter 17 **Auricular Surgery**

Gustavo A. Colon, M.D.
Clinical Professor of Plastic Surgery,
Tulane University,
New Orleans, Louisiana
Chapter 3 **Intraoperative Management**

Denton A. Cooley, M.D.
Clinical Professor of Surgery,
University of Texas Medical School;
Surgeon-in-Chief,
Texas Heart Institute;
St. Luke's Episcopal Hospital,
Houston, Texas
Chapter 9 **Selection and Care of Cardiac Patients for Plastic Surgery**

Stéphane Corriveau, M.D., C.M.
Silver Spring, Maryland
Chapter 24 **Head and Neck Cancer**

John A. Dean, M.D.
Ochsner Clinic of Baton Rouge,
Baton Rouge, Louisiana
Chapter 40 **Genital Surgery**

Tue Anh Dinh, M.D.
Plastic Surgery Resident,
Baylor College of Medicine;
The Methodist Hospital;
St. Luke's Episcopal Hospital;
Texas Children's Hospital,
Houston, Texas
Chapter 38 **Free Tissue Transfer**

Robert A. Ersek, M.D., F.A.C.S.
Assistant Clinical Professor,
School of Health Professions,
Southwest Texas State University,
San Marcos, Texas
Chapter 19 **Injection Surgery**

Jeffrey D. Friedman, M.D.
Assistant Professor,
Baylor College of Medicine;
Clinical Assistant Professor,
M.D. Anderson Cancer Center,
Houston, Texas
Chapter 33 **Hand Surgery**

Frederick M. Grazer, M.D.
Associate Clinical Professor,
Division of Plastic Surgery,
University of California, Irvine;
Clinical Professor of Surgery,
Penn State University;
Hershey Medical Center;
College of Medicine,
Hershey, Pennsylvania
Chapter 31 **Excisional Body Contour Surgery**

F. Parker Gregg, M.D.
Clinical Assistant Professor of Radiology,
Baylor College of Medicine;
The Texas Heart Institute;
St. Luke's Episcopal Hospital,
Houston, Texas
Chapter 29 **Mammography in Aesthetic and Reconstructive Breast Surgery**

Robert J. Hall, M.D.
Director of Education, Cardiology,
Texas Heart Institute;
St. Luke's Episcopal Hospital,
Houston, Texas
Chapter 9 **Selection and Care of Cardiac Patients for Plastic Surgery**

Clifton Hebert, M.D.
Director of Acute Postoperative Pain Service,
St. Luke's Episcopal Hospital,
Houston, Texas
Chapter 5 **Anesthesia for Plastic Surgery**

Howard Heppe, M.D.
Mary Washington Hospital,
Fredericksburg, Virginia
Chapter 28 **Nipple-Areola Reconstruction**

Terri L. Hill, M.D.
Clinical Instructor,
University of Maryland,
College Park, Maryland
Chapter 23 **Craniofacial Surgery**

Charles E. Horton, M.D.
Professor of Plastic Surgery,
Eastern Virginia Medical School,
Norfolk, Virginia
Chapter 40 **Genital Surgery**

Charles E. Horton, Jr., M.D.
Assistant Professor of Urology,
Eastern Virginia Medical School;
Sentara Norfolk General Hospital,
Children's Hospital of the King's Daughters,
Norfolk, Virginia
Chapter 40 **Genital Surgery**

Benjamin H. Johnson III, M.D.
Assistant Clinical Instructor,
University of Alabama,
Birmingham, Alabama
Chapter 27 **Breast Reconstruction After Mastectomy**

Fred B. Kessler, M.D.
Clinical Professor of Plastic Surgery,
Chief of Hand Surgery,
Baylor College of Medicine;
Plastic Surgery Division,
St. Luke's Episcopal Hospital;
Texas Children's Hospital,
Houston, Texas
Chapter 33 **Hand Surgery**

Tareq Obaid Khan, M.D.
Chief of Service,
Department of Anesthesiology,
St. Luke's Episcopal Hospital,
Houston, Texas
Chapter 5 **Anesthesia for Plastic Surgery**

Malcolm A. Lesavoy, M.D.
Chief, Plastic and Reconstructive Surgery,
Harbor General Hospital;
Professor of Surgery,
Division of Plastic Surgery,
University of California—Los Angeles Medical Center,
Los Angeles, California
Chapter 37 **Microsurgery**

William P. Magee, Jr., D.D.S., M.D., F.A.C.S.
Associate Professor,
Eastern Virginia Medical School;
Chief, Department of Plastic Surgery,
Children's Hospital of the King's Daughters,
Norfolk, Virginia
Chapter 24 **Head and Neck Cancer**

Christina Mathis
Certified Operating Room Technician,
Houston, Texas
Chapter 6 **Plastic Surgical Nursing**

John B. McCraw, M.D.
Professor of Plastic Surgery,
Eastern Virginia Medical School,
Norfolk, Virginia
Chapter 36 **Myocutaneous Flaps**

Paul K. McKissock, M.D.
Clinical Professor of Plastic Surgery,
U.C.L.A. School of Medicine,
Los Angeles, California
Chapter 26 **Reduction Mammaplasty**

John D. Milam, M.D.
Professor, Pathology and Laboratory Medicine,
University of Texas-Houston Medical School;
Medical Director, Laboratory Services,
Hermann Hospital,
Houston, Texas
Chapter 7 **Transfusion Therapy**

D. Ralph Millard, Jr., M.D., F.A.C.S.
Light-Millard Professor of Plastic Surgery,
University of Miami;
Jackson Memorial Hospital;
Miami Children's Hospital,
Miami, Florida
Foreword
Chapter 22 **Cleft Lip and Palate**

Richard A. Mladick, M.D., F.A.C.S.
Director, Center for Cosmetic Plastic Surgery,
Virginia Beach, Virginia
Chapter 32 **Lipoplasty**

John H. Moore, Jr., M.D.
Clinical Associate Professor of Surgery (Plastic),
Thomas Jefferson University;
Consulting Staff,
Magee Rehabilitation Hospital,
Philadelphia, Pennsylvania
Chapter 36 **Myocutaneous Flaps**

Ross H. Musgrave, M.D., F.A.C.S.
Clinical Professor of Surgery (Plastic),
University of Pittsburgh;
Executive Director,
University of Pittsburgh Medical Alumni Association,
Pittsburgh, Pennsylvania
Introduction

Lewis J. Obi, M.D., F.R.S.A.
The Obi Plastic Surgery Clinic,
Jacksonville, Florida
Chapter 2 **Preoperative Evaluation and Preparation**
Chapter 4 **Postoperative Management**
Chapter 18 **Chemical Peeling and Dermabrasion**

Donald H. Parks, M.D., F.R.C.S.(C.), F.A.C.S.
Professor and Chairman,
Department of Plastic and Reconstructive Surgery,
University of Texas Medical School;
Chief, Plastic and Reconstructive Surgery,
Hermann Hospital;
Lyndon B. Johnson General Hospital,
Houston, Texas
Chapter 34 **Burns**

John G. Penn, M.D., F.R.C.S.(Ed.)
Plastic Surgeon,
Winter Park Memorial Hospital,
Winter Park, Florida
Chapter 35 **Skin Grafts and Skin Flaps**

Arthur H. Rathjen, Sr.
Director, Medical-Professional Liaison,
Dow Corning Corporation,
Midland, Michigan
Chapter 10 **Medical Photography**

Thomas D. Rees, M.D.
Clinical Professor of Surgery,
New York University Medical Center;
Chairman Emeritus, Department of Plastic Surgery,
Manhattan Eye, Ear, & Throat Hospital;
Attending Surgeon,
University Hospital—Bellevue Medical Center,
New York, New York
Chapter 14 **Eyelid Surgery**

William B. Riley, Jr., M.D., F.A.C.S.
Clinical Professor of Surgery,
University of Texas Health Science Center;
Baylor College of Medicine;
Houston, Texas
Chapter 13 **Wound Healing and Problem Scars**

Franklin A. Rose, M.D.
Private Practice,
Houston, Texas
Chapter 2 **Preoperative Evaluation and Preparation**

Richard C. Schultz, M.D.
Clinical Professor of Surgery,
University of Illinois College of Medicine at Chicago;
Active Staff,
Lutheran General Hospital,
Chicago, Illinois
Chapter 21 **Maxillofacial Injuries**

Jack H. Sheen, M.D.
Clinical Professor of Plastic Surgery,
University of Southern California;
Clinical Associate Professor of Plastic Surgery,
University of California,
Los Angeles, California
Chapter 16 **Rhinoplasty and Mentoplasty**

Saleh M. Shenaq, M.D.
Professor of Plastic Surgery,
Chief of Microsurgery,
Baylor College of Medicine;
The Methodist Hospital;
St. Luke's Episcopal Hospital,
Houston, Texas
Chapter 37 **Microsurgery**
Chapter 38 **Free Tissue Transfer**

Scott L. Spear, M.D.
Professor of Plastic Surgery,
Director, Division of Plastic Surgery,
Georgetown University,
Washington, District of Columbia
Chapter 28 **Nipple-Areola Reconstruction**

Thomas Ray Vecchione, M.D.
Clinical Associate Professor of Plastic Surgery,
University of California,
San Diego, California
Chapter 12 **Lacerations**

William Dixon Wiles, J.D.
Attorney,
Dallas, Texas
Chapter 11 **Medicolegal Considerations**

S. Anthony Wolfe, M.D.
Clinical Professor,
Department of Plastic and Reconstructive Surgery,
University of Miami,
Miami, Florida
Chapter 23 **Craniofacial Surgery**

W. Graham Wood, M.D.
Clinical Assistant Professor of Surgery,
Division of Plastic and Reconstructive Surgery,
University of Southern California,
Los Angeles, California;
Medical Director,
Corona del Mar Surgery Center, Inc.,
Corona del Mar, California
Chapter 31 **Excisional Body Contour Surgery**

To Doctors D. Ralph Millard, Jr., Denton A. Cooley, Paul K. McKissock, Michael E. DeBakey, Melvin Spira, and the late Sir Hedley Atkins, K.B.E., who taught me surgery and inspired me in life,

and

to Julia, Beverly, Julie, Audrey, and Bart—each a source of great joy and happiness.

Foreword

In all surgery, and particularly in plastic and reconstructive surgery, patient care is vital.

The presurgical preparation and planning are often as important as the surgery itself. Before any sound plan of treatment can be outlined, it is essential that the plastic surgeon gain insight into the patient's true desires. This may be accomplished during the first consultation or it may require additional meetings with the patient. Of course the "ideal, beautiful normal" is usually the desire of the patient and the goal of the surgeon, but this end point is not always a possibility. Once the surgeon understands the patient's desires, the surgeon can estimate the probability of success of the surgery from personal experience. It is important that the surgeon discuss this carefully with the patient.

The postoperative follow-up can mean the difference between success and failure. Too often this care is partially ignored or taken for granted. Many of the great surgeons that I had the privilege of training with in my early years left the postoperative dressings or splint to the resident surgeon. I never do, and our residents are taught to apply their own. It is felt that the pressure dressing or the nasal splint are almost as important as key sutures and should be applied personally to make certain they are not only placed correctly but are also accomplishing the aid to healing that is their prime purpose.

Bernard M. Barrett, Jr., has focused the center ring light on preoperative, operative, and postoperative patient care—subjects often relegated to side rings. With the skilled whip hand of a circus master, he has collected an impressive array of temperamental stars: Lipizzaners, Kodiacs, lions, tigers, cheetahs, and Chihuahuas. We are indebted to Dr. Barrett for getting so many experts together and for coordinating them so their contributions bring close and instructive scrutiny of the *art of patient care.*

D. Ralph Millard, Jr., M.D., F.A.C.S.

Foreword *to the First Edition*

In all surgery and particularly in plastic and reconstructive surgery, patient care is vital. The presurgical preparation and planning are often as important as the surgery itself. The postoperative follow-up can mean the difference between success and failure. Too often this care is partially ignored or taken for granted.

Bernard M. Barrett, Jr., with the combined charm, gall and acumen of a whip-handed circus master, has adroitly corralled into one large side tent an astonishing array of temperamental star performers—gymnasts, riders, trainers, Lipizzaners, Kodiacs, lions, tigers, cheetahs, and Chihuahuas. We are all indebted to him for getting so many experts together and keeping them from biting each other or him. Obviously it has not been easy. Here are just two random reports of his many ploys to edit a winner.

1) As 12 players had received emergency medical care during the regular season Houston-Pittsburgh game, when they travelled to Pittsburgh for the play-offs, Barrett accompanied the Oilers as a "suture between rounds" consultant. Being unlicensed in Pennsylvania, he prevailed on the Steelers No. 1 plastic surgery fan to arrange hospital privileges in case of an emergency. There were no emergencies and as the Steelers annihilated the Oilers in 25-degree weather with snow, slush and ten inches of watery ice on the field, the No. 1 Pittsburgh fan could not find it in his heart to add insult to injury. He agreed to write an introduction on judgment.

2) When one of the California stars was requested to contribute a chapter he puffed on his cigar and refused explaining he was writing his own text, lecturing all over the world and just too busy. He did admit his only scheduled relaxation was planned in Hawaii. Barrett immediately volunteered to meet him in Kona Village with a tape recorder. In fact he extracted the chapter in a thatched hut with the surf breaking in the background. The dictation was interrupted occasionally for a sortie on to the tennis court, where Barrett gracefully accepted several early game losses in order to keep another of his star performers contentedly performing.

Barrett is to be commended for turning what is often unfortunately relegated to sideshow status into a fully lighted center ring event and thus directing our attention to important aspects in patient care which can mean all the difference to us and our patients.

D. Ralph Millard, Jr., M.D., F.A.C.S.

Preface

Our purpose in writing *Patient Care in Plastic Surgery,* second edition, is to offer the reader practical advice for preoperative, operative, and postoperative care of plastic and reconstructive surgery patients. These recommendations for treatments have proved successful for each of the authors during many years of medical practice and teaching.

It is not intended that this book be an encyclopedia or attempt to set standards for plastic surgery care but rather that it provide guidelines and suggestions for physicians, nurses, and medical staff involved in the broad speciality of plastic surgery, ranging from lacerations to craniofacial surgery, burns to face-lifts, microsurgery to transfusions, medical photography to medicolegal considerations.

It is hoped that the appeal of this text should be not only for plastic surgeons, especially younger surgeons and physicians in training, but also for many other physicians and health professionals who deal with the ever-expanding range of included topics.

The distinguished contributing authors all possess special expertise in patient care and have contributed extensively to medical literature. A number of them have published texts of their own. Selected references, many of them texts written by the contributing authors themselves, are listed at the end of specific chapters for those desiring enhancement of their knowledge of plastic and reconstructive surgery.

The plastic surgeon, perhaps more than other physicians, should use unlimited imagination, skills, and judgment to achieve an ideal result for each patient. Plastic surgery patients appreciate our attention to subtle detail. I hope this second edition will provide each of its readers with more helpful information for obtaining safety and near perfection in patient care.

B.B.

Acknowledgments

My special thanks to each of the 53 outstanding contributing authors who generously gave their valuable knowledge in plastic surgery care for the second edition of this book.

Fortunately, each of the actively practicing plastic surgeons who contributed to the first edition of *Patient Care in Plastic Surgery* as primary chapter authors graciously repeated their efforts to make the second edition even more comprehensive and up-to-date.

Amongst the brilliant stars who contributed to this text are three presidents of the American Society of Plastic and Reconstructive Surgeons: Bill Riley, Jerry Adamson, and Ross Musgrave. Ralph Millard has served as president of the American Association of Plastic Surgeons; Millard, Charlie Horton, and Mal Lesavoy have been presidents of the Plastic Surgery Educational Foundation. Tony Wolfe and Richard Schultz have each served as president of the American Society of Maxillofacial Surgeons. Charlie Horton, Tom Rees, Tom Baker, and Jim Baker are all Aesthetic Society presidents; Gus Colon is president-elect. Gus Colon and Fred Grazer have each been president of the American Association for Accreditation of Ambulatory Plastic Surgery Facilities. Dick Mladick is a former Lipoplasty Society president.

Amongst our contributors are three honorary fellows in the Royal College of Surgeons: heart surgeon extraordinaire Denton Cooley, Ralph Millard, and Charlie Horton. Julia and I were fortunate enough to be present at the White House luncheon ceremony when Denton Cooley received the Presidential Medal of Freedom, America's highest civilian award, from President Ronald Reagan.

A very special thanks to Jacksonville's Lew Obi, who authored three chapters for this text and offered many helpful suggestions throughout its production. Thank you Sal Shenaq and Joe Agris for authoring two chapters each.

The 26 new contributing authors to this second edition are all talented surgeons and teachers. They are carrying forward the proud traditions of the original authors, including four colleagues who passed away: Reed Dingman, Paul Natvig, Jerry Klingbeil, and Jaime Caffarena. Amongst the several authors who no longer practice surgery today are "giants" Tom Rees, Paul McKissock, Jerry Adamson, and Ross Musgrave.

Acknowledgments

A sincere debt of gratitude is expressed to the men who inspired and guided my surgical education and to whom, along with my family, this book is dedicated. My father, Bernard Barrett, Sr., and grandfather, Mozart Lischkoff, were both exemplary physicians and early role models for me while growing up in Pensacola, Florida.

Kathy O'Brien Adjemian deserves a special thank you for skillfully editing both this edition and the original. Kathy worked heroically with diligent focus while undergoing surgery, radiation, and chemotherapy to conquer breast cancer. She is an inspiration to all of us.

Very special recognition and appreciation are also extended to Teri Duncan and Teri Carstens who typed, retyped, and rearranged these pages. Each contributing author had a personal team of office assistants to help with the chapters—to these individuals I express my sincere gratitude.

Fourteen contributing authors are Texas Medical Center colleagues in Houston. St. Luke's Hospital radiology chairman Milton Gray coordinated with Parker Gregg for a specialized radiology chapter. Outpatient surgery director Ale Temple provided material for sections on outpatient surgery.

I am especially grateful to Mosby Executive Editor Robert Hurley for publishing this second edition of *Patient Care in Plastic Surgery.* Associate Developmental Editor Christine Pluta helped keep this project moving forward. Special thanks to Dottie Martin, production editor; Amy Buxton, designer, for her terrific cover design; and Cindi Harwood Rose, who skillfully created the silhouette that appears on the cover. Retired editor Fred Belliveau is deeply appreciated for suggesting that I write the first edition and this second of *Patient Care in Plastic Surgery.*

Finally, my sincere thanks to my medical colleagues and patients whose ideas, ideals, and examples have provided valuable material for this text.

B.B.

Introduction: Plastic Surgical Judgment

Ross H. Musgrave

While an old Pennsylvania Dutch expression asserts "we grow too soon old and too late smart," some long forgotten sage wrote along the same line "experience comes with age, which is the time it does you the least good." In almost all areas of endeavor, experience can and frequently does compensate for talent or for book knowledge or for specialized training, whether this be for a football letterman, a 747 pilot, a gourmet chef, or even a plastic surgeon. Approximately 35 years ago, a close surgical colleague visited some primitive hospitals in Africa and observed young surgical technicians (originally, male nurses) who had been taught to do technically good surgery in months rather than the years of internship, residency, and fellowship training common in most civilized areas of the world. He observed that these bright native youths were taught "how to," but not much attention was given to "when to" or even more important, "when *not* to" operate. (These decisions were made by a supervising chief of surgery.)

Unfortunately, in most of the residency programs in plastic surgery, much of the time is spent in teaching the young trainee how to handle tissues properly, how to apply a dressing, how to suture, how to graft, how to delay a flap and transfer it, but very little time is ever spent on patient selection. It is just assumed that the newcomer to the field of plastic surgery will somehow absorb this from the seniors and that with the passage of time, he or she will have gained sufficient experience to pick out good candidates from the bad, select those elective surgery patients whose chances for a good result are better than the borderline patient-candidate, and somehow develop a sixth sense for spotting potentially troublesome patients. Unfortunately, residency programs are frequently so jam-packed with both private and semiprivate patients that the eager resident, dealing with a lesser volume of clinic patients, is willing to gamble that a certain otherwise borderline patient will somehow get a decent result and be a satisfied man or woman. The same surgeon, 5 years later, would in many instances turn down an identical borderline patient. How does all this change in attitude come about? Does the maturing surgeon have to make the same errors in selection that the predecessors did? I am not sure anyone has the finite answer, but for most practicing plastic surgeons, patient selection seems to become more conservative with each passing year.

Unfortunately, careful patient selection can sometimes take a distant backseat to the exigencies of a booming office practice. We all know surgeons who have developed such a burgeoning practice, constructing elaborate offices and operating rooms, adding associates and physician assistants, operating room nurses, cosmetic consultants, and business advisors ad nauseam, so that the surgeon-entrepreneur has to keep working like the squirrel on the perennial treadmill just to keep even with this gigantic financial overhead. When this occurs unfortunately some of the well-balanced conservatism that came with the physician's improving judgment in the first 4 or 5 years of practice all somehow goes out the window, and this overcommitted surgeon tends to schedule anybody who wanders in the front door.

It was disheartening to see and hear on television of the unfortunate patients who had been somehow gulled into plastic surgical procedures as a result of advertising by some less than completely trained but self-labeled "plastic surgeons." In these instances, patients were led to believe (by clever advertising) that their lives would be happier and brighter and success would be theirs if they only had a better nose or less jowl or larger bosoms. Unfortunately, even in the absence of enticing newspaper ads, word-of-mouth in certain social circles brings some of the same sort of less than ideal patients to the busy practicing plastic surgeon's office. It is always flattering for the surgeon to find from a prospective patient that Mrs. A and Miss B and Mr. C were all thoroughly delighted with the surgery they had received from him or her. Many patients are not above a little apple-polishing and cajoling to get the surgeon to agree to carry out a particular operative procedure for which the patient may not be a suitable candidate. If there is an opening on the schedule and the financial-overhead clock is ticking away, it can be ever so tempting to schedule the procedure and keep one's fingers crossed that the surgery *will* somehow turn out satisfactorily (with little attention paid to the possibilities of its *not* turning out so well) and that the patient *will* be satisfied.

When I was still a struggling resident more than 40 years ago, the late Gustave Aufricht told me one evening at a dinner party that the most difficult thing I would ever have to learn in plastic surgery was how to say "No." How right he was! It took me a number of years to realize that just because a patient had a "correctable deformity" and that I, the surgeon, knew how to do a procedure to correct it was no reason that I had to be the catalyst who would bring the two elements (sometimes cataclysmically) together.

In 1974 Mark Gorney wrote: "It is vital for plastic surgeons to understand that ours is a very unique situation. We are dealing with deformities which are inextricably linked with emotional factors, and the only possible improvement in our lot can come from thorough preoperative screening and patient selection." I couldn't agree more heartily with this statement. But how does one with limited experience decide which is the "bad" candidate for elective surgery? There is, of course, the time-honored trial-and-error method. There is the perceptor-preceptee method, wherein a young man or woman working with an older surgeon can observe at first-hand crafty and shrewd patient selection (which is frequently an art). (The older and more experienced plastic surgeon frequently will have developed a sixth sense as to which patient to turn down.)

Dr. Robert Goldwyn a few years ago published the following list of potential problem patients:

1. The perfectionist patient
2. The shopper
3. The plastisurgiholic: the seeker or bearer of multiple operations
4. The acquiescing patient
5. The paranoid or depressed patient
6. The patient with a recent loss
7. The patient in psychotherapy
8. The male patient
9. The patient whom you do not like
10. The special patient (a VIP in whose case surgical judgment may defer to status)
11. The patient who writes an excessively long letter to arrange the initial consultation
12. The rude or pushy patient
13. The unkempt patient
14. The patient who makes your office his or her home
15. The patient who praises you excessively and denigrates colleagues
16. The patient who hides the fact that he or she is under some form of treatment, either mental or somatic
17. The indecisive or vague patient
18. The patient with minimal deformity
19. The patient who refuses to undress for proper examination
20. The patient who does not wish to be photographed

That is quite a list. In addition to the patients whom Goldwyn described, I should like to add some other problem patients who I often feel should be turned down or at least approached with some skepticism. (For even the most inexperienced physician or resident, the obvious "crocks" are relatively easy to spot and reject, and so we won't devote space to them.) In the case of the shady, gray-zone patient, frequently an affluent person's or prominent official's wife, or even a physician's wife, the decision of whether to do or not to do elective surgery gets a little more sticky. Be extremely cautious about doing surgery to satisfy someone other than the patient. For instance, be cautious about doing a face-lift on an attractive elderly woman who is contemplating surgery only because her husband is distressed by her wrinkles and wants her to look like the gal he married 39 years ago and *not* because she particularly desires a face-lift. Likewise, be cautious about doing an otoplasty on the rebellious, belligerent lad whose parents are attempting to force this procedure on him because of their own inherent parental guilt feelings. Also be wary of the 17-year-old girl who really is not very upset about the little hump in her nose, but whose mother had had a rhinoplasty at age 17 and now insists that her daughter have a similar operation in order to make her, the daughter, more eligible in the current marriage market.

Also be very careful about the patient who is seeking elective cosmetic surgery in order to either save a marriage or a love affair. Remember: "The most skillfully wielded scalpel cannot overcome a once-sharp Cupid's arrow long since dulled by infidelity or boredom." This situation may be a little difficult to ferret out, but with a good interviewing technique, it often is right there, almost staring one in the face.

Be particularly wary of the patient who never lets you finish a sentence and keeps interrupting before you finish explaining a possible complication or a particular technique. Beware of the patient who only wants to hear "the good things" and does not want to hear about anything that might even be considered a possible complication. That patient has both selective hearing *and* selective cerebration!

Also be wary of the patient who is a plain Jane (particularly an older plain Jane), who wants to be tightened up in order to "look gorgeous." Most experienced plastic surgeons would candidly admit that a face-lift has never yet made anybody handsome or beautiful if they didn't have good bones and were handsome to begin with (unlike a rhinoplasty or a chin implant). If the patient is realistic and you, the surgeon, are completely candid, you probably will have no trouble, *but* be certain she knows that what you're about to do surgically will be making her appear less tired and less wrinkled but *not* necessarily beautiful.

Incidentally, there are particular surgeons who seem to attract borderline candidates for elective cosmetic surgery. After a recent presentation about patient selection in which I discussed most of the above items, a noted Hollywood plastic surgeon told me that if he were to eliminate the patients described above as troublesome or worrisome, he wouldn't have any practice left! This man is an extremely talented, experienced surgeon, and in a high percentage of cases perhaps can get away with an occasional less than smashing or less than satisfactory result by later explaining to the patient that he or she wasn't particularly a good healer, or turned out to have poor muscle tone, or had had an unexpected infection, or an unfortunate amount of edema. Not every surgeon has *his* charisma or fame.

Surprisingly, there seem to be surgeons, not only in plastic surgery but in other areas, who seem to get a little extra thrill out of living on the brink of disaster. They get a certain vicarious thrill from pulling off successfully a procedure or operation that some of their colleagues would have eschewed. This practice of living dangerously, although frequently exhilarating and more frequently financially successful, cannot begin to compensate for the certain percentage of failures (albeit a small percentage) that are bound to happen when the patient selected for elective surgery was ill chosen and that particular procedure ill advised. Perhaps a subconscious "macho" self-image makes any number of plastic surgeons literally *unable* to say "No" to a prospective patient (particularly an affluent patient).

Several decades ago in the famed Rodgers and Hammerstein Broadway hit musical, "Oklahoma!," Ado Annie stopped the show each night by singing, "I'm Just a Gal Who Cain't Say No." But at least she wasn't charging—and in advance, yet! Unfortunately, we all know plastic surgeons who *are* Ado Annies!

I constantly tell my residents and young plastic surgeons with whom I come in contact that in the field of aesthetic elective surgery all plastic surgery is a trade-off. Furthermore, if the patients don't know what they are trading for, then they shouldn't trade. It is up to you, the surgeon, to inform them.

I, furthermore, have one additional aphorism that follows the same line of reasoning that I give the borderline elective surgery patients—"If in doubt, don't." It will really save you many headaches, add years to the life of your coronary vessels, and protect you from the trials and tribulations of patient dissatisfaction and either threatened or actual litigation.

I tell my residents that I earn my living by the patients I operate upon, but I earn my reputation by the patients I refuse to operate upon.

Contents

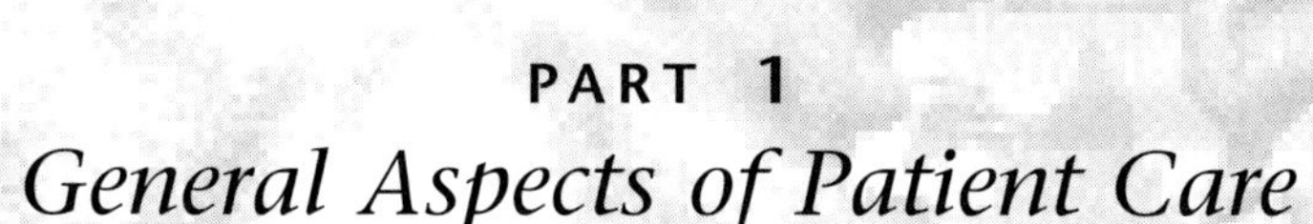

PART 1
General Aspects of Patient Care

CHAPTER 1

Patient Selection

Bernard M. Barrett, Jr.

Now more than ever, patients expect the results of surgical treatment to be aesthetically pleasing as well as functionally correct. Owing to this greater demand and growing patient expectations, plastic surgeons have become increasingly involved in providing an expanding variety of patient care. Carefully selected cardiac and cancer patients—who previously may have been denied the benefits of plastic surgery—are now being accepted as candidates for plastic surgery (See Chapter 9.). Decisions as to when, where, how, and upon whom to perform plastic and reconstructive surgery must be made logically, with the patient's well-being as the primary concern.

TRAUMA

Occasionally the plastic surgeon may be the only physician involved in the initial care of patients who have been victims of life-threatening emergencies. Patient "selection" does not realistically exist when the plastic surgeon is the only physician available to treat trauma. However, in most circumstances the plastic surgeon is an essential member of the critical care team, which usually includes general surgeons, neurosurgeons, orthopedists, emergency room specialists, and other experts of trauma. In both situations, the plastic surgeon should offer the expertise and special skills necessary to the immediate or delayed treatment of traumatic deformities.

Decision for Immediate versus Delayed Plastic Surgery

Depending on the severity and the etiology of the patient's injuries one can base a decision as to whether to perform immediate or delayed plastic surgery on the following considerations:

A. **Patient's general condition and prognosis.** The first step in making this determination is the taking of a complete health history and the performance of a thorough physical examination. When the patient's general condition is good and the prognosis is favorable for normal recovery, injuries such as lacerations should be treated immediately to lower the chance of infection and decrease morbidity (See Chapter 13.). When the patient's condition and prognosis are poor, nonessential surgery, such as the treatment of a simple nasal fracture, could reasonably be delayed.

B. **Severity and location of major life-threatening injuries.** A patient with multiple trauma who requires immediate, lifesaving surgery may benefit from simultaneous reconstructive surgery if it can be provided without interfering with the essential surgery. For example, when a patient with serious trauma in the thorax or abdomen responds well to treatment, lesser injuries on the face or extremities can be treated concomitantly.

C. **Reconstructive plastic surgery necessary to save patient's life.** A major head or neck injury obstructing an airway or causing severe hemorrhage must be corrected immediately if the patient is to survive. The first priority is the relief of an obstructed airway. Control of hemorrhage and maintenance of cardiac output follow closely in importance.

D. **Additional injuries that may benefit from immediate plastic surgery.** For example, a lacerated tendon could be repaired while the patient is anesthetized for treatment of another traumatic injury.

E. **Time interval from onset of injuries until treatment can be provided safely and effectively.** If many hours have elapsed and excessive edema or obvious infection are already present, it is better to delay nonessential plastic surgical repairs. Details are provided in the following chapters dealing with patient care in specific types of plastic surgery.

Procedures for Immediate Surgery

Once the decision is made to provide immediate plastic surgical care of traumatic injuries, the following steps should be taken:

- Irrigate and débride open contaminated wounds. Normal saline under pressure will mechanically remove gross and microscopic debris while lowering the bacterial count.
- Resect nonviable tissues. Dead tissue that has not been removed provides a ready culture medium for bacterial infection.
- Suture displaced tissues into normal position (an important Gillies and Millard principle). By lining up the normal anatomic landmarks, the surgeon can accurately assess what is missing and how it might be replaced.
- Stabilize fractures. As a rule, bone heals more quickly and accurately when the fragments are held together.
- Give appropriate antibiotic therapy. Initially, clinical judgment will dictate the use of either penicillin or a broad-spectrum antibiotic for prevention of streptococcal or other infections. Cultures of open wounds, with sensitivities, will specify the appropriate antibiotics.
- Provide tetanus prophylaxis. Tetanus toxoid, given at 0.5 ml, is the usual dose for children or adults. Tetanus immune globulin and tetanus toxoid should be administered to a patient who has not been immunized previously.
- Begin rehabilitation and physical therapy as quickly as possible. As specified in Chapters 4 and 33, early mobilization is essential for optimal return of function.

RECONSTRUCTIVE SURGERY

Reconstructive surgery is available for the later correction of congenital defects, traumatic deformities, or cancer disfigurements. Patient selection here is based on the following considerations:

Patient's Goals, Desires, and Prognosis

For example, breast reconstruction can be performed on a patient free of metastatic disease. A woman with liver or bone metastasis and failing health would benefit little from this operation (See Chapter 27.).

Family's Requests and Valid Expectations

For example, the parents of an infant with a cleft lip may urge the surgeon to make immediate surgical correction. The guidelines given in Chapter 22 should be followed to obtain optimal results. The family should be made to understand that multiple procedures often are required to achieve an acceptable result.

Surgeon's Judgment

The surgeon should estimate whether the possible gains from reconstructive surgery are greater than the possible losses that could result from complications. This is especially true when previous reconstructive procedures have been attempted and their results were less than ideal. The presence of old scarring or radiation injury with decreased blood supply can lead to further problems.

Surgeon's Technical Skills and Individual Abilities

This assessment is probably the most difficult to make. The surgeon must ask oneself, "Do I possess the special skills necessary for successful microsurgical anastomoses, or is it better for the patient's care to call in a more experienced microsurgeon?" An honest assessment of one's abilities must be the guiding policy.

AESTHETIC SURGERY

When the surgeon evaluates a candidate for aesthetic surgery, the following questions must be considered:

- ▼ Are there any medical contraindications to surgery?
- ▼ Does the patient have a realistic understanding of the anticipated surgical gains and a reasonable expectation of the desired results?
- ▼ Does the patient exhibit any psychologic or emotional problems that could interfere with a normal postoperative recovery?
- ▼ Is the request for surgery coming from the patient or from a relative or friend exerting undue influence? (Except for small children with deformities, operate only if the patient is the one who desires the surgery.)

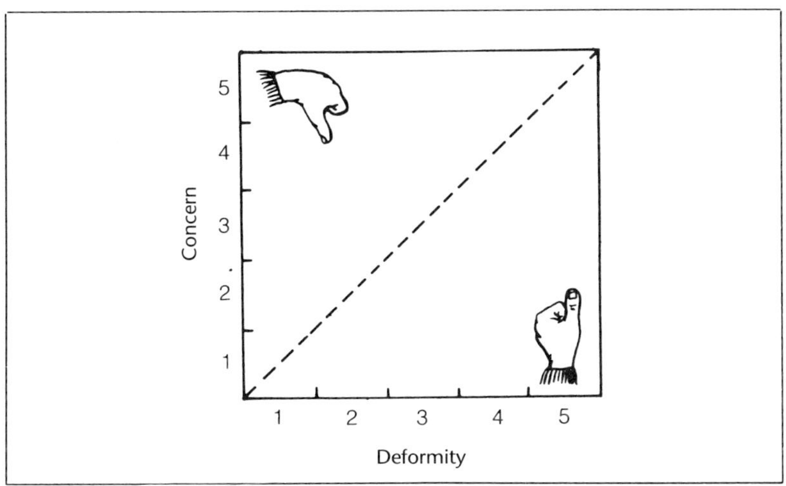

FIG. 1-1 *Gorney chart for selection of patients for elective surgery.*

▼ Does the surgeon have the technical expertise and artistic judgment necessary to satisfy the patient's desires?

Mark Gorney of San Francisco has devised a valuable graph for patient selection that measures the degree of patient concern against the amount of anatomic deformity (Fig. 1-1). The surgeon assesses the anatomic deformity on a scale of one to five. Five is the highest degree of deformity. The patient's concern about the deformity is then evaluated using the same scale. Five represents an unusual degree of concern. These two factors are plotted on the graph. If the patient has a high degree of deformity and a low degree of concern for the deformity, the patient is a good surgical candidate. A bad surgical candidate is one who has a high degree of concern about a small anatomic deformity. This patient may be displeased with any results from plastic surgery.

OUTPATIENT SURGERY

Quality of Surgery

A plastic surgeon with a general plastic surgical practice may perform more than 90% of surgery in an outpatient surgical facility because the quality of patient care and surgical practice are maintained with less time and inconvenience, and lengthy health history and physical examinations, hospital rounds, orders, and discharge summaries are reduced to a minimum. Growing acceptance of this practice by patients has significantly influenced the success of ambulatory surgical care. Surveys have found that more than 90% of patients are pleased with the outpatient surgical experience and that 95% prefer it to overnight hospitalization. There is little doubt that convalescence at home is less traumatic to pediatric patients and to many adults than is hospitalization. Insurance carriers have begun to realize the savings possible with outpatient surgery. Costs for a given procedure are often 40% to 60% lower when it is performed on an ambulatory basis.

Selection Criteria

For most patients, outpatient surgical selection is based in great part on the American Society of Anesthesiologists (ASA) physical status classification:

A. **Class 1:** Patients with no organic, physiologic, biochemical, or psychiatric disturbance (e.g., an inguinal hernia in an otherwise healthy patient)

B. **Class 2:**

   - Mild to moderate systemic disturbance caused either by the condition to be treated surgically or by other pathophysiologic processes, such as the presence of mild diabetes or essential hypertension
   - Extremes of age although no discernible systemic disease is present (e.g., neonates or octogenarians)
   - Moderately severe obesity or chronic bronchitis

C. **Class 3:** Severe systemic disturbances or pathologic processes from any cause, such as severe diabetes, moderate to severe pulmonary insufficiency, angina pectoris, or a healed myocardial infarction within six months

A patient in class 1 is acceptable for outpatient surgery. A patient in class 2 may be scheduled after consultation with, and approval of, the patient's internist or anesthesiologist. A patient in class 3 and beyond usually is not accepted for outpatient surgery.

POSSIBLE RISKS AND COMPLICATIONS

The surgeon should always inform the patient of possible risks and complications of surgery; these risks include, but are not limited to, bleeding, infection, severe scar formation, neurologic weakness, numbness, and death. Finally, when deciding whether to schedule a patient for surgery, one must ask oneself these two important questions:

- ▼ If I or a member of my family were in a similar circumstance, would I want this particular operation to be performed? (If the answer is no, do not operate.)
- ▼ Is the surgical candidate capable of coping with a complication if one were to arise? (If the answer is no, do not operate.)

The wise plastic surgeon is the one who knows upon whom *not* to operate. This statement is not meant to imply that surgical skills should be withheld from suitable candidates. Remember, however, when a question arises about the patient's need or desire for plastic surgery, it is wiser to wait (Gillies and Millard's last commandment).

CHAPTER 2

Preoperative Evaluation and Preparation

Lewis J. Obi, Bernard M. Barrett, Jr., and Franklin A. Rose

Evaluation and preparation of patients for plastic surgical procedures varies according to the type of procedure to be performed. Requirements for specific procedures are discussed in many of the chapters in Section II. This chapter discusses general aspects of preoperative evaluation and preparation. An organized approach to preoperative evaluation and preparation will provide the plastic surgeon with a basic rationale for managing each patient.

Safety, compassion, and empathy should be integral parts of the surgeon's handling of all patients anticipating surgery. Physicians should recall their psychologic state before any surgery they may have had to undergo. Regression to infantile behavior occurs in varying degrees in most preoperative patients. This regression is expressed in the form of anxiety, and it may be minimized if preoperative evaluation and preparation are well planned and smoothly executed. Favorable intraoperative and postoperative courses for the patient are determined not only by events during surgery but also by careful preoperative evaluation, screening, and patient selection.

PATIENT MOTIVATION AND EXPECTATIONS

Initial Meeting

The initial meeting of a plastic surgeon with the patient is one of the more important events of the surgeon-patient relationship. Both surgeon and patient are evaluating each other's conduct. The patient usually has a specific complaint or a set of complaints, and the plastic surgeon evaluates not only these complaints but also the general physical makeup of the patient. At the same time, the plastic surgeon should evaluate the patient's motivation for surgery and the psychologic makeup of the patient. These factors will determine whether surgery is indicated and agreed upon and whether the surgeon-patient relationship will be a successful one.

Evaluation

Like all medical practitioners, the plastic surgeon must elicit an accurate chief complaint and determine its duration. With an aesthetic patient, it is wise to have the patient point out the exact deformities causing the complaint. The appropriate features can be viewed by the patient with a hand mirror when describing the problem of concern to the surgeon. It is crucial that the area of patient dissatisfaction be described to the plastic surgeon accurately. The surgeon should ask the patient to state the results expected from surgery in a similar manner. Motivation for cosmetic surgery should be carefully assessed. Striving for personal improvement (i.e., self-motivation) is one of the prerequisites for a successful result and a satisfied patient. Even an outstanding result will not be satisfying to a patient with inappropriate motivation or unrealistic expectations. An attempt to salvage a faltering marriage through plastic surgery or an effort to correct a body-image disorder are examples of inappropriate motivations.

SPECIFIC COMPONENTS OF PREOPERATIVE EVALUATION AND PREPARATION

The most crucial factors in successful outpatient surgery are proper evaluation, selection, screening, and preparation of the patient. These factors should be considered according to the following phases:

Initial Patient Interview

A. **Appointments.** Most appointments are made by the patient using the telephone. This is the patient's first contact with a prospective plastic surgeon. Therefore only a well-trained and capable person should be allowed to answer the telephone and to make appointmens.

Quite often the patient may ask many questions pertaining to the operative procedure being considered, including various associated expenses. A good policy is to provide the patient only with general information regarding operative procedures and surgical expenses on the telephone. Specific information regarding consultation fees, office hours, and details of the individual consultation should be provided at this time. Patients seeking an appointment with a successful plastic surgeon may anticipate a waiting period of reasonable length before consultation can be given. However, if an appointment is made for a time in the immediate future, a statement such as, "We had a patient reschedule from Wednesday, so perhaps we can schedule you a little sooner than usual," may divert attention from the fact that a beginning plastic surgeon lacks experience or an adequate patient load. Personnel should avoid phrases such as, "We had a cancellation, so we can schedule you a little sooner." Certain words, such as cancellation, have a connotation of uncertainty that reflects directly on a plastic surgeon's image. No one, including a new patient, should be placed on hold on the telephone for more than a few seconds. If this occurs, it conveys to the patient that delays are likely in the future. An individual with a pleasant telephone voice should fulfill this important position in the plastic surgeon's office. Informational tapes may compromise the professional image of the plastic surgeon and therefore are not recommended to be given to a new patient as a marketing tool.

The patient's arrival at the office and the reception may affect any subsequent surgeon-patient relationship. The patient should be greeted warmly and promptly. An explanation regarding completion of any informational forms as well as any anticipated delays should be given at this time. Two waiting rooms allow for patient separation so that any loud children may be isolated from older patients. Scheduling policies may isolate new patients from postoperative or unsightly patients. Pleasant surroundings and decor not only provide for the patient's comfort, serenity, and sense of security but also reflect the personality and success of the plastic surgeon.

B. **Patient questionnaire.** Before the patient enters the consultation room, a preoperative questionnaire should be filled out concerning previous and current medical conditions, allergies, medications, operations (including previous plastic surgery) and other health history (Fig. 2-1). The questionnaire should also include information about health insurance and other administrative data. Completeness must be verified when these forms are returned to the receptionist. If there are any questions about the patient's medical background, the patient should have a complete medical workup before any elective plastic surgical procedure.

C. **Patient information brochures.** An example of the patient information brochure used in the Obi Plastic Surgery Clinic is provided in Fig. 2-2. Patient information brochures should be concise, personalized, and sophisticated. Procedure brochures inform the patient during the office waiting period just before consultation with the plastic surgeon. Generic but professionally prepared information brochures may be obtained from the American Society of Plastic and Reconstructive Surgery.

D. **Patient interview, health history, and consultation.** Because the initial meeting between a plastic surgeon and a patient is one of the most important periods during the surgeon-patient relationship, the meeting should be professional, private, and unhurried. Consultations with prospective cosmetic surgery patients are usually held in the plastic surgeon's private office. Consultations with other patients may be held in other areas of the office (e.g., examination rooms). During the consultation, the physician should ask about the patient's general health and, specifically, about the following:

- Allergies
- Serious illness, particularly, heart disease, respiratory problems, high blood pressure, and bleeding disorders. Also of significant concern regarding risks for the surgeon and the staff are acquired immunodeficiency syndrome (AIDS) and hepatitis.

(Text continued on p. 19)

Bernard M. Barrett, Jr., M.D., F.A.C.S. Franklin A. Rose, M.D., P.A.

CONFIDENTIAL PATIENT HISTORY

Date ______________ 199 ____ Date of Birth ______________ Age ______________

Name ____
(Last) (First) (Middle)

Address ____
(Street) (City) (State) (Zip)

Telephone ______________ ______________ Marital Status __________
(Home) (Work)

Social Security No. ______________ Employer ______________

Spouse's Name ______________

Name/Address of Person to Notify in Case of Emergency ______________

____

Name/Address/Phone of Insurance Company (if claim may be submitted)

____

Policy/Group No. ______________ Insured ______________ Social Security No. ______________

MEDICAL DATA

Allergies ______________________________
(List all allergies to medication and substances)

Medications ______________________________
(Taken in the past 6 months and dosages if known)

Do You Take Aspirin/Advil ____________ Date Last Aspirin/Advil Taken ____________

Aspirin and Advil cause bleeding. Do not take them 10 days before surgery. Tylenol (acetaminophen) is acceptable (no bleeding).

Previous Surgery (including plastic surgery and dates) ______________________________

____

Height ____________ Weight ____________

Family History of Breast Cancer? ______________________________

Serious Illnesses? ______________________________

Heart Disease? ____________ High Blood Pressure? ________ Bleeding disorder? ____________

General Health: Excellent Good Poor

Referred by: ______________________________

Fig. 2-1 *Example of preoperative patient questionnaire.*

GENERAL INFORMATION

The term *rhytidectomy* is derived from the Latin word *rhytid,* which means *wrinkle,* and *ectomy,* which means *removal of;* thus, rhytidectomy is the removal of wrinkles. These wrinkles can be related to age, hereditary or environmental factors. Not everyone ages at the same rate. A great deal of the aging process relates to your tissues and what you do to care for them.

Rhytidectomy is considered a major operative procedure. Like any extensive surgical procedure, operative incisions and complicated surgical stitching are required. Contrary to popular belief and despite some newspaper and magazine articles, this is *not* as simple as having your hair set or a facial. Also, contrary to some nonmedical reports, it is *not* possible to remove *all* the folds and eliminate *all* the wrinkles of the face, regardless of the treatment applied. You must accept the judgment of your plastic surgeon and realize that only the skin of the face that can be taken off safely and that is suitable for your particular facial contour will be removed. The face lift procedure is directed toward improvement and cannot in any way guarantee that each and every wrinkle and fold of the skin will be removed. The type of skin and age of the patient are important factors in the final result.

The most common question in regard to a face lift is "how long will it last?" This is impossible to state because there are many factors involved: amount of skin removed; age and general condition of the patient; type of skin as well as its condition and texture; amount of previous sun and wind exposure as well as healing ability. Skin aging continues after this operation even though the excess skin and wrinkles have been removed. On rare occasions, a minor secondary procedure may be advisable. The operation does *not* stop *nor* does it accelerate the aging process.

Frequently, in combination with a face lift, eyelid surgery or a lip peel or sanding will be performed. A lip peel or sanding minimizes fine line wrinkles on the upper lip. Crusting occurs after a peel or sanding is performed. After approximately 5 to 7 days, the crust separates, and the upper lip skin is pink and shows a distinctly different color than the surrounding skin. It is imperative to avoid sun exposure to this area for a minimum of 3 to 4 months. If suntanning occurs on this pink skin, permanent discoloration or blotching may result. The initial color change is easily covered by a liquid base makeup. When outdoors where sun exposure is imminent, a sunscreening product, such as Pre-Sun, Oval, or Sun's Screen Gel, may be used. Postoperative pain is minimal; however, the bandages may be uncomfortable.

PROCEDURE

The operation is usually performed in the clinic on an outpatient basis. Patients return home following the procedure providing they have a responsible adult to care for them the first 2 to 5 days.

OPERATIVE TIME

A rhytidectomy should take approximately 3 hours when combined with other procedures such as eyelid surgery, lip peel, or lip sanding.

FIG. **2-2** *Example of patient information brochure.*

ANESTHESIA
What type of anesthesia to use will be the surgeon's decision. Most commonly, a local anesthetic is used, and the patient is adequately sedated so that little or nothing about the actual operation is remembered. As a rule, rejuvenational surgery of the face does not cause the patient to have significant postoperative pain.

SURGICAL PROCEDURE
Beginning 5 days before surgery, the patient is instructed to wash the face and shampoo the hair with pHisoDerm daily. The incisions are within the temple area, in front of the ear, behind the ear and back into the scalp over the mastoid areas. After the incisions are made, the skin is advanced to a more youthful level in the proper lines of tension, and the excess is removed. Sutures are placed in deeper structures to assist in maintaining stability. The incisions are then closed with surgical stitches. The patient can expect some swelling of the face and eyelids, and some discoloration is common with any type of facial surgery. This is usually most notable on the second and third days and diminishes in approximately 5 to 7 days. This also depends on the type of skin, age, and healing ability.

POSTOPERATIVE CARE
Immediately after surgery, bandages are placed on the head and face for 24 to 48 hours. A scarf may be worn to cover the stitches until they are removed. The patient is encouraged to report to the surgeon any significant pain not readily quelled with pain pills or if minor bleeding, redness, or other drainage is noted around the incisions. It is not uncommon on the third to fifth day after any major surgery to feel some *postoperative depression.*

Any postsurgical questions should be directed to the SURGEON or SURGEON'S NURSE because it is unwise for a patient to accept advice from individuals who are not directly concerned with the operation. Call the surgeon if any medical problems arise.

You must remain within reasonable traveling distance of the surgeon's office for approximately 1 to 2 weeks.

MEDICATIONS
Take all medications *exactly* as ordered. You may be requested to take some medicines before surgery. DO NOT TAKE ASPIRIN OR ASPIRIN-CONTAINING COMPOUNDS FOR 2 WEEKS BEFORE OR 2 WEEKS AFTER SURGERY. Acetaminophen (Tylenol, Valadol, Tempra) may be used in place of aspirin. AT THE FIRST SIGN OF HIVES OR RASH, DISCONTINUE ALL MEDICATIONS AND CALL IMMEDIATELY.

POSSIBLE MINOR COMPLICATIONS
Some blood may accumulate under the skin. This can be removed by your physician. Occasionally, minor crusts will appear on the incisions; however, this is a temporary problem. Small areas of numbness may be noted around the ears, cheeks, and incision areas. It is unusual for this to be permanent. Infection and areas of skin or hair loss are possible but uncommon.

FIG. 2-2—cont'd.

SCARS
The surgical scars are permanent; however, they are placed so that they are barely discernible to normal visual observation after a reasonable period of time.

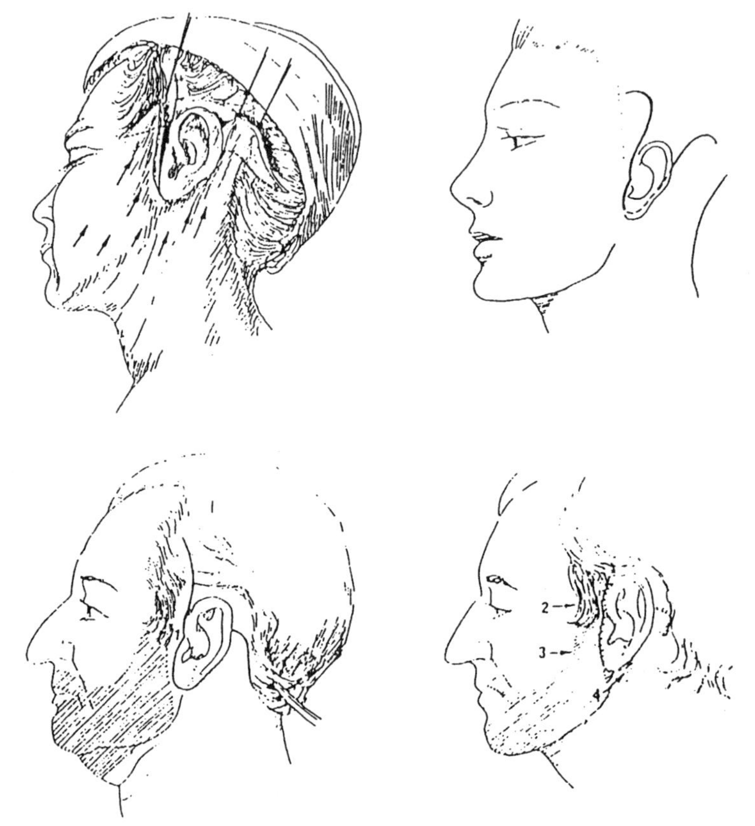

MAKEUP
Makeup may be applied over the skin of the face, up to the edge of the surgical scars, approximately 5 days following the surgery. Within 1 to 3 weeks after surgery, our makeup artist will coach you on skin care and makeup application.

SHAMPOO AND HAIR COLORING
No hair dye or stripping should be done until your surgeon approves. Other coiffure procedures may be carried out approximately 2 weeks following surgery. Do not permit any beauty operator to pull on your hair or roughly massage the scalp. A hair dryer, if used, should be set at medium to cool temperature. This is of utmost importance if any areas of numbness, especially around the ears or temples, are noted.

Fig. 2-2—cont'd.

BATHS AND SHOWERS
Cautious bathing and showering is allowed 24 hours after surgery.

SOCIAL ACTIVITY
Social activities should be limited for approximately 2 weeks. Strenuous exercise should be avoided for 3 to 4 weeks.
Do not wear earrings until sensation, if dimished, has returned to your earlobes.

FEE
The surgeon's fee includes all clinic services, but it does not include hospital or general anesthesia costs if these are required.
In compliance with the suggestions adopted by the American Society of Plastic and Reconstructive Surgeons, Inc., it is routine to request that fees for all cosmetic surgery be paid before surgery.

FIG. 2-2—cont'd.

- ▼ Medications the patient is taking, particularly aspirin or other drugs that may cause bleeding (See Chapter 7.). The physician should explain to the patient that aspirin and other drugs can cause abnormal bleeding during surgery and should be avoided for at least ten days before surgery.
- ▼ Previous surgery, including plastic surgery

After interviewing the patient and obtaining the health history, the patient is prepared for physical examination.

E. **Physical examination.** Examination of the patient regarding areas of chief complaint may have been initiated during initial contact with the patient. The completeness of the physical examination of all systems depends on details of the health history and on the age and apparent health of the patient, but special attention should be directed to the cardiorespiratory system. A complete examination should be performed by an appropriate assistant only in a well-lit, well equipped examination room.

After obtaining the health history and performing the physical examination, an attempt must be made to place the patient in one of the three anesthetic risk classes defined in Chapter 1. These physical status classifications are based on criteria established by the American Society of Anesthesiologists (ASA). Much of the anesthetic risk is reduced by eliminating the need for general anesthesia, except for procedures such as reduction mammoplasties, abdominal lipectomies and other major body contouring procedures.

Recommendation For or Against Surgery

Based on the results of the patient consultation and other pertinent data, an intelligent and objective decision regarding surgical feasibility is made. However, when any doubt exists regarding patient suitability for surgery, a second consultation should help facilitate this decision. The decision to operate must be made only after the following criteria have been met:

- ▼ The patient's motivation for surgery should be determined and deemed appropriate.
- ▼ The margin for surgical improvement should be adequate.
- ▼ The patient's expectations must be within the realm of the surgeon's capabilities.
- ▼ The surgical and anesthetic risks must be negligible. The patient should be in good health and free of infection or other disease processes before elective plastic surgery. Specific conditions detrimental to elective surgery must be corrected. For a patient undergoing face lift, augmentation mammoplasty, or other cosmetic procedures, one of the common potential risks is hematoma. Therefore any condition that increases the chance of hematoma formation should be corrected before surgery. These conditions include uncontrolled hypertension, cough, nausea, vomiting, and any disorder of the coagulation system.

Description of Surgery, Anesthesia, Potential Risks and Limitations of Surgery

When making the decision to operate, it is the surgeon's responsibility to inform the patient about procedures and risks of surgery and anesthesia. Careful and discriminate use of diagrams, photographs, and films may assist the surgeon in this important task. The patient must be allowed adequate time for questions during this discussion and also during at least one subsequent evaluation before surgery. A written consent for surgery should be signed by the patient on an appropriate operative consent form, such as that shown in Fig. 2-3. Imaging devices with projected printouts are not recommended to help inform the patient because an implied warranty may be a legal conclusion in case of litigation. Instructional films about surgical procedures are better received by patients if they are personalized, nonpromotional, and strictly informational. This may be achieved if the plastic surgeon produces the films.

Interview of Patient for Business Arrangements

Various logistic information, including scheduling and admission procedures is provided at this time by the secretary. At the same time, a business agreement regarding financial arrangements is concluded. It is customary for elective aesthetic surgery to be fully paid before the operation.

Interview of Patient by Surgical Nurse

Following the initial consultation or during a subsequent visit before surgery, the patient is interviewed by a nurse on the operating room team. This visit allows the patient to ask personal questions that he or she may have been reluctant to ask the plastic surgeon. Preparatory instructions regarding diet, showering, and other preoperative information are provided by the nurse before surgery. Occasionally a nurse may elicit information regarding surgical feasibility that the surgeon may have overlooked. This is especially true when female patients are being interviewed by female nurses.

Photographic Workup

Graphic documentation of all elective plastic surgery patients is important for many reasons. Photographs, slides, and videotapes can assist in definitive preoperative planning by the surgeon. Documentation of the patient's preoperative condition is also important from a medicolegal standpoint. Aesthetic patients can be given copies of their preoperative photographs following surgery. These may reinforce the

OBI PLASTIC SURGERY CLINIC

SPECIAL CONSENT TO OPERATION OR OTHER PROCEDURE

Patient: ______________________________

Date: ______________________ Time: ______________________

1. I hereby authorize Lewis J. Obi, M.D., to perform a surgical procedure known as: ______________________

   ____

   on ______________________________
   (Name of Patient)

2. The procedure listed in Paragraph 1 has been explained to me by the above doctor, and I completely understand the nature and consequences of the procedure. The following points have been specifically made clear:
   a. Where incisions are made a scar always results, but every effort will be made to make this scar as inconspicuous as possible.
   b. The same complications may follow plastic surgical procedures as may follow any other type of surgical procedure, such as inflammation, tenderness, swelling, discoloration, scar tissue, infection, hematoma, etc.

3. I recognize that during the course of the operation unforeseen conditions may necessitate additional or different procedures than those set forth above. I therefore further authorize and request that the above-named surgeon and assistants or designees of the surgeon perform such procedures as are, in professional judgement, necessary and desirable, including but not limited to, procedures involving pathology and radiology. The authority granted under this Paragraph 3 shall extend to remedying conditions that are not known to the above named doctor at the time the operation is commenced.

4. I consent to the administration of anesthesia to be applied by or under the direction and supervision of the above-named doctor or such anesthesiologists as shall be selected and to the use of such anesthetics as may be deemed advisable.

5. I am aware that the practice of medicine and surgery is not an exact science, and I acknowledge that no guarantees have been made to me as to the results of the operation or procedure.

6. I consent to be photographed before, during, and after treatment and that these photographs shall be the property of the above-named doctor and may be published in scientific journals and shown for scientific reasons. (Faces will not be shown of patients undergoing breast surgery, abdominal lipectomies, etc.)

7. I agree to keep the above-named doctor informed of any change of address so that I may be notified of any late findings, and I agree to cooperate with the above-named doctor in my care after surgery until completely discharged.

8. I have read the above consent and fully understand the same and do authorize the above-named doctor to perform this surgical procedure on me.

9. I am not known to be allergic to anything except: (List) ____________________

____

Witness: ____________________ Date ____________________ Date

____

If patient is a Minor, complete the following: Patient is a minor, __________ years of age, and we, the undersigned are the parents or guardians of the patient and do hereby provide consent for the patient.

____________________ ____________________

Witness Date Parent or Guardian Date

Fig. 2-3 *Example of patient consent form.*

benefits of surgery because many patients tend to forget what they looked like before surgery. Additionally, these visual aids assist in plastic surgery education.

Laboratory Tests

Appropriate laboratory tests can be ordered on the basis of the health history and physical examination. However, certain routine tests should always be performed before any elective surgical procedure.

A. **Blood studies.** A complete blood count (cbc) or a hemoglobin and hematocrit should be performed. Clotting studies such as prothrombin time (PT), partial thromboplastin time (PTT), and bleeding time should be done if the patient has any bleeding tendencies or recent use of drugs that interfere with clotting.
B. **Urinalysis.** Although routinely performed, a urinalysis is of questionable necessity. However, in older patients it is worthwhile to routinely perform urinalysis to evaluate for urinary tract infections or renal problems.
C. **Chest x-ray examination.** Patients with a long history of smoking or respiratory problems should have preoperative chest radiography.
D. **Electrocardiography.** Electrocardiography should be performed on men older than 40 years of age and women older than 45 years of age if they have a positive cardiac history.
E. **Other studies.** Blood chemistries and pulmonary function studies are other tests that can be performed in either routine or special cases. HIV testing is still a controversial and emotional procedure that could have great legal ramifications; therefore it cannot be done without the explicit consent of the patient.

Consultations with Other Physicians

Consultations with other physicians are requested for a patient rated in class 2 or higher of the ASA physical status classifications with the following characteristics:

▼ Mild to moderate systemic disturbances caused either by the condition to be treated surgically or by other pathophysiologic processes, such as the presence of mild diabetes or essential hypertension

- Extremes of age, although no discernible systemic disease is present (e.g., neonates or octogenarians)
- Moderately severe obesity or chronic bronchitis

Second Interview with Surgeon

Second interviews before surgery are indicated in most major cosmetic surgery patients. An elective patient can be seen for a second interview on request or if any doubt exists in the mind of the plastic surgeon or the patient following the preoperative workup.

Final Preoperative Preparation

Much information regarding preoperative preparation can be provided in various patient information brochures. Four types of preoperative preparations are considered:

A. **Skin preparation.** All elective plastic surgical patients are instructed to shower and shampoo with a bacteria-reducing solution (pHisoDerm) the evening before surgery. Whenever alloplastic materials are implanted, surgical scrubbing with a hexachlorophene type soap is started several days before surgery. If an infectious or inflammatory condition of the skin is present, this is treated with systemic and local antibiotics before surgery. Surgery is postponed until the inflammatory condition is resolved, except in an emergency. Oil-based soaps and solutions are to be avoided by a patient undergoing chemical peel.

B. **Diet.** Limitation of alcoholic beverages is recommended for 2 to 3 days before surgery. As a general rule, a patient undergoing surgery should refrain from eating or drinking after midnight on the night before surgery. This approach results in a lower incidence of nausea and vomiting for the patient. Any medication by mouth after a prolonged period of complete fasting tends to increase the incidence of nausea and vomiting. A patient with excess gastric acidity may also neutralize this with dry toast and antacids.

C. Medications to avoid and preoperative drugs.

- ▼ Drugs that interfere with the coagulation of blood are the foremost type of medication that a patient must avoid before surgery. These include salicylates, glycerol guaiacolates, vitamin E, alcohol, clofibrate (Atromid-S), and coumarins.
- ▼ In general, cardiac and antihypertensive drugs such as propranolol hydrochloride (Inderal) should be continued.
- ▼ If the patient has been on long-term diuretics, serum potassium should be checked during the week before surgery, and gradual potassium replacement therapy should be initiated when indicated.
- ▼ A patient requiring prophylactic antibiotics, such as one with a heart murmur or Barlow syndrome, should begin taking these the night before the scheduled surgery.
- ▼ A patient is given prescriptions to be filled before surgery so that medications will be on hand after surgery as needed for sleep, relief of pain (propoxyphene napsylate with acetaminophen [Darvocet-N 100]), and anxiety.
- ▼ Mild tranquilization 1 or 2 days before surgery with a medicine such as diazepam (Valium), 5 to 10 mg by mouth, may be indicated.
- ▼ Soporifics like pentobarbital (Nembutal) 100 mg by mouth, are prescribed the night before surgery. If necessary, a mild tranquilizer and narcotic potentiator such as hydroxyzine (Vistaril), 25 to 50 mg, may be taken with dry toast the morning of surgery.
- ▼ Most patients are medicated preoperatively with pentobarbital, 100 mg by mouth, on arrival at the outpatient clinic. Glycopyrrolate (Robinul) is administered by mouth as a drying agent. An intravenous pathway is started, and additional preoperative and intraoperative

GENERAL POSTOPERATIVE INSTRUCTIONS

Follow these instructions very carefully following surgery:

1. Before leaving, make sure you have received a copy of the discharge instructions that are specific to your surgery.
2. Because you may still be sleepy when you go home, you will need to have an adult family member or friend accompany you. You will also need a responsible adult to stay with you for 24 hours after your surgery.
3. When you get home, rest comfortably in bed, on the couch, or in a recliner chair. When you need to get up, move slowly and have someone walk with you at your side. Don't try to stand for a long time.
4. If you have received general anesthesia, begin eating slowly. Start with ice chips and clear liquids, such as apple juice, broth, gelatin, and soft drinks. Then, as you feel able or as your doctor advises, you may progress to a regular diet.
5. Don't drink any alcoholic drinks while you are taking medication for pain.
6. Do not plan to drive, use any type of machinery, sign important papers, or make important decisions for 24 hours after your surgery. You may still be sleepy from the medications you have received at the center.
7. If you are experiencing pain, take only medicine that your doctor has prescribed for pain. If you continue to have pain, contact your doctor.
8. Call your doctor if you develop a fever of 101°F or above, if you feel nauseated, or if you are vomiting.
9. If you experience any type of medical emergency, go directly to the nearest emergency room.
10. Call the doctor's office to schedule a follow-up appointment.

FIG. 2-4 *Example of general postoperative instructions.*

medication is given as needed. Diphenhydramine enhances drying of secretions, potentiates tranquilizing drugs, and counteracts nausea. Antipruritic and antihistaminic activities are additional benefits of this drug.

D. **General instructions for immediate postoperative period.** In the preoperative period, it is wise to give the patient, in writing, general postoperative instructions so that plans can be made. Fig. 2-4 is an example of written postoperative instructions. The physician or nurse should review the instructions with the patient when they are given to the patient.

E. **Admission to hospital or operating room facility.** The patient is generally accompanied to the hospital or outpatient surgical facility by an adult family member or friend. This person is responsible for driving the patient home, dispensing pain and sleep medications as instructed by the medical staff, and observing the patient for possible problems while away from the medical facility. After the patient is admitted to the facility, the final preoperative preparation is carried out. The outpatient is escorted to a dressing area where a hospital gown and slippers are provided. No makeup or body sprays should be applied following the preoperative shower and shampoo. Any residual facial makeup that may be present is removed before the patient enters the operating suite. Dentures are not removed for local anesthetic cases but are removed before general anesthesia is given. Preoperative patients are segregated in a holding area away from postoperative patients. Complete monitoring and resuscitative equipment must be available in the holding area in the event of adverse drug reactions to the preoperative medications.

CHAPTER 3

Intraoperative Management

GUSTAVO A. COLON

OUTPATIENT SURGERY

Outpatient surgery has grown rapidly because of the consumer need for less expensive health care that is both of excellent quality and convenience. More than half of all operations performed in the United States in 1992 were on an outpatient basis. The American Hospital Association predicts that by 1995, 75% of all operations will be performed in an outpatient facility. Like other types of surgery, plastic surgical procedures—aesthetic, reconstructive, and traumatic—are increasingly being performed safely and efficiently in an outpatient setting. Elective surgical procedures for aesthetic surgery lend themselves well to outpatient surgery with the only limiting factors being medical contraindications that require hospitalization.

Advantages of Outpatient Surgery

A. **Reduction of cost.** The major stimulus for the conception and maturation of outpatient surgery has been savings in health care costs, which are passed on to the patient. Studies conducted by the American Society of Plastic and Reconstructive Surgery, the American Medical Association (AMA), and the Joint Commission for Accreditation of Hospital Organizations (JCAHO) have shown that outpatient surgery, including office-based surgery, decreases the ultimate cost not only to the patient but to third-party payers. This is because often the outpatient surgical procedures can be global or total allowing both the patient and insurer to know exactly what the surgical procedure and costs will be. These costs are generally less than hospitalization because of smaller staffs, procedure-oriented operating facilities, elimination of overnight stays, and extended staffs within the facilities.

B. **Comfortable setting for patient and patient's family**
C. **Privacy**
D. **Streamlined health services and delivery of these services**
E. **More efficient use of surgeon's time**

Ensuring Patient Safety

Despite the advantages of outpatient surgery the overriding principle that must prevail is the intraoperative and postoperative safety of the patient. As the trend of office-based surgery was fueled by patients looking for cost savings and convenience, concern was expressed by governmental and professional agencies about the potential for substandard care. The potential for substandard care is cause for concern because doctors operating in their offices are out of sight of the "watchful eye" of hospital peer programs. Also, no formal standards exist to govern the outpatient facilities when possible dangers are obvious. The need for evaluation, accreditation, and inspection has been supported by three organizations: (1) the American Association for Accreditation of Ambulatory Surgical Facilities (AAAASF), which is the largest organization and has the most extensive expertise in setting the standards and accrediting office-based surgical procedures; (2) the American Association for Ambulatory Health Care (AAAHC); (3) and the JCAHO. Each organization has programs for accrediting outpatient facilities. The following *three classes of accreditation* have been established by these organizations:

- Class A: Centers that perform only minor plastic surgical procedures using local or regional topical anesthesia
- Class B: Centers that perform minor and major plastic surgical procedures using only intravenous (IV) or parenteral sedation and all dissociative drugs
- Class C: Centers that perform all types of surgical procedures using all types of anesthesia, including general anesthesia and external support of vital body functions as required

Because of the need for national standardization of office-based surgical procedures, the following recommendations were made to Congressperson Ron Wyden's Committee on Regulation of Outpatient Facilities by the AAAASF. However, because the major stimulus for ambulatory surgery is cost savings, the problem of entrepreneurism can affect the credibility and integrity of ambulatory surgery. Therefore the AAAASF recommended the following:

- National standards should be developed to govern both office-based surgical facilities and the surgeons who practice. These standards would consist of a core of generic criteria that requires standardization of monitoring equipment and procedures.
- A requirement should be established that these mandatory standards are enforced by nationally recognized accrediting organizations (i.e., AAAASF, AAACH, and JCAHO).
- Mandated peer review should be required for physicians practicing in office-based surgical facilities.
- Malpractice insurance should be required for all physicians operating in their offices in order to maintain and ensure truth in advertising requiring full disclosure of the physician's formal training, certification, and accreditation of the facility. These requirements would be mandated through national legislation and state statutes as necessary.
- Licensors should distinguish between hospital multispecialty and free-standing ambulatory surgical units. Licenses should be defined for unispecialty office facilities, such as plastic surgery or ophthalmology.
- The physician who practices or performs surgical procedures in the office should protect patients from non-trained physicians and require that physicians practicing in those facilities have the same surgical privileges in local hospitals.
- The appropriate staff, anesthesia, and operating room (OR) personnel should be required in office surgical facilities, and all such facilities should be equipped to handle the necessary medical and surgical emergencies. It is evident that office surgery is an area in which there

are no guidelines or controls. However, some offices have voluntary guidelines and controls that are promoted by specific accrediting organizations.

Licensed physicians are authorized to practice all types of medicine and surgery throughout the United States. However, tattoo artists, hairdressers, and manicurists need licensing or health board examinations to practice their *specific* art, while practitioners who decide to perform surgery in the office do *not* need licensing to perform any specific procedure. Because current advertising in all professions can be misleading, seductive, ridiculous, and fraudulent, it is obvious that office surgical facilities should not be created without meeting appropriate guidelines and standards. A system should be developed for approval of all ambulatory and surgical office units. Likewise, a system should be developed to ensure the quality of the facility and its medical staff and to create an appropriate peer review and evaluation. It is therefore the purpose of such mandated national guidelines to create an atmosphere of safety in office surgery in order to benefit the outpatient population.

STAFFING

Outpatient staff should consist of full-time and part-time employees. It is advisable that the office surgical facility have an arrangement with pool nurses who can supply the facility with a nurse, operating technician, or other staff on short notice because the usual staff in an operating facility is small, and gaps in personnel can disrupt an operating schedule. It is imperative that an outpatient ambulatory surgical facility in an office setting be run exactly as any other well-functioning and accredited OR, whether it be freestanding or a hospital. The requirements of the staff are less while the surgical delivery is much more efficient and streamlined. As always, patient care and safety are the most important concerns of the office surgical facility.

Anesthesia Staff

Anesthetic services can be contracted with an anesthesia group that supplies either an anesthesiologist or a full- or part-time certified registered nurse anesthetist (CRNA). Currently some office surgical facilities do not use anesthetists or anesthesiologists to monitor patients. The patient is instead monitored by a registered nurse (RN) who is a full-time employee of the surgeon. In either case, the patient should be carefully monitored by trained personnel other than the operating surgeon. (Chapter 5 discusses anesthesia in more detail.)

Nursing Staff and Technicians

A. **Operating room.** The regulations of the AAAASF require that an RN serve as a full-time nurse director of the OR. There should also be an OR technician or assistant who is trained in the appropriate surgical mechanics of an OR along with a circulating nurse.
B. **Recovery room.** The recovery room should have trained recovery room personnel, such as an RN, in order to have appropriate postoperative monitoring of the patient.

Other Staff

A contractual arrangement should be made with a janitorial staff that is hospital trained in cleaning ORs and with biomedical engineers from the hospital or from other service areas who can regularly check the biomedical equipment on a part-time basis. All pharmaceuticals, particularly narcotics, should be cross-checked by an outside pharmacist who can monitor and independently log all drugs that are used in the facility.

PAPERWORK

All procedures performed in an outpatient operating facility should be properly documented. The paperwork should be detailed, and the facility should have a complete record (Figs. 3-1 to 3-4) of the following:

- Preoperative evaluations
- Intraoperative care, including an operative note
- Anesthesia administered
- Postoperative nursing evaluation and postoperative recovery room information
- Documentation of discharge, including the condition of the patient at discharge and to whom the patient was discharged

Surgi–Unit RECOVERY ROOM RECORD

DATE: ____________ PROCEDURE: ____________
TIME IN: ____________ ANETHESIA: ____________
TIME OUT: ____________ ALLERGIES: ____________

POSTANTHESIA RECOVERY SCORE	IN	MINUTES 30	60	90	OUT	PAR
ACTIVITY move 4 extremities vol./command =2 " 2 " " " =1 " 0 " " " =0						200 180
RESPIRATION Deep breathe and cough freely =2 Dyspneic or limited breathing =1 Apneic =0						B P 160 V—V 140 Λ—Λ
CIRCULATION BP + 20 of Preanesthetic level =2 BP + 20-50 of Preanesthetic level =1 BP + 50 of Preanesthetic level =0						P 120 o—o R 100 X—X
CONSCIOUSNESS Fully awake =2 Arousable on calling =1 Not responding =0						80 60
COLOR Pink — Normal =2 Pale, dusky, blotchy, jaundiced, other =1 Cyanotic =0						40 20

DRESSINGS ____________
CHANGED ____________
DRAINS ____________
PACKS ____________
ICE PACKS ____________
CHANGED ____________

IV FLUIDS:
IN PROGRESS ____________
ADDED ____________
TOTAL ABSORBED ____________

MEDICATIONS:

NAME	DOSE	ROUTE	TIME	SIGNED

NURSES' NOTES:

____
____
____
____
____
____
____
____
____
____
____
____

____ VITAL SIGNS STABLE
____ SWALLOW, COUGH, GAG REFLEX PRESENT
____ N & V, DIZZINESS MINIMAL
____ ABSENCE OF RESP. DISTRESS
____ ABLE TO AMBULATE
____ ALERT AND ORIENTATED
____ RECOVERY SCORE ON D/C

DISCHARGE CRITERIA:

____ DRESSINGS DRY & INTACT
____ PT. VOIDED
GIVEN & UNDERSTANDS D/C INSTRUCTIONS
____ RESPONSIBLE ADULT PRESENT TO ESCORT PATIENT HOME

SIGNED ____________
RELATIONSHIP ____________
____ TAKE HOME MEDICATIONS

RECOVERY ROOM NURSE ____________

Fɪɢ. **3-1** *Example of recovery room record.*

Surgi–Unit NURSING ADMIT ASSESSMENT

PRE-OP INTERVIEW

INFORMANT: ____________

DATE: ______ TIME: ______ AM / PM

ROUTINE LAB: Hct

Hqt

Wght.

ADDITIONAL COMMENTS: ______

DAY OF SURGERY

APPEARENCE: ____________

CONSCIOUSNESS: ☐

AWAKE AND ALERT

OTHER: ____________

EMOTIONAL STATUS:

NPO: ☐ YES

SKIN:

UNREMARKABLE ☐

OTHER: ____________

HEAD:

UNREMARKABLE ☐

OTHER: ____________

NECK:

UNREMARKABLE ☐

OTHER: ____________

ABDOMEN:

UNREMARKABLE ☐

OTHER: ____________

GENITOURINARY:

UNREMARKABLE ☐

OTHER: ____________

EXTERMITIES:

UNREMARKABLE ☐

OTHER: ____________

VALUABLES: ☐ YES ☐ NO

DISPOSITION: ____________

SURGICAL CHECK LIST

ADDRESSOGRAPH PLATE↑	YES	NO
I.D. BANK ON		
SURGICAL PERMIT SIGNED		
HISTORY AND PHYSICAL		
ALLERGIES		
OPERATIVE AREA PREPPED		
PRE-OP MARKING		
NPO AFTER MIDNIGHT		
H AND H DONE		
BP AND TRP TAKEN		
VOIDED		
WIGS AND JEWELRY REMOVED AND SECURED		
HAIRPINS, MAKEUP, AND NAIL POLISH REMOVED		
CONTACT LENSES AND GLASSES REMOVED		
DENTURES REMOVED		
HOSPITAL GOWN		
NAME PLATE		
PRE-OP MEDICATION		
OTHER PROSTHESIS		

DATE ______ NURSE ______

Fig. 3-1—cont'd. *Example of recovery room record.*

PREMEDICATION

Sedatives

Premedication should be minimized or possibly avoided in an outpatient setting because it might prolong the recovery period. However, the use of meperidine (Demerol) 1.0 mg/kg with atropine 0.01 mg/kg does not necessarily prolong recovery after outpatient surgery. Diazepam (Valium) and even hydroxyzine (Atarax, Vistaril) also do not appear to prolong recovery. Nevertheless, these premedications can impair

Surgi–Unit

Ambulatory Surgical Facility
4204 Teuton Street Metairie, LA 70002

ANESTHESIA RECORD

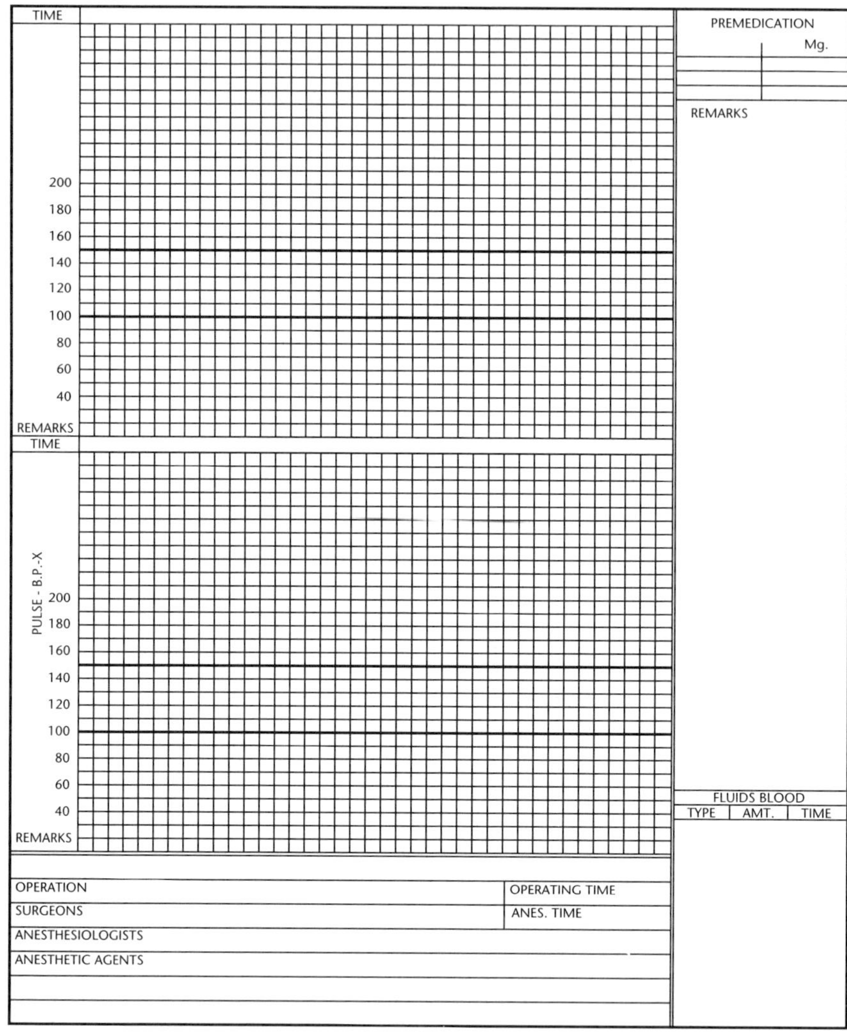

DATE

TIME

200
180
160
140
120
100
80
60
40
REMARKS

TIME

PULSE - B.P.-X
200
180
160
140
120
100
80
60
40
REMARKS

PREMEDICATION	Mg.

REMARKS

FLUIDS BLOOD		
TYPE	AMT.	TIME

OPERATION	OPERATING TIME
SURGEONS	ANES. TIME
ANESTHESIOLOGISTS	
ANESTHETIC AGENTS	

PATIENT'S RECORD

Fig. 3-2 *Example of anesthesia record.*

Surgi–Unit

4204 Teuton Street
Metairie, LA 70002

OPERATING ROOM RECORD

DATE: ______ SURGERY BEGAN: ______

OR #: ______ ENDED: ______

PT. NAME: ______ TO RR: ______

SURGEON: ______ COUNT: ______

	1st	2nd	
ANESTHETIST: ______	___	___	LAPS: ______
SCRUB NURSE: ______	___	___	RAYTEX: ______
CIRCULATER: ______	___	___	NEEDLES: ______
OTHER: ______	___	___	BLADES: ______

PREOPERATIVE DIAGNOSIS: ______

PROCEDURE: ______

POSTOPERATIVE DIAGNOSIS: ______

ANESTHESIA LOCAL: ______ LOCAL STAND–BY: ______ GEN: ______ MASK: ______ ENDO: ______

POSITION SUPINE: ______ PRONE: ______ FOWLER'S: ______ SEMI–FOWLER'S: ______

ARMS AT SIDES: ______ ARMS ON BOARDS: ______

SURGICAL PREP BETADINE: ______ PHISOHEX: ______ HIBICLENS: ______

DRAINS TYPE: ______ LOCATION: ______

PACKS: ______

BOVIE MACHINE #: ______ PAD LOCATION: ______ COAG: ______ CUT: ______

SPECIMENT SENT TO LAB: ______

IV FLUIDS:

______ UP ______ DOWN ______

______ UP ______ DOWN ______

______ UP ______ DOWN ______

MEDICATIONS:

NAME	DOSAGE	ROUTE	TIME	SIGNED

CIRC. NURSE: ______

FIG. 3-3 *Example of operating room record.*

PLASTIC SURGERY ASSOCIATES'
OPERATIVE NOTE

PATIENT'S NAME

ADDRESS: DATE:
TELEPHONE #:
AGE: SEX:

PREOPERATIVE DIAGNOSIS:

POSTOPERATIVE DIAGNOSIS:

PATHOLOGIC FINDINGS:

OPERATION: DURATION: ANESTHETIC: ANESTHETIST:
BY: DATE: AT: DATE:

DISCHARGE NOTE:

FIG. 3-4 *Example of plastic surgery associates' operative note.*

coordinative and reactive skills for anywhere from 5 to 12 hours so it is best to avoid these as routine outpatient premedications. Some of the newer sedative benzodiazepines such as midazolam (Versed), which is a rapid-acting water-soluble benzodiazepine, have the potential to be a good, quick intramuscular or oral premedication for outpatients. The judicious use of sedatives as premedicants in outpatient surgery usually relieves anxiety without prolonged recovery. Remember that premedication is given primarily as an anxiolytic rather than as a true intraoperative anesthetic.

Antacids

Outpatients have some residual gastric volumes postoperatively. Therefore the administration of an oral antacid such as ranitidine (Zantac) 300 mg, before outpatient surgery is recommended. Antacids help minimize postoperative vomiting with the possible risk of aspiration. Droperidol (Inapsine) can be given by IV at a dose of 0.25 to 1.5 mg to decrease postoperative nausea and vomiting and minimize recovery time.

MONITORING THE PATIENT

The monitoring system is only as effective as the person who is observing it. Therefore it is important that qualified and trained personnel observe and monitor the patient. Certain standards have been set for patient monitoring. These standards are warranted and adopted to reduce anesthetic complications and improve overall patient care. It is no longer sufficient to observe blood pressure, pulse, and color during surgery; noninvasive, affordable methods of monitoring oxygenation and respiration have become available. It is important in this medical-legal era that physicians not deviate from the appropriate standards for outpatient monitoring of surgical patients.

Basic Guidelines

Basic guidelines for the monitoring of a patient under general or sedative anesthesia follow:

- Oxygenation
  - Measure inspired gas with an oxygen analyzer.
  - Monitor blood oxygenation continuously. Conduct quantitative measure with a pulse oximeter.

- Ventilation
  - Evaluate adequacy of ventilation continously.
  - Use a CO_2 analysis, if appropriate.
- Circulation
  - Display an electrocardiogram (ECG) continuously with printout.
  - Evaluate blood pressure and heart rate every 5 minutes.
  - When general anesthesia is used, palpation of the pulse, auscultation of the heart sounds, or oximetry must be performed.
  - Continuously measure the patient's temperature.

Monitoring Equipment

Outpatients require the same basic equipment for delivery of anesthesia monitoring and resuscitation as is used for inpatients. The standard intraoperative monitoring equipment for routine outpatient surgery should be available for both general and MAC anesthesia.

A. **Monitoring circulation.** The methods of monitoring circulation have improved and now yield much more information. A number of ECG monitors combined with recorders and automatic tripping devices are available to provide a printout or trigger alarm when necessary. Many of these machines include noninvasive automatic blood pressure monitors that can be programmed with printout capability providing a permanent record. *Oximeters,* which are now being used, are highly reliable. They work by measuring the absorption and specific length, light waves reflecting the ratio of oxygenated to deoxygenated hemoglobin. The resultant relationship of quantity of oxygen to hemoglobin can be calculated and presented in a readout form on an oximeter. Oximeters do have limitations, however, because of the loss of signal when perfusion is poor and interference from electrocautery.

B. **Monitoring ventilation.** A method of ventilatory monitoring called *capnography,* which measures exhaled CO_2, is being used more now that a nasal-prong system has become available. The system measures endtidal CO_2 in the sedated patient who is awake and not intubated.

INTRAOPERATIVE EMERGENCIES

Emergencies can occur at any time during an operative procedure. The staff and the OR personnel must be properly trained to handle an emergency, and the OR should be equipped for any type of emergency.

General Requirements for Dealing with Emergencies

A. Personnel training

- ▼ Personnel must be familiar with all the ECG cardiac monitors and some of the abnormal parameters of pulmonary and cardiovascular physiology, which includes being well-trained in cardiopulmonary resuscitation (CPR) and advanced CPR.
- ▼ Emergency drills should be run for all cardiac and medical emergencies as well as nonmedical emergencies such as a fire or other problems that may arise during the operative procedure.

B. Equipment

- ▼ There should be appropriate backup generating equipment in case of electrical failure during operative procedures.
- ▼ An IV conduit should always be maintained on a patient undergoing any sedative or anesthetic operative procedure.
- ▼ Suction should be available not only for the surgical procedure but also separately for anesthesia. All the oxygen and anesthesia gases should have appropriate backup and reserve tanks.

Respiratory Distress

Respiratory distress can occur in any patient undergoing IV sedation. Therefore vigilant monitoring must be maintained in these patients. The signs and symptoms of respiratory distress may be difficult to distinguish from aberrant behavior of a difficult patient who may be restless, confused, or irritable. Hypoxia and hypercarbia can lead to increased heart rate, blood pressure and, if allowed to persist, arrhythmias. When confronted with a restless patient, the surgeon needs to decide whether to further sedate the patient or if the problem is caused by a lack of oxygen. Hypoventilation can be corrected by increasing the amount of oxygen concentration given to the patient. The use of narcotic antagonists, such as naloxone (Narcan), for hypoventilation because of narcotic-induced respiratory depression can reverse induced depression effectively. Its duration of action is only approximately 45 minutes, and the patient can easily be renarcotized after its effect wears off. Drugs such as morphine and demerol have a much longer duration of action. It is important that narcotic antagonists be used only in early recovery if at all. Administration in late recovery could prevent the patient from meeting the criteria for discharge.

Ventricular Fibrillation

Surgeons monitoring patients should be prepared for severe cardiac problems. Appropriate defibrillators should be available. New defibrillator-monitors have both modalities. Knowledge about defibrillators and when to use them is essential for both the surgeon and OR personnel. The staff should become thoroughly familiar with using defibrillators, and there should be periodic drills on their use, particularly in a CPR emergency.

Anaphylaxis

Anaphylactic shock can result from hypersensitivity to certain medications. Respiratory distress, which often accompanies anaphylactic shock, usually progresses to laryngeal edema or bronchospasm. Epinephrine is the drug of choice for initial treatment, and 0.5 ml of 1:1000 epinephrine in 10 ml of saline should be given IV for severe reactions. The dose can be repeated every 5 to 15 minutes if the latter response occurs. Airway maintenance is essential. Rapid infusion of IV is important because sizable losses of fluid from the intravascular space during anaphylaxis can occur as third space loss. Corticosteroids, such as dexamethasone phosphate, may be given IV 8 to 12 mg or an alternative of 500 mg of hydrocortisone can be used.

Convulsive Seizures

Convulsive seizures while a patient is on the operating table can be difficult and have dangerous consequences. However, convulsions most commonly occur in the recovery room. The convulsive spasm can override respiratory movement causing the patient to become hypoxic. Occasionally, convulsions may be secondary to hypoxia. Two medications commonly blamed for convulsive disorders in plastic surgery are lidocaine and cocaine. Although the toxic levels of these and related agents can cause convulsions, treatment for convulsive seizures is diazepam (Valium) or any other sedative that can be injected slowly by IV. Diazepam administered in slow IV doses of 5 to 25 mg may control the seizures and is usually effective in 80% to 90% of cases. The airway needs to be maintained, and the use of oxygen is crucial because hypoxia may be the cause of the seizures.

Hypotension

To treat hypotension, the surgeon has to make every effort to determine its etiology. Blood loss and hypovolemia are usually the cause of hypotension on the operating table, but this is rarely the cause in outpatients, unless the patient is undergoing a procedure such as liposuction in which a great deal of fluid volume is being removed quickly. To treat hypotension, IV fluids that expand the intra-vascular space should be administered. Vasopressors such as metaraminol (Aramine) may be needed to maintain blood pressure for persistent hypotension. Should hypotension persist in spite of IV fluid treatment, the patient will need to be transferred immediately to a hospital to determine if cardiac causes for hypotension are present.

Cardiac Arrhythmias

Surgeons must keep the electrophysiology of the heart in mind during surgery because certain cardiac arrhythmias can occur during an operative procedure without any stimulus.

A. **Sinus tachycardia.** This is due to an accelerated heart rate from overstimulation of a sinoatrial (SA) node, can be caused by both hypovolemic shock and inadvertent infiltration of anesthetic containing epinephrine.

B. **Sinus bradycardia.** This may be due to parasympathetic stimulation on the eye, carotid sinus, gastric distention, or even fear and anxiety (e.g., vasovagal reflex). It can be associated with hypotension, and the treatment of choice is 0.5 mg of atropine administered slowly by IV. This can be repeated every 5 minutes up to a total dose of 2 mg.

C. **Supraventricular arrhythmias.** These are due to one or more atrial or atrioventricular (AV) nodal ectopic foci stimulating one or more multiple premature beats. This condition usually is best left untreated. When symptoms are particularly severe 1 mg of propranodol can be given slowly by IV if necessary. This dose may be repeated with great caution up to a total of 3 mg.

D. **Ventricular arrhythmias.** These are usually caused by one or more ectopic foci within the ventricles that stimulate premature ventricular contractions (PVCs). Occasionally, PVCs are frequent. More numerous PVCs are of ventricular origin, causing these multifocal PVCs to require treatment. Ventricular ectopic foci can be stimulated by the presence of epinephrine, cocaine, or other common plastic surgical medications. Because PVCs are a common warning sign of hypoxia, one must not only check the airway but also make certain that the depth and rate of respiration are adequate. As a rule, the following are indications for the use of lidocaine given IV as a bolus of 50 to 100 mg:

- More than 6 PVCs per minute
- Multifocal PVCs
- Coupled PVCs with bigeminy or trigeminy
- Runs of ventricular tachycardia

HYPOTHERMIA

Hypothermia during cosmetic surgery is unintentional loss of body heat caused by extreme exposure. The loss of the temperature-regulating mechanism can occur occasionally with dry gases leading to heat loss and evaporation. Vasodilatation and heat loss from open wounds can be significantly helped by maintaining a warm temperature in the OR by using fluid warmers, warming the body surface, and humidifying inspired gases. Treatment of hypothermia includes using high inspired-oxygen concentration, surface warming, and suppression of severe shivering. Some drugs for the suppression of shivering, also called hypothalamic central stimulation, include chlorpromazine, droperidol, magnesium sulfate, and calcium chloride. Calcium chloride is effective in the treatment of shivering when given IV up to 1 gram.

MALIGNANT HYPERTHERMIA

Malignant hyperthermia is a potentially fatal disorder characterized by hypermetabolic response to one or more triggering agents. Mortality can be high. No reliable noninvasive testing can detect malignant hyperthermia, but the creatine phosphokinase (CPK) test may reveal patients who are susceptible to the disorder. Protocol should be developed that includes the use of dantrolene sodium (Dantrium) at 2 mg per kg. This is an expensive drug therefore a regimen should be arranged with the hospital for its availability. The Malignant Hyperthermia Association (M.H.A.E.U.S., P.O. Box 3231, Darian, CT, 06820) has a treatment protocol for malignant hyperthermia that includes flow sheets and wall posters, which are helpful in any surgical office facilities.

FURTHER READINGS

Abajian JC, Page P, Morgan M: Effects of droperidol and nitrazepam on emergence reactions following ketamine anesthesia, *Anesth Analg* 52:385, 1973.

Beesey L et al: Reduction of the psychoto-mimetic and circulatory side effects of ketamine by droperidol, *Anesthesiology* 37:536, 1972.

Bredlove B: *Successful management of ambulatory surgery programs,* Atlanta, 1985, American Health Consultants.

Coleman III WP, Colon GA, Davis S: *Outpatient surgery of the skin,* New York, 1983, Medical Examination Publishing.

Colon G: Office surgery. In Marsh JL, editor: *Current therapy in plastic and reconstructive surgery,* Burlington, Ontario, 1989, BC Decker.

Courtiss E: Office surgery, *Clin Plast Surg* 10(2), 1983.

Cunningham BL, McKinny P: Patient acceptance of dissociative anesthetics, *Plast Reconstr Surg* 72:22, 1983.

Erbguth PH, Reiman B, Klein RL: The influence of chlorpromazine, diazepam and droperidol on emergence from ketamine, *Anesth Analg* 51:693, 1972.

Fishman TG, Fishman JH, Colon GA: Office surgical anesthesia. In *PSFF Instructional Courses,* Vol 2, St Louis, 1989, Mosby.

Gallozzi E, Van Poznak A, Artusio J: Is there a place for the use of ketamine in plastic and reconstructive surgery?, *Ann Plast Surg* 4:85, 1980.

Goldsmith SB: *Ambulatory surgery,* Rockville, Md, 1977, Aspen Publishers.

McClean AG: Ketamine and diazepam in the adult patient, *Med J Aust* 2:338, 1971.

O'Donovan RR: Ambulatory surgical centers: development and management, Rockville, Md, 1976, Aspen Publishers.

Schultz RC: *Outpatient surgery,* Philadelphia, 1979, Lea & Febiger.

Trieger N, Newman MG, Miller JC: An objective measure of recovery, *Anesth Prog* 16:4, 1969.

Vinnik CA: An intravenous dissociation technique for outpatient plastic surgery: tranquility in the office surgical facility, *Plast Reconstr Surg* 67:799, 1981.

White P: Outpatient Anesthesia. In Miller R: New York, 1986, Churchill Livingstone.

CHAPTER 4

Postoperative Management

BERNARD M. BARRETT, JR. AND LEWIS J. OBI

That the aftercare is as important as the planning was stated as a basic premise by H. D. Gillies and D. R. Millard in *The Principles and Art of Plastic Surgery.* Planning, execution, and aftercare is a triad that must be dealt with repeatedly and successfully by the plastic surgeon. Each patient has a slightly different problem. To arrive at the correct solution to the challenges presented by all of these patients, one must undertake careful planning and precise execution and provide methodical postoperative care.

Postoperative care is actually conceived when the plastic surgeon sees the patient for the first time. By careful patient screening and preoperative planning along with a precisely executed surgical procedure, the surgeon will minimize the need for extensive postoperative care. Because the majority of plastic surgery patients undergoing elective surgery are healthy individuals, a significant number of such procedures may be performed with the patient under local anesthesia, either in a well-equipped and well-staffed outpatient facility or in the hospital. A reasonable approach to postoperative care is to assume that one is usually dealing with a basically healthy preoperative patient who will remain so during the postoperative period. A simplified but comprehensive approach to postoperative care lends itself to execution by a well-trained plastic surgery staff. The net result is that the patient is well cared for postoperatively and the plastic surgeon's time is conserved. If one is dealing with a sick postoperative patient, then a primary care physician—internist, cardiologist, or other specialist—frequently may be involved with the patient's care.

Postsurgical care can be divided into the phases of recovery room period, immediate postoperative period, and intermediate-to-late postoperative period.

RECOVERY ROOM PERIOD

Recovery Room Design and Equipment

The recovery room environment should be well planned, with consideration given to space, equipment, and patient requirements. Automatic blood pressure and cardiac monitoring devices channeled into a central nursing station enhance patient safety during the recovery room period. A defibrillator should be available not only for the recovery room but for the operating rooms (ORs) as well. An advantage of the outpatient surgical facility is that the design and decor of the recovery room can be planned to avoid a sterile hospital-type setting. Spacing of recovery room beds should provide for nursing accessibility as well as patient segregation. A quiet, private recovery room environment separated from any recovering seriously ill or recently extubated patients favors an uneventful and serene postoperative recovery period for the elective surgical patient.

Recovery Room Nursing

A well-trained recovery room nurse must be capable of caring for all of the patient's needs during the recovery room period. Both OR and recovery room nurses should be certified in cardiopulmonary resuscitation and advanced life support techniques. Early postoperative complications such as hematoma can be reduced or prevented by an attentive and well-trained recovery room nurse. Safety, compassion, and empathy should be an integral part of all phases of patient care, including postoperative care.

Transfer from Operating Room to Recovery Room

After surgery, the patient is transferred from the OR table to a stretcher when the following criteria have been met:

- Respiratory function is spontaneous, and perfusion color is acceptable.
- The vital signs are stable and within normal limits for the postoperative period.

The patient is then gently moved to a stretcher without abrupt changes in position or disturbance of the incisions. The head and neck are held stable and unstressed during this transfer. Sudden changes in the patient's position may led to hypotension or nausea. Inadvertent stresses to the wounds may lead to development of unwanted edema and hematoma formation.

Arrival in Recovery Room

Once the patient is in the recovery room, the vital signs are carefully monitored and the intravenous (IV) pathway is kept open. The IV conduit permits, when necessary, rapid treatment of pain, nausea, and drug reactions. Taking blood pressures with arm compression should be minimized or, preferably, avoided in a breast surgery patient because arteriovenous (AV) shunting to the axillary and thoracicoacromial areas may increase the chances of breast hematoma formation. It has been shown that postsurgical nausea following surgery is often relieved by the administration of nasal oxygen. Because nausea may occur secondary to hypotension, antiemetic drugs that greatly lower blood pressure, such as phenothiazines, should be avoided because they may enhance the hypotension.

Patient Discharge from Recovery Room

The time required for adequate recovery varies from patient to patient. A hospital patient returning to a well-supervised plastic surgical floor or outpatient recovery center can leave recovery sooner than an outpatient who is going home. Because good outpatient anesthesiologic practice recognizes that these patients must be reactive, normotensive, and ambulatory before discharge, drugs used for IV sedation ideally should be reversible and short acting. Only the necessary amounts of narcotics and other sedative drugs are given to outpatients. The use of short-acting anesthesics is one method of making outpatient anesthesia quick and comfortable.

Before being discharged, the outpatient is gradually placed in an upright position and then transferred to a wheelchair. Because a recovery period of several hours is usually required for outpatients, the danger of later hematoma formation is reduced. The nurse provides the person responsible for the patient following discharge with printed instruction sheets and an appointment card for the patient's return visit. All printed instructions are verbally reviewed with the patient at this time (Figs. 4-1 and 4-2).

The same criteria for discharge must be met if the patient is being transferred to the hospital or to an overnight facility. Trained medical personnel should accompany the patient during transfer with copies of the health history, physical examination findings, and postoperative orders to ensure patient safety. The outpatient surgical facility should be near a general community hospital, and a written agreement stating that the hospital will accept patient transfers as necessary after outpatient surgery should be made with the hospital administrator. This allows the surgeon to admit any postoperative patient should the recovery room period be prolonged unexpectedly or should an adverse reaction to surgery or anesthesia occur.

IMMEDIATE POSTOPERATIVE PERIOD

This period begins when the patient leaves the recovery room or outpatient clinic area, and it lasts for approximately 2 weeks. During this time, the incisions are carefully attended to, the sutures are removed, and daily activities of the patient are increased gradually. After discharge from the clinic, the first contact with the patient usually occurs within 24 hours when the recovery room or OR nurse telephones the party responsible for the patient's home care to confirm that the postoperative instructions are being carried out properly. Also, this call allows the person caring for the patient to have any additional questions or concerns addressed. In rare situations, the outpatient may experience pain or nausea that is not alleviated by the usual oral or rectal medications. One can admit the patient to a hospital or an overnight facility if this situation arises.

The patient's first postoperative office visit occurs 1 to 5 days after surgery, depending on the type and extent of surgery performed. Contact with the patient and family should be maintained during the intervening time. Face-lift patients return to the office the morning after surgery for drain

The following is a list of postoperative instructions and information pertaining to your surgery. Hopefully, it will answer many of the questions you may have. However, should you have any further questions, please feel free to call the office. In addition to this information, you will be given written instructions the day of surgery explaining what you need to do upon leaving the hospital or outpatient facility when discharged.

1. Eat nothing after midnight the night before surgery.
2. Carefully wash your body and hair with Hibiclens or Betadine the night before surgery. Avoid applying any makeup or body deodorant afterwards.
3. Wear comfortable and loose fitting clothing.
4. Your drains and dressings will be removed the day after surgery. A fresh dressing will be applied.
5. All sutures will be removed by the eighth postoperative day.
6. You will be unable to drive for the first week following surgery.
7. Depending upon the rapidity of your recovery, you will be allowed to return to work 1 or 2 weeks following surgery.
8. Avoid sun completely for 4 to 6 weeks, after which time you should take protective precautions with a large-brim hat and sunscreens.
9. A tight feeling on the face and neck is normal and will probably last for 2 to 3 months.
10. You may have your hair washed before and after all sutures are removed; however, you should not sit under a hot hair dryer. Hot air will provoke swelling. Hair treatments such as permanents or dyes should be avoided for at least 6 weeks.
11. You may start applying a limited amount of hypoallergenic makeup 5 days after surgery, and you may schedule an appointment with a makeup consultant after 10 days.
12. Your follow-up care schedule with the doctor is as follows:
    1st visit—day after surgery: drain removal and dressing change.
    2nd visit—3 days after surgery: partial suture removal.
    3rd visit—8 days after surgery: final suture removal.
    4th visit—4 weeks after surgery.
    5th visit—8 to 10 weeks after surgery: postoperative photographs are usually taken at this time.
    6th visit—6 months after surgery.
    7th visit—1 year after surgery.

IF YOU ARE NOT IN THE HOSPITAL OR RECOVERY CENTER, IT IS IMPERATIVE THAT YOU HAVE A RESPONSIBLE INDIVIUAL TO TAKE CARE OF YOU FOR THE FIRST 48 TO 72 HOURS FOLLOWING SURGERY. YOU ARE NOT TO REMAIN ALONE.

FIG. 4-1 *An example of postoperative instructions given to the patient before surgery.*

removal and dressing change. The patient is instructed not to leave home during the interval between surgery and the first office appointment. It is recommended that a pain medication or a tranquilizer be taken by the patient before

1. Remain in bed on the day of surgery with the face up.
2. Rest. No physical activity is allowed at all. Stay out of the sun and the heat.
3. Keep head elevated at all times on two or three pillows when lying down.
4. Do not remove pressure dressings. They will be changed at your appointment tomorrow.
5. An appointment for your first postoperative visit will be made before you leave the hospital or clinic.
6. Keep Hemovac drains compressed at all times.
7. Eat only liquids for 24 hours followed by soft foods that require little chewing.
8. Avoid showering the first few days.
9. Take medications as ordered for pain and sleep. Never take more than one type of medicine at the same time. Allow 45 minutes in between different types of medication. Medication on an empty stomach may cause nausea.
10. Do *not* take aspirin or aspirin-containing drugs such as Bufferin, Empirin, Excedrin, or others.
11. Take a pain tablet or tranquilizer 1 hour before leaving home for your first postoperative visit. Someone must transport you to and from the office for this visit because you are not to drive a car for a week following surgery.

FIG. 4-2 *An example of postoperative instructions given to the person responsible for the patient at the time of patient discharge.*

the initial office appointment and dressing change. Use of acetone helps make removal of adhesive easy and painless.

It is advantageous to both the patient and physician to avoid exposing the patient to any health delivery system that the surgeon cannot adequately direct and control. More complications, both physical and psychologic, occur when the patient is exposed to an inefficient and apathetic health care system as typified by some general hospitals. A paradoxical attitude of resentment toward cosmetic patients occasionally has been noted among some hospital personnel. Hospital staff caring for postoperative plastic surgery patients must be trained and motivated to provide proper treatment, otherwise cosmetic surgery patients may be paying premium hospital rates for care that is not provided. Frequently, better and more attentive care for patients is provided at a specialized recovery center or by a family member or friend who has been informed and coached by the plastic surgeon's

1. Facial swelling will be minimized if the head is elevated for 24 hours a day. A chin strap that exerts gentle pressure, such as a tennis head band under the neck, will minimize neck swelling.
2. Soft foods not requiring excessive mastication are permissable 1 or 2 days following surgery. Avoid excessive talking and neck motion because these lead to excessive swelling.
3. Ambulation in the house is permissable but avoid activities that may excite you or result in blood pressure elevation.
4. Before and after suture removal the hair may be gently washed and rinsed using baby shampoo. The hair should be washed by someone else and only as often as once daily. Washing the hair once a day for several days may be required in order to effect thorough cleansing of the hair. Gentle towel drying and room temperature blow drying may be used.
5. Coughing, sneezing, vomiting, hiccupping, and constipation all increase the chance of excessive swelling and hematoma formation (bleeding beneath the skin). Therefore these disturbances should be reported to the doctor's office at once so that appropriate treatment may be recommended. Fluids and milk of magnesia may alleviate constipation whereas tranquilizers and antacids may minimize the incidence of hiccups.

FIG. 4-3 *An example of postoperative instructions given to the patient during the first office visit after surgery.*

surgical staff. The patient's own home environment often makes for speedier recovery than do busy hospitals with staffs that are unresponsive to the needs of plastic surgery patients.

An additional patient care instruction sheet is given at the first postoperative visit to prepare the patient for the intermediate and late postoperative periods (Fig. 4-3). Sessions with a hairstylist or makeup artist enhance postoperative cosmetic results and help reduce the incidence and duration of the usual postoperative depression. Copies of preoperative photographs may be given to the patient after the cosmetic makeup session to reinforce the benefits of surgery in the patient's mind. Almost always the patient forgets the extent of the preoperative deformities after surgery. The lack of positive comments from family members may add to the patient's doubts regarding the surgical improvement. The psychologic aspect of the patient's personality should constantly be reinforced by every member of the plastic surgery team after surgery. All transient side effects of surgery as well as any complications that may arise should be recognized, treated, and explained to the patient promptly. Professional honesty is essential in preserving patient confidence and in minimizing the possibility of medicolegal difficulties (See Chapter 11.).

INTERMEDIATE-TO-LATE POSTOPERATIVE PERIOD

Assuming that planning, execution, and aftercare have been successful, this period of care from 2 weeks to 1 year postoperatively should require minimal expenditure of time. The usual schedule of appointments following each type of operation is given to the patient, usually involving visits at 4 weeks, 10 weeks, 6 months, and 1 year following surgery. This period is largely a time of long-term wound care, ancillary cosmetic enhancement (i.e., makeup, hairstyling, and dress), prevention of psychologic sequelae, and management of any complications or untoward side effects of surgery. Postoperative photographs are taken during this period. During the patient's last regular visit, generally 1 year postoperatively, the patient is told to return annually or whenever a future visit is necessary. It is explained to the patient that the original surgical fee includes all postoperative visits relative to the procedure. Patient records and photographs are cross-indexed and properly filed so that future retrieval is simplified. Each plastic surgeon must adapt the individual approach to postsurgical care so that the needs of the patients and practice are fulfilled. Although there is a tremendous heterogeneity among plastic surgeons and the patients treated, the common denominator of good patient care is the triad of careful planning, precise surgical execution, and effective postsurgical care.

MANAGEMENT OF COMPLICATIONS

For a discussion of the management of complications in the postoperative period, see Chapter 8 and those chapters dealing with specific types of plastic surgery.

CHAPTER 5

Anesthesia for Plastic Surgery

CLIFTON HEBERT AND TAREQ OBAID KHAN

ROLE OF THE ANESTHESIOLOGIST

The role of the anesthesiologist involved in plastic surgery is to maintain patient safety and comfort while accommodating the special needs of the plastic surgeon. Plastic surgery often presents challenging anesthetic management situations. A significant amount of plastic surgery occurs around the face and mouth, isolating the anesthesiologist from the airway, which is always the anesthesiologist's foremost concern. Bleeding, even in small amounts, can deleteriously affect the outcome of surgery. Therefore wide blood pressure swings, postoperative nausea, and postoperative vomiting must be minimized. Coughing and bucking should also be prevented.

Increasingly we can expect to see older patients requesting plastic surgery. These individuals may have one or more coexisting medical conditions that must be properly managed by the anesthesiologist. Also, patients desiring plastic surgery are sometimes in a psychologically vulnerable state, therefore the anesthesiologist must not only be sensitive to the physical concerns of each individual patient but also to the patient's emotional concerns.

The decision to use local anesthesia alone, monitored anesthesia with sedation, or general endotracheal anesthesia depends on many factors, among them patient and surgeon preference. What matters most is that the anesthetic be tailored to the patient. The anesthetic should also be attentively and deliberately managed with its goal being a safe and smooth perioperative course that contributes to the desired surgical outcome. To achieve this, the anesthesiologist must be adept, knowledgeable, and flexible.

PREOPERATIVE EVALUATION

The preoperative visit is the first crucial step in developing each patient's ideal anesthetic. This is a valuable time to discuss with the patient the anesthetic options that are available, the monitoring equipment, and any medications of concern. Any of the patient's questions should also be answered at this time. In these few moments, the anesthesiologist must allay the patient's fears and gain the trust and confidence of the patient. A thorough, well-managed preoperative evaluation including the following will contribute to the patient's sense of well being and give the anesthesiologist all the pertinent information needed to skillfully care for the patient during the intraoperative period:

- ▼ Prior anesthetics are discussed, especially with regard to complications or side effects (e.g., nausea and vomiting).
- ▼ A history of current disease states, medications, and allergies is obtained. In general, current medications should be continued until the day of surgery. Exceptions include monamine oxidase inhibitors, long-acting anticholinesterases, and platelet-inhibiting drugs such as aspirin.
- ▼ A complete physical examination is performed, with particular attention given to the airway anatomy and the pulmonary, cardiovascular, and neurologic status.
- ▼ Appropriate laboratory studies, including ECG and chest x-ray examinations, are performed and interpreted.
- ▼ A thorough assessment of the patient's psychologic state, especially the level of anxiety and acceptance of the proposed surgery, is done.

PREMEDICATION

Sedation

Not every patient requires sedative premedication; for many patients, the preoperative visit is calming and reassuring enough. However, most patients benefit from premedication. There are several options that will render the patient calm and sedated.

A. One hour before surgery

- ▼ Midazolam (Versed) can be given intramuscularly (IM) at a dose of 0.1 to 0.15 mg/kg approximately 1 hour before surgery. This dose is reduced by half for patients more than 65 years of age.
- ▼ A narcotic is another option. Morphine sulfate given at a dose of 0.1 to 0.15 mg/kg IM or meperidine (Demerol) given at a dose of 50 to 100 mg IM are often used in combination with an antiemetic such as hydroxyzine (Vistaril). Many other medications may also serve as well; the choice lies with the individual anesthesiologist and surgeon.

B. While in holding area or operating room. When the patient reaches the holding area or operating room (OR), an adequate intravenous (IV) line must be established. At this time, the anesthesiologist should assess the patient for level of sedation and decide whether to add to the premedication or wait to proceed to general anesthesia.

Aspiration Prophylaxis

Some specialists recommend aspiration prophylaxis for patients undergoing prolonged anesthesia. Typically this includes an H^2 receptor antagonist such as ranitidine and a nonparticulate antiacid such as sodium citrate. One should consider metoclopramide (a stimulant to gastric motility), which increases gastric clearance and lowers esophageal sphincter tone. Routine preoperative use of anticholinergics as antisialagogues is no longer recommended.

ANESTHESIA PROCEDURE

Local Anesthesia

Local anesthetics are drugs that provide a reversible blockade of nerve impulse conduction without damaging to the nerve. Local anesthetics fall into two groups based on their chemical structure: amides and esters. The most commonly used local anesthetics and their onset of action, duration of action, and maximum recommended dose are given below. Techniques for application of local anesthetics are discussed in chapters on specific types of plastic surgery.

A. **Specific anesthetic agents**

▼ Amides

■ Lidocaine. This is the most commonly used local anesthetic for infiltration. Its onset is rapid, and it has a duration of action of 45 to 120 minutes. The addition of 1:200,000 epinephrine will approximately double its duration of action. Lidocaine is extensively metabolized by the liver; thus, repeated doses are possible.

■ Bupivacaine. This drug is less commonly used than lidocaine, its onset of action is slower, but its duration is longer (240 to 480 minutes). The maximum dose is 175 mg.

■ Mepivacaine. This drug has a slow onset of action and a duration of action of 90 to 180 minutes. The maximum adult dose is 300 mg.

▼ Esters

■ Cocaine. The first local anesthetic discovered, cocaine is used when both anesthesia and vasoconstriction are desired (e.g., nasal mucosa). It is supplied in solutions of 4% and 5% for topical administration.

■ Chloroprocaine. This drug has a rapid onset and a short duration of action (30 to 45 minutes). The maximum dosage is 600 mg for a single dose.

B. **Side effects.** Side effects of local anesthetics are principally allergic reactions or systemic toxicity.

▼ Allergic reactions are quite rare. Cross sensitivity between esters and amides does not occur so a patient who has had an allergic reaction to a local anesthetic of one class may safely receive a local anesthetic of another class as long as it is free of preservatives.

▼ Systemic toxicity is related to plasma levels of the anesthetic and primarily involves the central nervous system and the cardiovascular system. Central nervous system toxicity is initially noted as tongue and circumoral numbness progressing to restlessness, vertigo, tinnitus, and difficulty focusing. With further increases in plasma levels, slurred speech and muscular twitching may occur. Muscle twitching may progress to tonic clonic seizures. Amide local anesthetics, especially lidocaine, may produce drowsiness before the onset of seizures. The cardiovascular system is more resistant to local anesthetic toxicity than the central nervous system. However, high plasma levels of local anesthetics may cause profound hypotension and myocardial depression. Significantly, bupivacaine if injected intravascularly may result in precipitous hypotension, cardiac dysrhythmias, and atrioventricular (AV) heart block.

Monitored Anesthesia Care

This is the technique whereby the surgeon administers local anesthesia while the anesthesiologist monitors the patient and adds supplemental IV sedation. Monitored anesthesia care (MAC) can be one of the most difficult but most satisfying anesthetic techniques. The patient must be adequately sedated to tolerate the procedure but not so sedated as to be uncooperative, or worse, unable to maintain and protect the airway. No magic formula exists for the necessary level of sedation; each patient requires an individualized technique. Careful titration of medication, constant communication with the surgeon, and vigilant observation of the patient will help the anesthesiologist to ensure success. It is important to inform the patient before the operation and again just before the actual injection of local anesthetic that some pain will be felt but that it will be transient.

A. **Patient selection.** Recovery from MAC is brief (1 to 2 hours), which makes it an excellent choice for outpatient procedures. Nausea and vomiting are less common following MAC than with general anesthesia. Remarkably, extensive procedures of the face and eyes, including face lifts and quadrilateral blepharoplasty can readily be managed with MAC. However, certain patients are not good candidates for MAC. Patients who are excessively anxious despite adequate preoperative explanation, patients with a history of significant neurosis or psychosis, patients with gastroesophageal reflux, and patients with marked chronic obstructive pulmonary disease (COPD) are frequently best managed with general anesthesia.

B. **Premedication.** Patients undergoing MAC typically receive a mild preoperative medication several minutes before the surgical procedure begins. Small incremental doses of a narcotic are often used (e.g., fentanyl, 25 to 50 mcg; alfentanyl, 100 to 200 mcg; benzodiazepine [almost exclusively midazolam] 1.0 to 2.0 mg). The narcotic provides some analgesia and a sense of well being, while benzodiazepine provides sedation and often amnesia. This combination can act synergistically to depress ventilation, especially in older patients therefore caution must be exercised.

C. **Patient monitoring.** Patients are monitored in essentially the same manner as patients undergoing general anesthesia:

- Blood pressure
- Electrocardiograph (ECG)
- Precordial stethoscope
- Temperature probe and pulse oximeter
- Nasal O^2 cannulae are placed before the surgical prep, then prepped in place. Recently, a nasal O^2 cannula with a capnography port to measure exhaled CO^2 has become available and has proven to be very useful.

The anesthesia machine and intubation and suction equipment should be checked to make sure they are ready for use.

D. **Anesthetic technique.** Used deftly, MAC is effective. Recent advances in pharmacology and infusion technology have spurred the refinement of the technique.

- A combination found to be effective is a propofol infusion, often used alone. An initial bolus of 0.5 to 1.0 mg/kg is followed by a constant infusion of 25 to 75 mcg/kg/min. The infusion pumps allow for boluses as needed and easy titration to effect. The patient can be sedated to a near ideal state: sleeping comfortably, easily aroused, and in control of the airway. The surgeon can infiltrate the operative field with local anesthetic usually with minimal discomfort to the patient.

- If propofol alone is inadequate or if the patient will be injected many times with local anesthetics, an infusion of alfentanyl in tandem with propofol is effective. The dose of alfentanyl is usually 10 to 15 mcg/kg/min. Patients on this regimen frequently have no recollection of intraoperative events, although amnesia is not assured and should not be promised in a MAC. Certainly, other pharmacologic combinations can be equally effective.

General Anesthesia

A. **Patient selection.** As previously discussed, certain patients are not good candidates for MAC and the following will require general anesthesia:

- Patients who are too anxious to accept any intraoperative awareness or mild pain should not be forced to undergo MAC.
- Patients whose surgical procedure involves extensive bone work are best managed with general anesthesia.
- Patients with coexisting medical conditions that predispose them to airway difficulty (e.g., sleep apnea or morbid obesity), hypoxia (e.g., COPD), or increased risk of pulmonary aspiration (e.g., symptomatic hiatal hernia or esophageal reflux) should have their airway protected by general endotracheal anesthesia.
- Patients undergoing surgical procedures that will be extremely long should be considered for general anesthesia because the necessary dose of local anesthetic agents may approach toxic levels and patients may also become agitated with prolonged immobility.

B. **Premedication.** Preoperative medications are similar to those for MAC. Narcotics are often given IV several minutes before the procedure to minimize the patient's hemodynamic response to laryngoscopy and endotracheal intubation. Among the most commonly used agents are the following:

- Fentanyl citrate is a synthetic opioid agonist that is 75 to 125 times more potent than morphine. Its onset and duration of action are shorter than morphine. When given doses ranging from 2 to 10 mcg/kg, it is used to blunt the circulatory response to intubation. Like other opioids, it is a powerful ventilatory depressant.
- Sufentanil is a thiamyl analog of fentanyl that is 5 to 10 times more potent as fentanyl. Its elimination half time is intermediate between that of fentanyl and alfentanil.
- Alfentanil is another analog of fentanyl with 10% to 20% of fentanyl's potency and one third its duration of action, making this a good choice for outpatient procedures.

C. **Induction.** Induction of anesthesia is usually accomplished with one of the following agents:

- Sodium thiopental. This barbiturate is the most commonly used induction agent in the United States. The induction dose is 3 to 5 mg/kg. The onset of anesthesia is rapid and smooth with mild cardiovascular depression in normovolemic patients. When combined with low to moderate dose narcotics, muscle relaxation, and a volatile agent (e.g., etomidate and propofol) in a balanced technique, thiopental provides excellent anesthesia for a wide variety of surgical procedures.
- Etomidate. This is a carboxylated imidazole containing compound chemically unrelated to other induction agents. The induction dose is 0.1 to 0.3 mg/kg. The onset of anesthesia is rapid and smooth, with less hemodynamic change than seen with thiopental; hence it is an alternative to thiopental for patients with an unstable cardiovascular system or in hypovolemic patients. Its clearance is more rapid than thiopental, making it a logical choice for outpatient procedures.

- Propofol. A substituted isopropylphenol, propofol is a rapid-acting intravenous anesthetic. It is virtually insoluble in water so it is solubilized in lecithin-containing compounds. It is lipid soluble, which accounts for its rapid onset. Awakening occurs in 4 to 8 minutes following the usual dose of 1.5 to 3.0 mg/kg. There usually is a more rapid return of preoperative cognitive function following propofol compared to barbiturates, and there is less likelihood of nausea and vomiting. Both of these characteristics make it desirable in the outpatient setting. There is a dose-dependent cardiovascular depression with propofol, similar to thiopental. Other side effects are rare but include pain at injection, involuntary muscle movement (not fasciculations), coughing, and hiccoughs.

D. **Endotracheal intubation.** Typically, patients receiving general anesthesia require endotracheal intubation. The endotracheal tube may be a standard low-pressure, high-volume cuff type or a preformed nasal or oral RAE tube that curves out toward the forehead or down along the chin. The type of surgery dictates the tube choice. Once the endotracheal tube is placed, most anesthesiologists mechanically control ventilation rather than allow spontaneous ventilation. Intubation is facilitated by muscle relaxation with one of the neuromuscular blocking drugs (listed). The hemodynamic response to intubation may be blunted with the following IV narcotics:

- Muscle relaxants
  - Succinylcholine chloride is depolarizing muscle relaxant with rapid onset and a short duration of action. Onset occurs in 30 to 60 seconds with a duration of 3 to 5 minutes following an intubating dose of 0.5 to 1.0 mg/kg. Succinylcholine is metabolized by plasma cholinesterase. The advantages of rapid and predictable onset, short duration, plasma metabolism requiring no reversal, and excellent intubation conditions ensure its continued use.
  - Vecuronium bromide is intermediate-acting, nondepolarizing muscle relaxant. The usual dose

is 0.04 to 0.07 mg/kg, with the onset of maximal relaxation in 3 to 5 minutes. Relaxation can be antagonized in 20 to 30 minutes. Metabolism is primarily hepatic. Vecuronium has few side effects, is predictable, and causes few hemodynamic changes.

- Atracurium is another intermediate-acting, nondepolarizing muscle relaxant. Its usual dose is 0.15 to 0.3 mg/kg with similar onset and duration compared to vecuronium. It is metabolized by Hoffman elimination and ester hydrolysis, which both occur in the plasma.

E. **Maintenance of anesthesia.** Typically this is accomplished with a combination of a volatile agent or propofol infusion, narcotic, and muscle relaxants. However, muscle relaxants may be eliminated in procedures involving dissection in the area of the facial nerve. It is prudent for the anesthesiologist to discuss the use of muscle relaxants with the surgeon preoperatively. Nitrous oxide may or may not be added to supplement intraoperative analgesia.

▼ Volatile agents

- Isoflurane is clear, nonflammable volatile liquid kept at room temperature with intermediate blood solubility and high potency. It provides the rapid onset of and quick recovery from anesthesia. Isoflurane produces a dose-dependent decrease in peripheral vascular resistance, thereby decreasing blood pressure. Used alone, it may cause an increase in heart rate 20% above baseline at 1 minimum alveolar concentration (MAC) and above. Isoflurane does not significantly lower cardiac output during normocapnic controlled ventilation. Currently widely used and effective, it is not an analgesic, but it is a good amnesic agent.

- Enflurane is also a clear, nonflammable volatile liquid with high potency and intermediate blood solubility. It provides rapid onset of and recovery from anesthesia. Enflurane produces a dose-dependent decrease in blood pressure, primarily by decreasing cardiac output. It produces a dose-dependent increase in heart rate at above 1 MAC. Like isoflurane, enflurane is not analgesic but is amnesic.

- Halothane is a halogenated, volatile liquid kept at room temperature. It has been associated with postanesthetic hepatitis and thus is less commonly used in the adult population than other agents.

F. **Emergence from anesthesia.** A smooth emergence from general anesthesia that is free of coughing, bucking, nausea, and vomiting is crucial to plastic surgery. Unfortunately, there is no fixed recipe or magic formula that guarantees a smooth emergence.

▼ One technique to ease emergence from anesthesia involves extubating the spontaneously breathing patient while the patient is still in relatively deep anesthesia. Deep extubation should be avoided in patients with a full stomach or an abnormal airway anatomy. It should also be avoided in patients in whom the intubation was difficult. When used in the proper patient population, this technique is effective.

▼ Another technique entails titrating moderate doses of narcotic throughout the operation so that at the end of the procedure the patient is comfortable, awake, and tolerates the endotracheal tube. The tube is removed once the patient is responsive and exhibits adequate reversal of neuromuscular blockade as determined by a nerve stimulator and sustained head life. To facilitate smooth emergence, many anesthesiologists administer lidocaine 1.0 to 1.5 mg/kg IV 3 to 5 minutes before the anticipated end of surgery.

▼ In patients with a prior history of postoperative nausea and vomiting, an antiemetic may be given intraoperatively. Commonly used medications include droperidol (1.25 mg IV) and metoclopramide (10.0 mg IV). More recently a new agent, ondansetron hydrochloride (Zofran), has been effective in controlling nausea and vomiting. The postoperative dose typically is 4.0 mg.

RECOVERY AND POSTOPERATIVE ANALGESIA

Patients who have had plastic surgery recover in a similar manner as other postsurgical patients. In addition to returning to clear consciousness and hemodynamic and hemostatic stability, patients must receive adequate postoperative analgesia.

- Narcotic agents. Traditionally, narcotics have been the mainstay of postoperative analgesia. Fentanyl in incremental dosages of 25 mcg repeated every 5 to 10 minutes up to 100 mcg is generally adequate for minor outpatient procedures. For more extensive procedures and for inpatients, morphine sulfate given in incremental doses of 2.0 to 5.0 mg IV in incremental doses is effective. Inpatients who will receive narcotics via IV patient-controlled devices should have their infusions started in the recovery room to ensure uninterrupted analgesia.
- Nonnarcotic agents. A recently approved nonnarcotic agent is ketorolac (Toradol), which is a nonsteroidal antiinflammatory agent that works by inhibiting prostaglandin synthesis. In the 30 to 60 mg IM range, its potency is similar to that of morphine sulfate 6 to 12 mg IM, with a duration of action as long as 6 hours. It does not cause ventilatory depression, and it causes less sedation, nausea, and vomiting than morphine. Ketorolac is useful in both the inpatient and especially the outpatient population.

CHAPTER 6

Plastic Surgical Nursing

CHRISTINA MATHIS

Plastic surgery is a diverse specialty encompassing the broad range of trauma, reconstructive, and aesthetic patients. The plastic surgical nurse serves a vital role in understanding the human element of the patient while the patient is most vulnerable. With the ability to "read between the lines," the nurse can assist the patient and inform the surgeon of the patient's special needs. When working together with the surgeon and the other medical staff, the plastic surgical nurse can contribute special skills to help make the surgical experience favorable for the patient and self rewarding.

INITIAL OFFICE VISIT

It is vital for the patient undergoing an elective plastic surgical procedure to feel confident with the surgeon and the office staff. The office setting is usually the patient's first impression of the surgeon. Although a patient may like a particular surgeon, the patient may be made to feel depersonalized or uncomfortable by that surgeon's office staff. Knowing that a major portion of the instruction, care, and solace would come from the surgeon's nursing and office staff, this patient may find comfort and treatment at another surgeon's office.

A skilled plastic surgical nurse can place the new patient at ease almost immediately when introducing oneself and explaining the nurse's function and the facts about the surgical procedure.

Answering Patients' Questions

After the patient has consulted with the surgeon, the nurse should ask the patient if all questions were answered by the surgeon. Often a patient will ask questions or express concerns with the nurse that the patient previously forgot or felt was too trivial to ask the surgeon. While building this initial rapport and trust, the patient will often reveal personal details or the reasons for undergoing a particular operation.

Evaluating Patients' Goals and Expectations

The nurse often helps in evaluating the patient's desired goals and expectations. A nurse's private and sensitive discussions with a patient can help ensure realistic results and honest expectations. Some patients seek surgery for social, sexual, or business approval. Some younger patients may desire to change an inherited trait. Some middle-aged patients seek restorative surgery because of competition in the workplace. Some older patients may want plastic surgery to help keep up with their grandchildren.

The nurse can, for example, evaluate the goals and expectations of a breast augmentation patient. The nurse can help a breast augmentation patient to determine the breast size desired by the patient. Initially a woman may say she does not want her breasts made "too big." The surgeon needs to determine what "too big" means to a particular patient. The nurse may talk in terms of brassiere size and encourage the patient to bring in pictures of women whose breast size she thinks is attractive. The nurse may also suggest that the patient go to a store to try on padded brassieres in the desired size. The nurse should also explain the type and approximate size of the brassiere to be worn after surgery and where it can be purchased. It is important to explain to the patient undergoing breast surgery that (1) it will take approximately 2 weeks for the breast swelling to return to normal and approximately 6 weeks for the breasts to loosen and appear more natural; and (2) at the first postoperative visit, the patient will be able to view the results of surgery, which is usually exciting for patients because they are usually instantly pleased.

Discussing Patients' Fears and Expectations

The patient often asks the nurse if the decision to have plastic surgery is appropriate. A patient discussing fears and expectations of surgery usually experiences less anxiety during surgery and requires less medication intraoperatively. The aesthetic surgical patient usually has different needs than a nonelective patient. Some patients may have a deflated self-image caused by the natural aging process, divorce, death of a spouse, or career difficulties. Improving one's appearance often enhances a patient's self-image, but regardless of a patient's expectations, plastic surgery will not "fix" a marriage or an unhappy life. A patient may receive varying reactions about plastic surgery from family and friends. For example, a husband may declare he loves his wife just as she is, implying "Please, do not change." Some spouses may be jealous or insecure, not wanting their spouse to look better than they themselves do. Others may elect to have plastic surgery after seeing their partner's happy results. Friends may not see the need for any change or may be jealous and say "I can't see any difference," or "I liked your old nose."

Reassuring Patients

Positive support from spouses, family, and friends undoubtedly helps achieve a smoother, uneventful operative and postoperative course. Considering that some patients lack such support, it is important to remember that plastic surgery patients need constant reassurance and understanding from the nursing, office, and hospital staffs throughout their entire surgical experience.

The nurse should reassure the patient that confidentiality is held in highest regard both in and out of the office setting. It is important for the medical staff to keep a patient's identity and surgery private, even though a patient may choose to discuss the situation with others. A patient who is concerned about seeing others in the office may be accommodated by coordinating a specific appointment time or by using a second entrance.

PREOPERATIVE VISIT

At the preoperative visit, which is scheduled a day or week before surgery, it is important for the patient to be able to express any remaining concerns and anxieties. By understanding the patient's level of anxiety, showing compassion, and encouraging open communication, the nurse helps build confidence in the preoperative patient.

Explanation of Procedure and Possible Complications

The nurse should explain what will happen the morning of surgery, knowing that some patients are frightened by too many details, while others are more comfortable knowing all the details. Both the physician and the nurse should explain again the procedure to be performed and ask if the patient understands. The risks of surgery are explained to the patient in a manner that informs the patient without being threatening. The nurse should explain that nothing in life, including plastic surgery, is without risk and that if a complication develops, it will be treated appropriately. At this time, the informed consent form, which allows the surgeon to perform the operation, will be explained in detail, signed, and witnessed.

Patients often inquire about scar formation. The patient should be told where the incision or incisions will be placed and approximately how long the scar will take to become less noticable. Knowing that it is normal for a scar to be red after surgery and that it takes several months to 1 year or more to completely heal not only informs the patient but also makes the patient more relaxed postoperatively.

Instructions for Preoperative and Postoperative Care

The nurse should give the patient instructions for preoperative and postoperative care, encourage the patient to ask questions, and make suggestions. Because patients are usually overwhelmed the week before surgery, instructions should be given to them in written form as well as orally. Some suggestions that the nurse can offer to make the postoperative period easier are listed below:

- ▼ Fill prescriptions before surgery so they are available when needed at home.
- ▼ Prepare meals in advance for several days after surgery (within usual postoperative nutritional guidelines).
- ▼ Plan postoperative care before surgery.

The nurse should explain to the person caring for the patient after surgery what care is needed and answer questions. At this time, the nurse may perceive whether or not the family member or friend feels comfortable caring for the postoperative patient. The patient and family member may opt instead to stay overnight in the hospital or an after-care facility with personnel trained to care for postoperative patients. This may also apply to patients from out of town or living some distance from where surgery is performed. The patient should be told that heavily sedated postoperative patients are not allowed to be discharged to home alone. The nurse should insist that a relative or friend stay with the patient for at least the first 24 hours. If this is not possible, arrangements can be made for a private nurse to stay at the patient's home.

Inquiry about Prior Surgeries and Medical Conditions

During the preoperative visit the nurse should again ask the patient about any prior surgeries performed and if any medications are being taken—either prescribed or over the counter. A patient may initially forget to mention a medication that was purchased without a prescription. The nurse should explain the importance of preoperative laboratory tests by informing the patient of specific abnormalities being screened for, such as prolonged bleeding time, increased white blood cell count, or low potassium level. With the increasing concern about the spread of the human immunodeficiency virus (HIV), many surgeons and hospitals are requiring HIV screening tests for surgical patients as part of the laboratory routine. The nurse should explain that all testing is confidential, and written consent should be obtained for HIV testing from the patient. A patient is less likely to complain about laboratory costs once the importance of these tests to normal recovery is understood.

DAY OF SURGERY

▼ The nurse should greet the patient cheerfully, confidently, and with ease. If a nurse is unsure of the job duties, the patient will sense it. By asking the patient how well he or she slept, one is able to assess the anxiety level and to provide an opportunity for expression of any misgivings. The skilled nurse can alleviate the fears and apprehensions of the preoperative patient by reassuring the person that what is being felt is normal. Often the patient needs reassurance that the decision to have plastic surgery is the right one. Although the patient has made the decision to have surgery, the patient still needs a professional to reinforce the decision. The nurse should refrain from making statements such as "You will look 10 years younger," or "You will have a perfect result," because this implies a guarantee and places the surgeon and nurse in a defensive position. *Elective surgery* means just that—the patient has decided to have surgery, not that the patient has been persuaded to have surgery.

- ▼ The nurse should check the patient chart for completeness, including laboratory values for all ordered tests, to help ensure promptness of the surgery starting time. Some preoperative prepping, such as trimming of hair, can be performed in the surgical holding area because it decreases actual operating room (OR) time. The anesthesia team may prefer to start intravenous (IV) medication in the surgical holding areas and administer some preoperative sedation.
- ▼ The OR should be set up for surgery before the sedated patient is brought into the room. The sight of all of the instruments and equipment can be frightening to a fully awake patient.
- ▼ After the patient is moved to the OR table, the nurse should explain each procedure as it is being done (e.g., placing cold monitoring leads, ground pad, and pulseoximeter lead). The nurse should reassure the patient that no one will do anything causing discomfort without warning the patient.
- ▼ The nurse should consider the patient's comfort during a long surgical procedure by applying foam padding, pillows, or a blanket as needed.
- ▼ Upon arrival in the OR, a patient often feels reassured in knowing that the surgeon is present. Having the surgeon say "Hello" and call the patient by name will help relax

an anxious patient. The anesthesia team will monitor the patient throughout the operative procedure and notify the surgeon of any irregularities or important changes in vital signs. The nurse is the patient's advocate at all times, and just holding the patient's hand is deeply appreciated by the patient. A patient may sense the nurse that gives extra and may be more able to relax throughout the OR experience. The surgeon can concentrate on the technical aspects of the operation while the nurse and anesthetist remain conscious of the patient's safety and comfort, always observing for restlessness, anxiety, or pain.

- After the patient is moved to the recovery room, the patient is carefully positioned and comforted again with pillows and blankets. The patient's vital signs and level of response are constantly monitored.
- Ice compresses are usually applied for nasal and eyelid surgery.
- The nurse may want to refrain from answering too many questions during the early recovery period because a patient is still sedated and usually will not remember the answers.

HOSPITALIZATION

During hospitalization, the aesthetic patient comes in contact with many different hospital personnel—admitting office staff, laboratory and x-ray technicians, housekeeping personnel, ward clerks, and nursing staff. The patient may feel the need to defend the decision for aesthetic surgery to each of these numerous hospital personnel. This defensiveness can be enhanced by well-meaning attempts by personnel to offer support with statements such as "You do not look like you needed surgery." Because the patient's need to defend the decision can be renewed with each staff member, it is advantageous to provide continuity of nursing staff whenever possible. This enables the patient to develop a relationship of trust with a few plastic surgery staff members. Such continuity with aesthetic patients will also allow the nurse to become comfortable with preoperative and postoperative requirements and needs of the plastic surgery patient.

DISCHARGE

- An outpatient should be discharged to the family or responsible adult only when fully stable and conscious. Before the patient leaves for home, the nurse should discuss again with the family the signs and symptoms to watch for possible complications of surgery. The nurse may show the person caring for the patient how to check the dressings and change the nasal drip pads or eyelid compresses. The nurse should explain that excessive swelling could be an indication of a hematoma, how painful it may be, and the necessity of calling the surgeon if abnormal bleeding or swelling occurs. The nurse should also clarify that some swelling is normal, and one should not be alarmed by some bruising and swelling.
- The nurse should explain to a breast augmentation patient how soft the upper breast is currently and describe how firm and painful the breast would become if bleeding were to occur.
- The nurse should reinforce diet, activity, and medications with the family. The dosage of pain medication is explained again. Sleeping medication is encouraged the first night after surgery to ensure rest. It is further explained that it is acceptable for the patient to remain somewhat sedated following surgery.
- The nurse should secure any drain reservoirs to the patient so that the patient will be comfortable overnight.
- The nurse or surgeon examines the patient before discharge. Outpatients leave by wheelchair because many feel faint when standing or walking.
- With nasal surgery, it is wise to anticipate postoperative vomiting if the patient has swallowed blood. Sending an emesis basin home with the patient may be appreciated by the patient.
- The patient is given an appointment for a return visit and assured that a physician is available day or night if needed.

- It is reassuring for the patient when the medical staff telephones later inquiring about pain, vomiting, swelling, and fever.

RETURN VISITS

Removal of Dressings

Dressings are removed on the first return visit. Even with the most thorough preparation, the patient may be upset by the appearance and should be reassured about discoloration and swelling. Some patients may experience varying degrees of postoperative depression, especially when looking in the mirror. They may recall that they came in feeling fine and now they feel terrible. It is important for the nurse, surgeon, and entire medical staff to be supportive and explain that this feeling is normal. Reassuring the postoperative patient that the swelling and bruising will subside in a few days and that hypoallergenic makeup can be worn soon helps the patient realize that the present appearance is only temporary. Personal care and gradually resuming normal activities should be discussed with the patient.

Viewing of "Before"Photos

Within a few weeks, the patient may view the "before" photos. Often the response is one of forgetfulness of the preoperative condition and appreciation of the new appearance. Slight displeasures concerning the results can be diminished at this time by the nurse's and the surgeon's reassurances that edema takes months to reabsorb and scars take as long as 1 year or more to mature. The nurse should explain to the patient that improvements after surgery will continue for several months to a year or more. Assurance is given that the surgeon will revise if necessary any long-lasting problem at the appropriate time. When the patient returns in 8 to 10 weeks for postoperative photos, the postoperative progress can be visually monitored.

CHAPTER 7

Transfusion Therapy

John D. Milam

Transfusion medicine refers to the treatment of certain disorders of blood, of the constituents of blood, or of the hematopoietic system. The objective of transfusion therapy is to improve the patient's status by using blood, blood components, blood derivatives, or pharmacologic agents. Issues associated with transfusion medicine relate to (1) supply, (2) safety, (3) cost, and (4) appropriate use of blood. In the last 15 years, our scientific and medical environment has changed primarily because of newly recognized infectious agents that can be transmitted by blood transfusion. Although blood transfusion is an essential part of the medical and surgical management of many patients, avoiding unwarranted transfusion of blood and any of its components that may cause adverse effects constitutes good medical practice. Despite the many measures that have been taken to reduce the risk of blood transfusion, it is not currently possible to provide a blood supply without risk. Physicians should be aware of the risks and benefits of transfusion therapy and should prescribe transfusion only when the expected benefits clearly outweigh the risks.

RISKS OF TRANSFUSION

Recognized risks of blood transfusion are listed in Table 7-1. Following are the primary reasons to avoid transfusion when possible:

- ▼ Risks of transmitting transfusion-associated infections will be avoided.
- ▼ The possibility of nonhemolytic (e.g., allergic, febrile, and bacterial), hemolytic, and delayed hemolytic transfusion reactions will be averted.

Table 7-1 *Risks of Blood Transfusion*

Immediate Adverse Reactions

Allergic reaction
Febrile reaction
Bacterial sepsis
Circulatory overload
Hemolytic transfusion reaction
Nonimmune-mediated hemolysis
Noncardiogenic pulmonary edema
Hypotension caused by prekallikrein activation
Hypothermia
Microaggregate transfusion
Metabolite toxicity
  Citrate
  Potassium
  Ammonia
Air embolism
Anaphylactic reaction

Delayed Adverse Reactions

Transfusion-associated infections

Babesiosis
Borrelia
Brucellosis
Cytomegalovirus
Epstein-Barr virus
Hepatitis (virus exhibiting tropism)
  A, B, C, D, E, and other forms of non-A, non-B
Herpes simplex
HHV 6
HIV
  Type 1
  Type 2
HTLV-1
Kala azar (*Leishmania donovani*)
Lyme disease (*Borrelia burgdorferi*)
Malaria
Human parvovirus B19
Syphilis (*Treponema pallidum*)
Toxoplasmosis
Trypanosomiasis (*Trypanosoma cruzi*)

Other delayed adverse reactions

Alloimmunization
Transfusion hemosiderosis
Graft-versus-host disease
Delayed hemolytic transfusion reaction
Posttransfusion purpura

HHV 6, Human herpes virus 6; *HIV,* human immunodeficiency virus; *HTLV-1,* human T-cell lymphotrophic virus, type I.

- The formation of blood-group alloantibodies, which are more significant in a patient who may require blood transfusion later and in a woman who may be alloimmunized and may subsequently experience hemolytic disease of the fetus or newborn during pregnancy, will be prevented.
- The formation of antileukocyte and antiplatelet antibodies, which may be significant after future transfusions or pregnancies, will be precluded.
- Practices that permit operations on a patient with religious opposition to blood transfusion will be promoted.
- Rare transfusion-associated complications, such as posttransfusion purpura and antiimmunoglobulin A anaphylaxis will be prevented.
- Blood shortages will be prevented.
- Costs will be reduced.

Most patients' concerns involve two issues: safety of the transfusion and diminishing thc risk of transfusion.

Transfusion-Associated Infections

Despite stringent measures for ensuring a safe blood supply, significant transfusion-associated infections still can occur.

A. **Hepatitis and human immunodeficiency virus.** The incidence of transfusion-associated hepatitis has decreased significantly with the availability of sensitive screening procedures. Transmission of the hepatitis C virus has been the most common serious complication of blood transfusion. However, the possibility of transmitting human immunodeficiency virus (HIV) has created the greatest public concern. Through the development of stringent procedures for donor selection and laboratory screening, the likelihood of hepatitis or HIV transmission by blood transfusion is remote. The risk of transmitting HIV by blood transfusion has been estimated to range from a ratio of 1:40,000 to 1:1,000,000 a unit. More recently the overall risk of transfusion-associated HIV infection is estimated to be a ratio of 1:225,000 a unit. The frequency of hepatitis C virus transmission is less than 1 in 3000 units of blood or components transfused, and the risk of transmitting hepatitis B virus is approximately 1 in 200,000.

B. Human T-lymphotropic virus, type I. Human T-lymphotropic virus, type I (HTLV-I) has been associated with adult T-cell leukemia and with tropical spastic paraparesis (HTLV-I associated myelopathy). HTLV-I is transmitted by sexual contact, by the infected mother to the fetus, by intravenous (IV) drug abuse, and by blood transfusions. Blood donors are screened by anti-HTLV-I and II testing, which detects antibodies directed against HTLV-I and II.

PREOPERATIVE EVALUATION

To achieve the goals of plastic surgery, avoidance of excessive hemorrhage and wound hematoma formation is desirable. The best way to detect bleeding disorders is to obtain the patient's complete medical history.

Medical History

A. Bleeding tendencies. Questions concerning the effect of trauma (mild to major), previous surgery, tooth extractions, small cuts, and bleeding gums help to detect abnormal bleeding tendencies. Petechiae and easy bruising may be of concern, although easy bruising is not uncommon in young women. The synthesis of prothrombin and coagulation factors VII, IX, and X depends on sufficient vitamin K availability. A patient who suffers from poor nutrition, alcohol abuse, or an impaired nutritional intake, even for only a few days, may show a tendency to bleed because of deficiency in one or more of the vitamin K-dependent factors.

B. Medications

- ▼ Aspirin and other drugs that may alter platelet function. Platelet function may be significantly altered by aspirin and other drugs (Table 7-2). The average life span of blood platelets is approximately 9 days. In general, a patient should not take medications that adversely affect platelet function for at least 5 days before elective surgery. Because many over-the-counter and prescribed medications contain salicylates, the facts regarding the effects of aspirin and other antiplatelet medications

Table 7-2 *Drugs that Adversely Affect Platelet Function*

GENERIC NAME	TRADE NAME
Aminophylline	Aminophylline
Amitriptyline	Elavil, Limbitrol
Aspirin	Numerous medications
Carbenicillin	Geocillin
Chlorpromazine	Thorazine
Clofibrate	Atromid- S
Dextran	Macrodex, Rheomacrodex
Dipyridamole	Persantine
Fenoprofen	Nalfon
Furosemide	Lasix
Glyceryl guaiacolate	cough syrups (e.g., Robitussin)
Heparin	Heparin
Ibuprofen	Motrin, Advil
Imipramine	Tofranil-PM
Indomethacin	Indocin
Mefenamic acid	Ponstel
Mezlocillin	Mezlin
Moxalactam	Moxam
Nitrofurantoin	Furadantin
Papaverine	Papaverine
Penicillin G	Penicillin G
Phenylbutazone	Butazolidin
Piperacillin	Pipracil
Promethazine	Phenergan
Propranolol	Inderal
Sulfinpyrazone	Anturane
Theophylline	Cough syrups
Ticarcillin	Ticar
Vitamin E	Vitamin E
Warfarin	Coumadin, Panwarfin
Antihistamines	More than 50 products
Local anesthetics	
Cocaine	Cocaine
Procaine	Novocain
Lidocaine	Xylocaine
Phenothiazine derivatives	Sparine, Temaril

should be emphasized to the patient well in advance of surgery.

- Coumarin. A patient on coumarin (warfarin) therapy, which interferes with vitamin K metabolism, may bleed excessively during surgery. When this patient is scheduled for elective surgery, the coumarin dosages should be reduced gradually for several days before surgery. The drug should not be discontinued suddenly because this may cause rebound hypercoagulability. When a patient who takes coumarin has a prothrombin time that exceeds the control value by 4 seconds, a mild bleeding tendency is generally observed. When a patient's prothrombin time is at least one and one half to two times the control value, hemorrhage often is significant. Clinically the risk of hemorrhage must be weighed against the benefit of anticoagulation and the need for surgery. Coagulation deficiencies are less problematic when pressure dressings can be applied.

C. **Liver disease.** The following coagulation factors are synthesized in the liver: factor I (fibrinogen), factor II (prothrombin), factor V (labile factor), factor VII (stable factor), factor IX (plasma thromboplastin component), and factor X (Stuart-Prower factor). In the patient with severe liver disease, one or more of these procoagulants can be reduced significantly.

Coagulation Tests

Depending on the type of surgery to be performed and the medical history of the patient, a battery of coagulation tests may be used to detect and define the bleeding tendency of the patient. No single test can disclose all coagulopathies. The most commonly used coagulation tests include the activated partial thromboplastin time, the prothrombin time, quantitative fibrinogen, and platelet count. Platelet function studies can help to identify platelet dysfunction.

Anemia

When detected preoperatively, anemia is a symptom of disease, and its etiology should be sought because the underlying cause may be significant. It is best to plan anemia therapy after its etiology has been determined. Using blood transfusion to restore the patient's hemoglobin and hematocrit to normal levels before elective surgery is rarely indicated. There is no unequivocally established hemoglobin level at which operative safety is increased or a level below which the risks of anesthesia and surgery are increased. A patient is evaluated objectively to determine if, based on clinical circumstances, there is a need for preoperative confusion. Clinical circumstances that indicate the need for preoperative transfusion relate to the patient's ability to physiologically compensate for reduced hemoglobin and hematocrit levels. Heart, lung, and cerebrovascular diseases are conditions that may compromise a patient's ability to compensate for decreases in hemoglobin.

AUTOLOGOUS DONATION OR TRANSFUSION

The term autologous transfusion or autotransfusion generally denotes the collection of blood from a donor/patient for subsequent transfusion in the same person.

Blood Collection

A. **Preoperative.** Preoperative autologous blood donation is the most common form of autotransfusion used in plastic surgery. The blood is collected preoperatively by means of predeposit phlebotomy for transfusion during or after surgery.

B. **Perioperative.** Blood also may be collected intraoperatively from an uncontaminated wound or body cavity or postoperatively by salvaging shed blood. Blood recovery with subsequent autotransfusion is commonly used in selected patients when blood loss is substantial and recovery of the shed blood may be feasible. Before transfusion, recovered autologous shed blood may be processed with saline solution wash in a computerized cell-washing instrument. This process eliminates significant particulate matter, thromboplastin activity, and other potentially detrimental factors. Intraoperative blood salvage and subsequent reinfusion has been effective and efficient in cardiovascular, trauma, and orthopedic surgery.

Advantages

When absolute patient and blood unit identification is maintained and when established guidelines are followed, autotransfusion offers significant advantages over the transfusion of allogeneic blood because of the following:

- ▼ It eliminates the risk of transmitting viral infections.
- ▼ It prevents the formation of blood group alloantibodies.

- It eliminates the risk of hemolytic transfusion reactions, delayed transfusion reactions, allergic reactions, and antileukocyte antibody responses.
- It precludes compatibility-testing problems.

Autologous transfusion is particularly advantageous in patients with chronic liver disease because viral hepatitis imposes a significant increase in morbidity and mortality in such patients. Furthermore, when autologous blood is stored frozen, 2, 3-diphosphoglycerate is preserved, which may enhance tissue oxygenation.

Identifying the Autotransfusion Candidate

Predeposit autologous blood donation should be considered for the patient who is scheduled or tentatively scheduled for elective surgery and who is likely to require blood transfusion. For example, many plastic surgical procedures are well suited for autotransfusion use because they are usually scheduled in advance and because blood loss is often less than the volume of two or three units of whole blood. For most plastic surgical procedures, one or two units of blood represent sufficient reserves to compensate for the blood loss encountered.

- Following appropriate discussion of the indications, advantages, and possible risks, the physician and patient should decide together if the patient will donate autologous blood. Autologous blood should not be collected or transfused indiscriminately, and it should not be requested for minor procedures or for a patient unlikely to require transfusion.
- Hemoglobin and hematocrit values should be 11 g/dl and 33% or greater respectively, although donors of homologous blood require higher values. There are no age limits required for autologous transfusion candidacy. Small children have tolerated autotransfusion when no more than 10% of their total blood volume has been withdrawn during each donation.
- The value of autotransfusion is limited in the patient who tends to be anemic. If a patient has a pre-existing anemia, the patient may not be a suitable autotransfusion candidate. A patient with bone marrow suppression,

iatrogenic or otherwise, may not be a candidate for autotransfusion. For example, a patient whose prophylactic chemotherapy is continued as adjunct therapy after mastectomy for carcinoma who is contemplating reconstructive breast surgery may not have responsive bone marrow that will permit serial blood donation for autotransfusion purposes.

Scheduling Blood Donation

Scheduling preoperative blood donation requires planning. Proper planning with the patient, the hospital blood bank, and the operating room (OR) personnel is not difficult to accomplish. Optimally, preoperative blood donations should be at intervals that allow for adequate red blood cell (RBC) regeneration and normalization of the patient's hemoglobin and hematocrit levels. Although the time required for restoring adequate hemoglobin and hematocrit varies somewhat from patient to patient, 1 week is a practical interval that allows for partial RBC regeneration. If time does not permit, the interval may be reduced to 3 days, but iatrogenic anemia will likely occur. Ideally, blood should not be drawn from the donor/patient within 72 hours of an operation.

Determining Type of Blood Storage

A. **Liquid storage.** Autologous blood may be stored in the liquid state, provided the collected blood is used within 35 to 42 days and depending on the type of anticoagulant-preservative solutions used. Therefore a patient who is expected to require one unit of whole blood during surgery can donate that unit 4 to 5 weeks preoperatively. In the past, with the use of citrate phosphate dextrose (CPD) or acid citrate dextrose (ACD) solutions, the time period allowed for liquid storage of the blood unit was 21 days. However, with the addition of adenine (citrate phosphate dextrose adenine), whole blood may now be stored for as long as 35 days. Red blood cell units may be stored for 42 days when using additive solutions (AS-1). Predeposit donation well in advance of surgical procedures for which autotransfusion is anticipated permits hematopoietic regeneration of RBCs and reattainment of acceptable hemoglobin and hematocrit levels before surgery. Once the intended time of usage has passed, unused autologous units may be released for another patient, provided that the autologous donor meets all the criteria for allogeneic donation. This practice is referred to as *crossing over.* However, some blood banks do not permit crossing over because they do not consider such a blood unit to be as safe as that of a regular volunteer allogeneic blood donor.

B. **Frozen blood storage.** The usefulness of frozen blood is well established, and its use is an important adjunct to autologous transfusion programs. Optimal circumstances exist when facilities are available for freezing and processing blood and when there is time to collect sufficient units of blood before surgery. When frozen, RBCs can be stored for years, although regulatory agencies generally restrict its storage to 10 years. If the scheduled time of surgery does not fall within the liquid-storage dating period, autologous blood may be frozen, although long-term storage without an anticipated medical need is not recommended.

Autologous blood units should be transfused only when the patient's condition warrants transfusion; these units should not be transfused simply because they are available.

Procedure

A. **Informing the patient.** When planning for autologous transfusion, the patient should be informed of the indications, advantages, and schedules. A patient tolerates single or serial blood donations better when the rationale is understood. The physician should obtain informed consent from the patient, or if a minor, from the patient's parent or guardian (Fig. 7-1). The autologous donor should be informed that, if not used at the intended time of surgery, the patient's blood units will not be stored for lengthy periods unless special arrangements are made. The patient also needs to know that on rare occasions, flaws in blood bags, equipment malfunctions, and other circumstances may render the autologous unit unsafe for use, in which case the blood unit can not be used.

TRANSFUSION MEDICINE SERVICE Request for Autologous Transfusion	
Patient's name:	Date of birth:
Address:	Social Security Number:
City: State: Zip:	Driver's license:
Telephone: (h) (w)	Medical records number:
I request that the above-listed patient have blood collected and stored for possible autologous transfusion. In my opinion, withdrawal of the number of units indicated below will not be detrimental, and I have discussed the procedure and its purpose with the patient.	
Diagnosis:	Contemplated surgery:
Anticipated date of surgery:	Number of units to be collected:
Comments:	
Requesting Physican (print):	Signature:

DATE(S) UNIT(S) TO BE COLLECTED	METHOD OF STORAGE (circle one)		BLOOD THAWED BEFORE SURGERY? (circle one)	
	Frozen Storage	Liquid Storage	yes	no
	Frozen Storage	Liquid Storage	yes	no
	Frozen Storage	Liquid Storage	yes	no
	Frozen Storage	Liquid Storage	yes	no

(To be completed by Blood Bank)

DATE OF PHLEBOTOMY	BLOOD UNIT NUMBER	TECHNOLOGIST	FINAL DISPOSITION

PATIENT'S CONSENT

My physican,____________________, has fully explained to me the need to donate my blood for my own use, if indicated. I realize circumstances may arise that would render my blood unit(s) unsafe or unavailable for my use. Also, I realize that if my blood is not used by me within a reasonable time following its intended time of possible use, the unit(s) may be released for another patient, if deemed feasible by the blood bank staff. I consent to testing of my blood as deemed appropriate to the Blood Bank, including those tests that may be indicative of HIV infection, hepatitis, and syphillis.

Patient's signature: ____________________ Witness: ______________________________

Fig. 7-1 *Example of patient consent form for autologous transfusion.*

B. Assuring donor safety. For the usual donation of allogeneic blood, the requirements relate either to the protection of the donor or to the protection of the recipient. When giving autologous blood however donor safety is the primary concern.

- Before donation, blood bank personnel should get an appropriate medical history from the patient. Patients with major cardiac, pulmonary, hepatic, renal, or systemic disease may not be acceptable donors.
- Vital signs and levels of hemoglobin and hematocrit are determined.
- The usual quantity of blood withdrawn is approximately 450 ml, unless the patient weighs less than 110 lb. In such a case, less than the customary amount may be removed, depending on the patient's size. The following formula may be used to calculate acceptable amounts of blood to withdraw:

$$\frac{\text{Amount of blood (ml)}}{450\text{ ml}} = \frac{\text{Weight of patient (lb)}}{110\text{ lb}}$$

When less than 300 ml of blood is removed from the patient, the blood bank personnel should adjust the amount of anticoagulant-preservative to prevent excessive anticoagulant solution. The patient, blood bank, OR personnel, and other involved physicians should be informed of the intended date of autologous transfusion. After final scheduling of surgery and admission to the hospital, confirmation of the time of surgery to the blood bank staff facilitates appropriate patient service.

- It is imperative to maintain absolute identification of both the autologous units and the patient from the time of donation to the time that the blood units are transfused (sample label for blood unit appears in Fig. 7-2). Because many patients do not have an assigned medical records number until admission to the hospital, the patient's name, social security number, date of birth, driver's license number, address, or other data may be required to ensure identification of the units. The patient may also be given a card that documents pertinent information concerning the autologous donation, such as assigned blood unit numbers. Such a card alerts

DO NOT REMOVE THIS TAG UNIT NUMBER MUST BE SAME AS BLOOD CONTAINER NUMBER	
AUTOTRANSFUSION	
Unit Number:	Do Not Use After:
PATIENT/DONOR	
Last Name:	
First Name: Initial:	
SOCIAL SECURITY NUMBER:	
MEDICAL RECORDS NUMBER:	
PATIENT'S PHYSICAN:	
DATE OF DONATION:	
DATE OF SURGERY:	

FIG. 7-2 *Example of autologous blood unit identification tag.*

hospital personnel that autologous units are available for the patient (Fig. 7-3).

Supplemental Iron

Using oral iron supplements during the donation period often helps the patient maintain suitable hemoglobin levels. In most cases, the autologous transfusion candidate initially will have adequate marrow iron stores, as well as normal hemoglobin and hematocrit values. Usually the objective is to provide the patient with iron supplementation only rather than to correct iron-deficiency anemia.

A. **Dosage and preparation.** Ferrous sulfate, 325 mg, taken orally three times daily is usually a plentiful supplement.
B. **Side effects.** Some patients may experience side effects with oral iron therapy, such as pyrosis, detecting a metallic taste, diarrhea, constipation, and dark

AUTOLOGOUS TRANSFUSION IDENTIFICATION CARD

(front)

TRANSFUSION MEDICINE SERVICE
Hermann Hospital
Texas Medical Center
Houston, Texas 77030
(713) 704-3640

Autologous Transfusion Identification Card

Please present this card each time you donate blood for autologous transfusion. When you are admitted to the hospital and have an assigned medical records number, please request members of the nursing staff to notify the hospital blood bank of your admission, medical records nember, room number, and intended date of surgery.

(back)

AUTOLOGOUS BLOOD DONATION RECORD			
PATIENT/DONOR NAME:			
SOCIAL SECURITY NUMBER:			
BLOOD UNIT NUMBERS	METHOD STORED	COLLECTION DATE	BLOOD BANK TECHNICIAN

Fig. 7-3 *Example of autologous transfusion identification card.*

stools. However, most patients experience few significant undesirable effects from oral iron supplements. Tablets that are not enteric coated should be specified when prescribing ferrous sulfate because iron is absorbed more effectively in the upper gastrointestinal tract. For greater absorption, the patient also should take iron between meals if it can be tolerated. The patient also need to be warned to keep iron medication out of reach of children because small children may ingest the tablets in amounts that could be toxic or fatal. Iron preparations that contain other hematinics, such as folic acid, are discouraged unless there are specific hematologic indications for their use. Sufficient folic acid is present in the normal diet to provide adequate RBC restoration, and its administration may mask latent pernicious anemia.

Processing the Autologous Blood Unit

When autologous blood units are intended for autologous transfusion only, certain tests must be performed. ABO blood grouping and Rh typing are conducted to help assure compatibility, and certain infectious disease marker testing is performed. In compliance with Food and Drug Administration recommendations, the autologous blood units must be tested for anti-HIV 1 and 2, anti-HCV, anti-HBc, HBsAg and a serologic test for syphilis must be performed if the unit collected is to be shipped to another facility, such as from the blood center to a hospital. A biohazard label should be placed on blood units that are confirmed to be reactive for one or more of the aforementioned infectious disease markers. If autologous blood units are used within the collecting facility and are to be transfused only to the autologous donor, the infectious disease marker testing is not required. If an autologous unit is positive for anti-HIV or reactive for HBsAg, it is recommended that the unit not be used because of potential exposure to health care workers.

Compatibility Testing and Transfusion

As a safety measure to prevent misidentification, it is recommended that compatibility testing be performed between the autologous unit and blood samples drawn from the patient after admission. Clerical error is a hazard of autologous blood transfusion, and compatibility testing helps to detect such errors. When all autologous units are transfused and more blood is needed, it helps to have blood samples available in the blood bank. With known ABO blood group and Rh type, as well as the results of unexpected antibody screen, compatible allogeneic blood units can be identified more quickly.

A. **Alloantibodies.** Detecting the presence of and identifying the significant alloantibodies in the patient are important parts of compatibility testing when the patient receives allogeneic blood and if significant blood group alloantibodies are present.

B. Frozen blood. When using frozen autologous blood units, it is important to consider the time required to thaw and deglycerolize (wash process) the unit. Usually not more than 1 hour is necessary to prepare a frozen unit. According to current standards, once the unit is thawed the storage period must not exceed 24 hours. Therefore frozen blood should not be thawed and washed unless it is likely to be needed for transfusion. The surgical staff needs to communicate to the blood bank staff whether the unit should be kept frozen or thawed and deglycerolized for immediate use. Many thawed, frozen RBC units are stored in a circular bag that is simple to use with a regular blood administration and filter set.

Forms and Records

The autologous transfusion program is enhanced by the use of preprinted forms and records that indicate appropriate patient data, clinical information, units to be drawn, methods of storage, and informed consent (See Fig. 7-1.). Figure 7-2 is an example of an autologous blood unit tag.

POTENTIAL USE OF RECOMBINANT HUMAN ERYTHROPOIETIN

Erythropoietin (EPO), a glycoprotein hormone that stimulates erythropoiesis, is produced mainly in the kidney in response to a low blood oxygen content. This hormone is present in plasma and is eliminated in urine. EPO may be produced in quantity by means of recombinant technology. Recombinant human erythropoietin (r-HuEPO) is used particularly in anemic patients with end-stage renal disease. It may be readily used to stimulate erythropoiesis, reduce the requirements for RBC transfusions, and enhance autologous donation and transfusion.

DESIGNATED DONORS

Because of concern about the safety of blood transfusion, some patients wish to provide their own donors. This tice is known as *designated* (or directed) *donations.* A patient who requests this method generally believes that the blood donated by friends and relatives is safer than that provided by the community volunteer blood banking system, but the data available do not support this belief. Blood from designated donors has not been demonstrated to be safer than blood from volunteers. The optimal time for a designated donor to donate blood is 5 days before the anticipated transfusion or a minimum of 2 working days before transfusion. This ensures ample time for processing the designated unit, which must undergo the same stringent testing as a regular allogeneic unit. One advantage of using a designated donor is that the individual can donate more frequently than a regular homologous donor. Also, all units may be reserved for the intended patient, which reduces donor exposure.

ALLOGENEIC (HOMOLOGOUS) TRANSFUSION

Before transfusion of allogeneic blood, immunohematology testing must be performed to help assure compatibility. Appropriate selection of the blood or blood component units is the physician's responsibility when transfusion is indicated.

Pretransfusion Study

When a patient has multiple unexpected autoantibodies or autoimmune antibodies (cold or warm), obtaining compatible blood on short notice can be a significant problem. However, with sufficient time and proper techniques, an experienced blood bank and transfusion service staff can resolve it. A short battery of tests can be used to avert problems that may occur when the transfusion is urgently needed.

A. **Short battery of tests.** This consists of the following:
   - ▼ ABO blood grouping
   - ▼ Rh typing
   - ▼ Antibody detection

B. **Unexpected antibody screen.** The unexpected antibody screen, a basic test used in compatibility testing, is a method of detecting blood group alloantibodies, some of which can cause hemolytic transfusion reactions. The test is routinely used for potential blood recipients and for donor units. Multiparous and previously transfused patients are more likely to have clinically significant alloantibodies than individuals who have not previously been exposed to RBC antigens.

- If the unexpected antibody screen is positive, antibody identification is performed. If the unexpected antibody test is negative, compatible allogeneic RBC units are readily provided; if multiple blood group alloantibodies are present or if an antibody to a high incidence blood group antigen is present, the task of obtaining compatible units may be time-consuming and complex. When indicated, compatibility testing is completed by mixing the donor's RBCs and the patient's plasma or serum and by observing for agglutination or hemolysis following incubation, centrifugation, and utilization of the indirect antiglobulin test.

BLOOD AND BLOOD COMPONENTS

In the last 30 years, emphasis has been placed on using blood components (e.g., RBCs, fresh frozen plasma, platelets, and cryoprecipitate AHF) for hemotherapy rather than transfusing whole blood units. Blood components represent the mainstay of hemotherapy in most clinical situations. However, there are circumstances in which whole blood should be transfused.

Whole Blood

A. **Indications for use.** Whole blood transfusion is indicated when there is a need to increase oxygen-carrying capacity and to expand blood volume. Whole blood reduces exposure to different donors when it is used in place of transfusing one unit of RBCs and one unit of fresh frozen plasma. Use of blood components has reduced whole blood transfusions significantly, but there has been an unjustifiable increase in the administration of fresh frozen plasma. Crystalloid solution, which may be administered readily as a volume expander with RBC transfusion is hypooncotic; therefore in massive transfusion, this solution can only be used in limited amounts. From a clinical standpoint, there is unquestionable justification for using whole blood in certain clinical situations.

B. **Drawbacks of whole blood.** To obtain whole blood units, approximately 450 ml of blood is drawn from the donor and mixed with a citrate anticoagulant-preservative solution that usually measures 63 ml. Because of the dilutional effect of this solution, the whole blood unit's hematocrit value will be less than that of the donor. Factors V and VIII are labile and are reduced during refrigerated storage. The reduced level of factors V and VIII in whole blood may contribute to coagulation factor deficiency states in patients who receive massive transfusions. However, the minimum level of factor V needed for adequate hemostasis is 15% to 25%. After approximately 24 hours of refrigerated storage, the platelets in whole blood units are no longer functional; therefore increments in platelet count are not achieved by transfusion of whole blood or units of RBCs.

Blood Components

To increase the efficiency and maximize the benefit of each donation, blood component production is used in transfusion medicine practices. When blood transfusion is indicated, the desired effect may be achieved more specifically with blood components than with whole blood. Blood component use is often the most efficacious form of hemotherapy. Preparation and use of the following blood components are reviewed: RBCs, frozen RBCs, platelets, fresh frozen plasma, cryoprecipitate AHF, and fibrin glue.

A. **Red blood cells.** Red blood cell units are prepared by centrifuging a freshly drawn unit of whole blood and expressing the plasma into a satellite bag. With anticoagulant-preservative solutions added to the RBC unit, the hematocrit will be between approximately 52% and 80%. This value also depends on the type of anticoagulant-preservative solution used. Transfusion of RBCs is the most effective form of hemotherapy when only increased oxygen-carrying capacity is indicated. Whole blood transfusion should be reserved for clinical situations in which immediate volume replacement is indicated and in which factor V and factor VIII are not needed.

B. **Red blood cells, frozen.** During the last 4 decades, refinement in techniques of cryopreservation (e.g., storing at low temperature and washing RBCs) and recognizing potential advantages of frozen blood use has resulted in selected use of frozen RBCs for transfusion purposes. Glycerol is used as the cryoprotective agent, and when the unit is thawed, it is washed with glucose-saline solutions.

- ▼ Advantages. The ability to store blood units for long periods of time has greatly enhanced autologous transfusion programs. It has also increased the availability of rare blood types and storage of phenotyped units, thus making available compatible blood units for patients with multiple blood group alloantibodies.
- ▼ Decision to thaw and deglycerolize. Once thawed, a unit of autologous blood has a maximum storage time of 24 hours. Therefore it should be transfused before using liquid-stored autologous units, which usually have longer dating periods. It is important to rank the transfusion sequence of blood units (e.g., frozen blood autologous units that are thawed should be ranked first, followed by liquid-stored autologous units and then allogeneic units). Communication with all members of the medical team, including anesthesiologists and nursing staff, is crucial to appropriate blood use.

C. **Platelets.** Platelets can be transfused by using pooled units of platelet concentrates that have been separated from a single unit of whole blood or by using units that have been prepared by plateletpheresis from a single blood donor.

- ▼ Preparation from single unit of whole blood
  - ■ Freshly drawn whole blood units are centrifuged at a controlled *G force* to permit separation of platelet-rich plasma from the infranatant RBCs.
  - ■ The platelet-rich plasma is expressed into a satellite bag, which is then centrifuged to separate

the plasma from the platelets. Platelets have a specific gravity of approximately 1.030 to 1.040, while the specific gravity of plasma is approximately 1.025 to 1.029. The specific gravity dissimilarities allow for separation by differential centrifugation.

- Following expression of most of the supernatant plasma from the bag, the pellet of platelets is resuspended in approximately 50 ml of residual plasma.

▼ Plateletpheresis. These units are prepared by hemapheresis where blood is drawn into a microcomputer-controlled cell separating instrument whereby platelets are separated and concentrated in the extracorporal circuit. Platelet transfusion from a single donor has the advantage of decreasing donor exposure because each unit is equivalent to approximately 6 units of platelet concentrates.

▼ The storage time is as long as 5 days from collection.

- The usual dose of platelets is one unit of platelet pheresis or a pooled dose of 6 units of platelet concentrates obtained from whole blood. Most platelet pheresis units should contain at least 3×10^{11} platelets, while each platelet unit prepared from whole blood should contain at least 5.5×10^{10} platelets and a small number of RBCs in approximately 50 ml of plasma.
- **Caution:** Platelets issued for a patient should be ABO blood group compatible and Rh compatible. Care should be taken that each unit of platelets is emptied completely, ensuring maximum benefit to the patient.

▼ Indications for Transfusion of Platelets

- Primary indications. Platelet transfusion may be indicated in a patient who is actively bleeding as a result of significant thrombocytopenia or dysfunctional platelets or in a patient who is undergoing massive transfusion if the platelet malady is likely to be causing or contributing to the bleeding. In the absence of a specific indication, such as severe thrombocytopenia or bleeding associated with platelet dysfunction, empirical transfusion of platelets in a patient undergoing major surgical procedures is not justified. If thrombocytopenia is the sole coagulation abnormality, it is unlikely that a patient with a platelet count of 50,000/µl or greater will benefit from platelet transfusion. Dilutional thrombocytopenia may occur in a bleeding patient who is receiving multiple transfusions, during which secondary generalized microvascular bleeding may develop, in which case platelet transfusion may be beneficial.

- Patient undergoing chemotherapy. Cytotoxic chemotherapy in a patient with a malignant disease often causes myelosuppression that leads to severe thrombocytopenia. Clinically significant bleeding may be averted in this patient by using prophylactic platelet transfusion. The critical level that indicates the need for such transfusion is medically debated; values of less than 20,000/µl are often considered critical. Both platelet function and number should be considered. If function is impaired, the need to transfuse may be greater.
- Patient with advanced renal disease. This patient commonly demonstrates impaired platelet function. In a uremic patient, correction of hemorrhagic tendencies and improvement of platelet function may be achieved by transfusing cryoprecipitate or by administering desmopressin (DDAVP). Conjugated estrogens have proved to be effective in treating uremic bleeding, but their mechanism is not known. When there is a history of bleeding or active microvascular bleeding, template bleeding time and platelet aggregometry can offer guidance with regard to platelet transfusions or other therapy for platelet dysfunctions.

D. Fresh frozen plasma. Fresh frozen plasma is prepared by removing plasma from fresh whole blood, freezing it within 6 hours of collection, and keeping it at minus 18° C or lower for up to 1 year. This plasma product contains all clotting factors but does not contain platelets. Plasma is thawed at 37° C once the patient's need is determined. The outdating time is changed to 24 hours from the time of thawing.

▼ Indications. The transfusion of fresh frozen plasma should be reserved for the patient in whom coagulation factor deficiencies are the primary cause for bleeding or a significant preoperative demonstrated deficiency justifies prophylactic transfusion.

- Fresh frozen plasma is used for replacement of isolated factor deficiencies, including deficiencies of coagulation factors II, V, VII, IX, X, and XI. It also contains factors I (fibrinogen) and VIII, but replacement of these factors may be achieved more effectively with cryoprecipitate AHF. In the patient who is bleeding or who requires surgery and who has a deficiency of one or more coagulation factors, coagulation factor replacement with fresh frozen plasma may be necessary.
- When a patient is actively bleeding or needs emergency surgery, fresh frozen plasma can be used to replenish the vitamin K-dependent coagulation factors (II, VII, IX, and X). If time permits, this goal can be achieved through parenteral administration of vitamin K. Proteins C and S, which also are vitamin K dependent, can be replaced through fresh frozen plasma transfusions.
- Fresh frozen plasma also may be indicated (1) during massive blood transfusion (e.g., one blood volume within several hours); (2) in a patient with antithrombin III deficiency; (3) as plasminogen replacement; (4) to treat immunodeficiency (although immune globulin for IV use has largely replaced fresh frozen plasma for im-

munoprophylaxis in the patient with immune globulin deficiency); and (5) to treat thrombotic thrombocytopenia purpura or hemolytic uremic syndrome.

- Contraindications. Because safer alternative therapies are available, there is no justification for the use of fresh frozen plasma as a volume expander or as a nutritional source. Crystalloid solutions, such as 0.9% sterile saline, or Ringer's lactate solution along with colloid solutions, such as albumin, plasma protein fraction, hydroxyethylstarch, and dextran solutions, are preferred to fresh frozen plasma for volume expansion. Total parental nutrition is the preferred method for nutritional support. Hydroxyethylstarch and dextran may be responsible for platelet dysfunction.

E. **Cryoprecipitate (cryoprecipitated antihemophiliac factor).** Cryoprecipitate is the cold insoluble portion remaining after fresh frozen plasma has been thawed between 10 and 6° C. Once prepared, cryoprecipitate is stored at minus 18° C or lower for up to 1 year. Cryoprecipitate contains factor I, factor VIII:C, factor XIII, von Willebrand factor, and fibronectin. Each unit is obtained from a single donor and contains 250 mg of factor I and approximately 100 units of factor VIII, as well as von Willebrand factor, factor XIII, and fibronectin in a volume of approximately 15 mL.

- Indications. Cryoprecipitate is used to treat deficiencies of factor I, factor VIII (hemophilia A), and factor XIII. It is used to treat von Willebrand disease (vWD) and to improve platelet function in the uremic patient. Cryoprecipitate is also used to prevent or stop bleeding in the patient with vWD. This disease, which is generally transmitted as an autosomal dominant trait, is a complex and varied defect that represents an abnormality of platelet-blood vessel interaction. Von Willebrand factor, a large multimeric glycoprotein, plays a key role in such interaction. In mild cases, the condition may be difficult to diagnose because of fluctuation in the levels of von Willebrand factor, especially during periods of stress, pregnancy, inflammation, and oral contraceptive use. Classification of vWD may be facilitated by electrophoresis of the patient's plasma in the presence of sodium dodecyl sulfate and by multimeric analysis of von Willebrand factor. Depending on the type and severity of the disease, the patient may have reduced factor VIII function (F VIII:C), von Willebrand factor, von Willebrand antigen, ristocetin cofactor activity, decreased platelet agglutination with ristocetin, or a prolonged template bleeding time. The intensity of perioperative treatment is related to the severity of the condition. Treatment involves the replacement of factor VIII and von Willebrand factor, which are present in cryoprecipitate. When indicated, preparation for the surgical procedure should include an initial transfusion of appropriate doses of cryoprecipitate, followed by evaluation of the template bleeding time. After surgery, cryoprecipitate should be transfused every 12 hours until bleeding is controlled. DDAVP, a synthetic derivative of the antidiuretic hormone, causes the release of von Willebrand factor and may be used in lieu of cryoprecipitate, although its use is contraindicated in type IIB variant of vWD because thrombocytopenia may develop. The patient with other subtypes of type II and with type III vWD often does not respond to DDAVP, but a patient with types IA and IB vWD usually does respond. DDAVP begins to work within 30 minutes after infusion. Certain platelet function disorders also may benefit from the use of DDAVP. These disorders include uremia, drug-induced platelet dysfunction, and myelodysplastic syndromes. DDAVP has also been used to reduce blood loss after cardiac surgery, but the benefit has been inconsistent.

- ▼ Dosage. An adult dose of cryoprecipitate usually consists of 6 to 8 units pooled together. Once pooled, cryoprecipitate has an expiration time of 4 hours. Cryoprecipitate should be ordered based on the factor activity required rather than in milliliters.

The following formula can be used to calculate the amount of factor VIII required for transfusion:

Plasma volume (PV, ml) = 40 ml × body weight (kg)

Factor VIII dose (in units) = PV (in ml) × [desired factor level in percent activity − initial factor VIII level in percent activity]

$$\text{Bags of cryoprecipitate} = \frac{\text{Factor VIII dose (in units)}}{100}$$

Factor VIII has an in vivo half-life of approximately 12 hours, and additional doses are necessary to maintain hemostatic levels for a hemophiliac patient in the postoperative period.

F. **Cryoprecipitated fibrinogen.** Cryoprecipitate fibrinogen (fibrin glue), either autologous or allogeneic, may be applied topically and mixed with thrombin (bovine) to produce a fibrin layer, thereby promoting surgical hemostasis. When dealing with capillary bleeding, the fibrin glue may help achieve hemostasis.

CHECKLIST FOR HEMOTHERAPY

The following guidelines can help obviate or minimize blood transfusion in clinical practice and can serve as a checklist for physicians who anticipate transfusing a patient or encountering hemostatic problems:

▼ If possible, preoperative anemia should be corrected with an appropriate medical regimen after a diagnostic workup. However, physicians should avoid using blood transfusion to preoperatively "correct" anemia if the patient's medical condition does not warrant transfusion and if time permits using specific therapy (e.g., iron, vitamin B_{12}, or folate).

▼ Blood transfusion during and after surgery is most often done to increase the oxygen-carrying capacity of RBCs. Allogeneic blood replacement should be used only when necessary. For most patients, mild to moderate anemia is not detrimental during the perioperative period. Extensive experience has shown that most surgical patients, including patients undergoing open-heart surgery, can tolerate postoperative hemoglobin values of 7 g/dl satisfactorily without blood transfusion. The decision to transfuse RBCs should be based on the following:

- Heart rate, respiration rate, blood pressure, and electrocardiogram tracings
- Serial hemoglobin and hematocrit determinations
- Sometimes, laboratory data (e.g., arterial blood gas values, mixed venous oxygen content, cardiac output, oxygen extraction ratio, and blood volume)

▼ To help prevent blood loss, the physician should make certain that the patient has a satisfactory coagulation status.

▼ Unless medically contraindicated, a patient should stop taking antiplatelet medication at least 5 days and preferably 10 days before surgery. Analgesic compounds that contain aspirin (e.g., Darvon compound, Empirin, and Percodan), as well as nonsteroidal antiinflammatory drugs (e.g., Nalfon, Motrin, and Indocin), can prolong the bleeding time. Other medications that interfere with platelet function are listed in Table 7-2.

▼ Blood loss should be appropriately counterbalanced by the infusion of crystalloid solutions. Loss of as much as 20% of the blood volume is well tolerated in most patients if the volume is maintained with crystalloid solution. In bleeding a patient, it is far more important to maintain a normovolemic status, which ensures good tissue perfusion, than it is to maintain normal hemoglobin levels.

▼ Transfusion of fresh frozen plasma should be reserved for a patient in whom coagulation factor deficiencies are seen as the primary reason for bleeding.

▼ If the platelet count is 100,000/µl or greater, platelet transfusion usually is not needed even in a bleeding patient, unless there is a coexisting platelet dysfunction. If the platelet function is good, and if thrombocytopenia is the only coagulation abnormality, a bleeding patient with a platelet count of 50,000/µl or greater generally does not benefit from platelet transfusion.

- Cryoprecipitate should be reserved for patients with hemophilia A or vWD, for a select group of patients with platelet dysfunction, and for patients with significant hypofibrinogenemia or dysfibrinogenemia. Cryoprecipitate also may be used effectively in the uremic patient with poor platelet function, although DDAVP often can be used to improve platelet function in such a patient.
- Autologous transfusion (using preoperative donation as well as intraoperative, and postoperative recovery of shed blood) is generally the safest form of transfusion, and it should be seriously considered.
- In select cases, oral iron supplements should be given preoperatively to make sure that there are enough iron stores present for hematopoiesis.
- Maintain normothermic temperature for the patient because a hypothermic patient tends to bleed. The optimal temperature for coagulation is 37° C.
- When clinical coagulopathies are detected, the physician should consider consulting the clinical hematology or laboratory medicine services. Consultation should be sought early to allow characterization of the disorder and the initiation of adequate preventative measures or treatment.

FURTHER READINGS

Aledort LM: Treatment of von Willebrand's Disease, *Mayo Clin Proc* 66:841, 1991.

Beck EA, Bove JR, Hogman CF et al: Which is the factual basis, in theory and clinical practice, for the use of fresh frozen plasma?, *Vox Sang* 35:426, 1978.

Blumberg N, Laczin J, McMican A et al: A critical survey of fresh frozen plasma use, *Transfusion* 26:511, 1986.

Collins JA: Hemorrhage, shock, and burns: pathophysiology and treatment. In: *Clinical practices of blood transfusion,* New York, 1981, Churchill Livingstone p. 425.

Consensus Conference: Perioperative red blood cell transfusion. *JAMA* 63: 869, 1988.

Cosgrove DM, Amiot DMI, Meserko JJ: An improved technique for autotransfusion of shed mediastinal blood, *Ann Thorac Surg* 40: 519, 1986.

Council on Scientific Affairs: Autologous blood transfusions, *JAMA* 256(17):2378, 1986.

Counts RB, Haisch C, Simon TL et al: Hemostasis in massively transfused trauma patients, *Ann Surg* 190:91, 1979.

Dodd RY: The risk of transfusion-transmitted infection, *N Engl J Med* 327:419, 1992.

Donahue JG, Muhoz A, Ness PM et al: The declining risk of post-transfusion hepatitis C virus infection, *N Eng J Med* 327:369, 1992.

Fredricks S, Milam JD, Dora JJ et al: Autologous transfusion and the preservation of frozen red blood cells, *Ann Plastic Surg* 8:486, 1982.

Holmberg L, Nilsson IM: Von Willebrand disease. In Ruggeri ZM, editor: *Clinics in hematology: coagulation disorders,* Philadelphia, 1985, WB Saunders, p 461.

Janson PA, Jubelirer SJ, Weinstein MS et al: Treatment of the bleeding tendency in uremia with cryoprecipitate, *N Engl J Med* 303:1318, 1980.

Kahn RA, Staggs SD, Miller WV et al: Use of plasma products with whole blood and packed RBCs, *JAMA* 242:2087, 1979.

Klein H, editor: Standards for blood bank and transfusion services, ed 16, Bethesda, Md, 1994, American Association of Blood Banks.

Larson CJ, Taswell HD: Human T-cell leukemia virus type I (HTLV-1) and blood transfusion, *Mayo Clin Proc* 63:869, 1988.

Liu YK, Kosfeld RE, Marcum SG: Treatment of uraemic bleeding with conjugated oestrogen, *Lancet* 2(8408): 887, 1984.

Livio M, Mannucci PM, Vigano G et al: Conjugated estrogens for the management of bleeding associated with renal failure, *N Engl J Med* 315:731, 1986.

Mannucci PM, Ruggeri ZM, Pareti FL et al: 1-Deamino-8-arginine vasopressin: a new pharmacologic approach to the management of hemophilia and von Willebrand disease, *Lancet* 1:869, 1977.

Mannucci PM, Canciani MT, Rota L et al: Response of factor VIII/von Willebrand factor in healthy subjects and patients with hemophilia A and von Willebrand disease, *Br J Haematol* 47:283, 1981.

Mannucci PM, Federici AB, Sirchia G: Hemostasis testing during massive blood replacement: a study of 172 cases, *Vox Sang* 42: 113, 1982.

Mannucci PM, Remuzzi G, Pusineri F et al: Deamino-8-D-arginine vasopressin shortens the bleeding time in uremia, *N Engl J Med* 308:8, 1983.

Mayer D, Zimmerman TS: Von Willebrand disease. In Colman RW, Hirsh J, Marder VJ et al, editors: *Hemostasis and thrombosis: basic principles and clinical practice,* Philadelphia, 1982, Lippincott, p 64.

Milam JD, Austin SF: Red cell salvage in open-heart surgery. In Barnes A, Jr, editor: *Hemotherapy in trauma and surgery: a technical workshop,* Arlington, Va, 1979, American Association of Blood Banks, p 67.

Milam JD: Blood transfusion in heart surgery. In Waldhausen JA, Biebuyck JF, editors: Surgery in the cardiac patient, *Surg Clin North Am* 63:1127, 1983.

National Institutes of Health Consensus Conference: Platelet transfusion therapy, *JAMA* 257: 1777, 1987.

National Institutes of Health Consensus Development Conference Statement: Fresh frozen plasma: indications and risk, *JAMA* 253:551, 1985.

Nusbacher J: Transfusion of red blood cell products. In Petz LD, Swisher SN: *Clinical practices of blood transfusion,* New York, 1981, Churchill Livingstone, p 289.

Oberman HA: Inappropriate use of fresh frozen plasma, *JAMA* 985(253): 556, 1984.

Pool JG, Hershgold EJ, Pappenhage AR: High-potency antihemophilic factor concentrate prepared from cryoglobulin precipitate, *Nature* 203:312, 1964.

Popovsky MA, Devine PA, Taswell HF: Intraoperative autologous transfusion, *Mayo Clin Proc* 60:125, 1985.

Ruggeri ZM, Zimmerman TS: The complex multimeric composition of factor VIII/von Willebrand factor, *Blood* 57:1140, 1981.

Sakariassen KS, Bolhuis PA, Sixma JJ: Human blood platelet adhesion to artery subendothelium is mediated by factor VIII-von Willebrand factor bound to the subendothelium, *Nature* 279:636, 1979.

Salzman EW, Weinstein MJ, Weintraub RM et al: Treatment with desmopressin acetate to reduce blood loss after cardiac surgery: a double-blind randomized trial, *N Engl J Med* 314:1402, 1986.

Schmidt PJ: Red cells for transfusion, *N Engl J Med* 299: 1411, 1978.

Shackford SR, Virgilio RW, Peters RM: Whole blood versus packed-cell transfusions: a physiologic comparison, *Ann Surg* 193:337, 1981.

Silbert JA, Bove JR, Dubin S et al: Patterns of frozen plasma use, *Conn Med* 45:507, 1981.

Silvergleid AJ: Autologous transfusions: experience in a community blood center, *JAMA* 241,2 1979. 724

Stehling LC, Ellison N, Faust RJ et al: A survey of transfusion practices among anesthesiologists, *Vox Sang* 52:60, 1987.

Vanderwoude JC, Milam JD, Walker WE et al: Cardiovascular surgery in patients with congenital plasma coagulopathies, *Ann Thorac Surg* 56:283, 1988.

CHAPTER 8

Prevention of Complications

JEROME E. ADAMSON

To reduce the incidence of complications in plastic surgery, the surgeon and staff must communicate clearly with the patient, perform a technically good operation, and provide superb postoperative care. The principles expounded by Ross Musgrave in the introduction *Plastic Surgical Judgment* and Bernard Barrett in *Patient Selection* (See Chapter 1.) relate directly to the material presented in this chapter on the prevention of complications. Individual steps to reduce unwanted complications are elucidated for specific plastic surgical procedures in Chapters 12 through 41.

GOOD PATIENT COMMUNICATION

Understanding the Patient

A. **Initial concerns.** In developing ideal patient communication, it is vitally important to clarify the initial concerns of the patient. Is the patient's initial complaint or primary request a reasonable one? Does the chief complaint reflect an anatomic problem that is present? If the patient requests correction of a deformity that to the surgeon's trained eye is not present, surgical attempts at correcting it obviously would be fruitless. Another approach is needed under these circumstances.

B. **Motives.** It is important that one determine the patient's motives for seeking an operative procedure, especially when one is dealing with patients who desire aesthetic surgery. If the patient's complaints do not relate to a clearly perceptible deformity, this should cause the surgeon to suspect the existence of excuses that are invalid reasons for surgery. One should be reluctant to operate on a patient whose motivation for the operation does not seem to the surgeon to be clearly defined or well founded, either in an anatomic or personal sense. Invariably these patients will be dissatisfied with any result or will strongly object to any minor deviation from the ideal result. The smallest complication becomes to them a major problem.

C. Psychiatric evaluation.

- ▼ Suspicious motivation. Correction of a physical deformity usually will not seem successful to the patient if it is undertaken as a somatic correction of a psychologic defect or if a major determinant is an interpersonal struggle (e.g., between husband and wife). Delve carefully into the patient's reasons for seeking aesthetic surgery. Even the best face-lift will fail to restore a crumbling relationship between an errant husband and his wife. In fact, this is a classic situation in which a minor complication or minimal scar may be enhanced in the mind of a dissatisfied individual into a major complication.
- ▼ Psychiatric referral. If it is obvious to the surgeon that some psychiatric imbalance is manifested by the patient's attitude, the patient should be referred for preoperative psychiatric evaluation before any surgery is scheduled. However, it is important that the psychiatrist to whom the patient is referred understands the basic problem and the possibilities for potential correction through plastic surgical techniques. The surgeon should establish good rapport with a psychiatrist who understands the capabilities and limitations of the reconstructive techniques used in plastic surgery. One should be wary of referral to a psychiatrist with whom the surgeon has had no professional involvement. Some psychiatrists do not understand exactly how plastic surgery techniques work or what realistic expectations are for plastic surgical reconstruction. If a patient is sent to a psychiatrist who is unfamiliar with or insensitive to plastic surgical procedures, problems that are already difficult may be compounded. Therefore the plastic surgeon *must* talk with the psychatrist before the referral.

- Recommendations. One should offer the patient an opportunity for treatment after a psychiatric evaluation has been completed. One should not destroy the hopes of a patient for improvement through plastic surgical reconstruction in the initial discussions by stating that one will not operate on the person unless a psychiatrist is seen first. Explain that the psychiatric evaluation is part of the plastic surgical workup and is essential in achieving the desired result. This is in fact the truth. One must not rashly deprive a patient of an opportunity for reconstruction, but one should let the psychiatrist respond with recommendations; these may vary from an injunction against surgery (e.g., in a schizophrenic individual) to a strong endorsement (e.g., "this patient would be an excellent candidate for aesthetic surgery").

Self-Evaluation

A. **Technical limits.** The surgeon also must be aware of personal capabilities. Is the surgeon capable of achieving the desired surgical reconstruction? If one does not have the technical capability, experience, or expertise to deal satisfactorily with the patient's problem, is it possible for others to do so? The time for referral of patients with technically difficult problems is soon after the first examination and not after one has spent a great amount of time and effort (and perhaps even operated on the patient) and then realized that the problem is one which does not fall within the surgeon's capabilities. One should refer early and not let the ego get in the way of sound judgment. This attitude will prevent complications from the outset.

B. **Personality conflicts.** In any busy clinical practice, the physician eventually will encounter a patient whose personality conflicts with the surgeon's own. This may be a temporary occurrence that can be resolved with further meetings. On rare occasions there will be patients whose attitudes conflict so basically with those of the physician that it is best not to attempt to develop any professional physician-patient relationship. This is the time for the patient to be transferred to an understanding colleague. It is always a wise decision to explain to the patient as delicately as possible this basic incompatibility and suggest that treatment be sought from "Dr. Jones across the hall" or "Dr. Smith, one of my partners." The longer a surgeon is in practice, the more the importance of developing good patient communications in order to obtain good results is realized.

Scheduling Interviews

A. **First interview.** One should make sure that sufficient time is allowed for thorough discussion of the problem with the patient. If the patient is anxious, the surgeon should wait until a later visit. If the surgeon is in a hurry, the patient should be scheduled at a less busy time. One must be sure that the initial information about the operative procedure and the evaluation of the patient's desires is unhurried and thorough. A hasty evaluation by the surgeon will invariably result in missing an important facet of the problem; this can lead to significant postoperative complications. One should make a strong effort to communicate well with the patient. The surgeon must be an educator. The surgeon must be able to inform the patient of the various aspects of the operative procedure and to define carefully the postoperative course and expectations. The surgeon should strengthen communication by repetition, the use of analogies, and multiple prospective interviews.

B. **Second interview.** This is valuable in establishing preoperative communication with the patient. In practically all instances involving major surgery, especially with the aesthetic patient, have a second interview with the patient at least 1 week before the scheduled procedure. At this time, much of the material touched on with the patient during the initial discussion is reviewed carefully. Invariably, repetition of original questions will occur, but fortunately in almost every instance, new questions arise. The raising of these new questions often reveals channels of misunderstanding that might lead to problems postoperatively. Providing a second interviewing opportunity for the patient is an important further step in developing ideal patient communication.

Complications

By establishing a good attitude and rapport with the patient about the possibility of complications (in most instances these events are not the surgeon's fault), when things do not go exactly right, a patient will understand and work with the surgeon in dealing with these problems. An *uninformed* patient who develops a complication, in the current medicolegal atmosphere, often will rush to indict the surgeon as the cause of the complication and work against the surgeon in satisfactorily dealing with the problem. An essential point in preventing complications is to educate the patient preoperatively.

A. **Operative risks.** One should assume that the patient knows nothing about the operative procedure and what happens during and after surgery. It is the responsibility of the surgeon to explain the risks of the operation. The potential problems with anesthesia must be reviewed with the patient.

   The surgeon should not perform elective surgery on a poor-risk patient but should wait until the patient is in better condition. The surgeon should be conservative in judgment not only for the best interest of the patient but also for the surgeon's own.
B. **Operative care.** The surgeon should reemphasize during the explanation about complications that support will be provided to the patient if any unfavorable events develop, and these points should be documented in the patient's record (in the presence of the patient) as they are explained. Review with the patient what will be done to prevent certain complications. For example, state that to prevent infection, meticulous preoperative skin preparation is carried out and careful attention is paid to sterile technique. Emphasize how potential complications will be prevented preoperatively by every possible mechanism, such as a complete medical workup. Explain how potential complications are prevented

during the operative procedure through cardiac monitoring, good facilities, ideal staff, multiple assistants, the use of drains, special dressings, and other measures. Discuss the need for special diagnostic studies (e.g., x-ray examination, blood typing and crossmatch) and the role that each plays in preventing or dealing with complications. Foster in the patient an attitude that complications may occur if certain steps are not followed. One should let the patient know that if complications do occur, the surgeon is equipped and readily available to deal with them.

C. **Scarring.** One should be concerned about operative scarring or defects that are produced by the operative procedure. Scarring must be explained preoperatively with all possible seriousness. For example, one should make it clear that when a split-thickness graft is used in reconstruction, there will be a donor site and that this site most likely will appear in a certain way, resulting in possible hypertrophic scarring. Such problems are not in most instances considered as complications by the patient if there has been a complete preoperative review by the surgeon about the potential for occurrence of scarring. The surgeon should assure the patient of a considerate follow-up and support if any unfavorable events occur.

Additional Aids to Communication

A. **Photographs.** A significant factor in preventing postoperative misunderstandings and enhancing communication preoperatively is obtaining high-quality, multiview, standardized, preoperative photographs. It is essential to use easily reproducible views that can be compared with postoperative photographs. Especially with the aesthetic patient, these can be used to help the patient appreciate the results.

B. **Printed information.** It is helpful in the initial and preoperative evaluations and discussions with the patient to provide patient information sheets regarding each operative procedure (See Chapter 2, Fig. 2-2.). Give instruction sheets either to the patient or a close family member preoperatively. See that their receipt is acknowledged. Be sure that these sheets are not merely something that has been obtained from another source. One should use the readily available commercial examples to develop one's own information sheets and be sure that they reflect the surgeon's personal attitudes.

C. **Office staff.** In some offices, an objective professional person is available for the patients to communicate with if they have questions that they feel embarrassed about or have forgotten to ask the physician. Through a scheduling clerk or other individual, this professional can express concerns that will then be dealt with either by office personnel or be reported to the surgeon, who can then formulate an appropriate response. This prevents postoperative problems not only in understanding the goals and purposes of the operative procedure but also in averting difficulties that might stem from misunderstandings regarding third-party financial coverage or from the financial obligations of the patient.

D. **Finances.** Many postoperative complications can be minimized if good patient communication has occurred preoperatively. One must make sure that the patient understands all costs of the operative procedure before the surgery is scheduled. Every experienced plastic surgeon knows that the patient who has a financial concern postoperatively may maximize a small complication in an effort to use it as a lever against the surgeon to reduce an unpaid fee. Communication in all areas includes careful explanation of the financial responsibilities of the patient as well as the potential or lack of such for third-party coverage.

E. **Professional relationship.** Plastic surgeons should do their best to establish superb professional relationships between their patients and themselves. One should try hard to make a sincere effort in this area in a thorough manner. The surgeon's job is to help the patient and not to see the patient only as an operative problem (i.e., "a nose" or a "carcinoma of the tongue" or as "that tendon graft") The surgeon should relate to patients as persons in need of help. The development of mutual trust between physician and patient can be mutually rewarding. The physician should keep this in mind. The surgeon should touch patients in an appropriate manner during physical examination as an effective way to reinforce this relationship. The development of ideal communications with the patient minimizes postoperative complications and establishes a strong and effective base for dealing with the patient in all situations.

A GOOD OPERATION

Preoperative Evaluation

Essential to a good operation is a good preoperative workup. A careful health history and good physical examination of the *whole* patient is absolutely essential in preparing for an effective operation. If one has questions about particular concerns, one should consult an appropriate colleague. With a patient who has a history of other medical problems, avoid jumping into the operative procedure without first communicating with the family physician or other specialists who have treated the patient in the past. Be conservative, thorough, and in many areas even overfastidious. Try to delve into all of the details of the patient's history and medical illnesses. Carefully question about previous operative procedures. Related operative procedures should be reviewed by analyzing the operative note and when appropriate discussing treatment with previous surgeons. Benefit from the experience and expertise of others.

Through this initial careful preoperative evaluation many problems can be dealt with effectively, and postoperative complications can be prevented. The worst thing a physician can do is to see a patient quickly, make a snap judgment, have the patient scheduled for an operative procedure, and then as the anesthesia begins occurring, attempt to review the basic problem and design an operation. It is too late at that point. A careful preoperative evaluation is essential in preventing complications and achieving the desired results.

Choosing the Procedure

One should fit the operation to the patient—not the patient to the operation. One of the joys of plastic surgery is that there may be many ways to deal with a given problem. Judgment is vitally important in this circumstance. Every operative procedure should be a good experience for the surgeon. The surgeon should feel rewarded by the knowledge that the the right operation has been chosen, that it has been performed well, and that the ideal result has been obtained.

It is best for the surgeon to use procedures that are familiar to the surgeon and that use the skills possessed by the surgeon. A new technique should be avoided unless long-term results have been seen, unless the author is known and respected, and unless every facet of the operative procedure is understood. The surgeon should not wait until the time of the operation to mentally review the various steps of the procedure. Instead the surgeon should sit down with an anatomy book and digest the description of the operative procedure at least the night before the operation. The surgeon should go over it multiple times to be sure that every angle and nuance of the operation is well fixed in the mind. This will then incubate through the night, and the surgeon will have an opportunity in the early morning to review any fine points that are not totally clear. This must be done before the operation and certainly not at the time one is scrubbing.

Preparing for Surgery

A. **Surgeon's self-evaluation.** The patient should be in as good condition as possible, and certainly the surgeon should also be in excellent condition. The surgeon should get plenty of rest before surgery. The surgeon should avoid excessive use of alcohol, abhor the use of drugs, and cancel procedures if not in ideal shape. Surgeons have performed formidable operations while sick with the flu noting how difficult the operation was. It is not fair for the surgeon to violate the trust of the patient who expects the surgeon to operate at 100% efficiency. One should develop an ideal frame of mind in dealing with patients in the operating room (OR) and should go into each operation with the idea of performing the best surgery of that particular kind one has ever done. The operative technique and the anatomy should be known completely and absolutely. The worst thing a surgeon can do is to "play it by ear." Upon hearing that phrase it is hard not to feel that the surgeon has abrogated the responsibility for careful preoperative planning. Occasionally, the results may be magnificent, but the surgeon should anticipate that most of the time less than ideal results and increased numbers of complications will occur. The surgeon should plan carefully, prepare oneself well, and perform each operation as if being judged for it alone.

B. **Planning the operation.** The operation should be carefully planned. The surgeon should measure, recheck, and ask assistants for their opinions. When in doubt, the surgeon should reevaluate. A "divine revelation" should not be expected to come at the time of the operation. Chances should not be taken with the result. A clearly formulated operative plan with steps carefully defined in the surgeon's mind should be developed before the patient ever comes to the OR. The surgeon should not wait for a final examination when the patient is asleep on the operating table. (This underscores the advantages of a second preoperative interview, at which time the patient can learn the answers to many questions and the physician can reevaluate the problem and have sufficient time to think about the operation before it is executed.)

C. **Preparing the operating room.** The surgeon or nurse should be sure that the OR is appropriately prepared. The special requirements for a particular procedure should be checked, and the supervisor should be informed well ahead of time so that there will be an opportunity to obtain what is needed. How many times has one been in an operation and seen the surgeon become impatient while waiting for a certain instrument that the surgeon knew all along might be needed during that particular procedure?

Technical Considerations

A. **Minimizing risk.** A general rule of doing as little as possible to achieve the best result holds for all facets of plastic surgery. One should try to minimize trauma, knowing that this will minimize scarring and morbidity and in most instances give a good result. The surgeon should avoid using an aggressive detailed operative procedure to gain an additional possible 2% improvement in the outcome if a simpler, less time-consuming technique that is time tried will achieve almost the same result.

At the time of surgery one should operate precisely, swiftly, and effectively, as if the patient were one of the family. Plastic surgeons should try to perform the best operation of their lives every time. Surgeons who dabble and diddle are individuals who for the most part have not planned carefully and are making motions with their fingers while their minds decide what to do.

B. **Reconstruction.** The basic rule of using like tissues for reconstruction whenever possible needs to be reemphasized. A full-thickness skin graft from the opposite upper eyelid used to reconstruct a lower lid defect will give a much better aesthetic and functional result than thicker skin from any other part of the body. The use of a full-thickness graft from any other portion of the body will provide a satisfactory technical reconstruction, but the overall result will be less than ideal, and an unnecessary complication of an additional donor site will occur.

C. **Operative support.** The author is a firm believer in getting the best operative support available to avert complications and obtain the best result. When performing emergency surgery in the middle of the night, this author believes that there is no way to perform an ideal operation with a surgical assistant, nurse attendants, and anesthesia team who are completely unfamiliar with what is planned or who have no insight into the surgeon the surgeon's techniques, or the operative procedure to be performed. The best support personnel that can be found should be demanded. One of the great joys of a practice is to have scrub nurses who go with the surgeon not only in the OR but who also see the patients with the surgeon preoperatively and postoperatively. These highly skilled nurses are an invaluable arm of the surgeon.

D. **Surgical instruments.** The best possible surgical instruments should be maintained and used. The rhinoplasty osteotomes and saws need to be sharp. One should have at least two sets of basic instruments, with extra sets of scissors, so that a set is always available while the other is away being sharpened or repaired. This same attitude carries over when performing an operative procedure such as augmentation mammoplasty. An augmentation with only one set of prostheses available should be avoided—always have a spare set. The day that one does not have that essential spare set will be the day that there is a mechanical defect, with rupture of one of the prostheses, or when what was planned as far as size is concerned is not really what the patient needs. Always have backups when implants are required.

E. **Actual technique.** Handle tissue carefully, using small delicate hooks or gentle fingers. The sutures should be delicate and only slightly stronger than the tissues they are to hold. Close all dead space. The surgeon should pay particular attention to suturing technique. One should avoid using cross-hatched sutures in the distal third of the nose, knowing that the thick nasal skin will invariably scar. One will recall that a running subcuticular suture in this area will be far more effective and leave minimal scarring. One should not take chances with blood supply because the fluorescein technique is available. Another specific deals with placement of sites of split-thickness grafts in children. Instead of taking skin from the anterior thighs and exposed areas of children, it should be taken from the lateral buttock where the skin is thicker. A deeper than anticipated donor site will result in hypertrophic scarring.

Reeducation

These thoughts reemphasize the need for continuing education of the plastic surgeon and all physicians. One must brush up on operative techniques and should reread the original operative procedures frequently. Surgeons should not let time rob them of valuable skills because of inattention to details or suffer the loss of a special technique with which they once were familiar but has now "rusted." One should keep abreast of recent developments. The plastic surgeon should ask questions of colleagues and not allow thinking to become insular. It is amazing what the youngest housestaff member will know that can be helpful at a particular time. The surgeon should go to meetings and analyze carefully what is presented. If a new operative procedure seems logical, follows sound principles, and the results shown are effective and long-term, one should think this through carefully and use the new technique if it is appropriate.

EXCELLENCE IN POSTOPERATIVE CARE

Immediate Postoperative Care

- Elevate hands postoperatively to limit edema.
- Use suction drainage when fluid accumulation may be a factor.
- The operator should personally perform or supervise the careful and precise application of all dressings. A poorly designed dressing may frequently attribute to the development of significant complications such as the shifting of skin or necrosis of tissue.
- Possible patient problems with anesthesia should be discussed preoperatively with the anesthesiologist. Be sure that the anesthesiologist sees the patient personally before the operative procedure. It is just not good medicine to pursue any other course.

Follow-up

The surgeon should follow the patient in the recovery room and postoperatively. No one knows better what has been done and what should be done with particular problem that may arise than the surgeon. Excellence should be developed in postoperative care. The follow-up is where many complications can be determined early and dealt with satisfactorily.

- If the surgeon does not write the postoperative orders and directions personally, be sure that they are checked and are appropriate for the care that has been ordered.

- Check positioning of the patient's extremities and head when there is a particular altitude that is essential for obtaining a good result. Be sure that the nursing staff clearly understands this special positional need.
- Use drains frequently. If hematomas occur, open the wound, evacuate the hematoma, and deal with the problem before it becomes a significant complication.
- Prophylactic antibiotics are not recommended except in instances in which there is an obvious contamination of the wound. Save antibiotics for the patient who needs them.
- Urinary catheterization performed routinely will produce a high rate of urinary tract infection. Early ambulation and bathroom privileges (with help) are effective in obviating the need for catheterization and reducing the complications of infection.
- Postoperative oxygen perfusion in the surgical patient diminishes nausea secondary to pain medications. Carefully monitored nasal or oral oxygenation is helpful in preventing hypoxia. If this area of treatment is not properly monitored, many problems can occur, including loss of the respiratory stimulus secondary to decreased carbon dioxide. Postoperative retching will produce more bleeding complications than any other single factor in all types of plastic surgery of the face.

Consultants

If a patient develops a problem postoperatively, one should use appropriate consultants before the situation becomes severe. Anticipation by the surgeon can prevent later trouble. Patients are grateful for this kind of care and become concerned when something unfavorable occurs.

Discharge and Home Care

To prevent complications, ambulate the patient early after surgery, and discharge the patient from the hospital as soon as possible. Be sure that the patient is reasonably over the affects of anesthesia before discharge. Keep a careful attitude regarding what the patient can or cannot do at home. Consider what type of home care is available. If a patient is in a situation in which the patient has to care for oneself after a rhytidectomy, it is better to leave the patient in the hospital a few days longer or to send the patient to an intermediate care facility. Outpatient nursing services are becoming more readily available. When these are used, be sure that the nurse who sees the patient understands the situation. Discuss the requirements preoperatively with the nurse personally, preferably in person rather than by telephone, and be sure that the nurse comprehends the patient's potential problems and needs.

Availability

The surgeon should be available to patients and their families. Do not hide behind a "communications wall." If problems occur, communicate readily and quickly with the family and the patient regarding the difficulty, what caused it, and what one plans to do about it. Explain the potential for relief of the problem.

To avert complications, practice the *art* of medicine. This includes using all of one's talents, education, and capabilities and fostering complete communication with the patient and the family. Anticipate complications to prevent their further development. When complications do occur, deal with them quickly and effectively in such a manner that the patient will be healed and gratified.

CHAPTER 9

Selection and Care of Cardiac Patients for Plastic Surgery

Robert J. Hall and Denton A. Cooley

Cardiovascular disease, a major health problem in the United States, is estimated to be present in more than 56 million Americans. Nearly 50 million Americans have high blood pressure; 6 million have coronary artery disease (CAD); nearly 3 million have had a stroke; and 1.3 million have rheumatic heart disease. More than 25 million patients require noncardiac surgery each year. Of these patients, 7 to 8 million had known or potential cardiovascular disease.

Plastic surgery and other types of general noncardiac surgery in the patient with known or suspected heart disease require the careful cooperative evaluation of the patient by the plastic surgeon, the anesthesiologist, and the cardiologist or primary care physician. The extent, severity, and magnitude of the contemplated surgery must be characterized. The type and severity of the concomitant heart disease must be identified, and the risks must be stratified to permit a rational decision regarding the advisability of elective surgery. The benefit to be derived from the planned plastic surgery must be clearly identified. Only then can an appropriate risk-benefit ratio be assessed. If an operation is deemed appropriate for the patient, it should be accomplished under the cooperation of the plastic surgeon, the anesthesiologist, and the cardiologist or primary care physician.

EFFECTS OF SURGERY AND ANESTHESIA ON CARDIOVASCULAR SYSTEM

Surgery and anesthesia place a burden on the normal cardiovascular system, depending on the following variables: (1) the magnitude, location, and type of surgery; (2) the duration of surgery and anesthesia; (3) the circumstances of operation (i.e., whether it is elective or emergent); and (4) other consequences of the operation, such as blood loss and volume therapy, extreme changes in blood pressure and heart rate, reaction to hypothermia, and shifts in intravascular and extravascular fluids. These changes result in increases in myocardial oxygen demand and decreases in myocardial oxygen supply and are well tolerated by a patient with a normal circulatory system. However, the burden of changes in myocardial oxygen supply and demand is proportionately less well tolerated in a patient with organic heart disease. The degree of tolerance relates to the type and severity of the cardiac disease. Thus when patients with cardiac disease undergo noncardiac surgical procedures, a close working relationship is required among the plastic surgeon, the anesthesiologist, the cardiologist, and the primary care physician to ensure the general well-being of the patient.

INDICATORS OF CARDIAC RISK IN NONCARDIAC SURGICAL PROCEDURES

Major Procedures

On the basis of an analysis in 1,001 patients, 40 years of age and older undergoing a major operative procedure, Goldman described a set of patient factors and operative characteristics that can be used to predict the development of life-threatening or fatal cardiac complications in the perioperative period. The indicators include the following:

- Preoperative recognition of a third heart sound or elevation of the jugular venous pressure
- Occurrence of acute myocardial infarction (MI) within the previous 6 months
- Presence of more than five premature ventricular contractions (PVCs) a minute
- Presence of a rhythm other than sinus rhythm or premature atrial contractions (PACs) on the preoperative electrocardiogram (ECG)
- More than 70 years of age
- Previous intraperitoneal, intrathoracic, or aortic surgery
- Emergent surgery

- Drop of 33% in systolic blood pressure for more than 10 minutes intraoperatively
- Important valvular aortic stenosis

These risk factors were confirmed in a prospective study of 1,140 patients by Zeldin in 1984 that showed that the risk of surgery is related to the severity of the underlying cardiac condition and the extent and magnitude of the surgical intervention. In a recent review by Mangano, the preoperative and intraoperative predictors of perioperative morbidity were analyzed in detail. In this report, recent MI and current congestive heart failure (CHF) were cited as the only predictors of perioperative cardiac morbidity.

Minor Surgical Procedures Performed with Patient Under Local Anesthesia

Backer and colleagues conducted a retrospective study of more than 9,000 cases in which ophthalmic operations were performed with the patients under local anesthesia, retrobulbar block, or both. In 287 cases, operations were performed on patients who had sustained a MI; most of these episodes had occurred 6 or more months previously. Not a single perioperative MI occurred, which demonstrates the general safety of using anesthetics while performing minor operations on patients who have sustained a MI.

OPERATIVE EVALUATION AND TREATMENT OF PATIENTS WITH CARDIOVASCULAR DISEASE

Ischemic Heart Disease

Ischemic heart disease is the most frequent type of heart disease found in patients older than 40 to 50 years undergoing anesthesia and surgery. Ischemic heart disease may be overt, as evidenced by prior MI, angina pectoris, CHF, or arrhythmias. In a candidate for elective or emergent surgery, ischemic heart disease may be occult.

A. **Basic evaluation.** The following evaluations are important in determining the condition of the patient:
    - Careful health history and physical examination
    - Review of the resting ECG

- Precise evaluation of the level of physical activity that can be tolerated without producing symptoms

B. Further evaluation

- Treadmill stress test. This may be required in less active individuals who are free of cardiac symptoms to elicit further information about the presence or absence of ischemic heart disease or to "risk-stratify" the patient with a known cardiac disease. In instances of baseline ECG abnormalities or in women, situations where the ECG treadmill test is less sensitive and specific, *stress testing combined with thallium imaging* of myocardial perfusion may be preferable to an ECG exercise test alone. In individuals who cannot exercise sufficiently in order to produce a valid stress test, dipyridamole thallium stress testing can be used as an effective alternative for stratifying risk before surgery.
- Coronary angiography. In some individuals, this is indicated to precisely evaluate the state of the coronary system and the consequent risk of planned surgery. Significant and critical coronary occlusive disease may require myocardial revascularization by either balloon coronary angioplasty or by coronary artery bypass grafting before another surgical procedure can be considered, especially when the extent of coronary disease is critical. Crawford and colleagues reported that noncardiac surgery is as safe in patients who have had successful coronary artery bypass surgeries as in patients without CAD. In addition, they reported a low risk of subsequent MI. The Coronary Artery Surgery Study (CASS) registry experience also supports the value of coronary artery bypass grafting in reducing the cardiac risk of major noncardiac surgery, especially in patients with known increased risk factors. Patients who have undergone coronary artery bypass grafting and who require noncardiac surgery should be evaluated according to the guidelines described for patients with ischemic heart disease.
- Postoperative electrocardiograph. This should be obtained from the patient with known CAD and

from the older patient presumed to be free of ischemic heart disease. Comparing the preoperative and postoperative ECG facilitates recognition of an intraoperative or perioperative MI, which is frequently silent.

Angina Pectoris

A. **Chronic stable angina.** Patients in the New York Heart Association (NYHA) functional class II who have chronic stable angina as the only cardiac risk factor are generally at low risk during noncardiac surgery. The patient who is on an effective antianginal regimen before surgery should continue treatment through the perioperative period. Even though patients are otherwise restricted to take nothing by mouth, they should continue to take nitrates and beta-adrenergic blockers through the morning of surgery. Nitrates are usually administered topically throughout surgery. When a long-acting beta-adrenergic blocker (e.g., atenolol) is taken the morning of surgery, its effect will usually persist until oral intake can be resumed, usually 12 to 24 hours after surgery. If required, a beta-adrenergic blocker (e.g., propranolol) may be administered intravenously (IV) (1 to 2 mg, every 6 hours) in the perioperative period. Nifedipine (10 mg), which can be given sublingually, is an effective antianginal and antihypertensive agent.

B. **Unstable angina or recent myocardial infarction.** Generally, a patient who has sustained an acute MI within the previous 6 months or a patient who has unstable angina pectoris should not be considered for elective noncardiac surgery.

Hypertension

A patient who has moderate hypertension may undergo noncardiac surgery with little additional risk. When blood pressure is stable and diastolic blood pressure is 110 mm Hg or less, no benefit is derived from delaying surgery to achieve better control of blood pressure.

A. **Preoperative evaluation.** Risk analysis should include assessment of other end-organ systems, such as the heart, brain, and kidneys. Serum electrolyte, blood urea nitrogen, and creatinine levels should be evaluated before surgery. There has long been a concern regarding potassium depletion and the need for urgent preoperative repletion in the patient on chronic diuretic therapy. Slogoff and colleagues have shown that hypokalemia is not associated with increased frequency of dysrhythmias, even when potassium levels are below 3 mEq/L. Thus surgery need not be delayed.

B. **Medications.** Antihypertensive therapy should be continued to the time of surgery and should not be abruptly withdrawn; this is especially true with clonidine and the beta-adrenergic blockers because of their association with withdrawal phenomena. The use of a long-acting beta-adrenergic blocker such as atenolol the morning of surgery will usually prevent reflex hypertension and tachycardia from the time anesthesia is induced and into the early postoperative period.

Cerebrovascular Disease

A. **Patients who have transient ischemic episodes or those who have had a cerebrovascular accident.** This patient should undergo a thorough neurologic evaluation before noncardiac surgery.

B. **Patients with asymptomatic carotid bruits.** The management of a patient with asymptomatic carotid bruits continues to be the subject of some controversy. This patient should undergo Doppler assessment of the extracranial carotid arteries. If evidence of high-grade occlusive disease is found, carotid angiography is indicated to precisely characterize the extent of disease. A high-grade carotid stenosis (90% or greater), even in the absence of symptoms, requires consideration of prophylactic cardiac endarterectomy if this can be performed in a setting where the surgical risk and morbidity are low.

Valvular Heart Disease

A. **Preoperative evaluation.** Patients with valvular heart disease should be evaluated by the following:

- ▼ Careful health history assessment
- ▼ Physical examination

- Chest x-ray examination
- ECG
- Two-dimensional and Doppler echocardiography should be used to confirm the clinical diagnosis and provide additional information about the condition of the valves and myocardial function. In the patient with valvular disease, the most important characteristic adversely affecting operative outcome is CHF. Therefore a patient in NYHA functional class III or IV should postpone elective general surgery until the valve has been surgically repaired or replaced or until the heart failure is brought under control.

B. **Asymptomatic valvular heart disease.** The asymptomatic patient with valvular heart disease generally has no difficulty with noncardiac surgery. However, to prevent infective endocarditis this individual should be given antibiotics, the choice of which depends on the intended surgical field.

C. **Stenosis**

- Severe mitral stenosis. A patient with severe mitral stenosis does not tolerate tachycardia well. Fast heart rates result in shortening of the diastolic filling period, along with evaluation of left atrial and pulmonary venous pressure, pulmonary congestion, and pulmonary edema. Sudden onset of new atrial fibrillation has similar consequences, usually resulting from both the rapid ventricular response and the abrupt loss of the atrial contribution to ventricular filling. Excessive fluid administration is also poorly tolerated by the patient with mitral stenosis and often leads to pulmonary edema.
- Severe aortic stenosis. In the patient with severe aortic stenosis, the mortality rate after noncardiac surgery approaches 13%, and aortic stenosis appears to be an independent risk factor. This patient has a fixed cardiac output (CO) that cannot increase in response to the stress of surgery. The patient with severe aortic stenosis poorly tolerates hypovolemia secondary to blood and fluid loss and may experi-

ence cardiovascular collapse in response to the vasodilation produced by spinal anesthesia or vasodilators. Careful monitoring of fluid balance is required and is often facilitated by monitoring the pulmonary capillary wedge pressure. Left ventricular hypertrophy associated with aortic stenosis results in increased ventricular stiffness and an increased dependence on atrial systole. Consequently, a patient with this condition also tolerates atrial fibrillation poorly. In general, a patient with severe aortic stenosis (aortic valve area of 1 cm^2 or less) should not undergo elective major noncardiac surgery until the valve has been repaired.

- ▼ Differentiating degenerative *fibrocalcific aortic sclerosis* from *hemodynamically significant aortic stenosis.* In the older patient this may be difficult based on clinical evaluation. A loud aortic systolic ejection murmur and the presence of angina, syncope, or CHF indicates significant aortic valve obstruction. Evaluating the degree of aortic valve obstruction by use of Doppler echocardiography is helpful in assessing this patient.

D. Aortic insufficiency or mitral insufficiency. A patient with chronic aortic or mitral insufficiency who is asymptomatic generally has no difficulty with noncardiac surgery. The operative risk appears to be related to the status of left ventricular function rather than the degree of regurgitation. The risk increases when the disease is more advanced, as evidenced by a third heart sound, pulmonary venous congestion confirmed by radiography, significant chamber enlargement confirmed by two-dimensional echocardiography, or reduced left ventricular ejection fraction. In general, this patient tolerates vasodilation well.

- ▼ Mitral valve prolapse. The patient with mitral valve prolapse (MVP), such as midsystolic click syndrome or floppy mitral valve syndrome, in the absence of major mitral regurgitation is not at increased risk from noncardiac surgery. *Antibiotic prophylaxis* is advised if any evidence of mitral valve regurgitation exists. This treatment is also recommended if the mitral valve is significantly deformed and redundant or if thickening is evident on two-dimensional echocardiographic examination. A patient with MVP commonly has palpitations and PACs and PVCs, which are usually benign and most often respond favorably to therapy with a beta-adrenergic blocker. Rarely a major prolongation of the Q-T interval is detected on the ECG. This prolongation predisposes patients to *malignant ventricular tachyarrhythmias,* and thus they require extensive evaluation before noncardiac surgery.

Prosthetic Cardiac Valves

A. **Asymptomatic patients.** The asymptomatic patient with prosthetic cardiac valve can be expected to do well during noncardiac surgery. However, most of these patients are on chronic anticoagulative therapy, an aspect of their treatment that must be properly approached. Knowledge of the patient's measured prothrombin time and its ratio to the control level, as well as the patient's sodium warfarin regimen, is essential. Generally the patient should discontinue taking sodium warfarin 2 to 4 days before surgery, depending on the index prothrombin time and the prothrombin time desired at the time of surgical intervention. The plastic surgeon must consider the vascularity of the surgical field, the need for a "dry" surgical field, and other problems that affect hemostasis.
B. **Patients with more complex valvular problems.** Patients with problems such as chronic atrial fibrillation, a large left atrium, multiple valve prostheses, a caged mitral valve prosthesis, or prior thromboembolic events, require hospitalization before surgery so they can receive continuous heparin therapy while the prothrombin time is allowed to return to normal. Heparin therapy should be terminated 6 hours before surgery. The process of normalizing prothrombin time can be accelerated by orally administering a small amount (2 to 5 mg) of vitamin K in one or several doses. Larger doses are rarely required and, postoperatively, may increase the

difficulty of reestablishing suppression of the prothrombin time with sodium warfarin. A patient on anticoagulants who requires emergent surgery may be given vitamin K intramuscularly or IV. In addition the prothrombin time can be restored to normal IV administration of fresh frozen plasma.

Anticoagulative therapy can usually be reinstituted 6 to 24 hours after most noncardiac operations. Simultaneous sodium warfarin by mouth and heparin by IV infusion should be administered to provide anticoagulative coverage until the prothrombin time has been restored to 1.5 to 1.6 times the control level.

Congenital Heart Disease

A. **Left-to-right shunts.** Patients with left-to-right shunts have little or no added risk from surgery and anesthesia unless they are in NYHA functional class III or IV. Nonetheless, elective noncardiac surgery is usually deferred until the congenital defect has been repaired. A patient with major elevation of pulmonary artery pressure and Eisenmenger's syndrome is at a considerably increased risk from surgery and anesthesia; thus elective surgery should be avoided. A patient with tetralogy of Fallot is sensitive to drops in systemic vascular resistance, which can result in greatly increased right-to-left shunting, hypoxia, acidosis, myocardial depression, and cardiac arrest.

B. **Right-to-left-shunts.** All patients with right-to-left shunting are susceptible to paradoxical air embolization to the systemic circulation, paradoxical thromboemboli, and septic emboli to the central nervous system from systemic venous sources.

Hypertropic Cardiomyopathy

A patient with hypertrophic cardiomyopathy has a wide spectrum of disease states and may have a resting or latent dynamic subaortic pressure gradient. The physical findings though variable are usually typical. Left ventricular hypertrophy can be detected through ECG and echocardiographic evaluation. The increased surgical risk associated with hypertrophic cardiomyopathy is related to an enhanced left ventricular outflow tract gradient, secondary to catecholamine secretion, and to factors that decrease left ventricular preload and afterload, (e.g., hypovolemia, venodilation, arterial hypotension, and spinal anesthesia). This group of patients requires careful assessment before elective noncardiac surgery. If an operation is undertaken, this patient must be managed skillfully during and after surgery.

Congestive Heart Failure

Surgery and anesthesia increase the risk of recurrence of CHF, but a patient with well-controlled CHF can successfully undergo cardiac surgery.

A. **Preoperative evaluation.** Careful preoperative evaluation is necessary. Attention should be given to the patient's health history and physical examination, especially assessment of the jugular venous pressure, the presence of basilar pulmonary rales, and the presence of a third heart sound at the apex. In addition, evidence of interstitial edema on the chest x-ray film may indicate CHF.

B. **Medications.** Medical therapy should be optimized before surgery and continued to the time of operation. Digitalis, unless required to control the ventricular response in a patient with atrial fibrillation, may be stopped for 1 or 2 days before surgery, with a resulting decrease in myocardial irritability and ventricular ectopy. The use of chronic vasodilator therapy to manage CHF is now widespread and should be continued into the operative period. If required, vasodilators, nitroglycerin, or nitroprusside can be given parenterally, but the patient's hemodynamic status must be appropriately monitored.

SURGERY IN PATIENTS WITH CARDIAC PACEMAKERS AND AUTOMATIC IMPLANTABLE CARDIOVERTER DEFIBRILLATORS

Because of the large variability in pacemaker programming, it is essential to know the type and model of the patient's pacemaker, as well as the most recent program setting. In

1985, Shapiro reported that at least 10 pacemaker companies were manufacturing more than 100 types of pacemakers. He stressed the importance of reviewing records regarding pacemaker function and programming, making available manufacturers' brochures regarding specifications and normal operating parameters, and having a manufacturer's representative available 24 hours daily to answer questions about pacemakers.

Intraoperative Management

The most significant problem during surgery in the patient with a demand cardiac pacemaker is the potential inhibition of the electronic pacemaker signal by the electrocautery signal. The risk is best minimized by (1) keeping the ground plate away from the pacemaker generator, (2) avoiding use of the cautery near the pacemaker if possible, (3) programming the pacemaker to a fixed-rate mode (most VVI pacemakers can be converted temporarily to the fixed-rate mode by placing a magnet on the skin over the pacemaker generator), and (4) limiting the duration of electrocautery to short, 1-second bursts, preferably 10 seconds apart. During electrocautery the ECG signal cannot be monitored, so cardiac rhythm should be checked by use of a finger "pulse oximeter."

Postoperative Management

After the surgical procedure, the function of the pacemaker must be analyzed to document the integrity and proper function of the unit. Automatic implantable cardioverter defibrillators (AICDs) are increasingly encountered in cardiac patients undergoing noncardiac surgical procedures. Device function can be altered by strong magnetic fields, which can result from using the electrocautery at a site near the device. Excessive electronic noise in the operating room may also interfere with device-sensing mechanisms. AICD can easily be inactivated by use of an external programmer or a magnet. Turning the unit off before surgery, then reactivating it at the completion of the procedure is advantageous. If an AICD is inactivated during surgery, the patient must be carefully monitored, and proper external defibrillation equipment should be available.

DRUG THERAPY

Antithrombic Drugs

The majority of patients with ischemic heart disease take aspirin or dipyridamole daily to protect themselves against intracoronary thrombosis. Many of these patients will experience increased bleeding during operation, which may be particularly detrimental to the outcome of cosmetic or reconstructive surgery. These agents must be discontinued for approximately 2 weeks before elective surgery to permit recovery of platelet function. There is no evidence to show that temporarily discontinuing aspirin or dipyridamole therapy is harmful to these patients.

Bacterial Endocarditic Prophylaxis

A. **Indications.** Endocarditic prophylaxis is recommended in (1) all patients with prosthetic heart valves, (2) patients with congenital cardiac malformations (except for an isolated secundum atrial septal defect), (3) patients with rheumatic or other acquired valvular dysfunction even after valvular surgery, (4) patients with hypertrophic cardiomyopathy, and (5) patients who have MVP with valvular regurgitation or who have associated thickening or redundancy of the valve leaflets.

B. **Contraindications.** Prophylaxis for endocarditis is not recommended in the patient who has coronary artery bypass graft surgery or in the patient who has a cardiac pacemaker or implanted defibrillator.

C. **Choice of antibiotic regimen.** The choice of a prophylactic antibiotic regimen should be based on the bacterial flora found near the operative region:

- Dental, oral, or upper respiratory tract surgery. The recently revised recommendation is amoxicillin. The patient should take 3.0 g, orally, 1 hour before operation and 1.5 g, orally, 6 hours after operation. A patient allergic to penicillin or its semisynthetic derivatives should take either erythromycin ethylsuccinate (800 mg, orally) or erythromycin stearate (1.0 g, orally) 2 hours before the operation, and half of this dose should be repeated 6 hours later. An alternative is to use clindamycin (300 g, orally) 1 hour before operation and half of this dose repeated 6 hours later.

- Procedures in genitourinary or gastrointestinal systems. For procedures in these areas, the antibiotic regimen includes IV or intramuscular administration of ampicillin (2.0 g) plus gentamicin (1.5 mg/kg, not to exceed 80 mg) 30 minutes before operation; 6 hours later, amoxicillin (1.5 g, orally) should be administered or alternatively, the parenteral regimen may be repeated 8 hours after the original dose. A patient allergic to penicillin or its semisynthetic derivatives should be given vancomycin (1.0 g, IV) over 1 hour, plus gentamicin (1.5 mg/kg, not to exceed 80 mg, IV or intramuscularly) 1 hour before operation. This regimen should be repeated once 8 hours later.
- Surgery performed in "clean" fields. Surgery in these areas results in little risk of infective endocarditis, in which case bacterial flora, including *Staphylococcus aureus,* coagulase-negative staphylococci, or diptheroids, are present. Prophylaxis is generally directed against staphylococci and usually consists of administering a "first-generation" cephalosporin immediately before operation and, depending on the type of surgery and the size of the surgical field, continuing cephalosporin administration at 6-hour intervals for 24 hours. Alternatively, vancomycin can be given IV immediately before operation then 12 hours later.

ACKNOWLEDGMENTS

Review of the contents of this chapter and constructive suggestions by Doctors Ali Massumi, Stephen Slogoff, Layne Gentry, Susan Wilansky, and Neil Strickman are gratefully acknowledged. We would also like to thank Christine Lanzisera for editorial assistance in the preparation of the manuscript.

FURTHER READINGS

Heart and stroke facts, 1994 Statistical Supplement, American Heart Association.

Mangano DT: Perioperative cardiac morbidity, *Anesthesiology* 72:153, 1990.

Goldman L, Caldera DL, Nussbaum SR et al: Multifactorial index of cardiac risk in noncardiac surgical procedures, *N Engl J Med* 297:845, 1977.

Goldman L, Caldera DL, Southwick FS et al: Cardiac risk factors and complications in non-cardiac surgery, *Medicine* 57:357, 1978.

Zeldin RA: Assessing cardiac risk in patients who undergo noncardiac surgical procedures, *Can J Surg* 27:402, 1984.

Backer CL, Tinker JH, Robertson DM et al: Myocardial reinfarction following local anesthesia for ophthalmic surgery, *Anesth Analg* 59:257, 1980.

Crawford ES, Morris GC Jr, Howell JF et al: Operative risk in patients with previous coronary artery bypass, *Ann Thorac Surg* 26:215, 1978.

Foster ED, Davis KB, Carpenter JA et al: Risk of noncardiac operation in patients with defined coronary disease: the Coronary Artery Surgery Study (CASS) registry experience, *Ann Thorac Surg* 41:42, 1986.

Weitz HH, Goldman L: Noncardiac surgery in the patient with heart disease, *Med Clin North Am* 71:413, 1987.

Hirsch IA, Tomlinson DL, Slogoff S et al: The overstated risk of preoperative hypokalemia, *Anesth Analg* 67:131, 1988.

Logue RB, Kaplan JA: The cardiac patient and noncardiac surgery, *Curr Probl Cardiol* 7:1, 1982.

Shapiro WA, Roizen MF, Singleton MA et al: Intraoperative pacemaker complications, *Anesthesiology* 63:319, 1985.

Dajani AS, Bisno Al, Chung KJ et al: Prevention of bacterial endocarditis, Recommendations by the American Heart Association, *JAMA* 264:2919, 1990.

CHAPTER 10

Medical Photography

Arthur H. Rathjen, Sr.

The plastic surgeon, along with other medical specialists, has long recognized the need and value of quality photographic documentation and standardization. If one is willing to learn and understand the basics of photography and to adapt them to the specific needs of a clinical setting, the result will be photographic documentation that is consistent, valid, reproducible, and of high quality.

EQUIPMENT: CAMERA BODY AND COMPONENTS

The photographic process begins with selecting the appropriate equipment and becoming familiar and comfortable with its use. Although a number of camera formats are available, it is generally acknowledged that the 35 mm camera is the most practical and versatile for the photographic needs of plastic surgery. The following factors should be considered when choosing a camera body:

- Camera body: level of sophistication necessary for camera body for use in office and operating room (OR)
- Light meter system: aperture or shutter
- Focus methods: manual or automatic
- Automation degree: metering and lenses, motor drive, databack
- Flash: dedicated; located on camera hot shoe or off camera
- Quality lens(es): most important camera feature

Any camera used in a plastic surgical practice should be a "concept system," which is defined as a camera system with integrated components and accessories. Unless the plastic

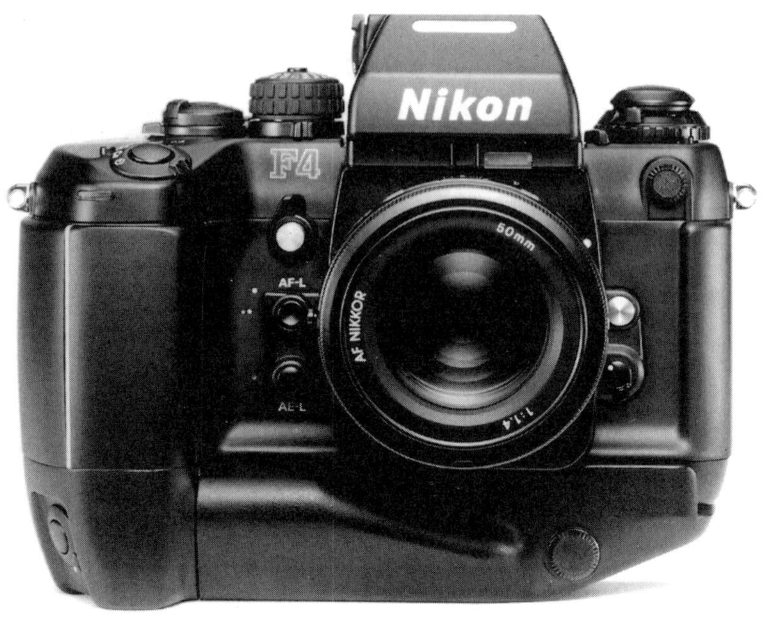

FIG. 10-1 *Nikon F4 35-mm camera.*
Any busy plastic surgery office with several surgeons or an office that routinely incorporates photography will require a reliable camera system that can withstand daily use and handling. This camera is not just an autofocus camera—it is a *professional* camera with the built-in option of a fast and reliable manual override. Professional characteristics include durability, size, use of all-Nikon lenses, several focusing modes, shutter speeds up to 1/8000 seconds, three metering systems, two program modes, and aperture priority or shutter priority. TTL flash exposure operates in all modes, has a built-in motor drive, and has interchangeable focusing screens. A less expensive but equally reliable camera is Nikon's M50.

surgeon and the staff are expert photographers who are knowledgeable enough to assemble a workable photographic system that consists of different accessories from multiple manufacturers, a good system should be invested in to eliminate possible frustration and poor photographic results. It is recommended to use the accessories that have been designed specifically for use with the chosen camera.

Camera Body

There are a number of quality manufacturers of single lens reflex (SLR) 35 mm cameras available. The author's personal choice is Nikon (Fig. 10-1), but camera manufacturers such as Leica, Canon, Minolta, Pentax, Olympus, Contax-Yashica,

Konica, and Ricoh also offer high quality. Certain principles of design and function are characteristic to all SLR 35 mm cameras. Each manufacturer has its own individual features and technical innovations, so it is up to the individual to decide what will best suit the needs of the plastic surgeon. Above all, the camera equipment should be simple to use. The following features should be a part of the camera body:

A. **Viewing system.** The viewing system should be *through-the-lens (TTL) viewing,* which means that when looking through the eye piece to focus, the actual image is seen as it passes through the lens and through the prismatic head of the camera. This differs from a range-finder camera that is similar to the many "point-and-shoot" cameras available today. The range-finder camera system incorporates a parallel method of viewing that can result in parallax error under certain conditions.

B. **Metering system.** The metering system for the camera should offer the choice of using either the aperture or the shutter. It is best if the "aperture preferred" setting is used. With this feature, the photographer can establish the depth of field by setting the aperture and letting the camera choose the shutter speed for proper exposure. For more than 95% of photographs, a flash will be used. When using a flash, the camera is usually calibrated for a shutter speed of 1/60th, 1/80th, or 1/250th of a second. The calibration is set by the manufacturer so that flash and shutter are synchronized. The best aperture setting is between f8 or f11. Most manufacturers and experienced photographers acknowledge that an aperture setting in this range results in the sharpest focus within the aperture range scale.

C. **Focus and viewing screens.** It is preferable to have a camera body with interchangeable focus and viewing screens. This author has for many years preferred a focus and viewing screen configuration that has a vertical and horizontal grid. The grid allows one to make specific visual references to anatomic landmarks on subjects and assists in the standardization of photographs. If the camera is designed for automatic focus, it should have the ability to manually override this function (Fig. 10-2). No automatic lenses that preset ratios are available.

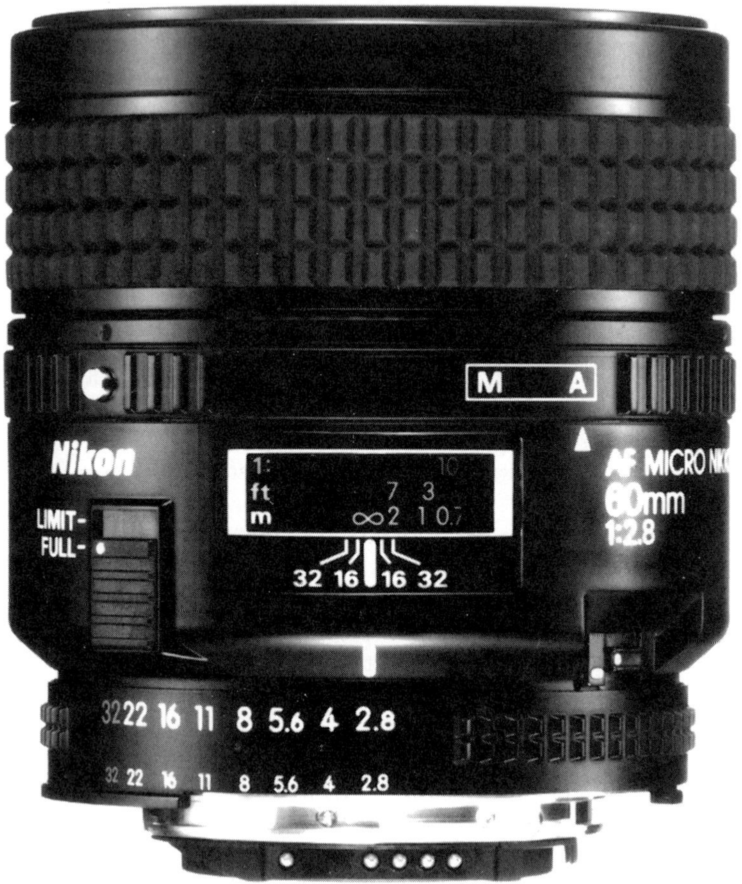

FIG. **10-2** *Nikon 60-mm f2.8 AF Micro Nikkor.*
This camera has the newest 60-mm micro autofocus lens that allows for manual override. Note white triangle that allows switch from A (auto) to M (manual). In viewing window, note the "1:" in upper left corner; this is the ratio scale that can be used in M (manual) mode.

Even with a camera as sophisticated as the Nikon F_4, the automatic focus must be manually overriden when a photograph requires ratios for anatomic areas such as full head and neck, eyes, ears, or breasts. The micro lenses have the ratio calibrations on the lens barrel. Once set, the photographer moves the camera forward or backward to put the subject in proper focus. A simple system with advanced technology in features such as metering and flash control is found in Nikon's N50 camera. This camera body offers two levels of exposure control: aperture or shutter priority and manual exposure. This uncomplicated camera is easy to understand and use for an inexperienced office staff.

Camera Lens

Camera lenses are identified by their *focal length.* The focal length of a lens controls the angel of view, degree of light transmission, image sharpness, and color reproduction, assuming that a quality lens is used. *Focal length* is defined as the angle at which a particular lens bends light rays. The focal length also has a direct bearing on image size (scale) perspective and depth of field; therefore the longer the focal length of a lens, the larger the image will be on the slide transparency or negative, regardless of film or camera format size.

I have used four specific focal length lenses which are capable of handling any and all of the needs in clinical plastic surgery. These lenses are (1) Micro 55 mm f/2.8, (2) 60 mm f/2.8 micro (See Fig. 10–2.), (3) Micro 105 mm f/2.8, (4) Micro 200 mmk f/4 IF. Each of these lenses can focus to one half life-size, and with the aid of a special extension adapter ring, each lens can also produce a full life-size (1:1) image. The functional difference between these lenses is the *lens-to-subject distance.* The higher the focal length calibration (i.e., 55 mm versus 105 mm), the further away from the subject the camera can be and still produce the same image (Fig. 10-3).

There are four definitions for image size:

- General photography: infinity to 1/10× (> 1:10)
- Close-up photography: 1/10× to 1× (1:10 > 1:1) (Macro)
- Life-size photography: 1× (1:1)
- Photomicrography: 1× to 10× (1:10 < 10:1)

With the exception of skin lesions and other small areas on the body that may require high magnification, the image sizes (ratio) will range from 1:25 (full body) down to 1:1 (fingernails).

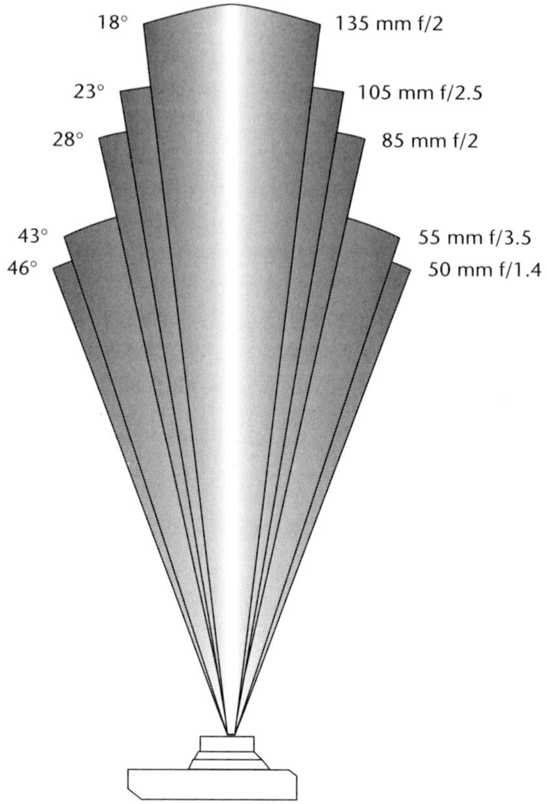

FIG. 10-3 *Angle of view for the most commonly used focal length lenses. The 55-mm lens is an excellent lens for full-body photographs. The 105-mm lens will nicely handle all other body views. Focal length determines picture angle, including field of view.*

A. Macro/Micro 55 mm f/2.8

- Focal length: 55 mm
- Aperture range: 5/2.8 to f/32
- Picture angle: 43°
- Distance scale to 9.5 inches
- Magnification scale:
    - Lens only 1:10 greater than 1:2 (one half life-size)
    - PK13 adapter ring 1:2 greater than 1:1 (life-size)

The 55-mm focal length lens is most practical when photographing the full length of the human body, (e.g., suction-assisted lipectomy). This lens, which is close to a normal angle of view, functions well without having to stand further than 10 ft from a subject. This lens is also practical when photographing close at 1:1 (e.g., skin lesions, birth defects, tissue specimens).

Reproduction ratios versus distance range:

SUBJECT DISTANCE TO FILM PLANE	RATIO	DISTANCE
Camera + lens	> 1:2	> 9.5 in
Camera + PK13 ring + lens	1:2 > 1:1	9.5 > 8.4 in

A 60-mm f2.8 automatic focus micro lens with a manual override is now available. See Figure 10-2.

B. Micro 105 mm f/4.0

- Focal length: 105 mm
- Aperture range: f/4.0 to f/32
- Picture angle: 23° 20′
- Distance scale to 1.55 ft
- Magnification scale:
  - Lens only 1:10 greater than 1:2
  - PN11 ring 1.2 greater than 1:1

For myself and many plastic surgeons, the 105 mm f4 or the newer f2.8 is the workhorse lens of plastic surgery (Fig. 10-4). Not only does it allow the photographer to stand further away from the subject while still getting the desired photographic ratio, but it also takes the guess work out of setting a desired ratio by providing ratio settings engraved on the lens barrel. The same is true for the 55-mm and 60-mm micro lenses. If the photographic area in the office is large enough, the 105 mm can be used for *all* photography, and—in my mind—the longer focal length is preferred.

Reproduction ratio versus distance range:

SUBJECT DISTANCE TO FILM PLANE	RATIO	DISTANCE
Camera + lens	> 1:2	> 1.55 in
Camera + PM11 ring + lens	1:2 > 1:1	18.6 in > 16.5 in

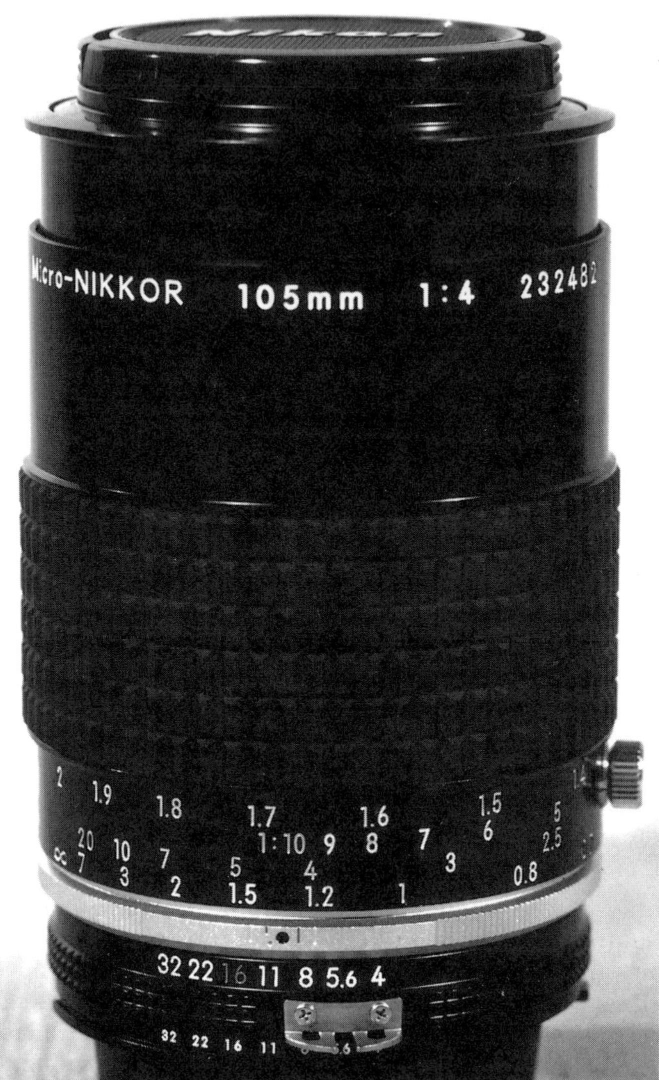

FIG. 10-4 *Micro 105-mm lens.*

Note ratio calibrations on midbarrel starting with 1:10. Lens also has locking nut, which prevents movement of barrel once ratio has been set. This lens allows a head-and-neck photograph that is in proper perspective (i.e., relationship of nose to rest of face with no distortion).

C. Micro 200 mmk f/4 IF

- Focal length: 200 mm
- Aperture range: f/4 to f/32
- Picture angle: 12° 20′
- Distance scale greater than 2.34 ft

The use of this lens in plastic surgery is for specialized photography such as in an OR where distance is a consideration. Having access to a 200-mm micro lens is an added luxury if the photographer plans to do a lot of OR photography. The 200-mm lens allows the photographer to stand well away from the operating table and the sterile areas and still take close-up pictures of the operating field while achieving the desired detail. This lens has little or no application in daily office photography. Several other references, listed at the end of this chapter, give more detailed specifications about lenses.

FILM

Unlike in the past, today's photographer has many different films from which to choose. For years, Kodak was everyone's choice, but there are now additional high-quality films such as Fugi from Japan along with film from Germany and Switzerland. For the sake of this chapter, only Kodak film will be addressed.

Film is used for many medical purposes. Film records the health history of a patient, and these photographs usually remain in the office files. Photographs are also used for teaching purposes, journal publications, and with matters of liability. Slides are used to make presentations at annual meetings of the American Society of Reconstructive and Plastic Surgeons (ASPRS) and the American Society for Aesthetic Plastic Surgery (ASAPS) or at state and local county meetings. Film types are used for different purposes, and all films are not the same. Each has certain characteristics including granularity, speed (ISO), and how the final photograph is made (i.e., color prints or slides, black and white, or instant prints like the Polaroid).

Reversal Film

The most commonly used film in plastic surgery is *reversal film*. All of the films available that use the suffix "chrome" are reversal film (e.g., Kodachrome, Ektachrome, Fujichrome, Agfachrome). These are all color slide films. However, these films have some characteristics of which one should be aware. The Kodachrome films (e.g., ISO 25, 64, 100) have a warm, reddish tint on the final slide. Ektachrome, unlike Kodachrome, renders a cooler, more bluish tint on the slide. The author has found that the new Ektachrome 100 HC film produces an excellent rendering of skin tones.

Negative Film: Color or Black and White

Unlike the above chrome reversal films, with negative film one (1) takes the photograph, (2) develops it into a negative, and (3) makes a print from the negative. There are some excellent negative films available, such as Kodak's Vericolor II and Vericolor III. Kodak's newest entry into the color negative field is EKTAR ISO 25 and 125. These are superb. The use of negative film for documents and record keeping has its merits; however, it is far more expensive to process and print. The developing and printing process is not as exact as the process used for chrome slide films. Prints made from negative film are more difficult to store, take up more room, and cost approximately twice as much as slide film.

LIGHTING

Correct exposure of film is absolutely necessary if one is to take a good photograph. It is unfortunate—but true—that correct lighting and the way it is used are the causes of more problems than any other aspect in plastic surgery photography. There are many ways to use lighting, beginning with a simple flash unit, which is connected to the camera's hotshoe, and graduating up to elaborate flash systems with utility track lights and large transformers such as the type one finds in commercial photographic studios.

Ease of Use and Size

One frequently asked question involves what lighting system to use that is easy and does the job without compromising space in a medical office. Before answering this question, it is imperative to understand one aspect about flash photography. What happens when one uses small flash units powered by AA-sized batteries? These camera-mounted flash units take either two or four batteries, and when in use, the flash indicates with the use of a "ready light" that the unit is ready to fire. It is unfortunate that in a busy medical office where the flash unit may be used all day, these batteries cannot maintain full power and begin to fatigue quickly. One will also find that the recharging and recycling time for these flash units gets longer and longer as the power quickly wears down. The use of 1.5 AA volt rechargeable batteries is not a good answer to the problem. These batteries may have a lower voltage rating than the standard alkaline battery, thus the flash with lower voltage will not provide the required light output resulting in underexposed photographs. The answer to that frequently asked question lies in using an AC adapter that connects to the flash or using a more sophisticated battery power system like the small Quantum Battery #1, which is a lead-type portable battery. If the AC adapter has a long enough cord, it will allow the necessary mobility to move around the patient while photographing. The AC adapter also assures a faster recharge cycle, and the flash will fire with maximum power every time.

Number of Light Sources

The ideal lighting system for a medical office should really consist of more than one light source that provides two or three flash units suspended from the ceiling or mounted on side walls. Almost all quality electronic flash units incorporate a thyristor circuitry. This innovation is designed to control and conserve the electrical power not needed to obtain a correct exposure. This type of circuitry also contributes to a faster recharging time between flashes. Most all modern camera units incorporate a TTL meter, which couples with a dedicated flash unit (Fig. 10-5), thus allowing a precise flash with adequate light transmitted through the lens and onto the film. All too often, the small camera-mounted flash units have a tendency to throw out a harsh light; they offer nothing to help alleviate unwanted shadows. Therefore some type of diffusion or filter material should be placed in front of the flash head in order to spread the light out and soften the effect on the subject. If one

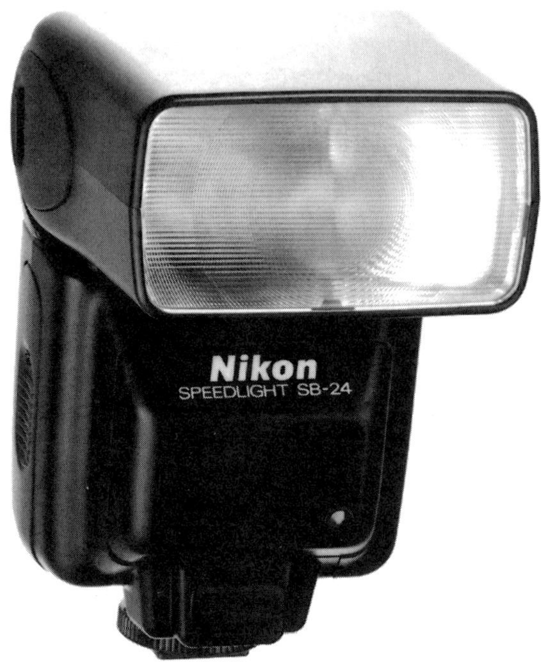

Fig. 10-5 *Nikon AF Speedlight SB-24*

This is an example of a dedicated flash unit that can be used on or off the camera. Off the camera requires a special but easy to use synchronizing cable, which allows all automatic TTL functions to perform. This flash with cybernetic controls synchronizes the camera's shutter speed and lens aperture for precisely controlled exposures. Nikon has recently introduced to the market a new power flash bracket unit (SK-6) designed to take the flash off the camera, thus offering movement of the light away from the camera. The bracket unit is designed to be used with Nikon's flash units, SB-25, SB-24, and SB-22.

wants to dramatically improve the photographs in the medical office, the flash or flash units should be moved off the camera and positioned above the subject being photographed so that the light is directed down at an angle of approximately 45°. Most light whether indoors or outside is directed from above, and that is the normal way we are used to looking at people and things. This control of light direction also drives shadows to the floor.

If one desires to use more than one flash, the units can be easily set up to be triggered from a small infrared unit (slave) mounted on the camera. These inexpensive units are available in better photography stores. A unit is attached to the existing contact points on the flash shoe, and then the photographer triggers one or more units with a small infrared cube that is coupled to the camera's hot shoe.

BACKGROUND COLORS

Those who have been involved with plastic surgery for many years have seen photographs presented at meetings that show patients standing in front of shiny highly varnished doors, bookcases, OR equipment, and other objects that are complete distractions from the subject being photographed. With little effort, a plain nonreflective background can be located in an office so that background shadows are eliminated and skin tones are more accurately recorded. Nonreflective backgrounds available include colored cloths of either sky blue, dark royal blue, gray, or black. If possible, a 4-foot wide background should extend from above the subject down onto the floor so that if a full body shot is taken, the baseboard and floor are eliminated from the photograph. This type of background can be purchased in any fabric store. One can also purchase rolls of heavy texture photographic background paper that can be attached to the wall, suspended from the ceiling, or pulled down onto the floor when photographing the patient, then rolled out of the way.

STANDARD PHOTOGRAPHIC POSES

To best illustrate certain anatomic areas of the human body, it is important to know when to use the vertical or horizontal camera format. Keep in mind that the final image on film measures 24 by 36 mm. If the camera is used horizontally, the photograph will be longer than it is high. If the camera is turned on its vertical axis, the photograph will be 36 mm high. A full body shot has to be photographed with the camera turned vertically or it will be virtually impossible to include the entire subject, head to toe, within the film frame at the desired ratio.

PATIENT POSITIONING: STANDARD PHOTOGRAPHIC VIEWS

One aspect of photographic documentation is consistency. There is leeway for one to develop personal photograph

Table 10-1 *Guidelines for Various Routine Photographs Taken Preoperatively and Postoperatively*

Body Part to be Photographed	Lens	Distance
Full body	55 mm	7-10 ft
Head, neck*	105 mm	Approximately 4-5 ft
Eyes, midface	105 mm	28-30 in
Nose	105 mm	28-30 in
Ear	105 mm	22-24 in
Upper extremities	55 mm	42-43 in
Breasts	55 mm	3 ft
	105 mm	6 ft
Abdomen	105 mm	5 ft
Hips, thighs	55 mm	4-5 ft
Pelvis, legs	55 mm	4-5 ft

**Young child or infant: ratio 1:7 to 1:8*
Adapted from guidelines of ASPRS Committee on Standards for Clinical Photography.

methods. Once these methods have been established, it is important to stay with the techniques so that one can develop a meaningful, reproducible record of the photographs that is consistent and accurately reproduces patient positions and views. The ASPRS Committee on Standards for Clinical Photography has published a set of guidelines for various routine photographs taken preoperatively and postoperatively (Table 10-1).

Full Body

Photography of the full body requires the use of a 50- or 55-mm lens with a lens-to-subject distance of at least 10 feet. One can further improve a photograph of the full body if the patient stands on a platform in front of nonreflective background material or if the photographer moves from a standing to a sitting position so that the focusing screen and lens axis are directed at the abdominal area (somewhere between the inframammary fold and the umbilicus). This is one of the few photographic positions where the photographer must estimate the ratio. It is generally considered that the ratio for a full body photograph is 1:25. The views for a full body photograph include frontal, 3/4° oblique left and right, profile, and back. Arms should be held off the body. It is important to take a photograph of a patient's back to be certain that there is no curvature of the spine that might contribute to asymmetry when viewing the patient from the front.

Head and Neck

This photographic series should incorporate the entire head including the neck down to the upper clavicular ridge. The desired ratio for the head and neck is suggested at a 1:9 ratio (1:8 for an infant or young child). When photographing a woman, any hair that masks the ears should be swept back so that the ears and forehead can be easily viewed (e.g., use of combs). Positions include frontal, 3/4° oblique left and right, and profile left and right. Be certain that the subject's head is level and that there is no undue projection of the chin that will distort the configuration and natural outline of the patient's profile. All head and neck photographs should be taken with the camera held vertically. With 45° angle oblique photographs left and right, the tip of the subject's nose should appear along the contralateral line of the opposite cheek.

Eyes Including Midface

For this series of photographs, the horizontal camera format is used. To maintain consistency, the lower margin in the focus-viewing screen should fall somewhere between the maxilla just below the nasal tip. A series of photographs should include eyes open, eyes smiling, eyes closed, and eyes open looking up without movement of the head.

Nose and Ears

The nose should be photographed with the camera in the vertical format. Take the routine frontal, 3/4° oblique left and right, and profile left and right. The photograph also should incorporate a "chin-up" view making certain that the tip of the nose is aligned with the eyebrows (i.e., displaying the nares, which Dr. Bernard Kaye refers to as the "Sign of the Golden Arches"). The ratio for a nose is generally 1:4 or 1:5. Once the ratio is established, continue to use it.

Photographs of the ears should be taken in the vertical format, along with a full face view, with any long hair combed or swept out of the way. The ear photographic series should include a close-up lateral view of each ear and a posterior view with the hair moved so that a full view is possible.

Lips, Mouth, Teeth, and Chin

This lower area of the face should include in its photographic series a full frontal view of the face, as well as 3/4° oblique left and right, and profile left and right views. Then using the horizontal format at a ratio of 1:4 or 1:5, photograph the lips and chin with the upper border of the photograph to include the tip of the nose and the lower border to include the underside of the chin. If for some reason it is necessary to photograph the teeth or the oral cavity, a dental speculum should be used. This is also one area in plastic surgery where the use of a flash ring light will improve the image considerably.

Upper Extremities

Photographs of the brachial area should be taken with the arms extended parallel to the floor and the hands rotated with the palms facing the camera with the thumbs pointing toward the ceiling. Where indicated, arms may be flexed at the elbow to illustrate muscle tone and skin turgor.

Breasts

When it comes to medical photography, this area of the anatomy seems to be one of continual controversy. Some plastic surgeons want all of their photographs to be in the vertical format; others only want the horizontal format. The patient should be photographed in the frontal, 45° oblique left and right and profile left and right. The image should border at the top along the sternal notch and at the bottom along the inferior border of the rib cage. The breasts may be photographed in three basic positions: arms at the side, arms akimbo (hands on hips), or arms raised and extended over the head. The ratio used is generally between 1:12 and 1:15.

Abdomen and Buttocks

Similar to other areas described, the abdomen and buttocks are photographed in the frontal, 3/4° oblique left and right, and profile left and right. It is preferred that the photographer use the vertical format and that the area of view incorporates the umbilicus at the upper border and the midthigh at the lower border. Where possible, legs should be slightly spread to reveal an accurate contour. This is particularly important with suction-assisted lipectomy. This same series of photographs also applies to the hips and thighs when photographed.

Lower Extremities

Positioning the camera in the vertical format, the camera lens should be down low with the focusing screen and the lens axis should be somewhere at the level of the knees. A good photograph will require the photographer to bend or kneel down, making sure that the lens axis is horizontal to the floor so that there is no distortion. The views of the lower extremities are similar to those noted earlier except that the rear view should also be taken with the thighs slightly separated. When photographing the lower extremities, it is also useful to position the leading leg either to the right or left and slightly forward.

FURTHER READINGS

Clinical Photography (Kodak data book), New York, 1972, Eastman Kodak.

Grazer M: *The atlas of suction assisted lipectomy in body contouring,* New York, 1991 Churchill Livingstone, p. 31.

Hedgecoe J: *The art of color photography,* New York, 1978, Simon & Schuster.

Nelson D, Drause JL Jr: *Clinical photography in plastic surgery,* Boston, 1988, Little, Brown.

Reeder, RC: *Source book of medical communication,* St Louis, 1981, Mosby.

CHAPTER 11

Medicolegal Considerations

William Dixon Wiles

Plastic surgeons in the United States must be aware of the legal aspects of practicing their specialty, which means that an introduction to the adversarial world of litigation has to infringe upon an otherwise scholarly discussion of surgical principles. Acceptance of the judicial facts of life and a willingness to understand basic principles of tort law may permit practitioners to operate more or less harmoniously in our litigious society. In some instances, knowledge of the legal system may improve the quality of patient care rendered by the plastic surgeon.

Minimizing the risks of litigation to plastic surgeons is the prime objective of the ensuing discussion, but real world considerations of insurance and the nature of medical malpractice litigation, once it arises, must be mentioned. It is improbable that plastic surgeons practicing their specialty today can avoid altogether our system of tort law and medical malpractice litigation. In the United States we have a dual system involving the federal government and the judiciaries of the 50 states and U.S. territories. Whether a lawsuit is filed in federal or state court, the law of the state in which the alleged malpractice occurred usually will be applied to the facts. The law of the state will include its statutes and its body of common law, formulated from opinions published by the appellate courts of the state. The laws of our 50 states and territories are not uniform, and it is beyond the scope of this chapter to detail the statutory and common law of each state. Certain principles of tort law will apply in most states, with some variation from state to state. When in doubt about the law in a particular jurisdiction, the plastic surgeon should consult an experienced medical malpractice attorney in that jurisdiction for specific advice.

BASIC PRINCIPLES APPLICABLE IN MEDICAL MALPRACTICE LITIGATION

Negligence

Most medical malpractice cases are founded on the theory of negligence. In essence, negligence involves the existence of a *duty* of care owed by one person to another and the *breach* of that duty, which is a *proximate* (i.e., foreseeable) *cause* of injury to another, resulting in *damages*. Some plaintiff attorneys will disdain the term "medical malpractice" because it implies evil or criminal intent and instead will speak of "medical negligence." The plaintiff's burden of proof in a civil case (preponderance of the evidence) is a lesser burden than is required in a criminal case (beyond a reasonable doubt), and plaintiffs understandably seek to avoid this semantic appearance of a heavier burden of proof. What this means in the context of a medical malpractice case is that a plaintiff must plead and prove by a preponderance of the evidence (defined usually as "the greater weight and degree of credible evidence") that (1) a physician-patient relationship existed (eliciting a duty of care), that (2) the defendant physician was negligent in some aspect of patient care, and that (3) the negligence proximately caused injury or damage to the patient.

In its simplest form, *negligence* is defined as the failure to use ordinary care. With respect to the practice of a plastic surgeon, this definition means the failure to do either that which a plastic surgeon of ordinary prudence would have done under the same or similar circumstances or the failure to do that which the same plastic surgeon would not have done under the same or similar circumstances. Negligence then can be either by omission or commission. The injury to the patient must be reasonably foreseeable to the surgeon as a consequence of the negligence. For example, if a surgeon severs an artery during surgery and fails to repair it properly, it is reasonably foreseeable that the patient may hemorrhage and sustain serious injury or even death.

A. **Recovery of damages.** The law permits recovery for *actual* damages that have occurred in the past or that will probably occur in the future (e.g., medical and hospital expenses, loss of earnings and earning capacity, pain and suffering, mental anguish, physical impairment, disfigurement, loss of familial or spousal consortium, etc.). If the negligence is found by a judge or a jury (generally a jury) to involve more than momentary inadvertence, that is, to constitute a willful or reckless disregard for the rights and welfare of the patient, it will be characterized as *gross negligence* and will evoke a claim for *punitive* or *exemplary* damages, whereby the jury is permitted to award "punishment" damages to penalize and make an example of the grossly negligent defendant.

B. **Proof of negligence.** Proof of negligence usually requires the testimony of an expert witness as to the applicable *standard of care* and the subsequent factual evidence of a violation of that standard. Plastic surgeons are specialists and thus are held to the standards of care applicable to their specialty. Like most disciplines in medicine, there is no compendium of "standards" reflecting acceptable or unacceptable practices in plastic surgery. Instead thc law permits plastic surgeons themselves to determine the standards of good medical practice, and considerable disagreement can exist among surgeons about what the standard of care actually is in a given circumstance. Other specialists who may be familiar with the type of procedure involved in the litigation in question, even though they are not plastic surgeons, can also testify about the standards of care. In a civil jury trial, the jury listens to conflicting evidence from multiple "experts" and ascertains for itself what the standard of care is and whether the defendant physician violated that standard. The judge will make a threshold determination whether a witness has sufficient expertise in a given discipline to render opinions on the subject matter of the case, but in truth judges are fairly liberal in permitting witnesses to render expert opinions. Hence, a general surgeon who claimed to be knowledgeable about reduction mammoplasty and who may even have assisted in several operations during training, might be permitted to testify against a defendant who is an experienced plastic surgeon in a case involving reduction mammoplasty. Certainly, trained plastic surgeons could also testify about the standard of care for reduction mammoplasty, but *other* specialists could be permitted to testify to the standards if the court believed that they possessed the requisite minimum knowledge or experience to offer some opinion. Physicians who claim to have expertise can be cross-examined by counsel, and their credibility can be impeached or even destroyed, but the jury will be the ultimate arbiter of the weight or credibility given to the testimony of a witness.

It was formerly the law in most states that the defendant physician was to be judged by standards applicable to the locale in which the physician practiced. The argument was made that physicians practicing in rural or remote areas, without the benefit of access to other specialists for consultation or without access to the latest in equipment and technology could not be expected to adhere to standards applicable to physicians practicing in urban areas or to physicians having access to the most current knowledge, expertise, and equipment. The realities of our advanced technologic society and the knowledge or information explosion have rendered this *locality rule* obsolete. In most jurisdictions, the locality rule has been abandoned. To the extent that the concept survives, it probably does so in the context of "same or similar circumstances." Thus physicians practicing in rural or remote areas will be held to the same standard of care as physicians practicing in urban areas, although there might be minor variations in standards when considering the same or similar circumstances confronting the defendant physician.

C. **Concepts of negligence.** Patients can pursue litigation against plastic surgeons if they can develop expert testimony of the existence of a standard of care that has been violated by the defendant physician. Such testimony is by no means conclusive, but it does permit the patient to create a "fact" issue that the jury will have to resolve. In virtually all cases, defendant physicians, either by themselves or by other expert witness testimony, must establish that a *different* standard of care is applicable and that there has been no violation of this standard. In some instances the experts will agree about the standards of care, but there will be a factual dispute as to whether there was a violation of the standard. Negligence cannot be inferred from a bad result, because physicians are not guarantors of cures. Most jurisdictions hold that a bad outcome is no evidence of negligence. With few exceptions, the jury or judge is dependent upon the testimony of expert witnesses to ascertain whether negligence has occurred and whether some act of negligence was a proximate cause of any injury or damage to the plaintiff (patient). The list of potential allegations against the plastic surgeon is limited only by the imagination of the plaintiff's attorney and ultimately by the willingness of the plaintiff's expert witnesses to testify that the standard of care required certain action that the defendant physician failed to undertake or that the defendant physician took some positive action that an ordinary prudent physician would not have taken under the same or similar circumstances. The following issues, which are commonly seen in medical malpractice cases, are illustrative only and are not inclusive.

- ▼ Plastic surgeons may be negligent during the preoperative period when selecting as a surgical patient an individual who is not an appropriate surgical candidate. A patient may express a desire to have a particular procedure performed, when in reality the patient does not require the procedure or does not meet necessary surgical criteria.
- ▼ Surgeons can also be negligent in their preoperative evaluation and workup of a patient, such as in failure to take a complete and thorough health history, failure to perform a complete and thorough physical examination, or failure to order appropriate diagnostic or preoperative laboratory tests.

One particularly important way in which a physician can be adjudged negligent in the preoperative period is the failure to obtain the patient's *informed consent.* This type of negligence is discussed in detail in the next section.

- Informed consent. The often quoted phrase by Justice Benjamin Cardozo remains as viable today as it did when he expressed it more than 80 years ago:

  "Every human being of adult years and sound mind has a right to determine what shall be done with his own body; and a surgeon who performs an operation without his patient's consent commits an assault, for which he is liable in damages."

  The patient, not the physician, is the final arbiter of whether a medical or surgical procedure will be performed. Once a physician appreciates the philosophic underpinnings of the doctrine of informed consent, the legal application becomes fairly clear. All adults of sound mind have the right to determine whether they will give or withhold consent for medical treatment. The integrity of an individual's *right* to choose or decline medical treatment is inviolate, even against reason, common sense, and good judgment. The physician's obligation is to explain the options and the recommended course of treatment and to advise of potential risks and hazards. It is *for the patient,* not the physician, to decide whether the patient will venture the risk.

  Since Justice Cardozo's opinion was written, the philosophic foundation of the principle of informed consent has endured steadfastly, but the legal theory has evolved gradually from one of "assault" to "negligence." In modern jurisprudence, the doctrine of informed consent is a negligence concept. Formerly the doctrine was viewed from the physician's perspective. Of what risks and hazards of an operative procedure would a reasonably prudent plastic surgeon inform a patient? Expert testimony to establish the local standard of care of physicians was required. If the standard necessitated that a physician inform the patient of a particular risk or hazard, the judge or jury had to decide from the evidence presented whether the physician in fact complied with the standard of care. There could be divergent testimony about the standard of care required to be disclosed to a patient. Most American jurisdictions have abandoned the physician perspective and now embrace the doctrine of informed consent from the patient's point of view. A physician or surgeon is required to inform a patient of such risks and hazards that could influence a *reasonable person* in deciding whether to give or withhold consent. Some courts have held that a risk or hazard, however slight or remote, must be imparted to a patient if the risk or hazard is inherent in the procedure and could influence the decision of a reasonable person. Thus a surgical complication that may occur even in statistically insignificant numbers must be disclosed to a patient if it could influence a reasonable person's decision. Logically *any* risk could influence this hypothetic reasonable person. The standard is thus really an objective rather than a subjective measure. In virtually all malpractice cases in which patients are claiming a failure of informed consent as a theory of recovery, they will testify that if they had known of a particular risk, they never would have consented. Fortunately the law invokes a broader appeal. Would a reasonable person, informed of the potential risks, withhold consent? Additionally the plaintiff must prove that the alleged unrevealed risk or hazard did in fact occur and that as a result the patient was injured.

- Provision for minors and other incompetent persons. In all jurisdictions special provision is made for minors and other incompetent persons who lack the legal capacity to give or withhold consent. The court may appoint a temporary or permanent guardian for the express purpose of determining whether to consent. Likewise, consent is implied in an emergency, and a surgeon need not be concerned about informing an unconscious or critically ill person, minor or adult, of potential risks or hazards. It is important for the surgeon to remember that in circumstances where consent can be given, it can always be withdrawn by the patient. The revocation of consent can be verbal or in writing.

- Signatures on consent form. Unfortunately, some surgeons make the mistake of assuming that they are legally protected and have met their obligations to the patient if the patient's signature appears on a written consent form. Some surgeons will delegate to a nurse the responsibility for obtaining the patient's signature on a consent form, without first having talked to the patient about the proposed procedure or its potential risks. The consent, to be effective, must be an *informed* consent. If the physician has failed to impart the information to the patient, notwithstanding the patient's signature on a written consent form, the physician has not obtained the patient's informed consent. It is important for the surgeon to view the doctrine of informed consent as a two-step process: (1) discuss the patient's options and operative procedure and the potential risks and hazards that could influence a reasonable person, (2) have the patient sign the consent form in the presence of a witness who will then date and time the consent form and countersign it. The witness acknowledging the patient's signature on the consent form should be someone other than the patient's surgeon. Routinely, nurses or physicians-in-training serve this function.
- Physician's liability despite informed consent. A physician will not necessarily be absolved of responsibility for the occurrence of a particular complication just because the

physician had warned the patient about the risk before surgery. For instance, hemorrhage may be a complication of a particular surgical procedure and the physician may inform the patient about that risk and have the patient acknowledge it by signing a consent form. However, if hemorrhage occurs and causes injury to the patient as a result of an error in surgical technique, the physician can be liable for this error in surgical technique even though the informed consent was properly obtained.

- Operative negligence. Surgeons can be liable for technical errors made in the course of performing an operative procedure. In most surgical procedures, the surgeon will use generally recognized methods and techniques with minor variation, depending upon the training and preference of the surgeon. There will be some intraoperative maneuvers that are not acceptable to surgeons practicing within the standard of care. Also there can be breaches of antiseptic protocol during the procedure that may result in an infection. Surgeons can also injure adjacent structures or organs, and the injury may or may not reflect a failure of the standard of care, depending upon the particular procedure being performed and the structure or organ injured.
    - Doctrine of *res ipsa loquitur.* On occasion, medical instruments, needles, or sponges can be left in the body cavity and may not be discovered until years later, or the surgeon may operate on the wrong part of the body. This kind of injury will invoke the doctrine of *res ipsa loquitur* ("the act speaks for itself"). Application of this doctrine permits a jury to infer that a physician was negligent if the nature of the injury is such that it ordinarily would not have occurred but for the physician's negligence in circumstances where the instrumentality causing the injury was under the physician's exclusive control. *Res ipsa loquitur* has limited application in most jurisdic-

tions in medical malpractice cases. The physician's negligence must be so obvious as to be within the comprehension of untrained laypersons. Applicability of *res ipsa loquitur* permits the plaintiff to avoid the introduction of expert medical testimony as to the standard of care. It does not compel a finding of negligence against the defending physician but shifts the burden of persuasion to the defendant surgeon to explain the patient's injury. Ultimately the jury will determine whether the defending physician has met that burden.

- Acts of other operating room personnel. Plastic surgeons may be alleged to be negligent in circumstances involving anesthesia complications. If anesthesia is to be administered by an anesthesiologist, then the anesthesiologist will be responsible for selecting the mode of anesthesia (unless dictated by the plastic surgeon), administering the preoperative and intraoperative anesthetics, explaining the proposed anesthesia to the patient, and obtaining the patient's informed consent for anesthesia.
    - Doctrine of "captain of the ship." Previously the courts adhered to the *"captain of the ship"* doctrine or approach to surgery, basically holding a surgeon liable for any misadventure in the operative suite. The theory borrowed heavily from nautical lore and likened the surgeon's skill and authority to that of a ship's captain. Nothing could be further from the truth, and enlightened jurisdictions have abandoned the captain of the ship doctrine.
    - Doctrine of "borrowed servant." Each participant in the operative suite is liable for his or her own conduct, although there are circumstances in which individuals who do not work for a surgeon can be considered a *"borrowed servant"* of the surgeon for a particular purpose. For example, a nurse

employed by the hospital, when acting on the instruction of the surgeon and at the surgeon's direction, may be considered a borrowed servant of the surgeon for that limited purpose, and the surgeon could be liable for the acts of the nurse who otherwise would be considered a hospital employee. The facts of each case have to be examined to determine whether the borrowed servant doctrine will apply.

To illustrate, a lawsuit might arise because a patient subsequently discovers that a sponge was left within the body. Typically the patient will sue the surgeon, the assistant surgeon, the hospital, and all participants involved in the operative procedure. The facts of the case may reveal that the surgeon was relying upon the nurses to give an accurate sponge count, and indeed the records and testimony may reflect that the surgeon requested a sponge count that was called "correct" by the nurses who were employed by the hospital. Under these circumstances, the hospital, and not the surgeon, would be liable for the retained sponge. Conversely, if the surgeon failed to request a sponge count and the matter was simply overlooked, the surgeon would be liable for failure to ascertain the correctness of the sponge count and the hospital might be possibly liable for failing to call it to the surgeon's attention. Therefore each case must be examined on its own merits.

- Risks with CRNAs. Plastic surgeons who operate with certified registered nurse anesthetists (CRNAs) who deliver anesthesia are at risk of being held vicariously liable for the negligent acts of the CRNA. A CRNA must practice under the direction of a physician, and without proof of any system for supervision by a physician anesthesiologist, the surgeon may be held responsible for the acts and omissions of a CRNA.

Additionally, surgeons can be vicariously liable for the acts of any of their employees, such as the surgeon's technician whom the surgeon employs and uses in operative procedures. Vicarious liability extends to all areas of tort law and is a concept that holds employers liable for the negligent conduct of their employees who are acting within the course and scope of their employment. The "status" of employer is sufficient to hold the employer liable under these circumstances for the negligence of the employee.

- ▼ Postoperative negligence
  - ■ Complications. Complications that develop during the patient's postoperative course may elicit allegations of negligent failure to diagnose, failure to timely diagnose the complication, or failure to refer the patient to another specialist for diagnosis or treatment. Despite preoperative warnings about the risks and hazards associated with a surgical procedure, some patients have a propensity to regard any complication, however transient, as a result of surgical or postoperative negligence. Litigation may ensue when a patient develops postoperative swelling, hemorrhage, hematoma formation, transient neurapraxia, breast contractures, skin slough, or infection. Greater care in explaining these complications to the patient in the preoperative period may assist in avoiding litigation when the complications develop postoperatively. For example, if a surgeon can anticipate that some tissue necrosis will likely occur after the procedure, it might be advisable to show the patient a picture of tissue necrosis before surgery so that the patient will be psychologically prepared for that temporary complication. Unexpected surprises are frightening to patients and often fuel thoughts of litigation.

- Patient communication. A common complaint against surgeons is that they fail to visit their patients postoperatively or to communicate with them effectively in the postoperative period. It is important that surgeons personally make rounds on patients and then carefully document those rounds in the patients' progress notes and doctor's orders, going so far as to time the progress notes and orders. Patients are often reassured by the presence of their surgeons and by the knowledge that they can have personal access to the surgeon to discuss their cases. When postoperative complications do develop, surgeons must explain to their patients the complications that have developed, document them carefully, and undertake a regimen to diagnose the source of the problem if it is not readily apparent.
- Surgical result. Plastic surgeons performing elective, aesthetic plastic surgery are probably more at risk for lawsuits than plastic surgeons who perform somewhat more urgent or emergent reconstructive surgery. Patients undergoing aesthetic procedures have certain expectations about the outcome of surgery, and failure by the surgeon to satisfy these subjective expectations can result in a hostile, litigation-minded patient. Some surgeons, in their zeal to reassure the patient about the efficacy and safety of the contemplated procedure, may actually be contributing to the patient's unrealistic expectations. Patients sometimes file lawsuits after breast augmentations or mammoplasty reductions because their breasts are not symmetrical after surgery. Well-qualified, trained plastic surgeons may view the patient's "before" and "after" photographs and remark on the excellent result obtained by the surgeon, but the patient will nevertheless pursue litigation, simply because she thought she was going to have symmetrical breasts. Surgeons could well avoid litigation by counseling their patients on the

limitations and the benefits of the proposed surgery.

D. **Legal defenses: statute of limitations.** Most jurisdictions have statutes or a body of common law that limits the time within which lawsuits may be brought. These are commonly referred to as *statutes of limitation,* and the precise nature of the statutes may vary from jurisdiction to jurisdiction.

- ▼ In most states, negligence actions have to be brought within 2 years from the date the cause of action arose or the date of the alleged negligent conduct. Statutes of limitations of various durations may be applied to particular kinds of claims. For example, a 4-year statute of limitations is often applicable to a contract claim, whereas a tort claim (such as negligence) must be brought within 2 years. If the lawsuit is not timely filed, the defendant must affirmatively assert the defense of statute of limitations. The fact that a lawsuit is filed untimely does not necessarily mean that it will be dismissed. The affirmative defense has to be urged and a ruling sought from the court.
- ▼ In some jurisdictions, the statute of limitations will be extended if the case involves an injury that the patient could not have discovered within the period of limitations. For example, 3 or 4 years after a surgical procedure a patient may become symptomatic, and subsequent diagnostic testing or laparotomy then reveals a retained sponge. In this instance, the patient could not have possibly discovered the retained sponge or perceived the negligence on the part of some health care provider within the 2-year period of limitations. States adopting the *discovery rule* maintain that the statute of limitations begins when the patient knew or should have known of the defendant's negligent act. The jury or judge will determine when the patient knew or should have known, and therefore a "fact" issue is raised for adjudication. Likewise the period of limitations will be extended if the physician or surgeon knowingly has concealed information from

the patient. Like the discovery rule, the doctrine of *fraudulent concealment* is a "defense" raised by plaintiffs to the defendant's assertion of the statute of limitations defense. Again, allegations and proof of fraudulent concealment create a fact question for the judge or jury to determine.

Product Liability Suits

Physicians involved in medical negligence cases may be surprised to discover that plaintiffs will sue product manufacturers or dealers in the same litigation with a physician. Plastic surgeons frequently use sophisticated medical instruments and products that, in addition to their beneficial aspects, can cause injury or harm to patients. Stories abound of instruments that break or fail during surgery, of prosthetic devices that fail after implantation in the body, or of Bovie units that cause burn injuries. Injuries that laypersons might associate with errors by the surgeon may, in fact, be caused by the failure of medical and surgical instruments or products or by design or manufacturing defects.

Manufacturers have a duty to warn surgeons about risks inherent in products, and the failure to warn can result in the manufacturers being held strictly liable for the damage caused by that failure to warn. Particular attention should be paid by surgeons to the manufacturer's instructions and package inserts, because they may avoid liability by proof that they used a medical instrument or product in accordance with the manufacturer's instructions. If in the exercise of judgment, a surgeon elects to use the product in a manner different from that recommended by the manufacturer, the surgeon must be prepared to offer proof that this use of the product is recognized and accepted within the surgeon's specialty. In an appropriate case, if the plaintiff patient failed to join a product manufacturer as a party defendant to the litigation when there was evidence of a product defect that caused injury to the patient, the defending physician can join the manufacturer as a "third-party defendant," although the physician will have the burden of proof on all allegations made against the manufacturer. Responsibility for the injury to the plaintiff may thus be shifted to the manufacturer of a medical instrument or product if it can be proved that a design or manufacturing defect caused injury to the patient.

PROFESSIONAL LIABILITY INSURANCE

Contract

Professional liability insurance is a contract between the physician (insured) and an insurance company (insurer) whereby the insurer, for payment of a specified premium, agrees to provide the insured physician with insurance coverage for injuries caused to others arising out of the professional services rendered to them by the physician. Different insurance policies will define the circumstances of coverage somewhat differently, but the concepts are the same. The individual physician may include the professional corporation, professional association, or partnership as additional insured under the policy. Typically the professional liability policy provides a maximum limit of liability for each occurrence and another maximum limit of liability for the aggregate of all occurrences during one policy period. The limits of liability will usually be found on the declaration sheet at the front of the policy or on a policy endorsement specifying the limits of liability. For example, a $500,000 or $1 million limit of liability means that the insured has limits of $500,000 for each occurrence, not to exceed an aggregate of $1 million in each policy period. A physician purchasing a policy of insurance is buying the following two important commodities:

A. **Indemnity.** In the event of a judgment against the physician for a covered loss or a settlement, the insurance company will pay the judgment or settlement or indemnify the physician up to the limits prescribed by the policy. In the example used previously, if a claim or lawsuit resulted in a judgment or settlement from $1 to $500,000, the insurance company would be responsible for paying it. If the judgment exceeded $500,000, the insured physician would be personally liable for the amount of judgment in excess of the policy limits. Recognition of the "limits" of indemnity may cause the physician to seek a settlement of a claim rather than risk an "excess" judgment. Indemnity payments will usually extend to the negligent acts or omissions of the physician's employees acting within the course or scope of their employment, because the physician or employer will be vicariously liable for the damages caused by their negligence.

B. **Cost of defense.** In addition to its obligation to indemnify the physician or pay the limits provided under the policy, the insurance company is obligated to pay the cost of defense, including legal expenses, investigation, expert testimony, court costs, and the expenses related to appeal, if any. The policy usually provides that the insurance company has the right to employ defense counsel and to control the litigation. An endorsement to the policy would be required if the physician negotiated the right to designate defense counsel. The insurance company is obligated to defend the lawsuit and pay for the cost of defense even if the allegations against the physician are not meritorious. Frequently, the cost of defense of litigation may exceed any indemnity payment for settlement or judgment. It is not uncommon, particularly in cases of birth injury, for the cost of defense to exceed $50,000 to $100,000. Not only is the time of the defense attorney involved, but the insurance company also has to pay for court costs such as deposition expenses, travel expenses for defense counsel and expert witnesses, or expert witness fees. If a case is brought by a plaintiff who is a minor, most courts will appoint a *Guardian Ad Litem* or *Attorney Ad Litem* to represent the interest of the minor child and may assess the defending physician (and the insurer) with Guardian Ad Litem fees, even if the defendant prevails in the lawsuit. The cost of defense is usually significant and is a valuable aspect of the professional liability policy.

Practical Considerations

In the face of escalating premiums, plastic surgeons frequently inquire about the benefits of being uninsured or *"going bare,"* and the amount of insurance coverage they should purchase if they elect to be insured. Hospitals frequently require some level of professional liability insurance as a prerequisite to staff membership, so for some surgeons, going bare is not an option. Owners and administrators of hospitals understand that in surgical malpractice cases, the hospital is likely to be named as a defendant together with the surgeon. It is in the hospital's best interest to require surgeons to be insured, so that the hospital does not find itself bearing the exclusive burden and risk of litigation. When going bare is a viable option for the surgeon, it needs to be weighed carefully.

A. **Uninsured plastic surgeon.** Certain consequences to the uninsured surgeon are obvious. The plastic surgeon, when sued, does not have the benefit of an insurance company to select competent counsel and to pay the cost of defense. Likewise, in the event of a settlement or judgment, the uninsured surgeon has no third party to indemnify, or satisfy the settlement or judgment. The uninsured surgeon would have to bear the entire cost of the litigation, which is not inconsequential.

   The lack of insurance produces more subtle consequences as well. Upon learning that a party is not insured and may not have the personal financial resources to satisfy judgment, the plaintiff's attorneys have a tendency to start looking for other individuals or entities whom they can join to the litigation. For strategy reasons, a plaintiff may elect not to sue certain individuals or entities, but may have a change of mind if the "target" defendant is uninsured. Likewise, an uninsured target defendant may encourage the plaintiff's attorneys to develop innovative theories of liability in an effort to include other potentially culpable parties.

   The common law is not static, and through time new legal theories are tested in the courts and some may gradually be accepted as doctrine. One such example is the expanding body of law in the area of corporate liability of a hospital. Another example is the fairly recent application to hospitals of an old legal doctrine known as *ostensible agency*. Emergency physicians and other hospital-based services, under some circumstances, are found to be the ostensible agency of the hospital, making the hospital liable for those physicians. Litigious creativity is encouraged when the participants most likely to be responsible for an alleged injury are uninsured.

Uninsured physicians are not only leaving themselves open to financial ruin by having to defend the lawsuit and by potentially having to indemnify a judgment, but they are also shifting the burden, risk, and expense of litigation to other insured physicians or entities, who often have to defend "strained" legal allegations. Remaining uninsured generally will not protect a physician from being joined as a party to a lawsuit. The physician will be sued and caused to incur defense costs, as will other insured individuals or entities who then become primary litigation targets. The plaintiff's attorney may seek to gain a tactical advantage over the insured physicians by offering to "deal" with the uninsured physician in an effort to develop testimony favorable to the plaintiff. The plaintiff's refrain is approximately like this:

> "I have to keep you in the lawsuit for appearances sake to the jury, or to prevent the remaining defendants from 'blaming' the events on you, or pointing the finger at the 'empty chair,' but I will not take a judgment against you after trial, or I will not execute on the judgment if you will testify in a way that is favorable to plaintiff's case. . . ."

Enormous pressure can be brought to bear on an uninsured physician who is at great economic risk as a result of being uninsured. As a practical matter, the plaintiff's counsel will seek to gain a tactical advantage using the uninsured surgeon's testimony at trial. The physicians who go bare and who are then sued usually see the advantage of carrying insurance and seek to obtain coverage after the unfortunate experience of bearing the cost of their own litigation. The "bare" surgeon may be shifting the burden of the lack of insurance to other innocent parties.

B. **Underinsured plastic surgeon.** How much insurance coverage is enough? The answer depends on (1) the plastic surgeon's ability to purchase adequate insurance, (2) the availability of a market for professional liability insurance, (3) hospital requirements for staff physicians to be insured, (4) the personal estate accumulated by the physician that is subject to execution to satisfy a judgment, (5) the litigation climate in the physician's state or community, and (6) the plastic surgeon's own tolerance for financial risk. Having some insurance may be better than having no insurance at all, and thereafter the amount of coverage needed will depend upon these variable factors. In many jurisdictions, $500,000 for each occurrence and $1 million aggregate will be sufficient, whereas in other jurisdictions $1 million for each occurrence may be considered the minimum "safe" amount of coverage.

Physicians should seek consultation with experienced defense attorneys in their own state or community regarding to the amount of coverage that may be necessary. Also, if surgeons elect to carry a minimum-limits insurance policy, they can find themselves in the uncomfortable position of contemplating settlement of a case simply because they cannot afford the economic risk of a trial. For instance, the facts of the case may be such that the surgeon has an 80% or 90% chance to win at trial, but the damage potential of the case, if the surgeon loses, is far in excess of the surgeon's policy limits. Under those circumstances, the surgeon will feel pressure to settle that case to avoid a potential adverse outcome.

There are circumstances in which physicians will want to settle a case but the insurance company will refuse. The insurance company and the physician may develop conflicting economic interests and in such an event, physicians should not hesitate to employ personal counsel to advise them of their rights against the insurance company in the event the insurance company fails to zealously protect their interests.

RISK AVOIDANCE

Why People Sue for Malpractice

If a plastic surgeon were to ask a hundred different attorneys why malpractice cases are brought, the surgeon would likely get a hundred different answers. The following list is based upon the experience over several decades of one defense attorney and is suggestive of why people bring malpractice cases:

A. **Medical negligence.** Medical negligence that causes injury to patients does exist. It would be subjective at best to suggest the percentage of cases that actually constitute medical malpractice, because the existence of a violation of the standard of care (i.e., negligence) is controversial and depends on the perspective of the expert reviewing the case. Nevertheless, in some instances, physicians do practice below the standard of care. It is undeniable that a number of liability suits are pursued because of substandard medical care that results in injury to patients. No reliable statistical data are available from which to extrapolate how many malpractice cases are "meritorious," but negligence does account for some degree of harm to patients. Likewise the practice of any learned profession (e.g., medicine, accounting, engineering, architecture, law) will involve some statistical incidence of negligence.

B. **Bad results.** Rarely will patients sue when they have experienced a good outcome. Under the law, negligence cannot be inferred from the occurrence of bad results, because, as was indicated earlier, physicians are not guarantors or insurers of good results or good health. Nevertheless, patients or their families who experience a less than favorable outcome may equate that outcome with negligence. Those patients or their family members should thus be viewed as candidates for filing lawsuits. Physicians should make special efforts to maintain close personal contact and rapport with patients and patients' family members when an unfavorable result occurs.

C. **Personal grievance against physicians.** Some patients will develop a personal dislike for their physician or surgeon and will look for the least excuse to file a lawsuit. Also, it is not uncommon for patients to transfer their personal dislike for one physician to another. For example, there are instances where patients may be angry with Dr. A but sue Dr. B because of some prior relationship with Dr. A that inhibits their litigiousness.

D. **Failure of surgeon to meet patient's expectations.** Patients often make assumptions about what kind of outcome they can anticipate, usually based upon information supplied by the surgeon. When the surgeon has failed to meet the patient's expectations, this frequently implies a failure from the outset for the surgeon and the patient to have a "meeting of the minds" about what the patient can realistically expect from medical treatment.

E. **Physician's poor bedside manner.** Some surgeons are brilliant technicians and scientists but lack good "people skills." These individuals are unable to develop rapport and a good professional relationship with their patients. This deficiency can often be corrected by spending more time with the patient or the patient's family to answer questions, express concern, and otherwise manifest interest in the patient's condition. The process of surgical treatment, even when successful, is traumatic and frightening to most patients. If the surgeon is unwilling or unable to talk to the patient about these basic human concerns or is not accessible to the patient, the patient will not be as reticent to instigate litigation.

F. **Health care providers make imprudent remarks against other health care providers.** The health care industry in the United States is a competitive industry, and not infrequently the competitive juices and egos of surgeons may result in one surgeon making comments about another that the patient interprets as critical. Attorneys defending medical malpractice cases can recite many instances in which patients pursued litigation because one doctor made an imprudent remark about medical treatment rendered elsewhere. For example, during depositions testimony from plaintiffs like the following is heard:

> "Don't they know how to do CT scans at that other hospital?"; or "The antibiotic that your other physician prescribed for you is really not very effective so I will prescribe another."

Patients may interpret a different regimen of treatment or therapy as a criticism of prior treatment or therapy, when it was otherwise not intended. Physicians must be careful in commenting on care rendered by other physicians, particularly when they are relying on patient history, which is often inadequate and inaccurate.

A significant percentage of malpractice cases are brought by individuals who work in the health care industry, or who have family members who are involved in health care. It is not uncommon to find as a plaintiff in a lawsuit a nurse or former nurse, a lab technician, or a relative of a physician, nurse, or other health care provider.

Recommendations for Avoiding Litigation

A. **Screen patients with great care.** Plastic surgeons need to evaluate patients very carefully to ascertain if they are good surgical candidates, both from a medical and psychologic point of view. There are certain medical contraindications to treatment that should raise concerns during the initial consultation or examination of the patient. It may be appropriate for a patient who is considering elective surgery for the surgeon to recommend against the procedure or even to decline to treat the patient. Likewise, surgeons should be alert to patient personality deficits and conflicts. Patients who seem overly concerned about money, or who are obsequious and flattering to the surgeon, or who criticize prior-treating physicians inordinately, or who express great reservation about the efficacy of surgical treatment and seem unsure if they should go forward with the treatment are probably likely candidates for malpractice litigation. The surgeon and the staff can learn to become more attuned to personality traits and attitudes that can adversely effect the physician-patient relationship.

B. **Focus attention on patient's expectations during initial consultation.** The surgeon should focus attention during the initial consultation on the patient's expectations of the anticipated procedure to ensure that those expectations are grounded in reality rather than in fantasy. There should be a "meeting of the minds" as to what the patient expects and what the surgeon reasonably anticipates as a surgical outcome.

C. **Explain graphically operative procedures and risks.** Plastic surgeons should graphically explain the operative procedure to their patients and detail for the patient risks and hazards that could influence a reasonable person in deciding to give or withhold consent. Schematic drawings or diagrams, which should be duplicated or referenced in the office records or progress notes, are often helpful to the patient in understanding what procedure will be performed. The surgeon should not minimize the seriousness of the risks or complications inherent in surgery, particularly in elective procedures, and should be candid and forthright about the potential risks.

There is a fine balance that the surgeon must maintain between informing the patient and frightening or discouraging the patient, particularly if the patient requires the surgical procedure in question. If the patient is not emotionally or psychologically well adjusted to handle the discussion of surgical options and procedures and the risks and complications of those procedures, the surgeon should reconsider whether the patient is an appropriate surgical candidate.

D. **Have patient execute informed consent form.** Once the patient has made a decision to have surgery, it is important that the requisite consent forms be executed *after* thorough discussion of the procedure, options, risks, and complications. The surgeon should if possible, have a witness present at the time the procedure and potential risks are explained to the patient. Nurses or resident physicians can serve as witnesses to these events, and the fact of their presence during the discussion can be recorded in office records or progress notes of the hospital. Likewise the consent form must be completely filled out in advance of the patient signing it, and then the form must be signed and dated by the patient. A witness, if available, should countersign the form and also note the time that the patient signed the consent form. Some states require that some disinterested person witness the consent form.

Patients sometimes allege in medical malpractice cases that they signed a consent form, but they allege that they were under the influence of preoperative medications at the time they signed the form and thus did not have the capacity to give their informed consent. A properly dated and timed consent form can dispel such allegations. Patients under the influence of drugs that alter their mental status should never be requested to sign consent forms.

E. **Keep detailed records.** In the trial of a medical malpractice case, the physician's medical records are literally placed under a microscope for the court and the jury to review. Often the records are enlarged and they are examined and reexamined during the course of trial for what they contain and what they do not contain. The plaintiff's attorneys are fond of quoting this axiom: "If it isn't in the records, it did not occur." Nothing could be further from the truth, of course, because most of what is done for a patient is not recorded in a medical record or hospital chart.

The surgeon should make a habit of recording significant events and including normal and abnormal findings of the physical examination. The physician and the staff should be trained to record the dates and times of any entries in the medical records, including patient "no shows" for office appointments, telephone calls to and from patients for follow-up, and similar occurrences. It is important also to remember that, in a litigation context, an expert witness will review the surgeon's records. Good consistent record keeping will imply that good medical care was rendered to the patient and may influence the plaintiff's reviewing expert to suggest that a lawsuit not be filed. Conversely, sloppy, incomplete, or inconsistent records imply commensurate medical care.

Physicians should never alter or change their records, whether in the office or in the hospital. If a correction in the records is required, the records should clearly reflect the old entry and the correction. Once the physician is notified of potential litigation, no entry should be made in the existing medical records. It is surprising how often patients will obtain copies of their records even before the physician is aware they have done so, and it can be disastrous to the defense of a case if two different versions of the same record are in existence.

F. **Practice within well-recognized standards of care.** There is no substitute for the practice of good medical care within the physician's specialty. In fact, the first line of defense in a medical malpractice case is that the physician practiced in accordance with the standard of care. Physicians should avoid recommending experimental procedures without having established an appropriate protocol through the hospital, and without having clearly (and in writing) communicated the fact of the experimental procedure to the patient.

G. **Communicate frequently with patient.** It is important for the plastic surgeon to communicate frequently and effectively with the patient. The surgeon should not use office staff as a barrier between the patient and the surgeon's time. Obviously, some screening mechanism is required to protect the surgeon's schedule, but the surgeon and the office staff should use good judgment in using the screening mechanism. Patients or their families who are anxious, or patients who have experienced complications, require access to their surgeons. Therefore surgeons should develop the practice of returning phone calls and should document them in the office and hospital record. In dealing with patients, it is important to listen to their complaints, their expectations, fears, and frustrations and to counsel patients on a human level. Treat patients with the dignity and respect with which you would want a member of your family to be treated. A surgeon who is sensitive to the needs and concerns of the patient and who is reasonably available to the patient is much less likely to be sued than a busy surgeon whom the patient never sees.

H. ***Never* guarantee a cure or result, verbally or in writing.**

I. **Train office staff.** Office staff members should be instructed to advise the physician of patients who have expressed anger or hostility toward the physician, or who have some concern that seems to be "out of the ordinary," or who have complained about the physician. However, staff members should be trained to avoid the appearance of practicing medicine without a license or attempting to diagnose a patient's complaints over the telephone. It is extremely important for staff members to develop rapport with a patient and to be courteous to the patient.

J. **Stay within area of expertise.** Plastic surgeons should not be reluctant to refer patients to other specialists when the need arises or to seek consultation with other specialists.

THE LITIGATION PROCESS

Physician's Involvement as Expert Witness for Plaintiff or Defendant

The physician's initial encounter with the litigation process may be as an expert witness for one side or the other in a malpractice case. In most jurisdictions, a malpractice case cannot go forward unless there is testimony by an expert witness of the standard of medical care and a violation of the standard of care by the defending physician. Therefore the litigation process in most instances requires the testimony of expert witnesses.

A. **Review of documents.** If you, as a plastic surgeon, are requested to serve as an expert witness for either plaintiff or defendant, make certain that you have reviewed all of the medical records, depositions, and documents furnished by counsel. If the records appear to be incomplete, you should request complete documents. Avoid making snap judgments without the benefit of all the information that the jury will have. Do not become so committed to any opinion or express an opinion so vehemently that it cannot be altered when confronted with other operative facts.

B. **Standard of care.** Considerable thought should be given by the expert witness to the standard of care. The negligence definition relates to doing or failing to do something that a plastic surgeon of ordinary prudence would have done or would not have done under the same or similar circumstances. The "same or similar circumstances" require a careful review. Do not require perfection of other plastic surgeons but only that they operate within the standard of care. Be realistic, not egotistical, about the standard of care. Likewise, do not gloss over substandard medical care. As an expert witness, it is important to take a balanced approach.

Physician's Involvement as Defendant in Medical Malpractice Case

A. **Notify insurance carrier (or attorney, if "bare") of any litigation threat.** Do not initiate correspondence or generate written documents until instructed to do so by the insurance carrier or attorney.

B. **Become active participant in defense of case**

- ▼ Inform attorney. Meet with the attorney and do not assume that the attorney has any level of knowledge or appreciation of the medical issues, unless you are familiar with the attorney. Do not attempt to mislead the attorney because that could ultimately be disastrous to the defense. The attorney-client privilege will protect confidential information that you give the attorney even if the attorney has been employed by an insurance company.
- ▼ Conduct literature searches. Provide literature to the attorney to assist with the education process, but do so only after getting approval from the insurance company or the attorney.

C. **Be objective about strengths and weaknesses of case.** When the lawsuit arises, it is no time for the surgeon to rail against the plaintiff attorney for questioning your treatment or judgment. Identify the problems in the case for the attorney, and be prepared to explain them in a deposition. If you can find the problems, so can the other side.

D. **Cooperate fully with insurance company and defense attorney.** They are on your "team," trying to represent your best interest. Failure to cooperate could result in the insurance carrier withdrawing its defense, although seldom does an insurance company invoke the "failure to cooperate" clause in the insurance contract. In reality, it is in your best interest to be cooperative. Occasionally, you will hear unpleasant news about the case, particularly as the discovery is unfolding. Do not ascribe ill will to the defense team, and do not assume that they are colluding with the plaintiff's attorney because they have informed you of bad news or of weaknesses in the case as they perceive it. That is part of their job. If your representatives are drawing improper conclusions from information reviewed, then explain in detail why the conclusions are inaccurate.

E. **Attend depositions of other witnesses when requested by attorney or when it might be important to be present.** Do not underestimate your instincts in ascertaining when your presence is required.

F. **When case has been adequately developed so that attorney can fairly evaluate it, ask for attorney's analysis; then carefully weigh attorney's assessment and recommendations.** Do not hesitate to employ at your own expense, personal counsel to review the case and give you a second opinion. This is especially true if you are facing exposure in excess of the limits of your liability policy or if you are being sued for damages not covered by your liability policy (e.g., punitive damages).

G. **Have attorney explain dynamics of trial.** You must understand that lawsuits are not always decided solely on the merits of the medical arguments. Other considerations may be involved, such as potential jury sympathy for the plaintiff or plaintiff's attorney or your attorney, whether you or any other witness will make a "good witness," the venue or jurisdiction in which the case is being tried, and the reputation of the judge. It is difficult for a plastic surgeon to weigh and evaluate these intangible variables, but an experienced defense attorney can analyze these factors and discuss them with you. Just as physicians cannot guarantee outcome, neither can attorneys guarantee or even predict outcome with any high degree of success. A jury trial relies upon the collective judgment and common sense of 12 laypersons (unless you are fortunate enough to have a physician qualify as a juror in your case).

H. **In deciding whether to settle a case or try it, be as objective as possible and try to make a good economic decision for you and your family.** If a decision is made to settle a case, it can almost invariably be done with language in the settlement documents stating that the settlement is not an admission of liability. You may need to consider other actions, such as the reporting of the settlement to a national data bank or to the State Board of Medical Examiners. You might also consider the effect on your insurance premiums in the future or whether your insurance may be canceled because of a settlement.

I. **If you decide not to settle a case, gird yourself for an experience that can be emotionally draining and physically strenuous.** Learn to listen to your attorney and follow the attorney's advice. It is important to remember that juries do not like angry, egotistical, and arrogant physicians. They do appreciate physicians who appear to be knowledgeable and confident, but who are also humble, sympathetic, and honest.

J. **When lawsuit is finished, try to put experience in perspective.** Litigation or the threat of litigation is often the price that must be paid to practice medicine. The more that you understand about the process and how the judicial system works, the better you will be prepared to avoid litigation and to deal with its vicissitudes if litigation should occur.

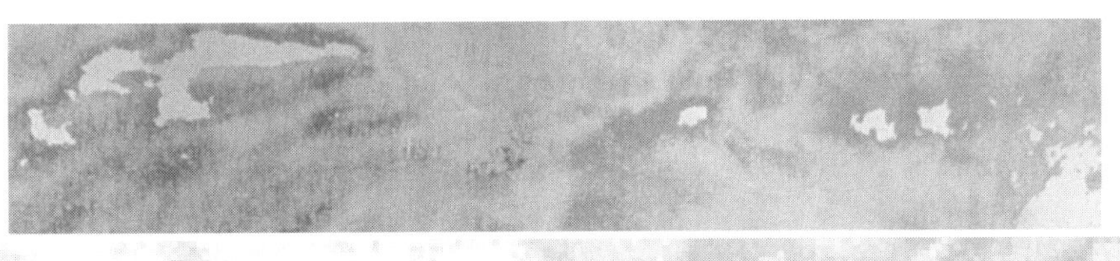

PART 2
Patient Care in Specific Types of Plastic Surgery

CHAPTER 12

Lacerations

THOMAS RAY VECCHIONE

The physician who performs the initial treatment and suturing of a laceration has the opportunity and the obligation to use sound techniques that result in normal healing. In repair of lacerations and wound closures, detail is the key ingredient. When small details such as removal of all foreign bodies and the careful placement of delicate sutures are overlooked, the result often is an aesthetically objectionable scar.

THE WOUND AS AN EMERGENCY

Priorities

In the presence of multiple injuries, the following priorities should be observed in patient care:

- Relieve airway obstruction.
- Control hemorrhage.
- Treat shock.
- Evaluate and plan for treatment of associated injuries.
- Repair lacerations.

When it is necessary to transfer a patient in an emergency situation, it is important not to increase the injuries but to stabilize them until definitive treatment can be performed. Hemorrhage must be controlled with pressure or vessel ligation. Gross debris should be removed, and wound edges should be unraveled before the final repair is undertaken. When they are available, temporary tacking sutures can be placed in the wound edges and a moist bulky dressing over the laceration as an initial treatment to reduce contamination from exposure. Elevation of the injured part helps reduce edema while transporting the patient for definitive treatment.

Timing

When necessary, lacerations can wait for as long as 24 hours for final suturing, with minimal compromise of the end result if bleeding has been controlled and the wound has been cleansed. When complete repair of the laceration cannot be done immediately, accurate initial approximation of soft tissues reduces exposure to bacteria and promotes a more acceptable end result. However, the sooner a laceration is repaired, the better. Edema makes tissues less pliable and harder to precisely approximate.

Preparation for Treatment

A photographic record of the injury should be made before definitive treatment is performed. Not only will this record help in explaining late wound-healing phenomena to the patient, but it is also of benefit to the surgeon in evaluating treatment techniques. Hair-bearing areas immediately adjacent to the lacerations, except for eyebrows or eyelashes, should be shaved to ensure thorough skin cleansing. Before an abrasion is scrubbed it can be covered with a lidocaine jelly-saturated dressing for 10 minutes. This will allow a more complete scrub to be performed without undue pain for the patient. When required, a second scrub and thorough irrigation can be performed after the local anesthetic has been injected. Materials accidently embedded in the dermis should be scrubbed vigorously and removed before they become fixed in the tissues. Embedded petroleum products, such as grease, can frequently be dissolved with small amounts of acetone or ether. When tattooing with foreign bodies is wide spread, general anesthesia may be required for adequate treatment.

Special Preparation for Children

Depending on the degree of sedation achieved with meperidine (Demerol), 0.1 to 1.5 mg/kg; promethazine (Phenergan), 0.1 mg/kg; and chlorpromazine (Thorazine), 0.5 mg/kg, physical restraint is frequently required before a laceration in a child can be treated. Commercially available infant-restraining devices employing adhesive straps are recommended for keeping injured areas immobile during laceration repair. As an alternative, an uncooperative child can be wrapped in a sheet and "mummified" or restrained by the physician's assistant.

Wound Toilet

Thorough cleansing of the wound is paramount in wound preparation before suturing of the laceration. A Water Pik-like device is ideal because it removes debris with the least amount of damage to normal adjacent tissues. Cleansing can also be performed with meticulous use of a nylon or wire brush, a high-speed dermabrader, a No. 15 scalpel blade, or by rubbing the wound edges with a moist gauze sponge. Copious irrigation of the wound with saline is important. Use of detergents such as pHisoHex or Betadine should be avoided in the depth of the wound because they have been shown to cause microscopic damage in the deep tissues. Some particles become enmeshed in the proteinaceous areolar edema and cannot easily be flushed from the wound. When gravel and grit debris are ground in and are not removable by the above methods, they must be sharply excised with a scalpel blade. Retained foreign bodies may be extruded later as the wound heals, but more frequently these undesirable foreign bodies remain in the subdermal position as unsightly foreign-body tattoos. To achieve cosmetic improvement of unwanted tattoos from incomplete initial wound toilet, dermabrasion or excision must be performed subsequently.

Instruments

In treating lacerations, proper surgical tools and adequate lighting are basic necessities for the surgeon in accomplishing delicate and precise tissue approximation with minimal trauma to dermal and epithelial edges. Five recommended instruments for laceration repair include the following:

- Smooth-jaw needle holder with a delicate tapered head
- Fine-tooth forceps
- Curved iris, tenotomy, or tissue scissors with sharp cutting blades
- Sharp scalpel
- Skin hooks

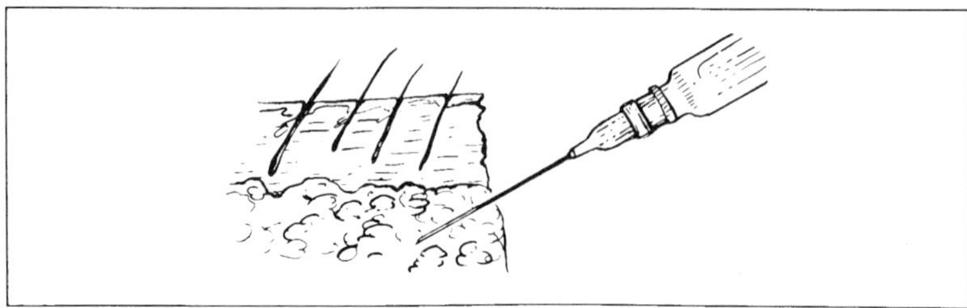

FIG. 12-1 *Anesthetic agent injected slowly into subdermal plexus with 30-gauge needle.*

These basic instruments are all that are usually required to perform a proper repair of most lacerations. The surgeon must use sufficient lighting and exposure to ensure that sutures are placed in the correct tissue planes, that minimal yet sound amounts of tissue are included with each sharp cutting needle bite, and that wound edges are everted when the knots are tied (Figs. 12-1 to 12-4).

Tetanus Prophylaxis

For patients who have been immunized a year or more before injury, 0.5 ml tetanus toxoid booster should be given intramuscularly (IM) if the wound contains seriously contaminated or crushed edges. A 1990 American College of Surgeons survey found that 65% of emergency room directors observed a 3-year or less interval for administering wound tetanus toxoid for tetanus-prone wounds and that 81% observed a 10-year or less interval for non–tetanus-prone wounds.

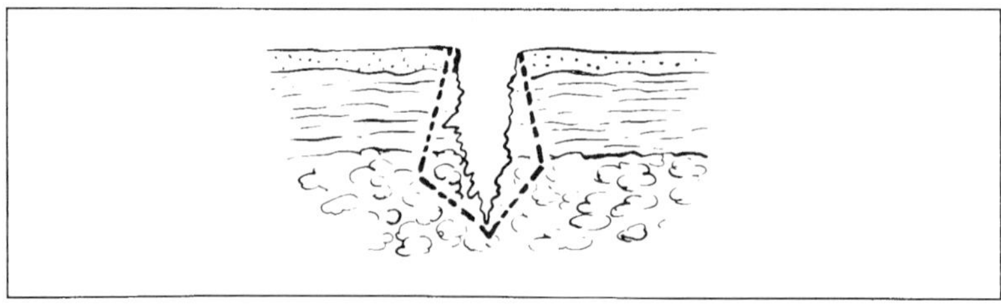

FIG. 12-2 *Wound debridement ensures healing with minimal tissue reaction.*

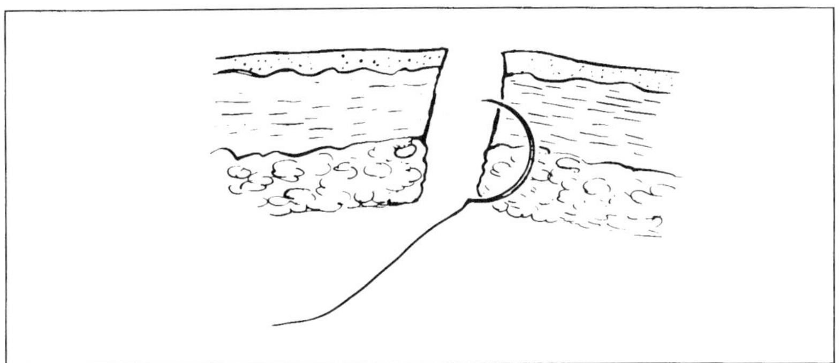

FIG. 12-3 *Approximation of subdermal fascia obliterates dead space and helps relieve tension at wound edges.*

The recommended prophylactic dose of tetanus immune globulin (human) [TIG(H)] in the United States is 250 U, with an increased dose of 500 U recommended for severe, neglected, or tetanus-prone wounds more than 24 hours old. The U.S. Public Health Service recommends administration of TIG(H) when only two doses of toxoid have been given, when the wound is not clean, and when the wound is more than 24 hours old. Nonwound booster immunization is recommended every 10 years unless the individual has shown a hypersensitivity to tetanus toxoid; thus individuals who have a uncontaminated minor wound will have some protection at all times against tetanus.

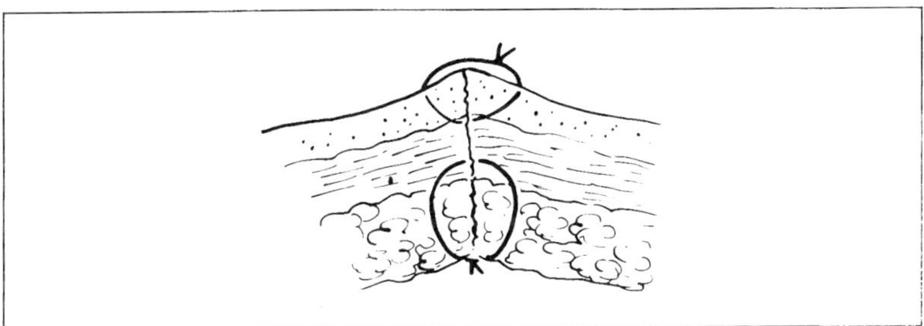

FIG. 12-4 *Correct placement of dermal and subdermal sutures results in clean, everted closure.*

EVALUATION OF WOUND TYPES

Puncture Wound

Sharp objects may drive foreign-body debris deeply through a small entrance wound. Tissue destruction, bleeding, and contamination can be present deep in the wound and covered by normal-appearing tissues. When clinical circumstances support a suspicion, puncture wounds either should be probed or opened and explored so that foreign bodies can be removed and deep damage can be repaired.

Sharp Dermal Divisions

Superficial or deep lacerations may result in significant wound spreading, which may or may not represent true tissue loss. Wound spreading is much more common in children and adolescents owing to the springy, elastic quality of the dermis, which is stretching over abundant subcutaneous fat. When underlying muscles have been lacerated and contraction occurs pulling tissues further apart, the appearance is of a much larger skin loss than is actually the case. This deceptive appearance is especially present in dog bite injuries of the cheeks and in forehead avulsions.

Tissue Avulsions

A glancing blow by a sharp object may dig into the skin and subcutaneous tissue, scooping it up and partially turning it over as an *avulsion*. The layers of dermis, subcutaneous fat, fascia, and muscle can be seen at various angles in an avulsed flap. These must be aligned correctly during suturing. Superficial avulsions may involve the dermis only. These may be manifested as partial thickness defects in the skin. If sufficient adnexal structures for epithelial regeneration remain in the skin, the wound can be treated in the same way as a partial thickness defect or split skin graft donor site (See Chapter 35.). This type of wound should heal by spontaneous epithelialization.

Crushing Injury

High-pressure injuries may result in the skin being compressed and split apart. Nonviable tissues may be present at the flap tips of this type of wound and must be sharply débrided with a scalpel or sharp tissue scissors. Irregular stellate lacerations are not uncommon in a crush injury, and these must be correctly aligned before being sutured together.

OPERATIVE CARE

Infiltration of Local Anesthetics

Individual sensory nerves to specific areas can be blocked with small amounts of local anesthetic such as lidocaine (Xylocaine) or bupivacaine (Marcaine) precisely placed in the correct location. One milliliter of local anesthetic placed at the foramen of the infraorbital nerve can block the ipsilateral upper lip. On the face, local nerve blocks also can be achieved in the supraorbital, nasal, maxillary, and mandibular regions. Excessive local infiltration should be avoided, because this distorts tissues and can cause misrepresentation of the correct anatomic landmarks. Important boundaries such as the vermillion lip border should be marked with methylene blue before anesthetic infiltration begins, so that anatomic mismatches will not be present when the edema subsides. As shown in Fig. 12-1, injection discomfort is lessened when the needle is introduced through the cut edge rather than through intact skin. No larger than a 25-gauge needle should be used to infiltrate the raw edges of an open wound. A minute amount of slow anesthetic infiltration negates the pain caused by rapid injection and tissue expansion. Thirty-gauge needles with dental syringes and Carpules are better for controlling the amount delivered, with pressure touch accuracy. Epinephrine, 1:200,000 or 1:400,000, should be used with local anesthetic, except around end arteries, such as in fingers and lower extremities.

Hemostasis

Time and pressure will stop the majority of small bleeding vessels, but small arterial pumpers may begin to pulsate as the wound is cleansed and débrided. Although precise cautery coagulation leaves the least amount of foreign body in the wound, arterial bleeders are sometimes best handled by fine suture ligature. High-frequency diathermy coagulation results in minimal adjacent tissue damage if only the vessel is grasped and the surrounding tissues are kept dry. Topical agents such as thrombin, fibrinogen, gel foam, and epinephrine solutions have been used with varying degrees of success in obtaining hemostasis.

Sutures

A. Types

- *Absorbable sutures,* such as collagen catgut or synthetic polyglycolic acid ordinarily are used to obliterate dead space in the muscular and subcutaneous layers and thus decrease the chance of blood or serum accumulation. Collagen catgut sutures, which are absorbed by phagocytosis, cause more tissue reaction than polyglycolic acid sutures, which undergo enzymatic degradation within 5 weeks. Most sutures are available with cutting needle swagged on one end (See Fig. 12-3.). It is recommended that nonabsorbable sutures such as nylon or stainless steel not be permanently buried near the skin surface, because some of them may work their way to the surface and cause a prickling sensation after the edema subsides and contraction ensues. Buried absorbable sutures should be placed in deep and subdermal tissue levels to relieve would tension at the superficial skin edges.
- *Nonabsorbable sutures,* such as prolene and nylon, or wire, or skin tapes can be used on the skin surface for wound approximation. Silk suture is preferred by some surgeons because of its accuracy in holding knots but increased tissue reactivity to silk dictates its early removal. Chromic or plain catgut sutures on the skin surface can be extremely inflammatory and should be used infrequently, as in treatment of nonaesthetic regions in children who would not easily tolerate suture removal. Multifilament sutures can be more reactive than monofilament sutures. Because of their low friction coefficients, nylon and prolene sutures can unravel if loose or carelessly tied knots have been placed. This should be remembered especially in treating children and active patients in whom an untied knot could result in unwanted wound edge separation.

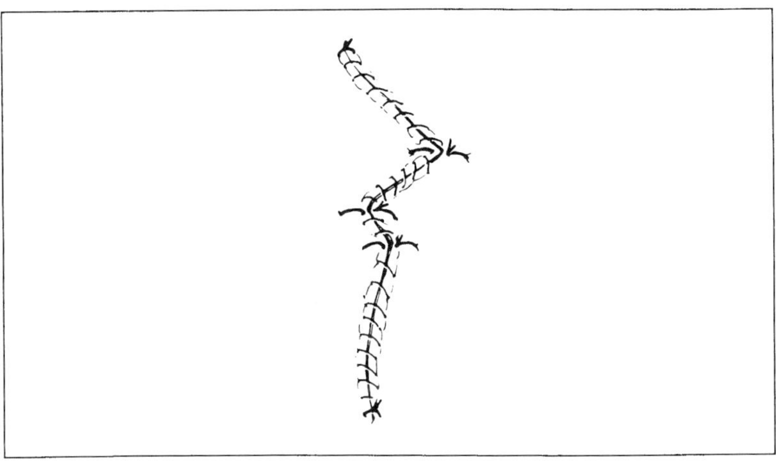

FIG. 12-5 *After subcutaneous sutures are placed, serially placed vertical mattress sutures begin edge eversion. Wound can now be closed with simple running suture.*

B. Placement of sutures. Lacerations are closed wither with running, interrupted, or subcuticular placement of suture.

▼ *Running sutures* involve over-and-over stitching tied at both ends of the laceration (Fig. 12-5). Eversion can be accomplished by angling back the direction of the needle 90° or more, which encompasses more deep than superficial tissues (See Fig. 12-3.). Running sutures can be placed with vertical mattress configuration (See Fig. 12-5.) or horizontal mattress placement (Fig. 12-6) to help hold tissue eversion.

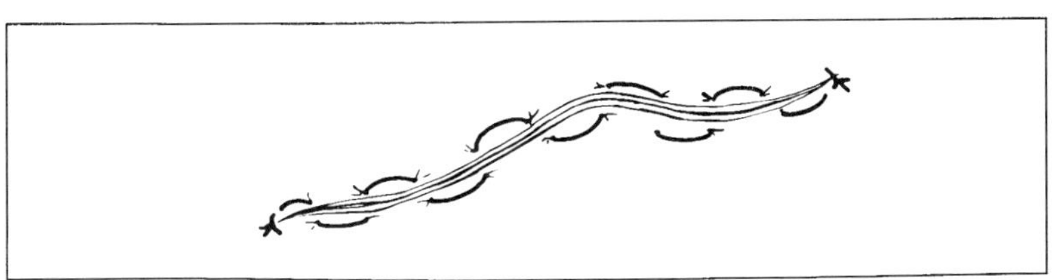

FIG. 12-6 *Running horizontal mattress suture ensures maximal tissue edge eversion on an extremity.*

- *Interrupted sutures* are placed and tied individually so as to coapt gently the edges of the wound in an everted position (See Fig. 12-4.). An interrupted vertical mattress suture (See Fig. 12-5.) begins farther away from the wound and then gathers 1 or 2 mm of superficial tissue on both edges. This type of suture helps obliterate dead space and brings together the underlying skin and subcutaneous tissues with epithelial eversion. Horizontal mattress sutures, half buried, are useful in holding skin flaps in position, with the knots being tied on the recipient side so that the flap is not damaged. This type of half-buried suture is recommended for approximating the tip of a pointed wound (Fig. 12-7).
- *Subcuticular sutures,* interrupted and buried, are placed in the subdermal region or in the subcutaneous fibrofatty layer to approximate wound edges and relieve skin tension. Knots are tied in the deep layer away from the wound surface (See Fig. 12-4.). Running absorbable or nonabsorbable subcuticular suture, used in the dermal layer to approximate the skin edges, has the advantage of averting cutaneous suture marks (Fig. 12-8).

C. **Gentleness.** Gentleness in tissue handling is paramount in obtaining aesthetically pleasing results with all suturing techniques. The basic principles of complete hemostasis, obliteration of dead space, avoidance of tension, and precise tissue alignment must be adhered to completely in treating lacerations.

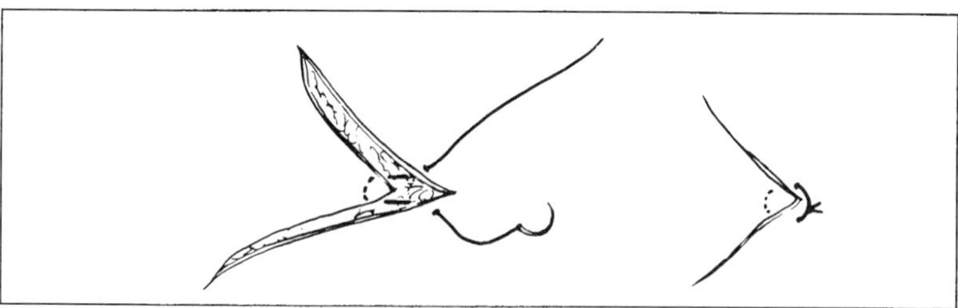

Fig. 12-7 *Half-buried angle corner suture helps keep tip of avulsed flap at proper level.*

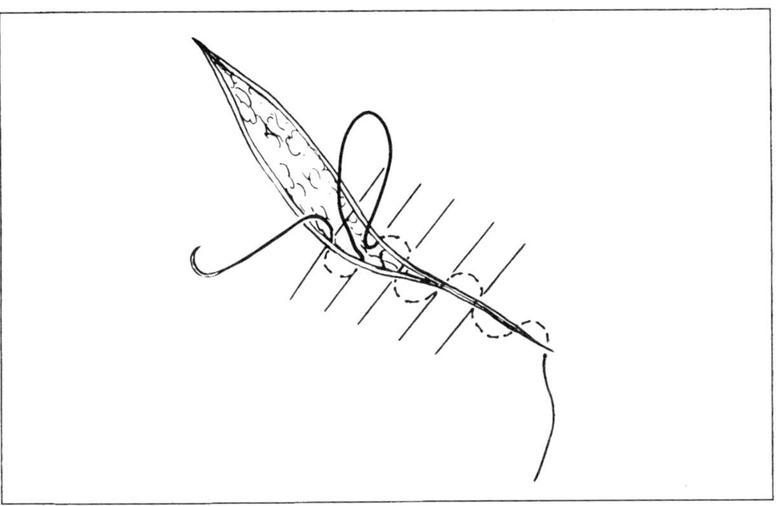

FIG. 12-8 *Subcuticular closure can be performed with buried absorbable suture or externally attached nonabsorbable suture, which can be pulled out in 1 to 2 weeks.*

APPROACHES TO WOUNDS

Simple Linear Laceration

A simple laceration can be closed with several interrupted deep sutures, bringing the skin edges together, and then approximating the skin surface with any of the suture techniques mentioned previously. Multiple fine sutures (5-0 or 6-0), which are interrupted, running, or subcuticular, should relieve tension and help prevent unsightly scar formation. The advantage of the subcuticular closure is that the suture can be left in place for a longer period of time without causing cutaneous crossmarks.

Beveled Laceration

Individual judgment and experience help dictate how much excision and recutting of a beveled skin edge is necessary to achieve the desired result. Partial-thickness skin edges may or may not require sharp excision to obtain an everted closure. Some surgeons feel that reapproximation of the avulsed tissue without sharp excision results in less noticeable scarring. Reapproximation of the partial-thickness skin edge over the avulsed dermis may result in a "softer-edged" scar, as opposed to that obtained with the straight 90° skin-edge line.

Semicircular Laceration

Use of half-buried horizontal mattress sutures has been advocated for semicircular lacerations to lessen the "trap-door" effect, which almost always evolves as wound contraction occurs. The need for later scar revision with serial Z-plasties or partial excisions will be inevitable in some cases of semicircular wounds, no matter what type of closure technique is used.

Triangular Flap Laceration

A half-buried suture should be used to repair the triangular flap laceration at its apex (See Fig. 12-6.). This type of suture allows the tip of the flap to be everted at the point. The suture passing through the flap tip must be precisely placed at the same level in the dermis as the adjacent tissues to avoid irregular tissue alignment. As an alternative, an elliptical excision of the sharp triangle will allow a curvilinear closure to be performed, reducing the potential of sharp point noticeability.

Stellate Laceration

After the nonviable edges of this type of laceration have been sharply excised, the stellate pieces should be carefully reapproximated with fine interrupted sutures. Often these wounds heal with better-than-expected results.

POSTOPERATIVE CARE

Dressings

Plain or petroleum-gel gauze or Telfa should be placed to absorb serum drainage from the wound edges. Depending upon the amount of drainage, the initial dressing should be changed in 24 to 48 hours. When no further drainage occurs, the dressing can be discontinued. Most wounds should be cleansed at 24 hours with dilute peroxide or saline to remove crusts and decrease eschar formation. Wound eschars left in place can result in subclinical wound infection and thus increase the amount and noticeability of deposited scar tissues.

Suture removal

A. **Timing.** Some of the factors contributing to the severity of suture marks are found to be the length of time a skin suture is in place, skin tension, proximity of the suture to the wound edge (the closer the suture to the skin edge, the less the amount of crossmarking), infection, and the location of the injury. Because of superb blood supply in the head and neck region, eyelid sutures can be removed in 3 days, and other facial sutures can be taken out in 4 to 6 days. Sutures should be left in place 1 week on the extremities and trunk. The back and feet, with less blood supply and potentially greater wound tensions, require suture retention up to 14 days. When sufficient subcutaneous suturing has been done, tension on wound edges is decreased so that skin sutures can be removed relatively early to reduce the chances of permanent stitch marks.

B. **Use of surgical adhesive tape.** Application of microporous surgical adhesive tapes (Steri-strips) provides the advantage of applying tensile strength to the wound after early suture removal. These tapes are no substitute for accurate deep and superficial suturing but can help to avert suture marks.

Healing Problems

In spite of meticulous suturing, careful wound care, and adherence to sound principles, some lacerations heal in a cosmetically objectionable fashion. The treatment of problem scars is discussed in Chapter 13.

CHAPTER 13

Wound Healing and Problem Scars

WILLIAM B. RILEY, JR.

The plastic surgeon ideally should be a wound-healing expert. Internist and surgical specialist alike look to the plastic surgeon to solve difficult wound problems in clinical practice. Successful management of such problems demands that the plastic surgeon combine basic principles of wound-healing biology with an armamentarium of technical skills and artistic finesse. Knowledge of basic mechanisms of wound healing in health and disease allow the plastic surgeon to make accurate diagnoses, formulate sound treatment plans, and obtain optimal functional and aesthetic results. Although technical considerations remain of paramount importance in analyzing and treating problem scars, the future holds the promise of pharmacologic manipulation of fibrous scar tissue. Indeed this promise now is an imminent reality.

BIOLOGY OF TISSUE REPAIR

All wounds heal by forming fibrous scar tissue. The basic mechanism that unites an abdominal wound or a broken bone also may produce a facial disfigurement or a cirrhotic liver. It is ironic that normal healing usually proceeds unnoticed. Only when abnormal healing ensues do the patient and physician become acutely aware of this amazing reparative process. Millard's admonition to first "know the normal" when solving artistic abnormalities is equally valid for healing abnormalities. First, know the normal.

Normal Repair

A. **Phases of healing.** The biochemical aspects of healing are best understood when considered in the following three different phases:

- Substrate phase. The substrate phase includes the first few days after injury. In this early period, hemostasis is achieved by a complex cascade mechanism that includes vasoconstriction, platelet aggregation, fibrin formation, fibrinolysis, and activation of the complement system. Complement products activate the platelet, causing degranulation and release of inflammatory mediators, fibronectin, and growth factors such as platelet-derived growth factor (PDGF), transforming growth factor β, (TGF-β), platelet factor 4 (PF4), and fibroblast growth factor (FGF). These mitogenic factors are also strong chemoattractants that recruit polymorphonuclear leukocytes, macrophages, lymphocytes, and fibroblasts into the wound environment. The macrophage is the crucial inflammatory cell orchestrating the repair process. Macrophages débride or "clean up" the wound and secrete substances that stimulate fibroblast replication (macrophage-derived growth factor or MDGF) and blood vessel ingrowth (wound angiogenesis factor or WAF). Endothelial and epithelial cells multiply, migrate, and effectively seal the wound. Fibroblasts proliferate and begin to synthesize type III collagen in the proteoglycan-rich fibrin matrix. The immature type III collagen is gradually replaced by the more mature type I collagen.
- Fibroplasia phase. The phase of fibroplasia continues through the third week; it is characterized by intense collagen synthesis and deposition in wounds healing by first intention. In open wounds healing by second intention, the processes of epithelialization and contraction proceed relentlessly with intense cellular activity. A moist environment and possibly topical application of vitamin A stimulate epithelialization, whereas scab formation, protein deficiency, and steroids retard the process. Histologically, an epithelializing wound displays increased mitotic activity in the basal cell layer and resembles a neoplastic process. Wound contraction is incompletely understood, but the contractile myofibroblast is probably essential to this process.

Wound contraction is inhibited by radiation, thick skin grafts, steroids, burns, and colchicine. It is important to distinguish between *contraction* and *contracture.* The latter term means loss of motion and usually represents the end product of wound contraction.

- Maturation phase. The maturation phase of healing begins in the fourth week and continues for many months. During this prolonged period, randomly oriented collagen fibers are cross-linked, broken, and recross-linked many times along lines of stress. This cross-linking involves the formation of chemical, electrical, and physical bonds within (intramolecular) and between (intermolecular) collagen molecules. The remodeling process results in scar tissue that more nearly approximates the appearance and function of the original tissue.

B. **Soft-tissue oxygen concentration.** Soft-tissue oxygen concentration is critically important in the healing process. Some hypoxia is a normal component of healing tissue, but ischemia imposes serious obstacles to repair. The astute clinician must distinguish between the two and prevent ischemia from occurring. Various tissue Po_2 monitoring devices are helpful in this regard.

C. **Healing of bone and cartilage.** Certain aspects of the normal healing mechanisms of bone and cartilage are of special interest to the plastic surgeon. Cortical (endochondral) bone provides superior mechanical strength for interpositional defects, whereas membranous bone used as onlay grafts for augmentation of craniofacial skeletal contour is superior to endochondral grafts in maintaining volume. Rigid fixation minimizes resorption of all types of bone grafts. In cartilage transplantation, viscoelastic properties, intrinsic forces, and immunologic privilege all affect healing. Cartilage deformed by external forces tends to return to its original shape unless the deformation is maintained for several months. Surgical carving alters the intrinsic tensile and expansive forces in cartilage and can cause both acute and delayed distortion in cartilage contour. Such distortion can be minimized by carving in balanced cross-section.

D. **Healing of nerves.** The normal healing of damaged nerves also involves different biologic mechanisms. Current concepts hold that a regenerating neural unit is guided distally by a combination of contact guidance and neurotropism. The growing axon sprout has affinity for laminin and type IV collagen. Nerve repair performed under tension will increase the degree of scar tissue at the suture line and decrease nerve function. Sensory reeducation significantly improves the functional results after all types of nerve repair and reconstruction.

E. **Cellular adhesion.** Another important aspect of all phases of normal healing in all types of tissue is mechanisms of cellular adhesion. The cells attach to surrounding extracellular protein matrix through structural receptors called *integrins*. The integrin-matrix bond can be inhibited by monoclonal antibodies directed against receptor subunits or by synthetic protein peptides. This inhibition of cell adhesion has important potential for cellular control of all phases of wound healing, malignant cell growth, and metastasis.

Abnormal Repair

A. **Unbalanced interactions between cellular and humoral components.** Normal healing is characterized by a delicate balance that exists between the complex interactions of the various cellular and humoral components described previously. If this balance is disrupted, healing abnormalities ensue. Of particular importance is the equilibrium among collagen synthesis, cross-linking, and degradation. In abnormal healing a disequilibrium exists; that is, most states of abnormal healing represent quantitative imbalances among collagen synthesis, cross-linking, and degradation, not production of qualitatively abnormal collagens.

B. **Oxygen-derived free radicals.** Abnormal repair may accompany production of oxygen-derived free radicals. These toxic metabolites cause tissue damage by lipid peroxidation of cellular and organelle membranes, disruption of intracellular matrix, and alteration of important protein enzymatic processes. Normal host defenses against oxygen-free radicals include oxygen radical scavengers, which are principally intracellular protective mechanisms. Oxygen-free radicals have been shown to perform important functions in inflammatory and ischemia-reperfusion disease states.

Fetal Healing

Much attention in recent years has been focused on mechanisms of fetal wound healing, which offers striking differences from adult healing. Primarily, closed fetal skin wounds heal rapidly and without scar formation; open fetal skin wounds do not contract. Amniotic fluid, rich in extracellular matrix components, such as hyaluronic acid and fibronectin, inhibit the wound contraction process. Fetal skin wounds are relatively hypoxic and neutropenic, are devoid of acute inflammation, and manifest minimal fibroblastic infiltration and proliferation. Fetal tissue repair may prove to be a process more closely resembling regeneration and growth rather than healing by fibrous scar formation. Later in gestation, fetal healing becomes more adultlike.

PRACTICAL POINTS AND CLINICAL APPLICATIONS

Certain aspects of healing in clinical practice deserve special attention. In some areas, basic principles have stood the test of time; in other areas, controversy has been resolved in the research laboratory.

Débridement and Irrigation

Meticulous removal of nonviable tissue is essential for uncomplicated healing, because wounds containing dead tissue usually become infected. Necrotic tissue is a good culture medium, and it places excessive phagocytic demands on wound leukocytes, thereby impairing their bactericidal capacity. In most wounds, there is no substitute for mechanical débridement with a scalpel and irrigation with physiologic saline. In situations in which such débridement is difficult or contraindicated, commercially available enzyme preparations are useful. Such preparations generally require a moist environment for enzyme activation and function and are ineffective if simply applied to a desiccated wound.

Antibacterial solutions containing iodine, alcohol, and certain other agents are toxic to delicate cells and rarely should be used for wound irrigation. Hydrogen peroxide also will lyse replicating cells, but when diluted with saline, it is an excellent and safe physical foaming agent for thoroughly removing clot remnants after hematoma evacuation.

Tissue Injury and Blood Supply

The manner and speed of handling tissues during surgery are more important than minor degrees of bacterial contamination. Ischemic wounds heal poorly and frequently become infected, whereas well-vascularized tissues heal well and rarely become infected even when contaminated. It has become axiomatic therefore that the rate and quality of repair is directly proportional to the blood supply.

Wound Closure

A. **Choice of suture material.** Although use of various tapes, tissue adhesives, staples, and clips has been advocated for primary wound closure, skilled use of suture material probably will endure as the method of choice for precise wound approximation. The primary indication for tape skin closure is to maintain wound approximation after percutaneous sutures or staples have been removed. The least reactive material for skin closure is stainless steel, followed closely by synthetic monofilaments, such as nylon and polypropylene. Because the latter offer an ease of handling not afforded by stainless steel, synthetic monofilaments have become the mainstay of skin closure for the plastic surgeon. A notable exception to this rule is the use of fine plain catgut for tension-free skin closure in children. Such sutures fall out after a few days before tissue irritation has become established. Tissue trauma associated with suture removal in young patients is thereby eliminated.

Another consideration in the choice of suture material is strength. Metallic sutures are strongest, and natural sutures, such as silk, are weakest. The strength of the synthetic materials is in between the metallic and the natural sutures. The synthetic materials are usually selected for plastic skin repair, because suture strength is relatively less important in wounds that have been properly closed in layers, resulting in no tension on skin edges. Plastic skin closure rarely demands sutures stronger than 5-0 on the face and hand and 4-0 on the trunk and extremity. It is illogical to use sutures stronger than the tissue they are holding.

B. **Interrupted versus continuous sutures.** Perhaps the most controversial aspect of skin closure involves the use of interrupted versus continuous suture lines. Continuous sutures have the advantages of speed and even distribution of tension. The old adage that interrupted sutures are superior, because if infections develop, a few sutures can be removed, has resulted in untold numbers of inadequately treated wound infections. In most infections, the most efficient drainage of pus, rapid resolution of inflammation, and optimal aesthetic result are obtained by removal of all skin sutures and delayed skin closure. Furthermore, if a properly placed continuous suture breaks, the entire suture does not unravel and result in wound dehiscence. Most linear closures lend themselves to continuous-suture technique; conversely, stellate and multidirectional wounds are best managed by interrupted-suture technique. In general, the closure technique employed for a given wound should provide rapid, precise approximation of edges with the least tissue trauma. The importance of meticulous hemostasis, atraumatic handling of tissues, and avoidance of dead space cannot be overemphasized as prerequisites for uncomplicated healing.

Suture Removal

When layered closure has been performed and skin edges have been apposed without tension, skin suture removal should be performed early to minimize suture marks, cysts, and microabscesses. *Early* means 3 to 5 days on the face, slightly longer on the trunk, and 7 to 10 days on the extremities. In healthy patients, it is unnecessary to leave sutures in place more than 10 days. In wounds closed under tension (e.g., in a facelift), the risk of both dehiscence and suture marks can be minimized by cutting sutures early and leaving them in place for a few more days. Tape may be used in a variety of ways to reduce tension on wound edges after suture removal.

Regaining Tensile Strength

During the maturation stage of healing, wounds regain tensile strength slowly over many months as collagen fibers are degraded, recross-linked, and realigned along lines of stress. Injured skin, tendon, and fascia never regain their normal, or uninjured, strength.

Resutured Wound

If a recently sutured wound is reopened and resutured, it will heal faster than the original wound; that is, the healing process does not return to the day of wound infliction. This effect is called the *secondary wound phenomenon,* and it is maximal in the second and third weeks after initial wounding. Because the cellular elements responsible for repair are concentrated within a few millimeters of the wound margins, the secondary wound effect is lost if a recent wound is excised, rather than reopened.

Epithelialization

A. **Dressings.** Epithelialization is the mechanism of healing in split-thickness skin graft donor sites, dermabrasions, and partial-thickness burns. Because the process is enhanced in a moist environment, saline or emollient dressings are beneficial. Dry dressings should also be avoided in partial-thickness wounds because regenerating epithelial cells are easily stripped away during dressing changes.
B. **Use of chemicals.** Many claims have been made regarding the superior healing effect of various chemicals impregnated in split-thickness skin graft donor site dressings, especially scarlet red. Studies have failed to show that any chemical can significantly increase the

rate of epithelialization. Topically applied vitamin A will reverse the inhibitory effect of steroids on epithelialization. Some evidence suggests that both topical and systemic use of vitamin A can accelerate normal epithelialization, but further clarification is necessary.

C. **Neoplasia.** The plastic surgeon also must remember that the process of epithelialization involves intense mitotic activity that resembles neoplasia histologically. Prolonged loss of epithelial integrity, such as in chronic ulcers and particularly in old burn wounds, must always evoke the question: Has this wound become neoplastic? Biopsies of such suspicious wounds are indicated.

Wound Contraction

A. **Difference in rates.** Wound contraction, the process whereby open wounds shrink, does not proceed at the same rate in all regions of the body. In unfavorable regions, such as scalp, anterior neck, anterior chest wall, and the extremities, contraction is slow and usually unsatisfactory for obtaining final wound closure. In favorable areas, such as back, posterior neck, abdomen, buttocks and perineum, contraction proceeds more rapidly and may be used to great advantage by the surgeon.

B. **Effect of steroids.** Steroids inhibit the process of contraction. Whereas the steroid-induced inhibition of epithelialization can be reversed by vitamin A, administration of that vitamin will not reverse the steroid-induced inhibition of contraction.

Hemodynamics

Much has been written about the deleterious effects of altered hemodynamic homeostasis on the healing process. Many variables such as hypovolemia, hypoxia, increased blood viscosity, low flow states, and anemia have been implicated in delayed healing. Wide variations in experimental models and design have contributed to clinical confusion. Healing is generally unaffected however if hematocrit levels are not less than 15 g/dl and normal blood volume is maintained.

Nutrition

Protein depletion inhibits all phases of healing, particularly fibroplasia and collagen synthesis. Deficiencies of specific vitamins and minerals however affect different aspects of the repair process.

A. **Vitamin A.** Vitamin A is a lysosomal labilizer (stimulates inflammation) and is important in maintenance of epithelial integrity. Vitamin A counteracts steroid inhibition of epithelialization and is effective topically.

B. **Vitamin B.** Elements of the vitamin B complex serve as cofactors in important enzyme systems, and deficiencies inhibit antibody formation and the bactericidal function of leukocytes.

C. **Vitamin C.** Vitamin C is a necessary cofactor in the synthesis of collagen (hydroxylation of proline). Vitamin C deficiency (scurvy) modifies the inflammatory reaction, inhibits collagen synthesis, and interferes with leukocyte function.

D. **Vitamin D.** Vitamin D is essential for calcium homeostasis.

E. **Vitamin E.** Vitamin E is a lysosomal stabilizer (inhibits inflammation) and enhances the absorption, storage and use of vitamin A. The steroidlike antiinflammatory action of topical vitamin E is probably responsible for its reportedly beneficial effect on reactive scars, but definitive data are not available. Use of parenteral vitamin E for the treatment of cystic mastopathies has stimulated a renewed research effort into the basic mechanisms of action and expanded the clinical applications of this important vitamin.

F. **Vitamin K.** Vitamin K is required for synthesis of clotting factors VII, IX, and X. The routine administration of vitamin K to healthy patients before elective surgery to minimize bleeding has no scientific basis.

G. **Minerals.** Minerals such as calcium, magnesium, copper, manganese, iron, and zinc function as enzyme cofactors. Although specific deficiencies must be corrected to ensure normal wound repair, there is no evidence that above-normal levels of any mineral result in accelerated healing. Iron, like vitamin C, is essential for the hydroxylation of proline, and copper is necessary for normal cross-linking of collagen. Plasma zinc levels less than 100 mg/dl result in delayed healing, altered intracellular bactericidal activity, and decreased host resistance. Healing of recalcitrant leg ulcers in an Unna boot plaster may be related to topical zinc applied to the wound through zinc oxide in the plaster. Fatty acid deficiency also results in diminished host resistance.

Impaired Healing

A. **Causes.** Impaired healing may be associated with certain diseases, such as diabetes, in addition to drugs, radiation, hypothermia, and hypovolemia.

- Disease states. Poor healing has been implicated in a wide variety of disease states, but *malnutrition* is probably the most important common denominator or contributing factor. For example, decreased neovascularization in jaundiced tissues and decreased collagen deposition in uremic patients are probably of secondary importance to the deleterious effects of the malnutrition accompanying these conditions. The malnutrition of cancer and chronic systemic infection is usually the principal factor when delayed healing complicates patient management.
- Acute infection. This however is specifically from gram-negative organisms, is associated with significant depletion of many components of the complement cascade and decreased chemotaxis. Virulent infections of greater than 10^5 levels of bacteria result in depressed capillary migration, decreased phagocytosis and intracellular killing, increased angiogenesis and granulation tissue formation, decreased epithelialization, increased collagen metabolism, increased glycosaminoglycans (GAG) deposition, and decreased wound contraction.
- Healing in diabetic patients. The well-known healing difficulties in diabetics reflect a variety of etiologic factors in the following complex pathophysiologic process:

- Regional ischemia caused by large vessel occlusive disease
- Local ischemia caused by increased blood viscosity secondary to increased red cell rigidity, aggregation and stagnation
- Soft tissue hypoxia resulting from increased affinity of glycosylated hemoglobin for oxygen
- Progressive and poorly understood diabetic neuropathy
- Impaired phagocytosis secondary to altered opsonic capacity
- Abnormal polymorphonuclear leukocytes, macrophages, and lymphocytes

▼ Current evidence has exploded the myth of diabetic microangiopathy and confirms that there is no condition as arteriolar occlusive disease or "small vessel disease" in the diabetic patient. Indeed, greater understanding of the wound-healing aberrations in diabetes mellitus has provided a more optimistic approach to wound closure in these patients. Amputations can frequently be avoided by combining the skills of the vascular surgeon in distal revascularization procedures and the plastic surgeon in aggressive flap closure of indolent ulcers.

▼ Drugs. Healing may be impaired by certain drugs.

- *Steroids* are lysosomal stabilizers (inhibit inflammation) and can retard epithelialization and contraction at any time. Steroids inhibit normal fibroplasia, collagen synthesis, and neovascularization. These observations are clinically significant and can result in major healing problems, such as dehiscence, if steroids are administered perioperatively in high doses. Low-dose regimens usually do not affect healing clinically.
- *Drugs used for cancer chemotherapy,* especially alkylating agents, such as nitrogen mustard, retard inflammation and adversely affect tissue repair.

- *Lathyrogens* represent a special group of compounds that interfere with the cross-linking of collagen. (β-Aminopropionitrile) prevents the first step in the cross-linking process by inhibiting the enzyme lysyl oxidase. Penicillamine prevents the second step of cross-linking by interfering with the spontaneous aldol condensation reaction. Both agents have been applied successfully to specific clinical problems, demonstrating thereby the potential for pharmacologic control of connective tissue metabolism and the repair process.
- *Colchicine,* developed and used primarily for the treatment of gout, is being reinvestigated as a connective tissue modifier. Colchicine slows cellular collagen transport, suppresses epithelialization, retards contraction, and yet has no effect on collagen deposition.

▼ Radiation. Radiation inhibits all aspects of healing and has a maximal effect if administered 36 hours after wounding. The principal mechanisms of radiation injury are the destruction of replicating and differentiating stem cells and the initiation of a progressive obliterative endarteritis. Such pathophysiologic disorders in radionecrotic ulcers result in an ill-defined zone of injury and demand wide excision with introduction of tissue with permanent blood supply for successful treatment.

▼ Hypovolemia. The untoward effects of hypovolemia have been discussed previously, however the importance of maintaining normal blood volume cannot be overemphasized. Hypothermia impairs healing but is of relatively little clinical importance.

▼ Smoking. Plastic surgeons have developed a large body of clinical experience indicating that smoking impairs healing. Deleterious effects are particularly striking in flap procedures wherein extensive areas of tissue necrosis may ensue after otherwise routine, safe, reconstructive, or aesthetic surgery. Although the precise mechanisms for these effects are not yet understood, both nicotine and carbon monoxide are strongly implicated. The untoward effects of smoking may be minimized by cessation of smoking at least 2 to 3 weeks before surgery and 1 to 2 weeks after surgery. Laboratory evidence is accumulating to corroborate these empiric recommendations. Many of the commercially available products, such as chewing gum to assist a patient to stop smoking, contain nicotine or similar substances that impair healing as significantly as the tobacco products themselves.

B. Methods of Promoting Healing

- Growth factors. A rapidly evolving area of applied research involves growth factor technology. A new process has been developed to extract growth factors from platelets, isolate them from the patient's blood, resuspend them in a buffer solution, and apply them topically to open wounds. The growth factors interact directly with cell receptors in the wounds, stimulating active growth of granulation tissue, capillaries, and epithelium. Initial results with this new technology suggest that type-specific growth factors may become available for different types of wounds. For example, epidermal cell-derived factors (EDF) might be utilized in wounds with a preponderance of proliferating granulation tissue, whereas a fibroblast-stimulating factor (TGF-β or PDGF) would be selected for an indolent ulcer deficient in connective tissue. Although the impact of such new technology is encouraging, it is important to recognize that growth factors only enhance cell growth. They do not correct low perfusion, edema, soft-tissue infection, osteomyelitis, or pressure abnormalities. In chronic wounds with multiple causes, each abnormal component must be analyzed and corrected to obtain a healed wound.
- Hyperbaric oxygen therapy. The use of hyperbaric oxygen therapy is increasingly perceived as a useful therapeutic adjunct in oxygen-deficient wounds, such as lower extremity ulcers, extensive burns, and ischemic skin flaps. Hyperbaric oxygen is also a strong stimulus for angiogenesis. Elevation of arterial

Po_2, however, cannot improve an ischemic wound environment if perfusion is inadequate. Although indications for hyperbaric oxygen therapy continue to be predominantly empiric and are based on clinical observations, laboratory data are accumulating to corroborate its efficacy in the appropriately selected patient.

- Methods for immunosuppressed patients. The immunosuppressed patient poses special challenges. The function of cytokines and lymphokines in normal repair has particular clinical implications in the management of these patients. The availability of biologic skin substitutes has expanded the armamentarium of the plastic surgeon in the management of extensive burn wounds. Epidermis can be replaced with tissue-cultured autogenous sheets of keratinocytes. Evidence indicates that the new epidermis directs the differentiation of the subjacent collagenous tissue into an architecture resembling a capillary and reticular dermis. Several methods are being evaluated for the direct replacement of the dermis, including use of cadavers, collagen-GAG matrices, and fibroblast-impregnated collagen gels.

Accelerated Healing

The secondary healing, or resutured wound, phenomenon has been discussed previously. The rate of healing in such wounds is actually normal, not accelerated. Many drugs and other biologic preparations, such as cartilage powder, have been reported to accelerate the rate of normal healing. To date however no such "superhealing" agent has survived rigorous scientific scrutiny. It has been well documented both experimentally and clinically however that correction of chemical deficiencies, such as trace metals, will restore delayed healing to normal.

PROBLEM SCARS

A *hypertrophic scar* is an exuberant scar that remains within the limits of the original wound. A *keloid* is an exuberant scar that exceeds the boundaries of the original wound. Controversy continues regarding histologic distinction between the two types of scars and is of more interest to the dermatopathologist than the plastic surgeon. The plastic surgeon however should conceptualize such scarring as components of the same spectrum of fibrous connective tissue metabolism. Biochemically, exuberant scars represent a disequilibrium in a local hypermetabolic state. Both collagen synthesis and degradation are increased, but synthesis exceeds degradation. The activity of certain inhibitors of collagen degradation is also increased in keloidal tissues. It should be emphasized that it is the rate of collagen turnover (metabolism), not the collagen itself, that is abnormal.

Etiology

The biology of fine-line scar formation and the pathophysiologic causes of problem scar development remain mysteries. Hypertrophic scars and keloids are more commonly observed in dark-skinned men and women and in children of all colors. They are found in regions of skin tension (deltoid, presternal, upper back, knee), in wounds with retained foreign bodies (earlobes), in wounds complicated by inflammation and infection, and in families with a history of bulky scars in several family members.

Treatment

Several modalities are used currently to treat hypertrophic scars and keloids: surgery, pressure, steroids, and radiation.

A. **Surgery.** Surgery may be useful in reducing the size of certain scars and thereby rendering them more amenable to other treatment modalities. The primary function of surgery, however, is alteration of scar polarity.

B. **Prolonged pressure.** Prolonged pressure greater than 22 mm Hg (capillary hydrostatic pressure) will flatten and soften exuberant scars. The various custom-made Jobst garments maintain such pressure effectively, but maximal benefit can be obtained only if the patient is fitted early and wears the garment almost constantly for many months. The patient should always have a spare garment to allow for regular laundering. Replacements must be ordered promptly when the compression delivered by the garment diminishes with time because of stretching or reduction in scar volume. The application of soft Silastic sheeting on recalcitrant hypertrophic scars beneath the garment enhances the maturation process. Delicate areas of unstable epithelium must be monitored closely and compression temporarily discontinued if breakdown occurs. Indirect evidence suggests that pressure alters collagen metabolism by decreasing synthesis, increasing degradation, and stimulating remodeling along lines of stress. Traction prevents, and in many cases reverses, joint contractures by a similar process.

C. **Steroid injection.** Direct injection of steroids, such as triamcinolone, will result in atrophy, depigmentation, and telangiectasia of both scar and normal tissues. Steroid injection therefore must be accurately localized within the offending scar tissue. Intralesional triamcinolone injections are helpful in relatively small hypertrophic scars and keloids. When such scars have become bulky or pedunculated, multiple triamcinolone injections will result in softening and relief of itching but will be inconsistent in size reduction. The recommended safe maximal dose of triamcinolone is 40 mg for infants and children aged 1 to 5 years and 80 mg for children aged 6 to 10 years. Up to 120 mg may be administered to an adult every month for large (10 cm^2) scars, although much smaller doses suffice for most lesions. A good rule of thumb is to continue injections at increasing intervals (weekly, biweekly, monthly) for several months until the desired response has been obtained. Slow, controlled injections until the lesion blanches rather than dilution of triamcinolone with lidocaine minimizes patient discomfort. Steroids are maximally effective when administered in the early phase of healing (e.g., when sutures are removed from an excised keloid) and should be used in conjunction with compression whenever possible. Although steroids inhibit inflammation and fibroplasia, evidence also suggests that steroids reduce local collagenase inhibitors (i.e., increase collagenolysis).

D. **Radiation.** Radiation kills replicating stem cells and produces an obliterative endarteritis. Superficial, low-dose (approximately 1000 rad) radiation may be safely administered by an experienced radiotherapist to bulky, recalcitrant keloids, but possible complications outweigh potential therapeutic gains in most patients. Radiotherapy for all benign conditions is contraindicated in children.

E. **Combinations of surgery, pressure, and steroids.** Combinations of pressure-triamcinolone or surgery-pressure-triamcinolone currently offer the best chance for success in the treatment of hypertrophic scars and keloids. Individualization of treatment plans and regular monitoring of the response to treatment, not rigid protocols, will achieve optimal results. Pharmacologic agents that interfere with various steps in the metabolism of collagen also hold promise for expanded clinical applications in the near future. Compounds, such as colchicine (stimulates collagenolysis and inhibits collagen secretion) and β-aminopropionitrile (inhibits cross-linking) have been thoroughly studied experimentally, but deleterious side effects have precluded their use clinically.

SCAR REVISION

In analyzing any scar for possible surgical revision,the plastic surgeon must first obtain a "scar history" and gain insight into patient motivation:

- How, when, and where did the wound occur?
- Was initial wound care optimal?
- Was a meticulous closure performed?
- Did the wound heal by first or by second intention?
- Did crushing contusion, infection, or retained foreign body complicate healing?
- Has the scar become painful or pruritic?
- Has the patient previously formed problem scars?
- What is the patient's attitude about the functional deformity?
- Is there a secondary gain aspect?

- Is litigation pending?
- Are patient desires reasonable?
- Are patient education and acceptance possible?

If the answers to such questions translate into a satisfactory profile for potential success, the surgeon may proceed to technical considerations.

Techniques

The objective of surgical revision is to camouflage the scar. Such camouflage may be accomplished by (1) altering scar polarity or direction to coincide more closely with relaxed skin tension lines (RSTL), (2) dividing a complex scar into smaller components, (3) leveling contour deformities, and (4) lengthening tight scars. The concept of reorienting as much of a problem scar as possible to conform to RSTL is essential for obtaining optimal results. Facial RSTL are illustrated in Fig. 13-1.

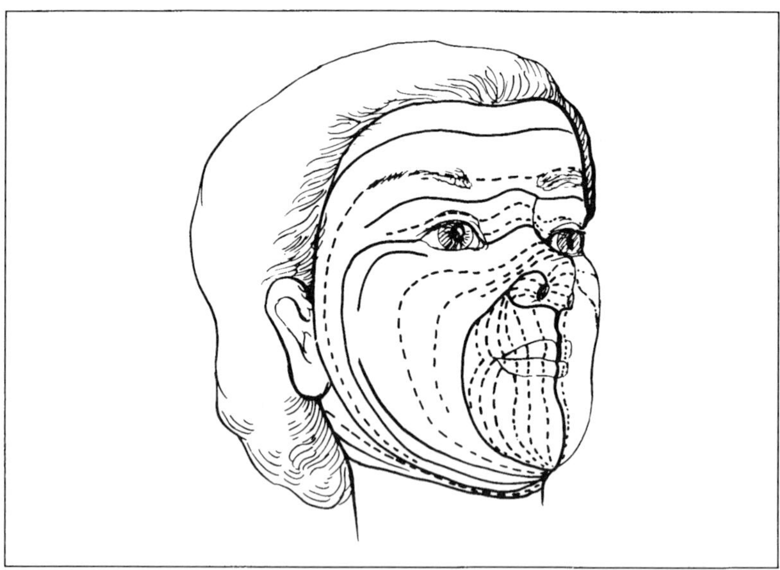

FIG. 13-1 *Facial relaxed skin tension lines (RSTL).*

If the scar history reveals suboptimal conditions, associated with original wound closure, a simple linear or fusiform revision is indicated, particularly if the scar is oriented favorably along RSTL. If a problem scar has resulted despite acceptable initial wound management, closure, and healing, or if the scar is unfavorably oriented along RSTL, then alteration of scar polarity is indicated. Scar polarity is most commonly altered by Z-plasty.

A. **Z-plasty.** With the Z-plasty, length is gained at the expense of width.

- ▼ Indications. The Z-plasty is useful for the following:
  - ■ Anti-RSTL scars on the eyelids, nose, lips, nasolabial folds, and nonfacial regions
  - ■ Scars on the forehead, temples, cheeks, and chin if the anti-RSTL angle is less than 35°
  - ■ Depressed anti-RSTL scars in any region
  - ■ Short anti-RSTL scars
  - ■ Regions with multiple, complex scars
- ▼ Procedural guidelines. A properly performed Z-plasty should conform to the following guidelines:
  - ■ The diagonal should lie on the scar
  - ■ The diagonal and two limbs should be equilinear
  - ■ The limbs should be as close to the RSTL as possible but no more than 60° from the diagonal. On the face, limbs of 1 to 1.5 cm are appropriate. In multiple Z-plasties, limbs should not be less than 1 cm, because of the tendency of small flaps to heap up or "trap-door"

B. **W-plasty**

- ▼ Indications. The W-plasty requires tissue excision and is indicated for long scars on the forehead, temples, cheeks and chin if the anti-RSTL angle is more than 35°. The stair-step W-plasty is useful for scars inclined 60 to 35° from the RSTL. Because a W-plasty requires excision of tissue, this technique cannot be used if significant tissue was lost at the time of original injury or if other factors have resulted in tension along the scar margins.

- ▼ Procedural guidelines. A properly performed W-plasty incorporates the following guidelines:
  - The base of the last triangle at each end should be at right angles to the scar.
  - The tip or corresponding angles should also be in a line at right angles to the scar.
  - The angle should be approximately 55 to 60°.
  - The length of the segments varies from 5 to 7 mm depending on the size and location of the scar.
  - The final few segments at both ends should be progressively less than 6 mm to prevent formation of dog ears or long anti-RSTL terminal components.

C. **V-Y plasty.** The V-Y plasty has limited application in lengthening certain scars and in altering polarity, but this technique ranks far below Z-plasty and W-plasty for overall utility.

D. **Dermabrasion and dermaplaning.** Dermabrasion and dermaplaning are effective methods for leveling the elevated components of contour deformities. These methods are most commonly applied to acne scarring, but they may be equally effective if contour deformities persist in a scar after maximal benefit has been obtained from realignment procedures. The most common complications associated with these techniques are temporary milia formation, eczematization, and hyperpigmentation.

E. **Skin grafts or flaps.** If significant tissue loss occurred at the time of original injury, skin grafts or flaps are usually necessary in ameliorating dysfunction and disfigurement. When using such methods, the surgeon must attempt to restore complete aesthetic units (Fig. 13-2). Violating aesthetic units and resurfacing isolated defects comprising subtotal units produce a poorly camouflaged result with a patchwork appearance. Because such an

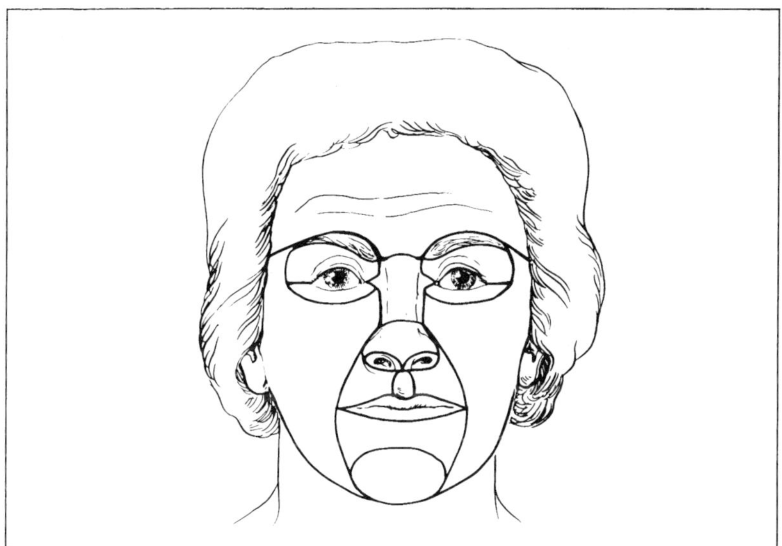

FIG. 13-2 *Facial aesthetic units.*

approach may demand sacrifice of varying amounts of normal tissue, aesthetic-unit resurfacing should not be undertaken by the inexperienced surgeon. Precious full-thickness donor sites, such as the postauricular region, must not be squandered before definitive revision-reconstruction is performed. When split-thickness skin grafts are required for coverage of keloid excision sites, the keloid tendency is minimized at the donor site by limiting the thickness of the graft to 0.001 inches.

F. **Methods used for trap-door scars.** U-shaped, heaped-up, or trap-door scar deformities are produced by incompletely understood biophysical phenomena. Significant improvement is usually obtained by fusiform revision of smaller scars and multiple Z-plasties or W-plasties for larger scars. Thinning or debulking seldom improves such scars and may even compound an already difficult problem. Abnormal pigmentation in mature scars may be managed successfully with the assistance of professional makeup consultation. Newer modalities, such as laser beam therapy, are currently being tested in clinical trials (See Chapter 39.).

Timing of Scar Revision

Regardless of the method employed for scar revision, surgical intervention should not be considered for at least 6 months after injury unless critical structure function is threatened by scar contracture. Softening and fading of reactive color herald advanced scar maturation and indicate that revision may be undertaken.

Principles that Maximize Changes for Successful Revision

- Judicious undermining
- Respect for tissues
- Meticulous technique
- Elimination of dead space
- Use of clear suture material near skin surfaces
- Subcuticular closure wherever possible

Postoperative Care

Postoperative care should incorporate the following:

- Hydrogen peroxide cleansing of suture lines
- Application of a lubricating ointment
- Early removal of sutures and splinting when appropriate
- Early pressure applied to scars in sites with a predilection for hypertrophy
- Normal bathing (i.e., "getting the stitches wet") is permitted 2 to 3 days after surgery, but suture lines must not be allowed to macerate.
- Cosmetics may be applied when all crusting of serum has ceased, usually after 7 to 10 days.
- Many regimens have been proposed for the care of split-thickness skin graft donor sites and freshly dermabraded skin. Silvadene cream seems to promote rapid healing and minimize patient discomfort and inconvenience.

CHAPTER 14

Eyelid Surgery

Thomas D. Rees and Daniel C. Baker

PREOPERATIVE EVALUATION

Ophthalmologic History

A thorough ophthalmologic history followed by an ophthalmologic examination will expose any preexisting eye problems. The ophthalmologic history should include specific questions about major ocular diseases such as glaucoma, detached retinae, cataracts, corneal abrasions, epiphora, and dry-eye syndrome. This review should also probe for a health history of thyroid disease, allergies, diabetes, and cardiovascular disease because these conditions in particular may affect the eyes and adnexa.

Physical Examination

Examination of the eye should include a visual acuity test and an examination of the adnexal structures, the bony orbit, and the extraocular muscles. An ophthalmoscopic examination for lenticular opacities or obvious retinal pathology should also be performed.

A. **Visual acuity.** A miniature, portable *Snellen's chart* is convenient for testing visual acuity, and each eye should be tested separately. A patient may be unaware of amblyopia, poor vision, or blindness in one eye before surgery, and if these defects become apparent postoperatively, the plastic surgeon could incorrectly be held responsible.

B. **Direct examination of eye and related structures.** Examination of the extraocular muscles is important in determining the existence of paresis or paralysis, which could lead to troublesome or even serious postoperative consequences. Paralysis of the superior rectus (e.g., with an absent Bell's phenomenon) could promote desiccation and lead to ulceration of the cornea because temporary lagophthalmos after blepharoplasty is not uncommon. Although spasm of the Müller's muscle is normal in some individuals, it can signal early thyrotoxicosis or expanding intraorbital lesions long before other symptoms occur.

A sign of levator spasm is a staring look caused by a scleral "show" above the limbus of the cornea. Spasm may or may not be associated with exophthalmos. Such eye signs can precede the symptomatology of hyperthyroidism and even the changes in protein-bound iodine fractions by many months. A slight bulging of the globes, known as *normal exophthalmos* or *proptosis,* occurs in some persons without thyroid disease or ocular pathology. This can be a genetically inherited family trait. Asymmetry is also common. Unilateral exophthalmos may suggest occult orbital lesions. Investigations of the orbit by tomography may be indicated if suspicion of a space-filling lesion or bony deformity exists.

Thyroid disease can produce localized signs in the eye and orbital regions in addition to exophthalmos, including excessive edema, which can occur in both the hypothyroid and hyperthyroid states.

It has been found that a computerized axial tomography scan (CAT) of the orbits is diagnostic for thyroid ophthalmopathy. The extraocular muscles, especially the medial recti, appear enlarged and swollen from the presence of edema and inflammatory infiltration. When thyroid ophthalmopathy is suspected but cannot be confirmed by other techniques, a CAT scan is indicated to confirm the diagnosis.

Edema and Allergy

Intermittent eyelid edema in women is often related to cyclic hormonal influence. Many women are prone to collection of periorbital edema during the immediate premenstrual days of their menstrual cycle. Fluid retention is common with interruptions of the normal hormonal balances at menopause. Periorbital edema related to hormonal influence often can be identified by a health history. The patient should be informed that swelling of the eyelids will continue even after a successful blepharoplasty with the removal of redundant fat and skin.

Allergy may manifest not only as allergic dermatitis of the eyelid skin but also as recurrent episodes of intensive periorbital edema. An unusual but typical localized edema can occur over the malar eminences, just below the bony infraorbital rims without involving the eyelid skin itself. This small, saclike area of edema is usually intermittent and eventually may result in subcutaneous fibrosis. It is typical and, once recognized, never forgotten. Because this type of edema is unlikely to be ablated by blepharoplasty, it may be a source of misunderstanding between the patient and plastic surgeon unless it is identified preoperatively. The patient should be advised of this condition. It is helpful to positively point out to the patient this localized area of edema formation on the preoperative photographs.

Dry-Eye Syndrome

Minor or subclinical forms of dry-eye syndrome are more prevalent than is commonly believed. When fully developed, the syndrome is called *keratoconjunctivitis sicca* or *Sjögren's syndrome,* which can result in blindness from corneal opacities. Diminution in tear production occurs normally as an individual ages. It also may be hereditary or occur as a consequence of certain systemic diseases such as thyrotoxicosis. A history of recurrent bouts of irritation of the eyes, with burning and itching often combined with a slight protrusion of the globe (exophthalmos), is suggestive. *Schirmer's test* is then advisable preoperatively to determine the amount of tear production. A small strip of absorbent paper is inserted into the inferior fornix. Tear production is measured in millimeters over a given time. Schirmer's test is unnecessary in every potential blepharoplasty patient, but it can suggest the diagnosis of dry-eye syndrome when positive.

The dry-eye syndrome can be complicated and exacerbated by eyelid surgery because of normal wound contracture with the slight lagophthalmos and ectropion that frequently occur during the healing period. A patient with slight exophthalmos, a dropped lower eyelid, and a scleral show before surgery is particularly prone to these mechanical forces of wound healing that can aggravate the symptoms. A patient with such contours should be questioned carefully about irritative eye symptomatology.

Cosmetic blepharoplasty is not necessarily precluded because of diminished tear production, but extreme caution should be exercised in the surgical approach. It is crucial to remember that skin and fat excision must be conservative. If the surgeon and patient elect to proceed with the surgery, a two-stage procedure is advisable: (1) operating on the upper eyelids first and (2) operating on the lower eyelids 1 week later. Levator fixation of the upper eyelids in such a patient is probably unwise. Some surgeons have advocated a partial resection of a prominent lacrimal gland if such is present at the time of blepharoplasty. Because diminution in tear production occurs normally with advanced age, the aesthetic improvement gained by this procedure does not seem to warrant the possible medicolegal consequences of postoperative dry-eye syndrome.

PREOPERATIVE DISCUSSION OF POSSIBLE COMPLICATIONS

As in other surgical procedures, it is incumbent on the plastic surgeon to inform the patient preoperatively of the likelihood of complications. Just how detailed such disclosure needs to be varies with each patient. Legal precedents exist, but they are controversial. Certainly a discussion of the more common problems such as edema, hematoma, eyelid lag, and pull-down (scleral show) is recommended. Rare complications such as extraocular muscle paresis or even blindness should be mentioned.

Complications following eyelid surgery occur most often during the immediate postoperative period. They may be mild or severe, temporary or persistent, and may or may not require definitive surgical correction. Because most of these complications are the result of surgical trauma or the aggravation of a preexisting condition, it is of utmost importance to reduce operative trauma to a minimum to obtain an accurate preoperative health history, and to perform a thorough physical examination.

INTRAOPERATIVE CARE

Anesthetic Technique

Anesthetic techniques vary according to the personal preferences of each anesthesiologist during the surgery.

A. **Local anesthesia.** Whether using general or local anesthetics, eyelid surgery is facilitated by the injection of a local anesthetic such as 0.5% procaine (Novocain) or lidocaine (Xylocaine) containing epinephrine 1:200,000 to help delineate tissue planes and promote hemostasis.
B. **Supplemental intravenous drugs.** Because adequate removal of intraorbital fat requires considerable traction on deep sutures, which causes pain that is difficult to block with local anesthetic alone, supplemental intravenous (IV) narcotics and tranquilizers are usually required (See Chapter 5.).
C. **Monitoring.** Pulse monitoring and preferably cardiac monitoring of the blood oxygen saturation is mandatory and provides the most accurate measure of the general status of the patient during the administration of anesthesia, whether local, monitored IV, or general.

Operative Technique

The design of incisions to correct palpebral defects must take into account all the different and distinct morphologic factors that constitute the deformity. The natural beauty and shape of the eye, which are important to individual expression, are camouflaged by the *total* defect. The most important factors to consider include the following:

- Degree of ptosis of the brow
- Amount and degree of wrinkling of the excess skin of upper and lower eyelids
- Amount and location of protruding orbital fat in both eyelids, with particular attention paid to the medial fat of the upper eyelid and the lateral fat of the lower eyelid

- Amount and configuration of redundant orbicularis muscle in both upper and lower eyelids
- Associated factors such as pigmentation and senile degenerative changes in the skin, the conformation of the bony orbit, the degree of ptosis of the lacrimal gland, and the presence of irritative signs of the conjunctiva

Each person has various combinations of these defects in varying degrees of severity. To vary the operative approach appropriately, it is important to analyze this combination and to define the role of each factor.

Incisions

A. **Evaluation for brow ptosis in planning incisions.** Before planning the upper eyelid incisions, it is important to determine if much or all of the problem associated with the upper eyelids is the result of ptosis of the brows. In a patient with significant brow ptosis, a forehead or brow lift, with or without upper eyelid blepharoplasty, may be required. Brow elevation is a relatively simple procedure requiring a coronal incision in the scalp behind the hairline. If brow elevation is necessary, it should *always* be done before upper eyelid blepharoplasty because elevation of the brows may negate the necessity of removal of a redundant cuff of skin and muscle from the upper eyelids. An important part of the preoperative examination is to carefully examine the degree of brow ptosis and the relationship of the brows to the upper eyelids. Surgical elevation of the brows is commonly performed today in conjunction with blepharoplasty.

B. **Trimming of skin in lower eyelid surgery.** With surgery of the lower eyelid, accurate determination of the exact amount of skin to be trimmed is imperative to avoid an ectopion resulting from an overambitious resection.

   - Patients under local anesthesia. If the operation is being performed with the patient under local anesthesia and the patient can cooperate, two maneuvers can help the surgeon avoid the removal of too much skin. The patient is asked to rotate the eyes upward to elevate the eyelid margin to a "safe" position. The undermined skin can then be draped over the wound edge, and the excess can be removed. Safety is further facilitated by having the patient widely open the mouth to duplicate the forces of an extrinsic ectropion, which is often seen in face burns.

- Patients under general anesthesia. If the patient is under general anesthesia or is unable to cooperate, gentle downward pressure applied to the globe results in an upward elevation of the lower eyelid allowing the skin to be safely draped over it and excised while the eyelid is in an elevated position.

A patient with considerable excess skin or muscles of the lower eyelids may sometimes have folds extending to the cheeks. This requires wide undermining, which may extend to the infraorbital margin itself. True cheek pads cannot be corrected by blepharoplasty.

The efficacy and safety of the skin-muscle flap as compared with wide skin undermining is not entirely established. Many surgeons use the skin-muscle flap in all cases; other surgeons prefer skin undermining in all but younger patients with tight skin. Both groups of surgeons claim equally good results.

Sutures

A. **Placement.** The surgeon's placement of the suture line of the standard upper eyelid excision is critical. The lowermost line of the ellipse, which becomes the final suture line, should lie between 7 and 12 mm above the ciliary margin in the midpupillary plane, depending on the morphology of the individual patient. The final scar should fall naturally into the supratarsal fold.

The lateral extension should lie in a crow's foot. Because the final suture line tends to rise upward, it should be drawn at a level lower than its intended destination.

B. **Type of sutures.** The upper eyelid wound is best sutured with a subcuticular suture of fine nylon, which can be left in place 4 or 5 days. This type of suture is most helpful in preventing troublesome epithelial funnels or inclusion cysts, which easily form around interrupted sutures after 48 hours.

When a subcuticular suture is used, it is important either to cut the medial end where it emerges from the skin so that the cut end can retract beneath the skin or to remove this suture by the fourth postoperative day. Otherwise, for unknown reasons, a pustule forms at the site of the skin entrance, resulting in an unsightly nodule of scar tissue requiring many months to absorb. The suture line in the upper lid can be further reinforced by several fine interrupted sutures, which are removed at 24 hours or 48 hours at the latest.

Prevention of Corneal Injury

It is better to prevent injury to the cornea rather than treat it after it occurs. The following techniques should help prevent corneal injury:

- Abrasive gauze sponges should be replaced with atraumatic absorbable synthetic sponges.
- A protective corneal shield can cause an abrasion if inserted improperly.
- It is important to prevent desiccation of the cornea during surgery because drying can result in abrasion that can, because of avascularity of the cornea, progress to ulceration. Frequent irrigation with sterile saline during the operation is therefore a good practice, particularly during suturing when the eyelids are likely to be open and the cornea is exposed.
- At the conclusion of the procedure, a bland lubricating ointment should be applied liberally to the incisions and the conjunctival sac to protect the cornea during the first few hours after surgery until muscular closure is reestablished.
- Thorough irrigation of the conjunctival sac at the end of the procedure helps remove foreign matter, such as

pieces of suture. Foreign material can cause corneal abrasion, an uncomfortable and painful condition.

POSTOPERATIVE CARE

Bandaging

Bandaging of the eyes after operation is not essential. Theoretically however a moderate pressure dressing for the first few hours after surgery is beneficial to help control oozing, edema, and hematoma. It provides added insurance against reactive bleeding during the immediate recovery phase. Every surgeon has experienced the development of a hematoma or active bleeding from the wound edges in a patient who has vomited or retched after general anesthesia (despite the excellence of the anesthetic technique) and sometimes even after local anesthesia.

A. **No use of bandages.** If bandages are not used, it is important to make sure that the cornea is well lubricated during recovery from anesthesia. For this purpose, liberal instillation of a bland ophthalmic ointment, such as Lacrilube (white petrolatum and mineral oil), is recommended. Application of iced sterile compresses as soon as possible, preferably beginning in the recovery room, is important for the same reasons as pressure bandages.

B. **Use of bandages.** If bandages are used, only moderate pressure is necessary. It is essential that the eyelids be in proper position under such dressings. This is especially true for the lower eyelids, which must be maintained in their normal position and not depressed in a caudal direction by the upper eyelid or by the bandage. Such depression of the lower eyelid can result in adherence of the skin flap to the wound in the orbital septum or to a lower than normal level on the muscle bed. Either occurrence can result in ectropion and eversion and must be treated by immediate reoperation and adjustment of the skin flap. Proper positioning of the skin flaps and eyelids can be provided by a temporary lid occlusal suture, which is placed through the gray line of the eyelid, and by the careful application of a wraparound dressing over two eye pads placed on each eye.

If dressings are applied, they are removed the following morning along with the eyelid occlusal sutures. Application of ice compresses is then begun and continued for the next 2 days.

Eye dressings may cause some patients to experience severe claustrophobia. When this is the case, sedatives or tranquilizers may be helpful in alleviating the patient's anxiety. The dressings are removed at once however if the patient's anxiety cannot be controlled by these medications.

Monitoring

Whether or not dressings are used, it is important to monitor the patient closely during the first few hours after blepharoplasty because retrobulbar bleeding resulting in a hematoma most commonly occurs during this period. Retrobulbar hematoma results in protrusion of the globe and carries the risk of temporary or permanent impairment of vision. Early recognition of this complication results in prompt treatment with diuretics and sometimes surgery. Pain and bulging of the globe along with discoloration are diagnostic and require the immediate attention of the surgeon or an ophthalmologic consultant.

Suture Removal

Most interrupted sutures, including the subcuticular suture, are removed by the fourth postoperative day. Sutures left longer than this often cause the formation of epithelial tunnels or sinuses. Wound agglutination can be ensured, even when sutures are removed at this early time, by the application of small sterile strips of paper adhesive across the tension lines of the incision. Paper adhesive has proved to be virtually nonreactive in most patients, and it is extremely effective in maintaining apposition of the wound edge during the period of maximal weakness.

Follow-up Care

- ▼ All crusts and scabs are gently cleansed away from the wound at the end of the first week.

- A bland eyewash such as Balanced Salt Solution (BSS) is sometimes beneficial if the patient complains of irritation, scratchiness, or marked itching.
- Some patients find the intermittent application of ice compresses to be soothing even several days after the operation, and they are encouraged to continue using them if they are helpful.
- Exercising of the orbicularis muscles by intermittent squeezing of the eyelids closed is helpful in reducing edema and regaining mobility after the first week.
- The use of oral or parenteral enzymes generally has *not* proved effective in the control of postoperative wound edema.
- Women may apply eye makeup on approximately the tenth postoperative day, but it is advisable to remove it thoroughly and carefully after each use. Oiled eye pads are recommended for this purpose.

CHAPTER 15

Face- and Neck-Lift

BERNARD M. BARRETT, JR.

INITIAL CONSULTATION

As emphasized in Chapter 1, it is essential that one critically select the correct patients for surgery. Adherence to the following guidelines for the initial consultation will help assure proper patient selection.

Patient Questionnaire

The surgeon should review the completed patient health history with the patient to obtain vital details about serious medical illness, allergies, medications, previous surgery, and other important information (See Chapter 2.). It is essential to determine the patient's general health, especially regarding heart disease, high blood pressure, or bleeding disorders. Because aspirin and other drugs can cause abnormal bleeding during surgery it should be stressed that these drugs must be avoided 7 to 10 days preoperatively.

Patient Interview

In the interview with the patient, a good place for the plastic surgeon to start is by asking a potential face-lift patient why he or she has come for a consultation. Answers such as "I would like to look better" or "I would like to have some of these extra tissues removed from my face and neck" are indications that the patient may be a suitable candidate for the procedure. But an answer such as "I do not like my face" or "I would be a happier person if I had a face-lift" should cause concern to the physician. The realistic face-lift patient will usually point to the excessive tissues of the face, neck, and eyes and state to the plastic surgeon that the reason for the office consultation is "to find out about having these extra tissues in my face and neck removed. . . with a desire to look better." Any patient who directly or indirectly suggests that a face-lift is sought because of the feeling that it will change the quality of life or solve living problems has an unrealistic view of what the procedure can do and is a poor candidate for plastic surgery. It should be emphasized more than once during the initial interview with the patient that a face-lift operation removes the extra tissues and usually restores a more youthful appearance, but it is not a special passport to success and happiness in life.

Informing Patients of Possible Complications

Following questioning of the patient about the motivation for wanting a face-lift, the patient should be informed of the possible complications of facial surgery, including but not limited to bleeding, infection, bad scar formation, neurologic weakness, numbness, blindness, and death. Death and blindness are extremely rare, but they have been reported and therefore should be mentioned because of the medicolegal responsibility to acquaint the patient with the worst possible results from surgery. While the incidence of complications varies and is usually in the range of several percent, incidence is increased in the patient who is too active after surgery, has uncontrolled high blood pressure, drinks alcohol excessively, or has preexisting infections.

Whether the surgeon should show the patient representative "before" and "after" photographs of other cases is a controversial point. Legal experts argue that showing a new patient photographs of a previous good result may imply a guarantee of a similar result. However, photographs, especially those of complications, can substantiate an informed operative consent. Chapter 10 covers these points more specifically.

Informing Patients of Operative Procedure

In addition to explaining the possible complications and their frequency of occurrence as well as discussing (or showing photographs of) successful surgery without complications, the plastic surgeon should also explain the following to the patient in some detail:

- Operative and anesthetic procedure
- Plan for dressing and suture removals
- Sequential stages in terms of general facial appearance

- Time required for hospitalization if the patient is to be admitted as an inpatient
- Type of anesthesia used: Patient is informed that face-lift surgery usually is performed using local anesthesia with sedation, monitoring, and usually with an anesthesiologist or nurse anesthetist nearby.

Further details, such as the specifics of the usual operative and anesthetic procedure, timing of dressing changes and suture removal, and the length of the average hospital stay are discussed by the surgeon and the office personnel. Costs and scheduling are usually discussed privately by the patient with the office patient coordinator. Some surgeons prefer however to discuss these matters with the patients themselves. In concluding the interview, the surgeon should ask, "What other questions do you have?" The surgeon should then answer such questions for the patient.

Health History and Physical Examination

If the patient has not fled in fear after learning about complications and other details, the health history and physical findings for the permanent office record are dictated in the patient's presence. The patient's height and weight are recorded. When the weight is greater than ideal, which is often the case, the surgeon should then explain to the potential patient that weight loss before a face-lift operation is beneficial not only for improvement of appearance but also for betterment of health. Weight loss after a face-lift can result in development of undesirable loose skin on the face and neck. At this point, the overweight patient frequently promises to lose a reasonable amount of weight before surgery. It is explained that weight loss is not essential for the slightly overweight patient, but if weight loss is anticipated, this ideally should occur before undergoing face- and neck-lift surgery. For obese patients, it is recommended that no facial surgery be performed until an agreeable amount of weight is lost by dieting and exercise. When necessary, the patient is referred to a behavior modification program under the direction of a physician for specific weight loss instructions and supervision.

In performing the physical examination of the face and neck, it is important to palpate the skin for assessment of turgor and to feel the bony structures of the mandible and zygoma. It is essential to note the excessive contents of the face and neck and to assess whether the tissues causing the deformities are primarily cutaneous, adipose, or muscular in origin. If the submental and submandibular regions contain excess fat, it should be either excised directly or suctioned. Prominent bony structures in the face and neck will help give a pleasing contour when the excess skin is excised and repositioned. It is typical that almost all patients who request face-lift surgery require some type of neck-lift surgery as well.

Recommendations

It is best to dictate the final recommendations in the presence of the patient because the patient immediately learns the surgeon's opinion at this time. Recommendations fall into the following categories:

- *Category A:* This person should benefit from face- and neck-lifting and can be scheduled for surgery when convenient.
- *Category B:* The patient is a reasonable candidate for face- and neck-lift surgery, provided the primary physician (internist or general practitioner) feels that the patient is a reasonable medical risk. A patient in this group may be taking medications, such as antihypertensives or diuretics, or may have a medical history that requires special medical or surgical attention. This patient must ask the personal physician whether or not elective surgery is contraindicated. The plastic surgeon does not care to know whether the personal physician thinks that the patient should have a face-lift. Invariably, the internist or the general practitioner will tell the patient, "You really don't need that face-lift." This is of course true; no one *needs* a face-lift.
- *Category C:* This patient should not have elective aesthetic surgery because of medical or psychologic contraindications. It is explained to the patient why, in the surgeon's opinion, the patient is not a good candidate for plastic surgery. If the patient insists upon having plastic surgery, the internist or psychiatrist involved should be called, and the situation should be discussed frankly. The insistent patient is invited to return later for

a second consultation after discussions with the primary physician have taken place.

INSTRUCTIONS TO PATIENTS BEFORE SURGERY

A patient scheduled for face- and neck-lift surgery should receive the following instructions:

- Take no aspirin or drugs that cause bleeding from this point forward. Aspirin can cause abnormal bleeding with surgery. Tylenol is acceptable.
- To reduce bruising, take vitamin K, 5 mg twice a day, for the week before surgery. To enhance wound healing, take multivitamins, especially vitamin C, for the week before surgery. (Some physicians do not believe in vitamin therapy, but this author feels that it is beneficial.)
- Optimal weight loss before face- and neck-lift surgery is beneficial even if the weight is partially regained later.
- Fees should be paid in full 2 weeks before surgery. Surgery is subject to cancellation if the fees are not paid when due.

SECOND CONSULTATION BEFORE SURGERY

A patient upon whom surgery is to be performed should be seen again within several days of surgery. The patient and chart are reviewed completely, and a preoperative list is checked to ensure that the following have been completed:

- Satisfactory resolution of any questionable medical situations
- Special instructions have been followed: avoid aspirin and other platelet-damaging drugs; light or no alcohol; vitamins by mouth as prescribed
- Patient understands the surgery planned and its possible risks and has signed an informed operative consent form
- Preoperative photographs are of good quality

PREOPERATIVE TESTS AND EVALUATION

The day before surgery, the following evaluations are performed:

- Complete blood count, prothrombin time, partial thromboplastin time, urinalysis
- Electrolytes, if the patient is more than 40 years of age or taking diruretics
- Human immunodeficiency virus testing (requested at some institutions) with the patient's signed permission
- Electrocardiograph, if the patient is more than 40 years of age or has a health history of heart disease
- Plastic surgery resident performs own complete health history and physical examination if surgery is at a teaching affiliated hospital
- Anesthesiologist responsible for the local standby evaluates the patient separately; if any problems are detected, such as hypokalemia in a patient taking diuretics, the plastic surgeon and anesthesiologist should consult about the necessary treatment before surgery.
- Chest x-ray examination obtained if general anesthesia used or if there is a question about pulmonary or cardiac function; most patients who have had recent chest x-ray examinations do not need another one performed at this time.

PATIENT PREPARATION

The following should be performed the night before surgery:

- Shower and shampoo with a surgical solution (e.g., Betadine or Hibiclens). One should avoid getting Hibiclens inside the ears, eyes, nose or mouth because it has been reported to be toxic in these areas.
- Sleeping medications should be taken by mouth after shower and shampoo, between 9:00 and 10:00 PM the night before surgery.

PATIENT CARE DURING IMMEDIATE PREOPERATIVE AND INTRAOPERATIVE PERIOD

The patient often is less tense when elective surgery is performed early in the morning and the patient has not waited half the day to arrive in the operating room.

Preoperative Medication

The preoperative medication, usually midazolam (Versed) without a drying agent, is administered in the holding area. It may be advisable to avoid scopolamine with local anesthesia. This drug often makes the patient confused and irritable on the operating table.

Hair Shaving

To prevent hair from falling on the operating table, the central temporal scalp and posterior cervical scalp (where incisions will be made), are shaved while the patient is on the stretcher. Adjacent hair is taped back with masking tape.

Positioning

The patient is placed on the operating table with the head elevated, a pillow under the knees, and soft restraints around the hands. Sitting on a soft, comfortable, rolling stool makes the surgeon's job easier and less stressful.

Eye Protection and Facial Preparation

Boric acid ointment is inserted to protect the patient's eyes before one begins the facial preparation. A light solution (e.g., Betadine, benzalkonium chloride, and saline) is preferable. The heavy yellow color of iodine-containing solutions occasionally obscures the detection of ischemia when facial skin has been pulled too tight. If an iodine-containing solution is used for facial preparation, its application should be followed with vigorous saline irrigation so that no distorting color remains on the skin.

Placement of Drains

Suction drains (usually soft Silastic or Synder Hemovac) are used by this author for 24 hours postoperatively in a face-lift patient. These drains do not prevent hematoma formation, but they do remove serosanguineous fluid and partially reduce facial edema.

Dressings

Dressings consist of antibiotic ointment on the suture line, fluff gauzes around the ears, Surgipads, Kerlex, and a 3-inch bandage (e.g., Ace wrap) placed loosely around the face (Fig. 15-1).

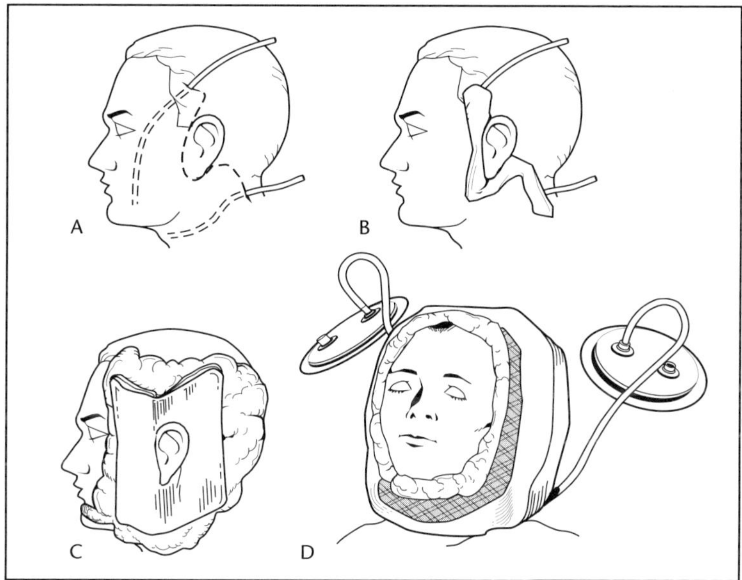

FIG. 15–1 *Face-life dressing.* ***A,*** *Small Hemovac drains in place.* ***B,*** *Antibiotic ointment and petroleum gauze applied to suture line.* ***C,*** *Fluffed gauze and Surgipad with an opening for the ear applied.* ***D,*** *Face and neck loosly wrapped with Kerlix and 3-inch bandage wrap. Drains connected to closed, self-contained suction.*

RECOVERY ROOM CARE

The patient is positioned in the recovery bed with the head elevated 30° and the knees flexed. Depending on the degree of sedation, the patient remains in the recovery room for several hours after the face-lift is completed. When the patient is reasonably alert and can tolerate clear liquids, the patient is returned to the room, postoperative care facility, or home with a responsible adult.

POSTOPERATIVE CARE

The following postoperative orders are recommended:

- Elevate head of bed 30°; this helps decrease facial edema.
- Discontinue intravenous (IV) solution after nausea has been controlled. Patients feel more comfortable taking

nourishment by mouth. The sooner the IV needle is removed, the less the chance of subcutaneous fluid infiltration.

- ▼ Clear to full liquids by mouth following surgery. Early chewing can cause facial bleeding.
- ▼ Mechanical soft diet the following morning. The patient should avoid excessive masticatory motion to promote early healing.
- ▼ Bed rest; bathroom privileges with help. Intraoperative and postoperative medications often make the patient unstable on the feet.
- ▼ Ambulate with help the morning following surgery. This helps avert embolism and phlebitis and restores a feeling of well-being.
- ▼ Meperidine, 50 mg, with hydroxyzine, 25 mg, given intramuscularly (IM) every 3 hours as required for pain when hospitalized. Hydroxyzine is an effective antiemetic and potentiates the pain-relieving properties of the narcotic meperidine.
- ▼ Darvocet N-100 or acetaminophen-codeine tablets (Tylenol #3), 1 to 2 by mouth every 3 hours as required, for moderate pain (Darvocet N-100 is preferred if the patient develops nausea with codeine). IM pain medications cannot safely be administered at home. The sooner the patient is comfortable with oral medications, the more quickly the patient can go home.
- ▼ Dalmane, 30 mg by mouth at bedtime, for sleep. It is often difficult for the patient to sleep at night with a facial dressing in place without first taking a sleeping pill.

DISCHARGE

Timing

Most face-lift patients go home late the day of surgery or the day after surgery. When blepharoplasty, rhinoplasty, or another procedure has been performed with the face-lift, the patient may choose to remain in the hospital or recovery facility for an additional day.

Predischarge Procedure

Inpatient's drains are removed the morning following surgery before the discharge time. When the drains are removed, the dressing is changed. At this time, the external auditory canals are thoroughly cleansed with saline or hydrogen peroxide. Blood clots and other exudate inadvertently left in the ear canals can cause otitis.

FOLLOW-UP

Short-Term Follow-up

A. **Three to 4 days after surgery.** The patient returns to the office for partial suture removal and another dressing change.
B. **Eight days after surgery.** All remaining sutures are removed. Patients may go from my office to an experienced professional hairdresser in the same building for a careful hair wash and dry before or after suture removal.

Long-Term Follow-up

A. **Four weeks after surgery.** The patient is reexamined in the office. Sometimes a previously undetected suture is removed.
B. **Eight to 10 weeks after surgery, follow-up photographs are taken.**
C. **Six months and 1 year after surgery.** Additional follow-up examinations are performed. The plastic surgeon explains that there should be a gradual improvement in facial appearance the first year after surgery and also points out that during the coming years the face and neck skin will gradually loosen again. After years of loosening, the patient may consider having a secondary face- and neck-lift operation performed. The majority of patients it seems is content to age naturally after one operation because the clock has already been turned back by the face-lift and neck-lift surgery.

CHAPTER 16

Rhinoplasty and Mentoplasty

Jack H. Sheen

Success in rhinoplasty comes to the plastic surgeon from sincere respect for the procedure (which may appear deceptively simple), from an honest assessment of results, and from sound patient care. Augmentation mentoplasty may be suggested by the plastic surgeon to the rhinoplasty patient as a means of achieving the desired profile symmetry and natural balance among the chin, nose, and forehead.

PATIENT SELECTION

Motivation

As with all aesthetic surgery candidates, the rhinoplasty patient must truly want a change in appearance. The teenage girl or boy whose parents are urging nasal surgery should be operated upon only when the patient expresses a desire for correction and projects realistic goals. Many patients seen in consultation for the first time are unaware of the profile improvement that can be obtained with augmentation mentoplasty or a segmental sliding advancement osteotomy. When the chin profile recedes significantly behind a vertical line dropped from the glabella through the upper lip, the plastic surgeon may inform the patient about mentoplasty as an option.

Timing

Rhinoplasty can be performed in mature adolescents. Hormonal changes such as the beginning of the menstrual cycle in the adolescent girl and facial hair growth in the adolescent boy should be present before rhinoplasty is undertaken. These characteristics are usually evidence that no further nasal growth is anticipated. Nasal maturity often occurs at age 14 to 15 in girls and at age 15 in boys. Although women frequently bleed more from their surgery when rhinoplasty is performed during their menstrual periods, this author has never deferred an operation because of uterine bleeding nor has any special attempt been made to schedule surgery around a particular time of the month.

Old age in the presence of good health is no contraindication to rhinoplasty. A patient who has undergone a face-lift or other procedures to look younger may benefit from the removal of excessive or dropping nasal tissues as well.

PREOPERATIVE PREPARATION

Examination

A. **External nasal examination.** During external nasal examination, the physician notes the anatomic characteristics of the nose. These include the following:
   - ▼ Thickness of nasal skin
   - ▼ Length of nasal bones
   - ▼ Presence of excessive bone and cartilage in the hump
   - ▼ Quality of alar cartilage and thickness of nasal tip
   - ▼ Length of nose
   - ▼ Nasolabial angle
   - ▼ Position of alae
   - ▼ Other individual characteristics of the patient

B. **Internal examination.** An internal examination of the patient should be performed with adequate lighting, a nasal speculum, 5% cocaine solution to shrink the mucosa, and bayonet forceps to determine whether airway obstruction is present because of a deviated septum, hypertrophied turbinate tissue, or previous nasal fracture. Either a reflecting mirror or a fiberoptic headlight is preferred for complete visualization of the internal nasal anatomy.

Photographic Documentation

Photographic documentation of the physical findings is essential for each rhinoplasty and mentoplasty patient.

These photographs should include frontal, lateral, both left and right obliques, and basal views, plus any additional angles necessary to document specific deformities. Good photographic records are not only beneficial to the surgeon in formulating and reviewing the operative plan but are especially helpful in explaining the recommended surgical changes to the patient.

Health History

As explained in Chapter 2, a complete health history (including medications taken and drug allergies), physical examination, and normal laboratory profile must be obtained before any type of surgery is performed.

Explanation of Risks

Risks of rhinoplasty and mentoplasty must be explained to the patient, including the possibilitly of infection and rejection of the alloplastic chin implant. A written consent form for surgery must be signed by the patient (See Chapter 11.).

Patient Instructions for Preoperative Preparation

Because patients frequently forget what the physician tells them, it is helpful to give them written instructions detailing the preoperative preparation. These instructions should include the following items:

A. Restrictions

- ▼ Avoid all medications containing aspirin 7 to 10 days before surgery.
- ▼ Avoid sunburn 2 weeks before surgery.
- ▼ Avoid vitamin E 7 days before surgery (increases capillary bleeding).
- ▼ Avoid alcohol for at least 1 day before surgery and preferably longer.

B. Night before surgery

- ▼ Wash face and hair thoroughly with a hexachlorophene soap (e.g., pHisoHex).
- ▼ Apply no makeup after washing.
- ▼ Eat and drink nothing after midnight.

- ▼ Begin antibiotics (erythromycin, 250 mg 4 times a day or 1 g/day) by mouth if an alloplastic material is to be used for the chin or maxilla. I do not use alloplastic substances in the nose.

Preoperative Medication

For the patient receiving local anesthesia, preoperative medication not only relieves the patient's apprehension but also serves as an indicator of the amount of drugs that will be required during surgery. Morphine, 15 mg given intramuscularly (IM) for a 55- to 80-kg patient, or 10 mg for a 45- to 55-kg patient, is given 1 hour before surgery. Morphine is preferred because of its clinical safety, the feeling of euphoria it provides for most patients, and the low incidence of associated nausea.

OPERATIVE CARE

Anesthesia

Most rhinoplasty and mentoplasty patients tolerate local anesthesia well. An endotracheal tube placed during general anesthesia distorts the patient's mouth, limits free positioning of the patient's head, and visually obstructs part of the face. However, general anesthesia may be used when emotional or physical factors dictate.

A. **Local anesthesia and sedation.** Rhinoplasty performed with the patient under local anesthesia is easier for the surgeon if the patient is relaxed and cooperative and if the entire nose is well anesthetized.

   - ▼ Procedure

     - ■ An initial dose of diazepam (Valium), 2.5 mg, is given intravenously (IV) after the patient is on the operating table, a cardiac monitor is attached, and IV Ringer's lactate solution (500 ml) is flowing. Depending on the patient's response as measured by slurring of speech and slowed respirations, an additional 5 to 20 mg of diazepam is given for a 5- to 10-minute period.

     - ■ Meperidine (Demoral), 100 mg, is added to the IV solution and is allowed to flow at 60 drops (1 mg) a minute.

- Lidocaine (Xylocaine), 50 mg of a 1% solution, is mixed in a sterile glass with 0.5 ml of 1:1,000 epinephrine, making a solution of 1:100,000 lidocaine with epinephrine. A 10-ml glass syringe with a 27-gauge, 1 1/4-inch needle is used for infiltration; usually 8 ml is injected for rhinoplasty.
- After local infiltration, the IV drip is slowed and given as needed during surgery. This titration method provides excellent contact with the patient, who frequently is in need of reassurance from the operating surgeon. If a patient becomes too deeply sedated with meperidine, this state can be quickly reversed by the administration of naloxone hydrochloride (Narcan), 0.4 mg IV.

▼ Place of Injection. Local injections begin at the radix, with placement of approximately 0.5 mg of solution into the soft tissues. Direct injection of local anesthesia into nasal tissues to obtain hemostasis is recommended; some surgeons prefer regional blocks, avoiding direct infiltration into the dorsum and tip. In either case, the final injection, 0.5 mg, is placed near the infraorbital foramen on each side.

B. **General anesthesia.** With general anesthesia, local infiltration of lidocaine with epinephrine is recommended to provide hemostasis.

Cleansing and Packing

▼ The vestibules are cleaned meticulously with povidone-iodine (Betadine) on cotton-tipped applicators, with special attention paid to the apices and the area to the level of the internal valve.

▼ Next, the vibrissae are shaved close to the vestibular skin with a No. 15 scalpel blade, followed by a second cleansing with povidone-iodine.

▼ Sterile cotton and 4 ml of a 5% cocaine hydrochloride (200 mg) are placed in a sterile medicine glass. No epinephrine is added because this increases the potential for cocaine toxicity. After cocaine-soaked cotton packs are inserted in each nasal vestibule, complete facial preparation and draping are carried out.

Operative Position

The plastic surgeon may find it easier to operate while in the sitting position, with the patient flat on the operating table; however, it is sometimes necessary to stand. Some surgeons prefer to have the patient's head elevated and extended during rhinoplasty. A strong fiberoptic headlight is required. Overhead operating lights are turned off when the surgeon is observing deep nasal structures.

Instruments

In selecting operating instruments for rhinoplasty, one should remember the following steps:

- ▼ Separation of soft tissues from the skeleton
- ▼ Preliminary modification of bony and cartilagenous parts
- ▼ Modification of tip cartilages, osteotomy, final contouring of all parts
- ▼ Fixation of soft tissues
- ▼ Reconstruction of the internal valve
- ▼ Septoplasty

Instruments used for each of these steps must be sharp, delicate, and well aligned:

A. **Foman rasp.** A sharp, coarse Foman rasp is recommended for lowering the bony dorsum, because it is easier to control the amount of lowering with this than with a saw. The rasp should be fine enough not to avulse the upper lateral cartilages. The chance of avulsion decreases by gently rasping on the bias and placing as little pull as possible on the cartilage-to-bone attachments.
B. **No. 11 scalpel.** To lower the cartilagenous dorsum, a No. 11 scalpel blade with the tip broken off is used, and mucosal continuity is preserved whenever possible.
C. **Bone rongeur.** A double-action bone rongeur is used to resect part of the spine.

D. **Bone wax.** This may be used if bleeding from cut surfaces is excessive.
E. **Osteotome.** It is important to begin the osteotomy as low as possible in the pyriform aperature with a sharp, guarded, curved osteotome, finishing high at the cephalic end when the tapping tone changes. If a high-to-high osteotomy is done, a step deformity with an unattractive formation of the bony pyramid will result.

Procedure for Septum

The rhinoplasty surgeon often must use septal cartilage as a graft or must partially remove septum to correct airway obstruction. Except for specific harvesting, only the obstructing septal parts should be excised because septal cartilage is a valuable material that should not be wasted. Surplus septal fragments should be replaced into the septal pocket and crushed with a Cottle cartilage crusher if necessary so that the patient has the double benefit of aesthetic improvement as a result of the cartilage grafts and a rigid straight septum. To obtain adequate anesthesia, a 22-gauge, 3.5-inch needle is used to inject 1% lidocaine with 1:100,000 epinephrine into the septal mucosa. The cartilage separates readily from the perichondrium when the solution is injected subperichondrially. When septoplasty is done for obstruction, the initial incision is made parallel to the caudal border of the septum, just caudal to the deviation and into, but not through, the cartilage.

Knight scissors are recommended for harvesting septal material because they cut through the osteochondral junction, providing a sizable piece of nasal cartilage and bone for grafting. Care must be taken to leave intact at least a 1-cm width of dorsal and caudal septal cartilage for support. At least one mucoperichondrial flap must remain intact to avert perforation of the septum. When the surgeon anticipates the need for a future septal cartilage graft in nasal surgery, the septal cartilage can be banked in the patient's scalp. A short incision is made in the occipital area of the scalp at the hairline, and a pocket is dissected large enough to comfortably accept the septal specimen, which becomes a readily available source of graft material.

Procedure for Turbinates

The treatment of airway obstruction caused by turbinate hypertrophy can be undertaken effectively at the time of rhinoplasty. The superior and supreme turbinates usually do not cause airway obstruction because of their location. The middle turbinate, which principally secretes mucus, has little or no control of nasal airflow. Recurring sinusitis and turbinate headaches are often associated with middle turbinate hypertrophy or malposition. The inferior turbinate contains venous lakes and has an erectile capacity. It can change mass rapidly, and it functions to control delivered air volume. The inferior turbinate is sensitive to such stimulants as alcohol, smoke, air pollution, air conditioning and emotion, and it responds by hypertrophy. The inferior turbinate ceases to function normally if it obstructs the airway. This leads to hyperplasia and polypoid degeneration. In this author's experience, the best long-term treatment is partial resection of the offending turbinates using Gruenwald forceps. Crushing, steroid injections, and topical agents have proved ineffective with time. Local anesthesia is provided with a 22-gauge, 3.5-inch spinal needle after cocaine packs have been removed. In turbinate surgery, the incidence of postoperative bleeding is slightly higher than in rhinoplasty alone, but it usually can be controlled by careful packing.

Procedure for Mentoplasty

Augmentation mentoplasty may be performed at the time of rhinoplasty to better achieve facial symmetry when dental occlusion is acceptable. Aesthetic surgeons should critically consider both the lateral and the frontal facial planes, keeping the line along the mandible to the point of the mentum as smooth as possible after mentoplasty. I tend to underaugment when doing a chin procedure so that notching is avoided at the implant-mandible interface.

- ▼ The lower labial sulcus is thoroughly prepped with aqueous Zephiran, and local anesthesia is injected.
- ▼ The intraoral approach, making a perpendicular incision well above the labial sulcus, is recommended. A pocket is dissected over the mentum, just large enough to accept the Silastic chin implant, which is modified to the desired shape by carving with a No. 10 scalpel blade.

- The implant is soaked in antibiotic (e.g., lincomycin) before insertion.
- The incision is closed with several layers of absorbable suture (4-0 plain catgut to muscle, 5-0 plain catgut to mucosa).
- When the pocket is made in the correct anatomic position and is only as large as the chin implant, migration is not a problem. An Elastoplast pressure dressing over a Telfa or gauze sponge helps hold the implant in place.

POSTOPERATIVE CARE

Nasal Packs and Splints

- Nasal and oral airways are thoroughly suctioned to remove clots at the completion of the operation.
- Packing is minimal when no septal or turbinate surgery is performed. Adaptic gauze, measuring 3 by 3 inches, is cut diagonally, and this triangle is placed in both vestibules to ensure good tissue approximation. The pack is removed after 24 hours.
- When septal or turbinate surgery has been done, a 6-inch No. 18 clear plastic suction catheter is positioned in each vestibule, just anterior to the posterior pharynx. Adaptic strips, 1 by 9 inches, cut lengthwise from the 3- by 9-inch package, are impregnated with bacitracin ointment and inserted around the breathing tubes. The positioned tubes are then trimmed flush with the nares and sutured to the packing. Four days after septal surgery, the packs and tubes are removed; they remain 7 days when turbinate surgery has been performed.
- The external dressing begins with 0.5-inch paper tape placed in overlapping layers from the radix to the supratip. A V-notch is cut in the tape, which goes around the nose as a sling under the tip.
- A layer of cloth tape is placed over the paper tape to serve as a base for the plaster cast.
- Four-ply quick-setting plaster of Paris is cut at the level of the radix, dipped in warm water, and folded back on itself to make an eight-ply cast in the central nose. Tape

is applied from the cheeks to hold the splint in place for 1 week.

- ▼ Gauze, 2 by 2 inches, is placed under the nostrils with 0.5-inch paper tape and changed whenever it becomes saturated.
- ▼ The tape and plaster splinter are extended onto the forehead if a radical resection of the radix and frontal bones has been carried out.

Discharge from Hospital

A. **Timing.** A rhinoplasty patient often is discharged at 5:00 PM on the day of surgery and should be ambulatory by 24 hours after surgery. A patient who experiences excessive bleeding or has had turbinate surgery remains in hospital overnight. The patient is instructed to continue to apply ice compresses to the eyes for at least 24 hours and to keep the head elevated.

B. **Discharge medications.** These include something for pain (e.g., acetaminophen, 300 mg, with codeine, 30 mg), sleep (e.g., flurazepam hydrochloride [Dalmane], 30 mg), and an antibiotic (e.g., erythromycin, 250 mg 4 times a day) for a chin implant patient. Antibiotics are not routinely given to the rhinoplasty patient.

C. **Instructions for patients and their families**

   - ▼ Cool clear liquids may be consumed in the first 24 hours, and a mechanically soft diet should be eaten for the first week.
   - ▼ Family, patients, and nursing staff are warned to expect hematemesis and excessive drainage after turbinate resection. The moustache dressing should be changed frequently, approximately every 15 minutes , or as necessary.
   - ▼ A rhinoplasty patient should avoid hot foods, hot baths, washing the hair, alcohol, and aspirin during the week following surgery. After 3 weeks, the patient can play tennis, but more vigorous activities should wait 6 weeks, and contact sports should wait 3 months. Because of the insensitivity of the nose postoperatively, snow and skiing should be avoided for 3 months to eliminate the chance of frostbite.

- Direct sunlight should be avoided for 6 weeks, and sunscreens or a mechanical device should be used to protect the nose for 3 months.
- If mentoplasty has been performed, the patient should refrain from excessive talking or laughing in the first 10 days to lessen edema. Antibiotics (e.g., erythromycin, 250 mg 4 times a day) are given for 1 week. The patient is encouraged to irrigate the mouth frequently with a Water Pik, saline, peroxide, or mouthwash to lower the intraoral bacterial count.

Suture and Splint Removal

- External alar base sutures are removed 3 to 4 days postoperatively. Internal nasal and labial sulcus sutures are absorbable and rarely require removal.
- The splint is carefully removed at 7 days using Metzenbaum scissors to cut through the tape at the tip and along the dorsum. The surgeon strips away the tape toward the maxilla, avoiding distraction of the nasal skin and ensuring that the skeletal parts and skin remain adherent. Acetone can be used to cleanse the skin of adhesive.
- The patient is instructed to use cotton-tipped applicators gently with normal saline spray to remove excessive dry mucus from inside the nose; the patient should refrain from blowing the nose for 6 weeks after surgery to prevent crepitance under the skin.
- Transient bleeding can be experienced after splint or pack removal, especially when turbinate surgery has been done. A piece of 0.5 by 3-inch Telfa saturated with phenylephrine (Neo-synephrine, 0.25%) and placed on the floor of the nose and against the inferior turbinates almost always controls bleeding. When bleeding is severe, a posterior nasal pack may be required for an additional 7 days.

Supratip Swelling

If elevation of the supratip area is noted 2 weeks after surgery, the patient is warned that small amounts of steroids may be required. At 16 or 17 days, if the supratip swelling persists, 0.02 ml of triamcinolone (Aristocort Forte, 40 mg/ml) is injected with a tuberculin syringe in the deep subdermal layer. This treatment is repeated in 10 days to 2 weeks if supratip swelling persists. After four times, treatments are stopped whether or not supratip fullness is responsive.

Bone Position

The patient should not touch the nose after surgery because the nasal bones should be separated from the maxilla after a complete osteotomy. If nasal bones begin distracting laterally secondary to edema, the surgeon should place the thumbs along both sides of the nose and bring the bones back toward midline with gentle pressure. This procedure is repeated every 4 days until the edema has subsided and the bones are in their correct position.

SECONDARY RHINOPLASTY

One should not abandon the unhappy rhinoplasty patient. A forthright discussion of postoperative problems is required. The surgeon's approach should be honest and supportive. Have the patient talk about and point out specific deformities; document these with photographic records. Minor revisions, which are inevitable in every practice, can be taken care of by using the patient care principles previously described. However, secondary rhinoplasty has inherent limitations of tissue damage, tissue deficit, and scarring; thus good judgment must be followed in deciding whether, when, and by whom secondary rhinoplasty should be performed. Expert consultation may be advisable.

Ground Rules

In caring for postsurgical nasal deformities, the following principles have proved invaluable:

- ▼ Defer surgery until there is final resolution of the tissues (at least 1 year).
- ▼ Make a proper diagnosis, as described under Preoperative Preparation.
- ▼ Follow proven aesthetic concepts.

- ▼ Limit the surgical dissection to what is *necessary.*
- ▼ Use only autogenous material in the nose.

Harvesting Ear Cartilage

As mentioned earlier, septal cartilage is the primary source of reconstructive material. When this is not available or when a smooth, convex surface is required, conchal ear cartilage can be harvested. As described by Burt Brent, total resection of the concha through an anterior approach leaves minimal deformity. The skin and perichondrium are injected with 1% lidocaine with 1:100,000 epinephrine, with anterior elevation of the perichondrium. After the cartilage graft is taken, a 19-gauge butterfly infusion set is made into a drain by notching holes along the distal inch. Through a small inferior conchal stab incision, the drain is placed in the donor site and the butterfly needle is inserted into a vacuum blood-collecting tube. Petroleum gauze is gently packed in the concha, and the ear is dressed with eye pads, fluffs, and circumferential Kling dressing. The drain can be removed after 24 hours and the ear dressing discontinued after 1 week.

CHAPTER 17

Auricular Surgery

Burt D. Brent

Reconstruction of the external ear offers both emotional relief to afflicted patients and a creative challenge to the reconstructive surgeon, who must put forth a dedicated effort to gain the experience necessary to obtain consistently good results. Sound patient management is a must throughout any surgical reconstruction.

Ear prostheses have no practical value for children, but they may be desirable in older patients who have undergone extensive cancer ablation. Ear prostheses often give rise to problems such as glue irritation, fear of their dropping off, and loss of color match as a result of climatic changes.

PATIENT SELECTION

Timing

The ear is approximately 85% full grown at 6 years of age. Ideally, deformed ears should be corrected when a child becomes aware of the problem and personally acknowledges the wish to undergo surgery. The author prefers to begin correction of microtia at age 6 because rib cartilages then are large enough to fabricate an adult-sized framework, and the child's deformity only then begins to cause psychologic distress.

Consultation

During consultation, a patient with auricular deformity must be self-motivated to ask for surgical correction. Limitations in ear reconstruction or any surgical correction must be emphasized to the patient or the parents before a realistic perspective can be reached via photographs showing the surgeon's results. Unrealistic expectations by the patient or family can be a reason to avoid surgery. Other contraindications to surgery are severe medical problems or excessive scarring and inadequate circulation as a result of previous attempts at surgical correction.

Discomforts and possible complications, including pain in the rib donor site, pneumothorax, and loss of skin or cartilage graft secondary to infection or hematoma must be discussed with the patient and family. It should be emphasized that several operative stages usually are required to correct an ear deformity.

PREOPERATIVE PREPARATION

Planning

A. **Ear reconstruction.** Before attempting any total ear reconstruction, each surgeon should become proficient at fabricating a good ear framework from cadaver cartilage using a replica of a normal ear as a model. Before surgery, a reverse photograph of the opposite normal ear can be printed in addition to the usual preoperative frontal, lateral, and posterior ear photographs. During preoperative examination, an x-ray film pattern is traced from the contralateral ear, and a framework pattern is designed several millimeters smaller in all dimensions to allow for the auricular-mastoid flap's thickness. These templates are sterilized and used as patterns during surgery. Remembering that the axis is roughly parallel to the profile of the nose, one determines the reconstructed ear's location by placing the above film template at the reconstruction site and comparing the proposed new ear with the normal opposite ear.

B. **Otoplasty.** Before contemplating an otoplasty, one should be aware that an ear's protrusion commonly results from an undefined antihelic fold or from pronounced conchal depth. In the same individual there may be a difference in the size and shape of each ear. One should structure the surgical plan to each specific deformity and follow principles outlined by Mustardé, Stenström, Furnas, Crikelair, and others.

Hearing Testing

Although the majority of otoplasty patients have normal hearing, the microtic patient deserves special consideration. Auditory perception should be tested before surgery, and if any question arises about hearing, a competent otologist should be consulted. Middle ear surgery is generally reserved for a bilaterally microtic patient with severe bilateral hearing deficits. In this patient, the external ear reconstruction should be performed first at age 6 and followed by a team approach to middle ear surgery.

Surgical Prepping and Draping

- ▼ The night before auricular surgery, all patients are asked to wash their hair with antiseptic shampoo (e.g., Hibiclens).
- ▼ Parenteral cefazolin sodium (Kefzol) is given before (as well as during and after) surgery when a rib graft is taken.
- ▼ When necessary for exposure, hair is removed with a hair clipper rather than a razor so that the skin is neither traumatized nor subjected to bacterial contamination.
- ▼ Only the chest is initially prepped and draped. Ten minutes before the framework is completed, the auricular region is prepped. Clear plastic Vidrapes are applied, with the nose and eyes as visible landmarks.

OPERATIVE CARE

Anesthesia

Local anesthesia is preferred for an otoplasty, unless the child is too young or the operative procedure is too involved. Use of epinephrine is avoided when one is placing an auricular framework, so that the surgeon can realize if blanching occurs that the skin pocket is too tight. However, local anesthesia with a vasoconstrictor (1:200,000 epinephrine) is preferred for otoplasty. General anesthesia is used when a rib graft is taken and later when the ear is elevated.

Complications

The two possible complications that can occur when taking a rib cartilage graft are *pneumothorax* and *dropping the framework onto a nonsterile area.* The latter is remedied by thoroughly irrigating the cartilage framework with antibiotic-containing saline solution before insertion. A pneumothorax is treated by inserting a small chest tube, completing the chest incision closure, fully expanding the lungs, and evacuating air via a large syringe that is connected to the chest tube; thereafter the tube is withdrawn. A portable chest x-ray examination is taken in the operating room (OR) while the patient is still anesthetized.

Trauma

A. **Otohematoma.** Otohematoma, a common contact sports injury, must be treated aggressively to prevent recurrences. Needle aspiration alone is followed by recurrent fluid collection. The hematoma must be evacuated via a small incision inside the posterior conchal wall or scapha and then dressed with pressure gauze bolsters on the ear's anterolateral and posteromedial surface. The bolsters are held with horizontal mattress sutures (4-0 nylon) for 7 to 10 days.

B. **Ear amputation.** Because replantation of the ear without augmentating the vasculature usually is not successful, dermabrasion of the amputated part, followed by reattachment and temporary "pocketing" below a retroauricular flap has been proposed by Mladick. Baudet suggests removing the ear's posteromedial skin and fenestration of the cartilage in an attempt to increase the recipient vascular surface of the replanted ear. Microvascular replantation is only occasionally successful because of the tiny ear vessels.

C. **Traumatic clefts and keloids.** Traumatic earlobe clefts are treated by rolling an adjacent skin flap (as advocated by Pardue) into the apex of the wedge repair thus allowing continued use of earrings. The earlobe keloid seems to respond favorably to pressure. An earring device that applies constant pressure to postexcisional keloids is helpful in preventing recurrences.

Drains

A small suction drain is placed beneath the implanted cartilage framework to remove fluid and minimize the risk of flap necrosis. Silicone drains are best, but one can fashion a drain by cutting several small holes into the end of a No. 19 butterfly catheter, which then is attached to a rubber-top vacuum blood-collecting tube. Fluid output is monitored closely; the drain is removed when serous fluid is insignificant, which is usually in 72 hours.

Packing and Dressings

Antibiotic petroleum jelly gauze packing is placed in the new ear's convolutions. Dressings are applied without pressure because the drain provides both fluid removal and skin adherence. Eye patches, fluffs, and lightly wrapped 3-inch Kling wraps complete the ear dressing. A similar dressing is employed for an otoplasty patient (without the drains).

POSTOPERATIVE CARE

Patient Positioning

After surgery, the patient is positioned in bed with the head elevated. The patient is instructed not to lie on the reconstructed ear and to sleep on a soft down pillow. Although a head dressing is applied for 10 to 14 days, protective head gear is not needed thereafter.

Preventing Complications

- ▼ The reconstructed ear's rim is observed closely for any signs of infection or vascular compromise.
- ▼ Cephalosporin antibiotic (Kefzol), which is begun the night before surgery is given intravenously (IV) every 8 hours for 2 days and is followed by oral cephalexin (Keflex 250 to 500 mg 3 times a day) for 5 days.
- ▼ Local erythema, edema, fluctuation, and drainage are early signs of ear infection and may precede pain or fever. An irrigation drain should be placed under the ear flap when infection is suspected, and continuous drip irrigation antibiotic should be given as indicated by wound cultures and sensitivities.

- Necrotic skin is excised, and exposed cartilage is covered with either fascial flap and skin graft or a transposition skin flap.
- For the patient who has undergone rib grafts, breathing exercises are encouraged each waking hour with a Triflow spirometer, which inflates the lungs and prevents atelectasis.

Discharge from Hospital

Assuming the patient has no fever or other complications, reconstructive a patient who has had rib grafts generally is discharged 2 days postoperatively. The drains are removed several days later in the office or in the ward. Otoplasty patients, and those who had less involved reconstructive procedures, are either discharged the day after surgery or undergo surgery as an outpatient.

Follow-up Care

Patients are seen in the office on the sixth postoperative day for removal of sutures, dressing, and the petroleum jelly gauze packing. A fresh protective dressing is applied for an additional week. It is recommended that an otoplasty patient wear a tennis headband to held the ears (2 weeks during the day and 6 weeks while asleep at night). To prevent stenosis, a patient who has had reconstruction of the auditory canal should wear an acrylic mold obturator for 3 to 6 months.

Activities

The patient can wash the hair within 10 to 12 days after ear surgery, depending on the rapidity of healing. The patient can swim several weeks thereafter. However, the patient must avoid sunburning the ears for 6 months by using a protective sunscreen (e.g., Eclipse with para-aminobenzoic acid [PABA] or Solbar Plus 15). Vigorous activities should be avoided for 6 weeks by those who have had rib grafts. These precautions are discussed with each patient. Children can play baseball at 6 weeks without special protective gear. The parents are instructed to treat the child as a normal child and not to restrict the child unduly. There is no further need for parents to call attention to a corrected "deformity."

CHAPTER 18

Chemical Peeling and Dermabrasion

Lewis J. Obi and Thomas J. Baker

The process of *chemical peeling* of the skin, also known as dermapeel, chemosurgery, chemerasure, skin peeling, chemexfoliation, and chemical face-lifting, is used in the treatment of fine facial wrinkling, hyperpigmentation problems of the face, and other facial skin problems. Recent advances and the introduction of trichloroacetic acid (TCA) and the alpha-hydroxy acids (AHA) have extended the use of chemical peeling to practically all skin types and many additional body areas.

Surgical planing, or *dermabrasion,* is a procedure involving the removal of the epidermis and a portion of the dermis. Reepithelialization without visible scarring occurs from the remaining epidermal adnexae. Surface irregularities are minimized, because the high points or elevations are sanded down to a level closer to the low points of the skin. Improvement is achieved because the thinned dermis cannot regenerate its thickness.

As with any other operative procedure in plastic surgery, the care of patients undergoing chemical peel or dermabrasion begins with proper patient selection and preparation. The patient's expectations should be well within the range of the surgeon's abilities. Benefits should far exceed the probability of complications, and the patient must always be fully informed. A sample of our TCA peel information sheet included under the TCA peel section is only one of our many efforts to inform and educate patients.

CHEMICAL PEELING

Chemical Peeling Agents

The variety of chemicals commonly used as peeling agents includes phenol peels, TCA peels, TCA-Jessner solution peels, TCA and carbon dioxide peels, and AHA peels. Today the two most common peel techniques use the Baker-Gordon phenol formula and the TCA formulations. This chapter will therefore focus on these two peeling techniques.

A. Phenol

- Baker-Gordon formula: Phenol USP 88%, 3 ml Tap water, 2 ml croton oil, 3 drops hexachlorophene soap (Septisol) 8 drops
- Chemistry. Phenol (carbolic acid) is an aromatic hydrocarbon derived from coal tar. Unlike other organic acids, phenol does not contain the carboxyl (COOH) group. The hydroxyl group (OH) indicates it is an organic alcohol more than an acid.
- Local action. In high concentration, phenol is a protein precipitant, but in more dilute solutions such as those used in the formula for the peel, proteins are denatured without being coagulated. When the solution containing phenol is applied to the skin, a gray to white pellicle of precipitated protein (frost) that may subsequently turn to a grayish-pink is formed. The ensuing penetration of phenol to the sensory nerve endings exerts a local anesthetic effect after the initial feeling of heat and tingling. The superficial layer of the skin then sloughs in a few days, leaving a red and pink cutaneous surface, which gradually turns to white over weeks to months. The activity of phenol decreases when used in conjunction with soap. Croton oil is a vesicant and therefore increases the depth of phenol peeling. Occlusion with tape or petroleum jelly also increases the peel depth. If phenol is inadvertently applied to an area of skin where it is not desired, it can be removed effectively with 50% alcohol or even water, if it is done immediately.
- Systemic toxicity. The toxic oral dose of phenol for adults is 8 to 15 grams, which usually is fatal within

24 hours. The systemic toxic manifestations of phenol at this oral dose are evident after a few minutes and include muscular weakness, faintness, weak and irregular pulse, depressed respiration, constricted pupils, coma, and possibly death. Phenol is eliminated from the body by oxidation to hydroquinone and pyrocatechol, with approximately 80% excreted by the kidneys, either unchanged or conjugated to glycuronic and sulfuric acids. Blood phenol studies-performed on patients in whom 3 ml of a 50% phenol solution was applied to the entire face showed the blood phenol level rising to 0.68 mg/dl 1 hour after application to less than 0.1 mg/L after 4 hours. A case of phenol ingestion is reported in which the blood phenol level of the surviving patient rose to 25 mg/dl. When one compares this amount to the level recorded with the face peel (in practice less than half of the 3 ml used contacts the facial skin), it is obvious that the margin of safety is more than adequate.

Although reports of systemic toxicity with the Baker-Gordon formula are rare, myocardial changes such as premature ventricular contractions (PVCs) are not uncommon. According to Truppman and Ellenby, segmental and slow application of phenol in face-peeling would decrease the chances of producing cardiac arrhythmias or other systemic side effects. Allowing 60 minutes for the application of the peel solution permits detoxification and excretion to occur at a faster rate than absorption.

B. **Trichloroacetic Acid** TCA is the other commonly used peeling agent, which was recently introduced as a skin rejuvenator. TCA also denatures protein and is used in concentrations ranging from 20% to 50%. Although the depth of peeling that may be achieved with 50% TCA is comparable to 50% phenol, the risk of scarring is greater with TCA in this higher concentration. Penetration by TCA may be increased not only by occlusion but also by prolonged exposure and by mechanical methods (rubbing). Preoperative and postoperative preparation of the skin with tretinoin (Retin-A) or AHA enhances peeling with TCA. The patient should also be informed that an end result may require two or more peeling procedures spaced 1 to 3 months apart.

- Local action. The local skin response to TCA is similar to the frosting that occurs with phenol. Frosting occurs earlier and with more intensity if the patient has been prepared preoperatively with tretinoin. The frosting is also more intense with the higher concentrations of TCA. As with phenol, degreasing the skin with ether, acetone, or absolute alcohol enhances penetration of the peel chemical. The TCA is neutralized at the appropriate time with water or rubbing alcohol. The peeled areas are then coated with silver sulfadiazene (Silvadene), A&D ointment, or petroleum jelly (Vaseline).
- Systemic toxicity. Because there is no systemic toxicity of TCA when used in a concentration of 50% or less, it is considered safer for older patients and for patients with serious medical problems. There is no evidence that allergic reactions to TCA occur.

Patient Selection for Chemical Peels

A. **Gender.** The patient most suited for a phenol peel is a fair-skinned woman with moderate to deep rhytids who is willing to accept the skin lightening that results from phenol peels. Sun-damaged women may be candidates if there is neither excessive freckling nor sun darkening of the neck skin. Gender is not a factor with TCA peels.

B. **Skin type.** Phenol peels are less suitable for women with thick and oily skin. TCA peels are applicable to all skin types and both sexes with variable results.

C. **Skin conditions.** Age and environmentally induced wrinkling are still the common indicators of chemical peeling. The conditions that may be treated with chemical peeling listed in the order of favorable response are as follows:

- Fine (mosaic) wrinkling with dry, thin skin
- Diffuse facial keratoses with wrinkling
- Spotty or irregular areas of pigmentation with wrinkling

- ▼ Superficial acne scarring, especially in fair or ruddy patients
- ▼ Posttraumatic facial scarring

D. **Patient's Psychologic Makeup.** The psychologic make-up of the patient must be evaluated carefully before surgery. The patient's motivation for surgery, expectations regarding results, and willingness to endure the postoperative sequelae and restrictions are all important aspects of the patient's psyche, as was emphasized in Chapter 1. All patients must be informed not only of the limitations of chemical peeling but also of the risks. Prospective peel patients must agree to multiple peel sessions and to preoperative skin preparation.

Preoperative Consultation and Informed Consent

The entire preoperative and postoperative course and the actual procedure of chemical peeling should be explained in detail to the patient. An abbreviated list of important points to cover is given below. A more detailed check-off list provided by Norman Cole is routinely referred to at the time of initial consultation.

A. **Indications for peeling (previously listed under Skin Conditions).**

B. **Anticipated results.** Eschar formation, desquamation, and discomfort followed by erythema.

C. **Possible side effects.** Transient versus permanent: erythema, irregular pigmentation, skin edema, skin sensitivity, sun sensitivity, scarring, etc.

D. **Restrictions.** Short-term versus long-term restrictions. Diet, presentability, activities, sun exposure, work limitations, etc.

E. **Length of time required for healing.** In general, a patient may resume work and most social activities within 1 week after a TCA peel and 2 weeks after a phenol peel. Outdoor activities in a sunny environment are more restricted with a phenol peel patient. In Florida, a patient is allowed to resume outdoor sports within 4 weeks after a TCA peel.

F. **Photographic records.** It is imperative to keep a photographic record of the areas undergoing treatment as a basis of comparison at the conclusion of the treatment. Preoperative and postoperative photographs in color should be taken with and without makeup. The Yashica Dental-Eye II with autodrive, ring flash, and autolabeling provides outstanding and consistent photographic documentation. Early postoperative photographs (with edema and eschar) may be exhibited to certain patients in anticipation of recovery.

Preoperative Preparation of Patient

The phenol peel should be performed in a hospital or an adequately equipped and staffed clinic. Laboratory tests such as complete blood count (CBC) and urinalysis should be obtained for a patient undergoing a total facial phenol peel. This patient should be monitored for cardiac and blood pressure irregularities during and after the phenol peel. The plastic surgeon must be prepared to manage cardiac arrhythmias that may occur during or after chemical peeling. Neither elaborate systemic preparation nor monitoring is required for the TCA peel because there is no danger of systemic toxicity.

A. **Skin Preparation.** Minimal skin preparation is required for the phenol peel. Avoidance of oily soaps, makeup, and skin preparations is recommended before surgery. Degreasing the skin with ether, acetone, or absolute alcohol just before phenol peeling is important. More preoperative skin care and preparation is required before TCA peeling. Use of Retin-A (0.05%-0.1% Cream) for 1 month before TCA peeling results in a more uniform and successful peel with less risk of hyperpigmentation. Addition of 2% to 4% hydroquinone prepeel and postpeel also diminishes occurrence of hyperpigmentation. Acyclovir (Zovirax) should be started preoperatively in patients with any history of herpes.

B. **Pharmacologic preparation.** Prophylactic antibiotics may be used for peel patients (cephalexin 500 mg twice a day). Minimal preoperative sedation is required for a TCA peel patient. If large areas are to be peeled in an apprehensive patient, diazepam (Valium) 5-10 mg given orally and ketorolac (Toradol) 40 to 60 mg given intramuscularly (IM) can be administered preoperatively. All phenol peels are performed with preoperative and intraoperative sedation combined with careful monitoring. Preoperative sedation includes sodium pentobarbital 100 mg, diazepam 10 mg or Versed 2.5-5 mg, and glycopyrrolate (Robinul) 2 mg.

Intraoperative Management

A. Anesthesia and Analgesia

- TCA peels. Minimal to no analgesia is required for TCA peels. Fanning minimizes the burning discomfort, which may last a few minutes to an hour. When large areas are peeled with TCA, sedation and analgesia are administered orally and in some patients given parenterally. Partial TCA peels are performed in the office with no sedation.
- Phenol peels. Phenol peels are performed in the operating room (OR) with intravenous (IV) injection in place. The patient is well hydrated and titrated with midazolam (Versed) and fentanyl. Methylprednisolone sodium succinate (Solu-Medrol) 40 mg (or a similar steroid) and diphenhydramine (Benadryl) 25 mg are given empirically to patients peeled with phenol to help reduce postpeel edema.

B. Management of arrhythmias

- Prophylactic measures. Cardiac arrhythmias and other side effects related to phenol absorption may be minimized if the peel solution is not applied too rapidly. Plasma detoxification and more rapid renal excretion may be facilitated by rapid administration of IV fluids and adequate preoperative hydration. As indicated previously, systemic phenol toxicity is rare. However, myocardial changes in the form of arrhythmias, especially PVCs including bigeminy, are not uncommon. Some controversy exists regarding the management of these arrhythmias. Our approach is to minimize the risk of arrhythmias by minimizing the rate of phenol absorption and hastening its excretion. The absorption is decreased by peeling the face slowly and in increments. Excretion is hastened with adequate patient hydration and more rapid renal excretion. Good ventilation and oxygenation are ensured for the patient by avoiding oversedation of the patient while providing adequate analgesia. Nasal oxygen is routinely administered. These measures minimize cardiac irritability and therefore the incidence of cardiac arrhythmias.

- Treatment of patient with arrhythmias. Should PVCs occur during a phenol peel, a decision to treat must be made. If treatment is required, the patient is given a 50-mg bolus of lidocaine, and this is repeated at 5 to 10 minute intervals until the premature contractions subside (maximum dose is 150 mg). Blood pressures are monitored carefully before and after each administration of lidocaine. PVCs, bigeminy, and even ventricular tachycardia not responsive to lidocaine have been reported, especially in patients with Barlow's syndrome (mitral valve prolapse). Treatment of these patients with IV propranolol, not exceeding 1 mg/min, may be necessary.

C. **Taping.** Occlusive treatment (taping or petroleum jelly) increases the depth of penetration with phenol peels but not with TCA and the AHAs. The increased secretions with taping may initially dilute the concentration of TCA, thereby decreasing the depth of peeling. Skin surfaces treated with phenol are covered with loose-fitting waterproof tape, which is left in place for 48 hours. During this time skin edema and maceration occurs with significant swelling. The resulting wetness under the tape facilities removal. Tape applied too tightly can ulcerate through the dermis and result in permanent scarring. Some surgeons prefer petroleum jelly in place of taping as a means of occlusion.

Postoperative Management

A. Phenol peels

- Recovery room. After completion of the peel and taping, the patient continues to be monitored for cardiac problems, with frequent blood pressure checks. Burning pain, especially during the first 4 to 6 hours after taping, is to be expected. Increments of

10 mg meperidine are administered as often as every 15 minutes until the pain subsides. Head elevation and ice bags applied to the cervical region minimize swelling and discomfort. Blood pressure elevation is noted routinely for several hours after phenol peeling. However no treatment is required unless the patient is hypertensive or the degree of elevation is excessive. A systolic pressure greater than 160 mm Hg is treated with sublingual nitroglycerin, procardia, or IV promethazine.

- Postoperative days 1 and 2. If the home environment is satisfactory, healthy patients may be discharged after 3 to 6 hours in the recovery room; otherwise, the patient is kept in an overnight facility or hospital for 1 to 2 days. The tape is left on for 2 days. During this period, chewing and talking should be kept to a minimum. Visiting is discouraged while the tape is in place. To limit facial movements, it is recommended that a pad and pencil be used for communication and that a soft diet be followed. To minimize facial edema the patient's head should be elevated 30 to 45°; a diuretic (furosemide, 20 mg every morning with orange juice) should be prescribed; and the patient should be sedated adequately (diazepam, 5 mg 2 or 3 times a day).
- Postoperative days 3 to 14. After 1 or 2 days the tape is removed. The patient is sedated with 5 to 10 mg diazepam and given 25 mg meperidine IV (or Mepergan Fortis, orally) in preparation for tape removal. The use of a room humidifier augments the wetness that normally occurs beneath the tape and greatly facilitates the tape's removal. After tape removal, the patient's face is coated with thymol iodide powder for 4 days. At this time (postoperative day 6), the patient coats the dry crust with petroleum jelly. Crust separation is further hastened by encouraging sweating (warm room and warm beverages) beneath the petroleum jelly-sealed crust. That same evening, the patient is instructed to rinse the hair and face in a shower. Most of the crust

separates at this time. The patient is cautioned not to remove any adherent crust. Once the crust has separated, a burning discomfort or itching occurs. The patient is told that these symptoms can be treated with cool tap compresses, oral hydroxyzine, and mild analgesics. Ten to 14 days after the phenol peel application, the patient returns for a session with the skin care and makeup assistant. Proper skin care, makeup technique, and hairstyling instructions are instituted. The skin care brochure that was given to the patient preoperatively is reviewed at this time. This approach minimizes the demands on the plastic surgeon's time as well as the incidence and degree of any postoperative anxiety during this violaceous period.

- Late postoperative management. From 2 weeks to 6 months after phenol peeling patient management is primarily centered around appropriate skin care and protection from solar exposure. For more detailed instructions, refer to the late postoperative management instructions for TCA peels later in this chapter.

B. Trichloroacetic acid peels

- Recovery room. Sedation and recovery room care are only required for total face peels or if large areas of the extremities and trunk are being peeled. In these cases minimal monitoring and recovery room care are required. Upon discharge, verbal and written instructions are provided to the caretaker as follows:
- Day 1. A thick layer of A&D ointment or petroleum jelly is applied with gloved fingertips or cotton-tipped swabs several times a day. On the evening of the TCA peel, the patient may rinse the hair and face with lukewarm water in the shower. Baby shampoo may be used on the hair.
- Day 2. A patient undergoing a total facial peel should be seen in the office so that additional peeling of skin areas may ensure more uniform results. Before this visit the patient should clean the face with Cetaphil and rinse in the shower without

reapplying A&D ointment. After this visit, the patient should continue with A&D ointment and the medications as prescribed (Cephalexin 500 mg twice a day, Lortabs or Darvocet-N 100 every 4 hours as needed, hydroxyzine 25 mg every 4 hours as needed for restlessness, itching, and sleep).

- Day 3. Continue A&D ointment several times a day and shower at bedtime using either Cetaphil or Neutrogena soap.
- Days 4 and 5. Gently clean the face with Cetaphil and rinse with lukewarm water in the shower. Baby shampoo may be used for the hair. A second office appointment should be made for day 5 or day 6; during this visit patient is given instructions for future skin care. General instructions include the use of 1% hydrocortisone cream for itching and for areas of intense erythema. Photoplex sunscreen should be applied every morning or before leaving the indoor environment. Water-based makeup (Clinique, Clarens) may be used in areas where the peeling is complete. Hydroxyzine 25 to 50 mg may be used at bedtime for itching and insomnia.
- After day 5. The erythema may intensify until flaking subsides. Reepithelialization should be evident within 5 to 7 days. Within 1 week the erythema should resemble a light sunburn. Near complete fading of the erythema should occur within 3 weeks. During the period of erythema the patient is placed on a combination of skin care products as follows:

    - Hydrocortisone cream 1% twice a day
    - Fluocinonide (Lidex) or flurandrenolide (Cordran) cream if excessive erythema occurs or areas of eminent scarring appear
    - Neutrogena (SPF 17) chemical-free sunblock or comparable sunscreen with high skin protection factor (SPF), no para-aminobenzoic acid (PABA), and compatible with tretinoin, applied before sun exposure

- Retin-A cream 0.05% starts 7 to 10 days postpeel. Tretinoin stimulates reepithelialization and enhances the results from TCA peels. If the patient is intolerant to tretinoin, a glycolic acid preparation may be used as a substitute. Tretinoin is applied every second or third night depending on patient tolerability.
- Hydroquinone 4% with sunscreen (Solaquin Forte gel or cream) is started 7 days after TCA peeling. Prepeel and postpeel preparation with a hydroquinone product minimizes the risk of hyperpigmentation.
- Skin cleansers. Ordinary soaps are generally avoided. The patient is given a choice of cleansing agents (Cetaphil or Clarens) versus Neutrogena soap.
- Bleaching agents. Solaquin Forte containing 4% hydroquinone is routinely prescribed, especially in patients who develop excessive or diffuse areas of hyperpigmentation.
- Silastic sheeting. If the patient develops any areas of intense erythema associated with induration (eminent or early scarring), the areas are treated with Silastic sheeting applied 24 hr/day according to the manufacturer's instructions. Early treatment with Silastic sheeting usually prevents permanent scarring.
- Repeat peeling with TCA is performed within 1 to 3 months. No repeat peeling is normally required with phenol peels. If hyperpigmentation from the TCA peel is not responsive to conservative treatment (tretinoin, glycolic acid, hydroquinone, sunscreens, steroids), then a subsequent peel in 3 to 6 months may be performed with glycolic acid (50% to 70%), TCA, or in select cases, phenol.

▼ Late postoperative management. The late postpeel management of phenol patients is similar to the care provided for TCA-peeled patients. However, the resolution and recovery is more prolonged, and the protection from solar exposure is more strictly enforced. Milia are more likely to occur after phenol peeling and are avoided by restricting the use of moisturizers or oily skin care products (use of noncomedogenic products) during the period of erythema. Although secondary peeling of the face is not necessary with phenol peels, the neck and "V-line" areas may be peeled with TCA 3 to 6 months later. Occasionally areas of pigmentary demarcation (especially along the border of the mandible) may be minimized with TCA glycolic acid 3 to 6 months after phenol peeling of the face.

▼ Makeup technique. The patient may begin applying camouflage and makeup within 5 to 7 days after TCA peeling and within 10 to 14 days after phenol peeling. The first application is performed by a makeup artist under the supervision of the plastic surgeon. Generally, water-based, hypoallergenic (fragrance-free) products are recommended (Clinique, Clarens, Revlon Formula 2). Many products either include a sunscreening agent or may be applied over a sunscreen base. In addition, a lime-colored foundation may be used to minimize the noticeability of the cutaneous erythema. Makeup may be removed with a skin cleanser (Cetaphil, Clarens), cold cream, or Neutrogena soap. The patient should avoid contact with irritating chemicals such as hairsprays, perfumes, soaps, and astringents.

DERMABRASION

Patient Selection

Patient selection is based on the patient's facial skin pathologic findings, complexion type, and psychologic makeup.

A. **Skin pathologic findings.** The more common indications for surgical planning include acne scars and pockmarks, deep facial rhytids, facial scarring with surface irregularities, certain keratoses, rhinophyma, and certain diffuse tumorous conditions of the face (e.g., neurofibromatosis, hemangiomatosis, and certain pigmented lesions).

B. **Patient's complexion type.** As is true in chemical peeling with phenol, dark-skinned individuals do poorly because the treated areas often become darker. Patients who respond best to dermabrasion are those with moderate to superficial pitting irregularities.

C. **Patient's psychologic makeup.** As was explained previously, psychologic makeup and motivation must be carefully considered before surgery. A patient unable to accept the inconvenience of erythema, edema, and discomfort should be rejected for treatment. Sometimes the patient's expectations may be unrealistic with respect to results and potential risks.

Preoperative Consultation and Preparation

Preoperative management is largely the same as that for chemical peel patients. History and physical examination determine anesthetic and surgical techniques. Basic laboratory tests and photographs are completed before surgery. Dermatologic care to control acne formation is provided when necessary. As with TCA peeling, the patient's skin is primed with tretinoin and hydroquinone. Acutane must be discontinued for at least 6 months before facial dermabrasion or chemical peeling to reduce the incidence of hypertrophic scarring.

Anesthesia and Intraoperative Management

In addition to the usual preoperative drugs for relaxation and pain relief, this author prefers disassociative anesthesia with ketamine. Other surgeons may prefer general anesthesia for total facial dermabrasion. During the period of ketamine amnesia and analgesia, the entire face is anesthetized with 0.5% lidocaine containing 1:200,000 epinephrine. Segmental facial sanding with continuous saline irrigations can then be performed without pain or discomfort. If necessary, the patient may be titrated with midazolam (Versed) and fentanyl. In some patients chemical peeling is performed after dermabrasion is completed. Phenol or TCA can be used over the dermabraded face whereas TCA is applied to the neck and V-line if needed.

Early Postoperative Care (First Two Weeks)

On completion of the dermabrasion or peeling, the treated area is coated with an ointment such as Bacitracin, Silvadene, or gentamicin (Garamycin). In addition to preoperative administration of a steroid methylprednisolone (Solu-Medrol) and an antihistamine (diphenhydramine), facial edema may be minimized with head elevation, cold compresses, and diuretics.

A. **Postoperative days 4 and 5.** A topical ointment gentamicin (Garamycin or bacitracin) is continued for 5 days postoperatively. The patient is allowed to shower and rinse with baby shampoo. If excessive exudate develops, these areas may be gently cleansed with 3% hydrogen peroxide. Drugs prescribed during this postoperative period include Mepergan-Forte (meperidine with promethazine) every 4 hours as needed for pain; hydroxyzine 25 mg every 4 hours as needed restlessness or nausea; cephalexin 500 mg twice a day and flurazepam 30 mg every 4 hours as needed for sleep. Mastication and talking are kept to a minimum. The patient is cautioned not to remove any well-attached crust and not to irritate the face by scratching.

B. **Postoperative days 6 to 14.** After separation of the crust, the facial skin is kept free of oils. Topical steroidal creams, tretinoin, Neo-Strata gel (glycolic acid, hydroquinone) are resumed as tolerated. An appropriate nonoily sunscreen is prescribed, and sun exposure is restricted during the period of erythema. Tap water compresses, aspirin, and hydroxyzine are used to control burning and itching. A makeup session and more detailed skin care instructions can be provided by a trained makeup assistant. Continuous psychologic reinforcement and encouragement help to minimize the duration of postoperative depression during this period of unsightliness.

Late Postoperative Care (Two Weeks to One Year)

At this point, patient care includes treatment of the various sequelae that may occur after dermabrasion. Additional procedures may be performed to enhance results during the period of resolution. These ancillary procedures include additional dermabrasions (more localized), chemobrasion (TCA or phenol), scar revisions, collagen injections, fat injections, and skin care with the various products previously described. Some potential side effects and their management are as follows:

A. **Erythema.** Excessive erythema may be minimized by eliminating the use of refrigerants such as Freon. Proper makeup technique and skin care will decrease the degree of erythema, which may last 3 to 6 months. Potent steroidal creams (Lidex, Cordran, etc.) are applied to localized areas of intense erythema or areas of impending scarring.

B. **Milia or keratotic microcysts.** These are prevented or treated with proper skin care. This includes washing the skin with Neutrogena soap for oil skin with a loofah sponge. Larger cysts are punctured and evacuated with a needle. Excessive oiliness is also minimized with water-based cosmetics and the use of mild astringents. Moisturizers and oil skin lotions are avoided. Foods and drugs that increase skin oiliness are also avoided.

C. **Pigment alteration.** Hypopigmentation may be minimized by avoiding the use of refrigerants and reducing the depth of sanding. Hyperpigmentation occurs in 15% of patients after dermabrasion and may be reduced by avoiding exposure to sun during the period of erythema. Sunscreens, special makeup technique, and bleaching agents are used both before and after dermabrasions to minimize the risk of pigmentary changes.

D. **Pyoderma.** Pyoderma sometimes occurs; it is best treated with specific antibiotic therapy, warm compresses, and judicial surgical drainage.

E. **Hypertrophic scarring or keloid formation.** This sequel to sanding is usually caused by too-deep dermabrasions, keloid-predisposed skin, or pyoderma. Inadequate irrigation (abrasive burns), refrigerant burns and the use of Acutane can also be contributing causes. The early application of Silastic sheeting to eminent areas of scarring has been successful in prevention and treatment. Steroidal tapes, intralesional steroids, and Jobst pressure appliances may also minimize scarring. Surgical revisions should not be attempted for at least 1 year.

F. **Residual deformity.** Patients with deep surface irregularities must be warned preoperatively of the limitations of dermabrasion and peeling. Realistic expectations on the patient's part cannot be overemphasized. When treatment of these difficult patients is pursued, the need for additional dermabrasions, peeling, collagen, fat injections, long-term skin care or any combinations of these must be emphasized before any initial treatment. A good model regimen for this type of patient (diffuse facial scarring with multiple areas of deep acne scarring) may include the following:

- Stage I. Total facial dermabrasion with simultaneous chemobrasion (TCA versus phenol), scar revisions of the deeper scars, fat injections for contour irregularities
- Stage II (1 to 3 months later). TCA peeling plus additional fat injections, continue prepeel and postpeel skin care including tretinoin and Solaquin Forte
- Stage III (6 to 12 months later). Additional localized dermabrasions, peels, scar revisions, and fat injections as indicated

In older patients (35 years of age or older), rhytidoplasties of varying extent can significantly minimize deformities if facial scarring is associated with some facial laxity.

CHAPTER 19

Injection Surgery

Robert A. Ersek

HISTORIC BACKGROUND

The popularity of liposuction for subtraction of figure faults has rekindled interest in the idea of injection surgery to fill indentations. After Illous, Bricoll, and others first described the processing of autologous fat for injection in 1984 and a few early successes with the procedure were enthusiastically reported, many physicians throughout the world began injecting autologous fat to correct indentations from overzealous liposuction, glabella frown wrinkles, nasal labial folds, atrophic cheeks, and atrophic subcutaneous layer of the hands. These initial attempts were generally abandoned because of resorption of the injected fat.

In the 1970s the development of a purified bovine collagen used for injection created a interest in the intradermal placement of foreign substances to augment the skin or to eliminate wrinkles. Although the collagen did not last long (a few months or less), its initial effect was dramatic. Fibrel was an autologous source of collagen that was also used with similar results.

In the 1980s the development of textured breast implants that allowed some tissue ingrowth in the hostprostheses interface surface led to the miniaturization of these implants into tiny spheroids with a textured surface. Attempts to inject such microspheroids were possible only with the 1987 development of a biocompatible get carrier called *Bioplastique,* a biphasic copolymer consisting of fully vulcanized and polymerized, textured dimethyl siloxane microparticles (between 100 and 500 micrometers) suspended in a biocompatible hydrogel (Fig. 19-1). Once injected through a can-

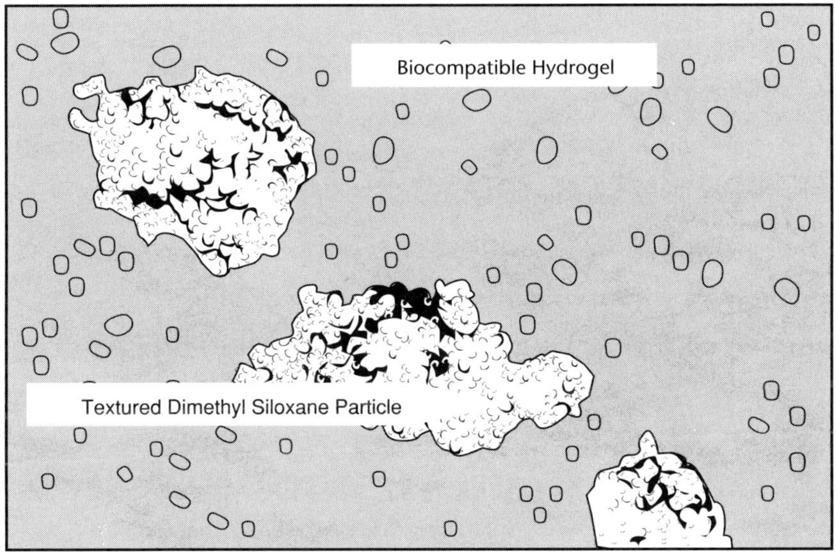

FIG. 19-1 *Biocompatible hydrogel acts as spacer so that microparticles have some distance between them. Here, microparticles are seen on a background of red blood cells (8 micrometers in diameter).*

nula as small as a 20 gauge, the hydrogel quickly disperses because of osmotic gradation and the pinocytosis method removes it from the body. (Fig. 19-2). Tissue fluid containing fibrinogen enters the space, and fibrinogen converts to fibrin. This fibrin holds the particles in place for a few days while fibroblasts secrete collagen fibrils in the space (Figs. 19-3, 19-4).

Clinical use of Bioplastique began in 1989. Since then, thousands of patients have been treated with this method throughout the world. Currently, 10 independent institution review board (IRB) protocols have been completed, and general use of the substance awaits formal approvals. Table 19-1 compares the various fillers that have been used for correction of facial scars and contour defects. The clinical experience supports the experimental evidence that Bioplastique has minimal complications and permanent benefits. This new technique of injection surgery enables permanent correction of a wide variety of small subcutaneous

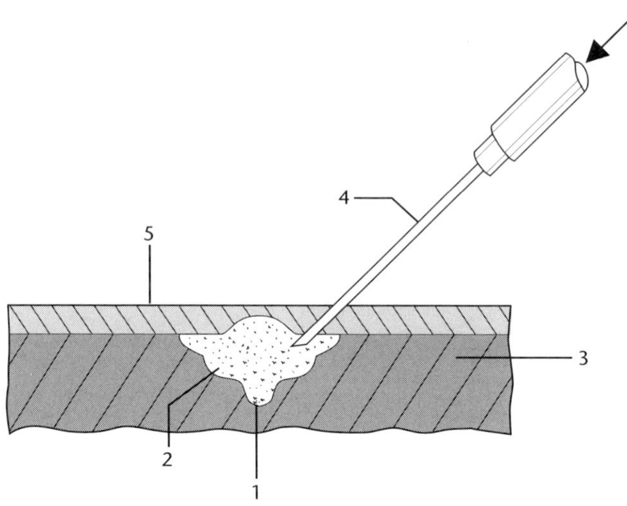

Fig. 19-2 *Microparticles in gel suspension (1) inserted under the skin into subcutaneous plane (2) well beneath the dermal surface (3). A 20-gauge (or larger) needle (4) used to pierce epidermis (5).*

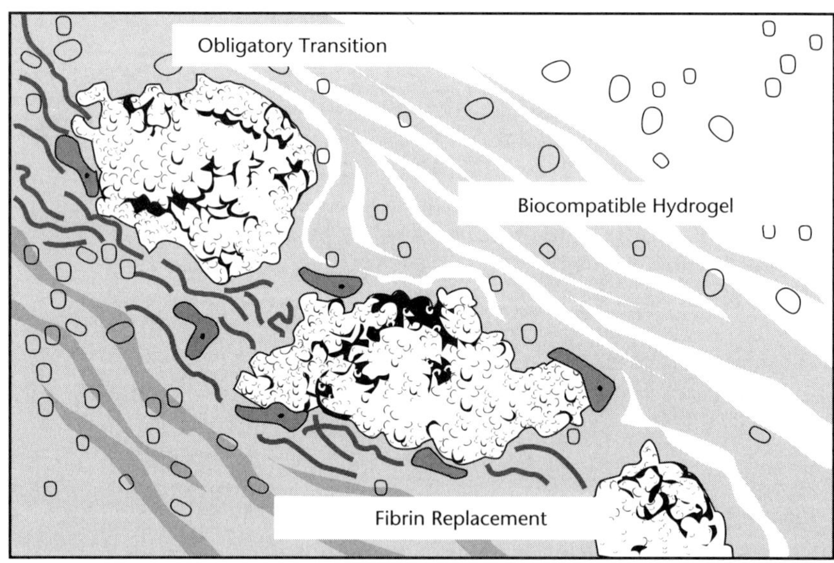

Fig. 19-3. *Because of an osmotic gradient, there is an obligatory transition so that the biocompatible hydrogel is removed by pinocytosis and replaced by host-tissue fluid, which contains fibrinogen. Fibrinogen converts to fibrin. This is a host gel replacement that holds particles in place for several days.*

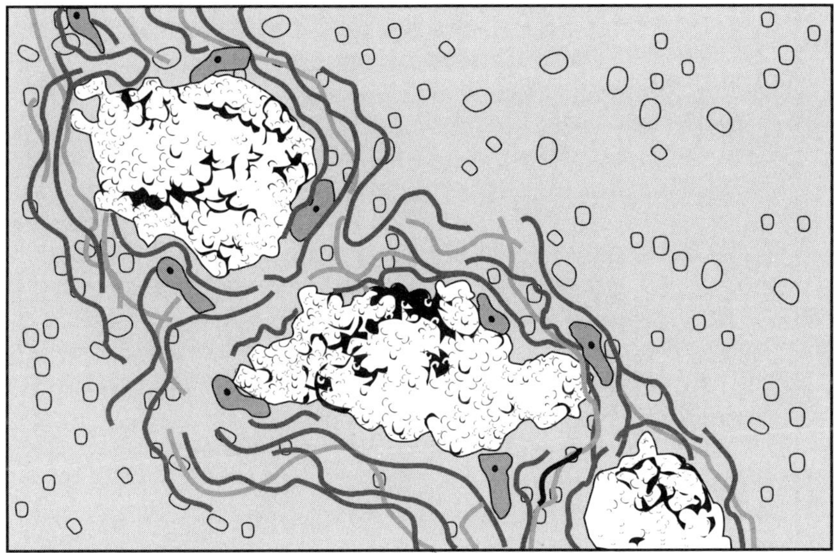

FIG. 19-4 *As inflammatory phase of wound healing subsides, host fibrin is replaced by collagen strands, thus anchoring all particles permanently in place.*

indentations of the skin, masal tip and dorsum elevations, and chin, cheek, and malar bone augmentations. The most useful application seems to be in chin and cheek augmentations. There have been some problems when too much material has been injected, especially in the lips, Injection of Bioplastique has now become the treatment of choice for ureteral reflux in children and urethral and bladder-neck incontinence in older women. For these conditions, a submucosal injection of a few milliters can immediately prevent ureteral reflux or bladder-neck incontinence. Augmentation of the vocal chords is another use of Bioplastique that is under investigation.

TECHNIQUE

General Approach

Defects as large as several centimeters in volume can be corrected by injecting Bioplastique, but special techniques are required to avoid lumping and bumping and blisters or blebs. If the biphasic copolymer is injected as a bolus, the

Table 19-1 *Comparison of Fillers Used For Facial Scars and Contour Defects*

Product	Indications	Procedural time	Procedure	Skin plane placement	Injectable needle/cannula	Anesthetic	Complications	Treatment visits	Efficacy
Bioplastique	Acne scars, deep wrinkles, contour defects	15-30 min	Prepackaged material injected through microcannula	Deep subdermal, subdermal	20-gauge micro cannula	Lidocaine, adrenalin	Redness, swelling (transient)	1-2	Permanent
Injectable Collagen (Zyderm-Zyplast) Purified bovine collagen suspension	Shallow to deep wrinkles, acne scars	15-30 min	Prepackaged material injected	High to middermis	30-gauge (thin) needle	Lidocaine included in syringe	Redness, swelling (transient)	1-4	6-20 months before correction subsides
Fibrel Plasma from patient's blood with bovine and porcine molecularly-altered collagen	Acne scars	60-75 min	Blood drawn from patient: plasma mixed with gelatin and reinjected into desired site	Dermis-subcutaneous (fat) juncture	20- or 21-gauge needle	Lidocaine	Redness, swelling (transient)	2-3	Not established for scar treatment because of small sample size; not tested for wrinkle treatment
Autologous Fat Patient's recycled fat	Atrophy, deep furrows	60-90 min	Fat withdrawn from donor site and reinjected into furrows	Subcutaneous (fat)	18- to 20-gauge (large) needle	Lidocaine	Contour irregularities infection (transient)	1	30% correction remaining at 1 year
Liquid Silicone synthetic polymer (source unknown)	Shallow to deep wrinkles, acne scars	15-30 min	Material is injected	Dermal-subcutaneous (fat) juncture	30-gauge (thin) needle	None	Redness, swelling (transient), inflammation (chronic), overcorrection (permanent), migration	6-12	1-3 years before correction subsides

particles may shift from one side of the bolus to the other during the healing phase, whereas if the biphasic copolymer is placed in a multitude of tiny tunnels (like fat suction in reverse), the host-prostheses interface and the surface-to-volume ratio greatly increases so that there is a vast active healing surface for a small volume of material. In this way, the encapsulation is uniform. Because infection of any kind could be devastating to the microimplants, surgical preparations and sterile gloves are required for safe injection surgery. Injections through multiple tunnels must be done through a remote puncture site because, if the entrance site were directly over the area of injection, any pressure within that area would cause oozing of the particles during the few days of instability. Presence of these particles at the skin entrance site results in a persistent lump and prevents healing. After placement, this surrounding area is splinted with stretch tape or microfoam to hold these particles in place for approximately 1 week.

Ten Steps for Safe Injection Surgery

The plastic surgeon should use the following steps to ensure safe injection surgery:

- Surgically prepare and mark the defect. Outline the defect carefully using a surgical marking pen.
- Wear sterile gloves to minimize any transcutaneous contamination because even minimal injection or inflammation at the time of implantation may distort the final results.
- Use adrenalin in the preoperative local anesthesia to maximize vascular constriction and minimize subcutaneous bleeding. Precise placement of Bioplastique in the tunnels and orderly dynamic substitution of the gel component with host fibrin depends upon minimal bleeding at the implantation site.
- Puncture remotely away from the intended augmentation site. This will allow precise placement of the microparticles and help avoid any seepage from the puncture opening. If a 20-gauge cannula is to be used, a 20-gauge sharp needle serves as a puncture-site lancet.
- Pretunneling should be done. If the defect is scar tissue, it is absolutely necessary that pretunneling be accomplished

with a blunt, pencil-pointed trocar or similar device The bluntness of the tip allows the tissue to be separated rather than cut thus bleeding is avoided. In the case of normal soft tissue, the blunt injection dissects through the subdermal plane to the tissue defect.

- ▼ Crisscross the tunnels, placing them in multiple planes of tissue. This allows for the greatest dynamic transition of the carrier gel with the host fibrin and allows the surgeon to correct larger defects evenly by making many small deposits.
- ▼ Inject only upon withdrawal after dissecting with the blunt cannula in soft tissue or into the pretunneling made in areas of scar. By carefully injecting on withdrawal and stopping as the cannula passes the defect, precise portions of Bioplastique can be placed within the tunnels, avoiding problems of subcutaneous splattering or particle migration.
- ▼ Place gentle pressure on the cannula tract between the puncture site and the injection site, and quickly remove the cannula. Rinse the entrance site with local anesthesia following injection. Rinsing prevents any of the Bioplastique from being deposited in the wound itself, which could result in visible and palpable eruptions of material.
- ▼ Splint the surrounding site with Suture Strips for several days after the procedure. This will immobilize the area until the vehicle gel is replaced with host collagen during the phase of dynamic transition.
- ▼ If undercorrection occurs, wait 6 weeks to reinject. At this time, all wound healing has been completed, and the defect should be in the final stages of collagen replacement. All host collagen has been converted to mature collagen. It is only at 6 weeks that final dimensions of the augmentation can be accurately assessed and the need for subsequent procedures can be determined.
- ▼ Never overcorrect because the biphasic copolymer will induce orderly and complete transformation between the carrier gel and the host collagen. However, if over-

correction does occur, Bioplastique and portions of its encasing collagen network can be removed with a micro-liposuction technique.

▼ Particulate injection must always be beneath the skin and never in the scar or dermis.

FURTHER READINGS

Allen O: Response to subdermal implantation of textured microimplants in humans, *Aesthetic Plast Surg* 16:227, 1992.

Chajchir A, Benzaquen I: Fat-grafting injection for soft tissue augmentation, *Plast Reconstr Surg* 87:219, 1991.

Ellenbogen R: Free Autogenous pearl fat grafts in the face: a preliminary report of a rediscovered technique, *Ann Plast Surg* 16:179, 1986.

Ersek RA: Molecular Impact Surface Textured Implants (MISTI) alter beneficially breast capsule formation at 36 months, *J Long-Term Effects Med Implants* 1(2):155, 1991.

Ersek RA: Transplantation of purified autologous fat: a 3-year follow-up is disappointing, *Plast Reconstr Surg* 87(2):219, 1991.

Ersek RA, Beisang AA III: Mammalian response to subdermal implantation of textured microimplants, *Aesthetic Plast Surg* 16:83, 1992.

Ersek RA, Beisang AA III: Bioplastique: a new biphasic polymer for minimally invasive injection implantation, *Aesthetic Plast Surg* 16:59, 1992.

Ersek RA, Beisang AA III: Bioplastique: a new textured copolymer microparticle promises permanence in soft-tissue augmentation, *Plast Reconstr Surg* 87(4):693, 1991.

Ersek RA, Stoual RB, Salisbury AV: Chin augmentation using minimally invasive technique and bioplastique, *Plast Reconstr Surg* 95(6) 985, 1995.

Hetter GP: *Lipoplasty: the theory and practice of blunt suction lipectomy,* Boston, 1984, Little, Brown.

Illouz YG: "The fat cell graft": a new technique to fill depressions, *Plast Reconstr Surg* 78(1):122, 1986.

Illouz YG: Origins of lipolisis. In Hetter GP (editor): *Lipoplasty: the theory and practice of blunt suction lipectomy,* Boston, 1984, Little, Brown, pp. 25-32.

Matsudo PKR, Toledo LS: Experience of injected fat grafting, *Aesth Plast Surg* 12:35, 1988.

Mladick RA: Twelve months of experience with Bioplastique, *Aesthetic Plast Surg* 16:69, 1992.

Planas J, Del Cacho C: 20 years of experience with particulate silicone in plastic surgery, *Aesthetic Plast Surg* 16:53, 1992.

CHAPTER 20

Surgical Hair Restoration

Martin L. Bell

The plastic surgeon has much to offer patients afflicted with male pattern baldness. Scalp reduction (staged excision of the bald scalp) and rotation flaps can greatly enhance the results previously obtained only by plug transplantation. Plug transplants, no longer the treatment of choice for vertex alopecia, still are crucial to front hairline reconstruction. They are also valuable in supplementing and augmenting the results of scalp reduction and flaps.

INITIAL CONSULTATION

Health History and Interview

A patient with male pattern baldness is approached by the plastic surgeon like any other person seeking cosmetic surgery. A thorough medical and psychologic history is obtained. Specific inquiry is made about bleeding problems or the use of aspirin or aspirin-containing products. Many patent medicines contain aspirin in disguise, so it is best to enumerate all medicines used. The anticoagulant effect of aspirin lasts several days after discontinued use of the drug.

Evaluation of Patient's Perception of Problem

After taking the health history, the patient's perception and understanding of the problem is then assessed. The patient is shown a chart depicting stages of baldness, as defined by Hamilton, and asked to identify the figure thought to be most representative (Fig. 20-1). Next the patient is asked to identify the baldest member of either side of the family. This will approximate the "worst case" prognosis if no reconstruction is undertaken. Finally, the patient should be shown that even the best reconstruction possible will bring the patient only as far as Class 3 to 3A. Currently a large

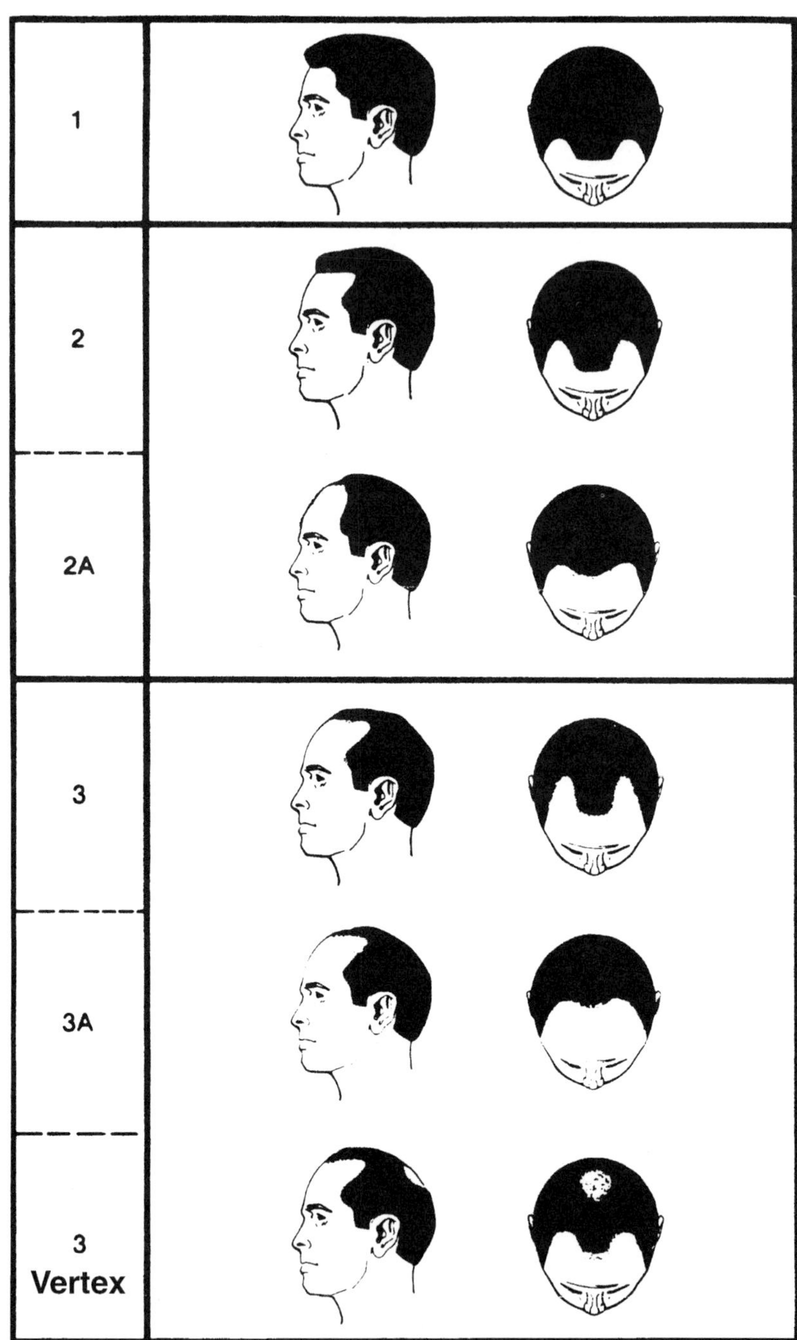

FIG. 20-1 *Classification of male pattern baldness.* (From Hamilton JB: Patterned loss of hair on man, *Ann Acad Sci,* 53:708, 1951.)

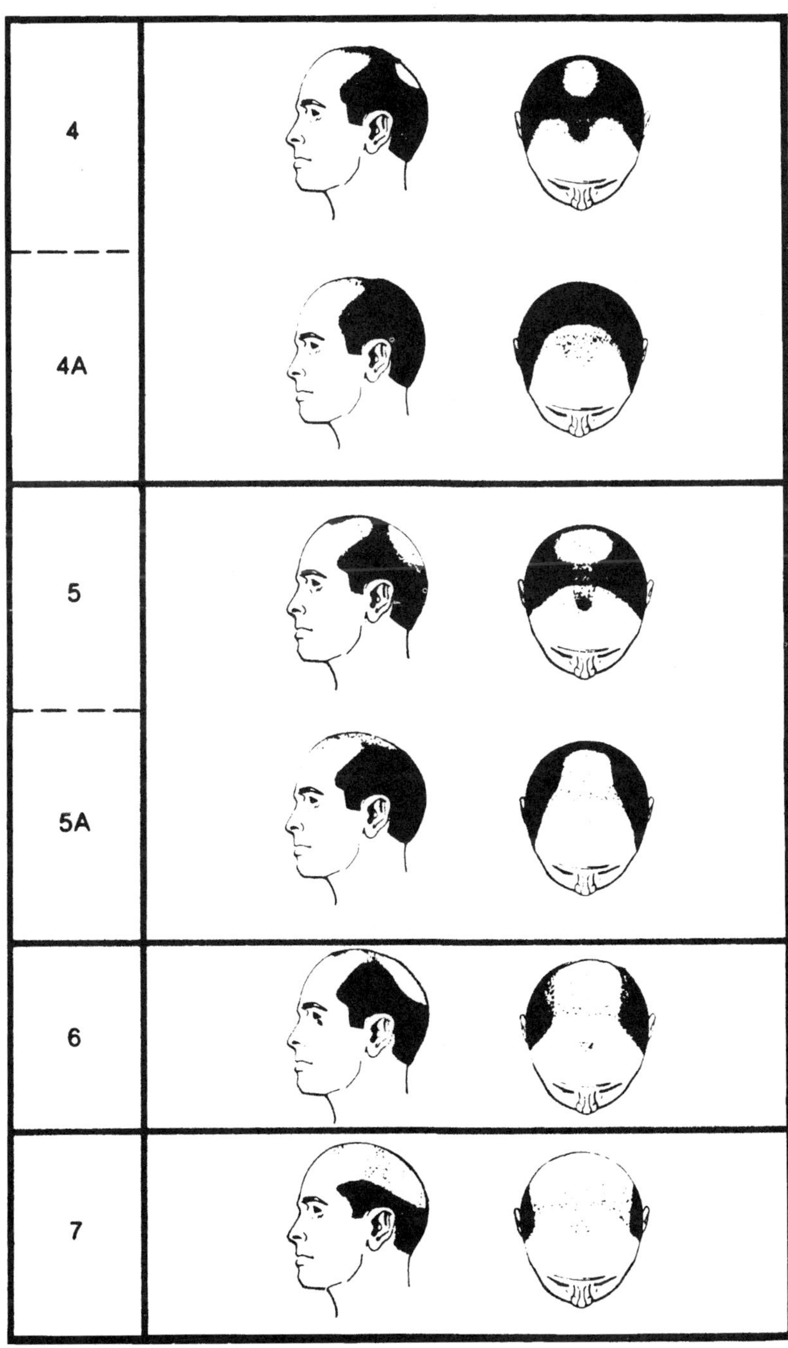

FIG. 20-1—*cont'd.*

percentage of patients may have tried minoxidil with disappointing results. A patients who wants to try topical therapy should be encouraged to do so for several months before surgery. This will dispel any notion that surgery was a mistake because good medical treatment was available. In this author's experience, a satisfactory result from minoxidil therapy has only occurred in the earliest stages of hair involution.

Scalp Examination, Formulation of Treatment Plan, and Patient Advice

A. **Candidates for scalp reduction.** This individual will fall between Class 3 vertex and Class 6. The principal variable here is *scalp flexibility.* Flexibility increases in proportion to age; however, there is a definite biologic or hereditary factor. On the ideal end of the spectrum is the relatively older person with intrinsically good scalp flexibility. On the other end is the younger person with a scalp that is tight. Experience suggests that only approximately 10% of patients need to be completely rejected because of poor scalp flexibility. However, a patient with a relatively tight scalp should be warned that more stages will be needed and the likelihood of complications at the suture line will increase. A patient with a moderate number of previous transplants generally falls into this category along with a long-term wearer of hairpieces. Faithful daily scalp massage, using a number of techniques, appears to significantly increase scalp flexibility. Scalp massage is recommended to intrinsically tight-scalped patients for 3 to 6 weeks preoperatively. The scalp should be checked for old laceration scars or other trauma. The shape and form of the permanent fringe should be measured and observed, and the density and quality of the remaining hair should be noted. Then, depending on the extent of alopecia, one to four staged excisions will be required.

B. **Candidates for scalp flaps.** This technique is most appropriate in the patient with a stable Class 3 pattern (no progressive baldness). Scalp flexibility must be sufficient to allow removal of a 2- to 3-cm wide flap from each temple without creating undue tension on the donor-site closure. Occasionally, a scalp reduction patient will have sufficient scalp flexibility remaining to allow anterior hairline reconstruction with flaps. Infrequently, a patient may be concerned only with the front hairline despite significant vertex alopecia. After careful explanation, the patient may choose flaps as primary therapy, thereby eliminating the scalp reduction option in most cases.

C. Hair transplants

- ▼ Indications. Plug transplantation is still the treatment of choice for minor degrees of temporal baldness, for anterior hairline reconstruction following scalp reduction, for augmentation of the results of scalp reduction at the vertex, and for camouflage of the scalp reduction scar. The quality, density and availability of donor hair must be suited to the desired result.
- ▼ Assessing and advising patients. The realism of the patient's expectations must be assessed by the plastic surgeon, and a realistic result must be conveyed.
  - ■ The tedious and time-consuming nature of the transplant process must be carefully explained to the patient, especially the delayed results. The common tendency of patients to abandon the process with incomplete results should be faced. In particular, the tendency of many physicians to perform hair transplants without patient sedation has created an inflated fear of pain in the public. This fear should be allayed because safe intravenous (IV) sedation with monitoring is now readily available.
  - ■ A suitable level for front hairline reconstruction is demonstrated to the patient. This is usually accomplished by using the "rule of thirds" (Fig. 20-2). This author believes a gently curved hairline is more natural than a "widow's peak" and makes better use of available donor hair. In any case, the proposed hairline is drawn on the forehead, and the patient's comments are invited by the surgeon.

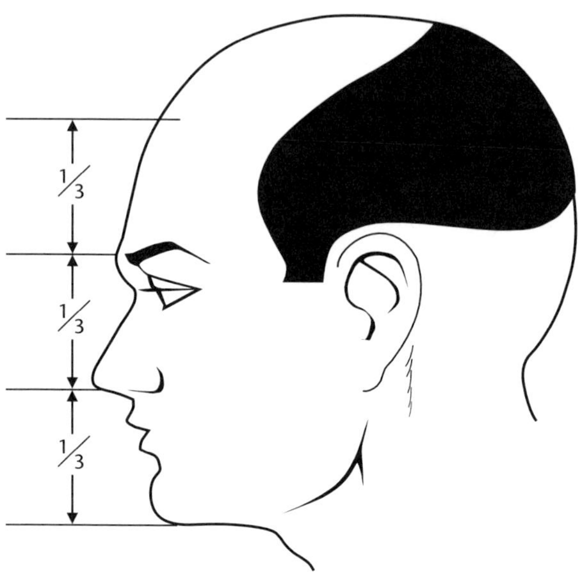

FIG. 20-2 *Rule of thirds used to reconstruct front hairline.*

- Available donor sites are discussed. The patient is reassured that full coverage of the donor site by surrounding hair will be possible and that donor site visibility after healing will not be a problem. Any anticipated donor site shortage is best addressed at this time.

Conclusion of Initial Consultation and Second Preoperative Consultation

- Upon conclusion of the initial consultation, a written brochure explaining the transplantation procedure is given to each patient, and a second preoperative consultation is arranged.
- At the time of the second consultation, additional questions are answered, a physical examination is done, and a hematocrit level is obtained. Written preoperative and postoperative instructions are furnished along with prescriptions for an analgesic and a prophylactic antibiotic of choice (cefadroxil [duricef] 500 mg by mouth 2 times a day) to be started 1 day preoperatively. Written informed consent is obtained from the patient.

INTRAOPERATIVE CARE

Sedation

IV sedation is essential for scalp reduction and flaps and is highly recommended for a hair transplant procedure involving more than 50 plugs. An identical technique is used for all three procedures. In my practice, sedation is administered by a qualified nurse anesthetist or physician anesthesiologist. A combination of midazolam (Versed) and fentanyl citrate (Sublimaze) can be used, supplemented if necessary with propofol (Diprivan). It should be emphasized that individual patient response to these agents is variable, and these agents should be titrated to effect by a practitioner skilled in their administration. A cardiac monitor and pulse oximetor are always used. If these agents are given too rapidly, the patient may have some respiratory depression requiring ventilatory support. Begin with the slow IV administration of midazolam, 2 to 5 mg, followed by fentanyl citrate, 50 to 150 micrograms (1 to 3 ml). During injection of local anesthesia, this may need to be supplemented with propofol 0.2 to 0.5 mg/kg.

Anesthesia

After IV sedation begin the administration of local anesthetic. Methohexital sodium in incremental doses of 10 mg may be given if needed to further sedate the patient. A ring block of the entire scalp is performed, using as much as 40 ml of 0.5 ml bupivacaine (Marcaine) with 1:200,000 adrenalin. The anesthetic is injected using 100 ml-finger tip-controlled syringes and 1 1/2-inch No. 25 needles. The block is kept well below any transplant donor or recipient sites or any scalp flap donor sites. For scalp reduction, a small amount of local anesthetic may be used to "balloon up" the area of scalp to be removed.

Scalp Reduction

The plan of excision must be individualized according to the baldness pattern and must take maximum advantage of scalp flexibility. Depending on the pattern, the supine, prone, or both positions may be used for the patient.

A. **Markings.** Generally, the center of a potential transplanted anterior hairline is located by the rule of thirds

(Fig. 20-2). Beginning three fourths of an inch behind this point, a midsaggital line is drawn extending approximately 1 inch into the permanent fringe. An anteroposteriorly directed ellipse is drawn with a maximum width of 3 to 4 cm, depending on the preoperative assessment of scalp flexibility (Fig. 20-3). Commonly there is a relative excess of permanent hair or especially good scalp flexibility or both in the occipital area. In such cases, a fishtail excision is added to the back end of the ellipse to allow greater advancement of hair. This is generally done only on the first scalp reduction. Subsequent reductions are done through the previous scar in similar fashion. Especially in Class 4 or 5 situations, the incision may be placed along the edge of one half to two thirds of the bald spot (Fig. 20-4). At the next stage, a contralateral approach is used. Finally, the remaining central scalp is excised.

B. Operative procedure

- ▼ The scalp reduction procedure is begun with an incision along one side of the pattern.
- ▼ Wide undermining is performed in the loose areolar plane between the galea and the periosteum. Undermining should be extensive laterally, less so anteriorly, and minimal posteriorly. Care should be taken to minimize bleeding by close avoidance of origins of the frontalis and occipitalis muscles. Multiple parallel incisions in the galea are rarely helpful in gaining additional advancement of scalp. The undermining of the other side of the pattern is done through this single incision.
- ▼ Excision of the pattern is begun anteriorly, and closure with traction sutures of 2.0 silk is begun several centimeters in front of the excision (Fig. 20-5). By performing excision and closure in simultaneous sequence, one does not commit oneself to the width of excision until the last possible moment. In this way, a maximum width consistent with reasonable tension on the closure can be excised.
- ▼ A layer of buried 2.0 absorbable suture is placed in the galea, and a running locked 4.0 nylon is placed

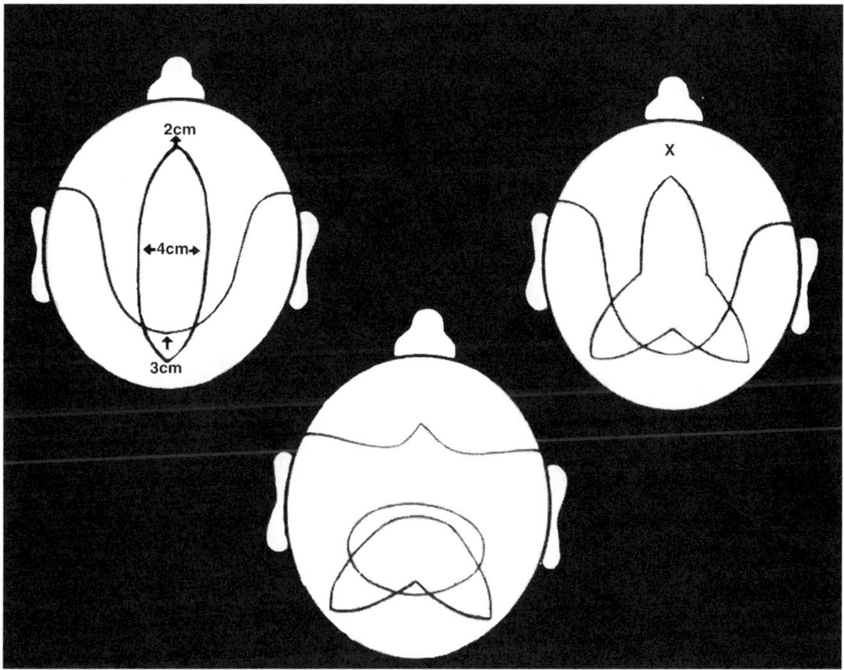

FIG. 20-3 *Commonly used patterns for scalp reduction.*
(From Bell ML: Role of scalp reduction in the treatment of male pattern baldness, *Plast Reconstr Surg,* 69:272, 1982.)

in the skin. An absorbent compression bandage is applied for 48 hours, then the patient usually removes the bandage and washes the hair.

C. **Follow-up.** The patient returns for suture removal in 10 days. After maximum benefit has been obtained by scalp reduction, plug transplants may be added for density at the vertex, to camouflage the scar, or for anterior hairline reconstruction.

Scalp Flaps

I prefer staged unilateral temporal flaps of the design described by Elliott and Stough (Fig. 20-6). Surgical delay is not routinely necessary for flaps of sufficient length to reach each other in the midline.

A. **Markings.** A front hairline is established by the rule of thirds described previously (See Fig. 20-2.).

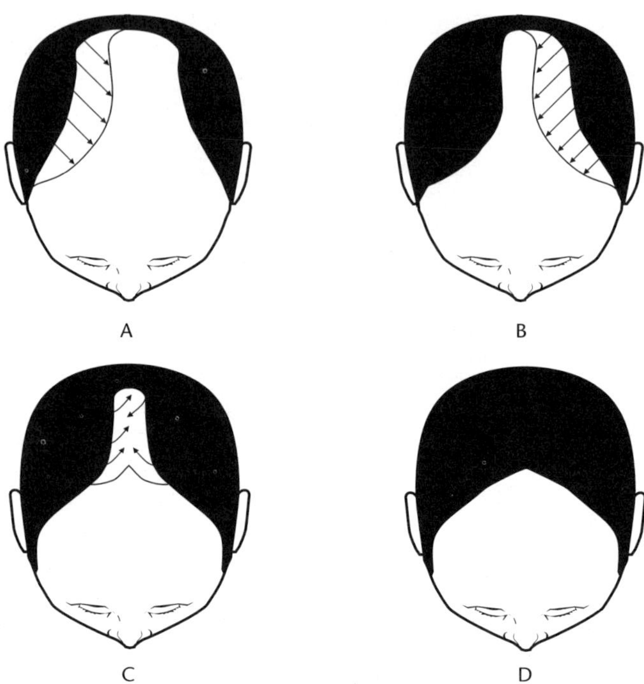

Fig. 20-4 *Incisions placed along edge of one half to two thirds of bald spot.*

B. **Operative procedure.** The design of the flap is illustrated in Figure 20-6. The width is kept uniform at 2 cm, and the length is 7 to 10 cm. The flap is raised beneath the galea, and the donor site is closed by undermining, mostly superiorly. The surgeon places a 2.0 interrupted Vicryl suture in the galea and a running locked suture of 3.0 nylon in the scalp.

- ▼ The flap is laid along the previously drawn anterior hairline, and an excision of bald scalp of comparable width is made. The flap is sutured anteriorly with a subcuticular 4.0 Prolene and posteriorly with interrupted 4.0 nylon. A "dog ear" is almost inevitable and often requires division and inset of the flap pedicle in 3 to 4 weeks.
- ▼ A similar absorbent dressing beneath a compression bandage is applied for 48 hours. Then the flap is checked, and the patient may wash the hair.

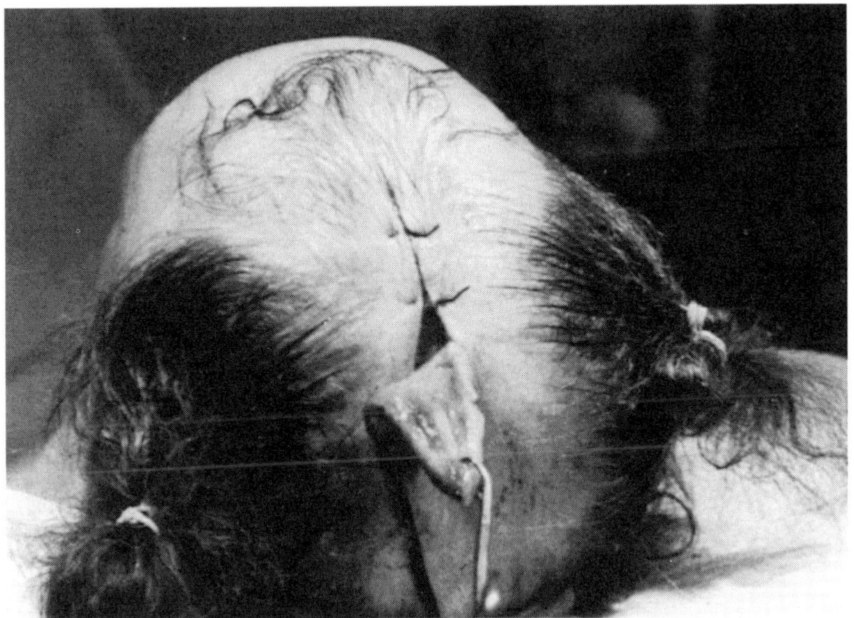

FIG. 20-5 *Simultaneous excision and closure is best way to avoid closure under undue tension.*
(From Bell ML: Alopecia reduction: complications of alopecia reduction and their management. In Unger WP (editor): *Hair transplantation,* ed 2, New York, 1988, Marcel Dekker.)

- Sutures are removed in 10 days. Any eschar formation is managed conservatively. Initial hair loss is unusual, but when it occurs a wait of 2 to 3 months for hair regrowth is prudent.
- In patients with exceptional scalp flexibility, the flaps may be done simultaneously without creating undue donor site tension. Ordinarily an interval of at least 6 weeks is advisable.

Hair Transplantation

The procedure is now used primarily for front hairline reconstruction and for added density and scar camouflage after scalp reduction on the vertex.

A. **Markings and operative planning.** The front hairline is established using the "method of thirds" (See Fig. 20-2.). A close estimate of the number and location of

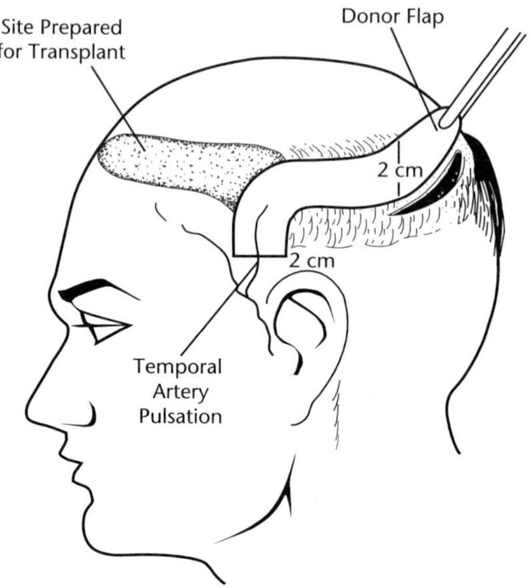

Fig. 20-6 *Unilateral temporal skin flaps.*
(Redrawn from Stough III DB, Cates JA: Transposition flaps for the correction of baldness: a practical office procedure, *J Dermatol Surg Oncol* 6(4): 286–289, 1980.)

plugs is obtained by making dots with gentian violet. Two to three transplant sessions are generally planned to allow adequate spacing of the plugs (Fig. 20-7). Mostly 3.0 mm plugs are used in the first two sessions giving way to mostly minigrafts and micrografts in later sessions. The proposed procedure is demonstrated to the patient in front of a mirror to gain approval. Surgical expenses are then explained. A donor site is chosen as high on the occiput as possible to maximize density and leave adequate surrounding hair to facilitate easy camouflage.

Whenever possible donor plugs are harvested in linear fashion, from one side of the occiput to the other, in two to three tightly spaced rows. This way the entire donor site may be excised. The excised scalp is used to make minigrafts and micrografts, and the donor site is sutured with running locked 4-0 Vicryl. The temporal scalp is a less desirable donor site for plugs but is often a preferred donor site for minigraft and micrografts.

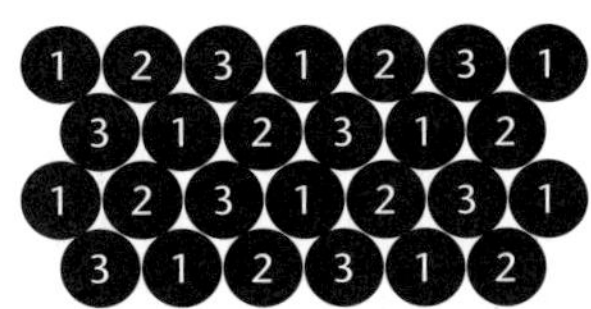

FIG. 20-7 *Orentreich method of filling in alopecia in three stages.*

B. Operative procedure

- ▼ It should be reemphasized that IV sedation, followed by ring block of the entire scalp, is required for reasonable patient comfort and to avoid abandonment of future procedures caused by operative pain. Once the block is in place, the sedation is usually allowed to wear off so that the patient can easily turn from the supine position to the prone or vice versa, as required.
- ▼ Plug recipient sites are prepared and donor plugs are harvested using sharp punches mounted on the Bell electric hand engine. The plug recipient sites are prepared first to allow maximum time for bleeding to subside before placement of the plugs. Recipient sites should usually be 3 mm in diameter. When they expand as a result of natural scalp elasticity, a 3.25-mm plug fits properly. Hemostasis is accomplished by direct pressure. Occasionally, topical thrombin spray is needed. Minigraft and micrograft recipient sites, mostly anterior to and between plug sites, are prepared later just before graft insertion by making 2- to 3-mm slits with a No. 15 scalpel blade.
- ▼ The patient is usually turned prone for harvesting of donor plugs. The donor site is ballooned out under pressure by injection of 50 to 100 ml of normal saline. This gives plump firm plugs, which are more easily trimmed, and it also helps hemostasis. Plugs are drilled parallel to the hair follicles and deep enough to come out with a generous pad of fat, well deep to the bulb of the hair shaft. Donor-site hemostasis is accomplished by pressure, but 3.0 Vicryl mattress sutures may be required. The plugs are placed in cool normal saline.

- The patient is then returned to the supine position if anterior grafts are to be placed. I clean all the plugs myself because this is the most critical aspect of the whole procedure. This is done under magnification to ensure that the bulbs at the base of the hair shafts are not exposed. A tiny pad of yellow fat must often be left behind to protect the bulb. As the plugs are cleaned, one or two assistants place them in recipient holes. Orientation of plugs is critical to ensure a natural direction of hair growth. Minigrafts and micrografts are prepared from strips of scalp by removing the epidermis and creating dermal strips containing two to six hair follicles using a No. 11 scalpel blade. These are laid out in rows of 10 onto a gauze pad wet with normal saline. When finished cleaning all the plugs and preparing minigrafts, I check the position and orientation of the plugs and place the minigrafts and micrografts. The latter is done by making slits with a No. 15 scalpel blade. As the blade is removed, an assistant places the tip of a Coddle elevator into the slit and turns it 45°. The graft is picked up gently by its dermal end with smooth tipped forceps and placed subcutaneously as the Coddle elevator is removed. Gentle pressure is momentarily applied with a cotton-tipped swab.
- Xeroform gauze is placed snugly over the plugs and also on the donor site. Finally, absorbent fluffed gauze, Kling, and an Ace wrap are applied.
- Postoperatively the dressing remains 4 to 5 days. Careful dressing removal in the office minimizes the danger of losing plugs in the bandage. The hair is gently washed with bland shampoo (Johnson's Baby Shampoo) and gently blown dry. The patient is reminded that any hair in the plugs will likely fall out after approximately a week and will not regrow for 2 to 3 months. The hair plug procedure may be repeated every 4 to 6 weeks until the patient and the surgeon are both satisfied.

CHAPTER 21

Maxillofacial Injuries

Richard C. Schultz

Every physician who attends patients with multiple system injuries should be familiar with the early management of facial trauma, even though a plastic surgeon may ultimately become responsible for the definitive treatment. An understanding of the needs of both the patient and the plastic surgeon relative to such trauma will give the physician the best perspective on the allocation of priorities.

A high percentage of patients coming to the emergency room (ER) with multiple system injuries will have sustained them in automobile accidents. Approximately 54% of these patients will have significant facial trauma. Typically, there will be soft-tissue injuries and facial bone fractures.

The early management of facial injuries is important in the outcome of those injuries, but the extent of the early treatment is dependent on the nature of such injuries. Even after the most competent management, sometimes complications occur after facial injury treatment, and these complications may eventually require complex multistaged reconstructive procedures.

TRIAGE

With respect to timing, definitive treatment of most facial injuries ordinarily deserves low priority in the total care of the patient with multiple injuries. With the exception of animal bites and accidental tattoos, treatment of soft-tissue trauma can usually be safely delayed for as long as 24 hours if the wound is given proper preparatory care. Most facial fractures are best treated several days after resorption of edema. Whether the delay is mandatory or elective, any neurologic, abdominal, thoracic, orthopedic, and urologic injuries should be given priority.

EMERGENCY MANAGEMENT

The priorities of early management for a patient with extensive facial trauma are the same as for a patient with any other trauma. They are (1) ensurance of a clear airway, (2) control of hemorrhage, (3) treatment of shock, and (4) evaluation of associated injuries. After these measures have been taken, the facial injuries can be evaluated, and when appropriate, treatment can be initiated.

Ensurance of Clear Airway

The causes of airway problems after facial trauma are varied. Obstruction from dentures, bone fragments, blood, or vomitus should be treated immediately by manual removal or aspiration. Although tracheostomy is often suggested for the patient with extensive facial injury, it is seldom indicated unless associated injuries of the head, neck, or chest are present. Occasionally the mandibular arch of a patient with a bilateral mandibular fracture will collapse, causing retrodisplacement of the tongue and subsequent airway obstruction, but such occurrence can usually be relieved by placing the patient in a sitting position, allowing the arch to fall forward.

Control of Hemorrhage

Hemorrhage from facial trauma usually will be diminished by the time the patient arrives in the ER. In most instances, persistent bleeding can be controlled by pressure alone; however, major vessels may have to be clamped and ligated through the wound. If so, care should be taken to avoid injury to important adjacent structures such as the facial nerve, parotid duct, or lacrimal sac.

Treatment of Shock

As with any other patient sustaining extensive trauma, shock must be treated aggressively. Blood loss from the facial injury alone is seldom of sufficient magnitude to cause hypotension; therefore, the shock is more likely to be due to neurologic or other associated injuries. Primary attention should be directed toward the facial injuries only after establishing that no other life-threatening injury needs immediate care. Although the relatively low priority of definitive facial injury treatment is stressed, it must also be emphasized that early evaluation cannot be ignored.

Evaluation of Injury

The facial injuries should be evaluated at the initial x-ray examination together with other system injuries. A minimum number of facial x-rays are required to supplement the plastic surgeon's clinical evaluation of facial fractures.

A. **Water's view (occipitomental).** This is the most valuable x-ray film for studying the maxilla, the zygoma, and the frontal sinuses.
B. **Oblique views.** These give the most information about fractures of the lower third of the face.
C. **Panorex view.** This view of the mandible may be included when available, for a more sophisticated view of the entire mandible on a single film.
D. **Computerized axial tomography.** This provides the most advanced radiographic evaluation of facial fractures. In complex cases of lost bone, volume three-dimensional computerized imaging may provide additional graphic representation of the extent and precise location of the defect.

The early taking of proper facial x-ray examinations should be stressed. If these are not taken early, difficult situations may develop later. For example, the plastic surgeon may be called to the operating room (OR) for concurrent treatment of facial injuries while a craniotomy, a laparotomy, or an orthopedic procedure is being performed. In this circumstance, the plastic surgeon would be treating the facial injuries without the necessary information that could have been available. Another problem is presented by the patient who has been set up in balanced orthopedic traction on the ward; the dilemma then is when to put the patient through the ordeal of a second trip to the radiology department to obtain the facial films.

The importance of routinely obtaining cervical spine x-ray films during the initial x-ray examination for the facial injuries must be emphasized. In a series of 400 patients with facial injuries of varied extent, 4% were found to have cervical spine fractures, many of which were asymptomatic.

SOFT-TISSUE INJURIES

Early Treatment

After hemostasis, the most important early treatment of soft-tissue injuries is cleansing of the wound. To cleanse the wound, wash the surrounding skin with soap or an antiseptic preparation (Betadine, pHisoHex or Hibiclens). Be careful to avoid soaking the wound itself with the solution. Irrigate the wound with saline solution by using a bulb syringe or a jet lavage. Solutions other than normal saline can be injurious to wounds and do not provide any significant antibacterial effect.

Injury Evaluation

In addition to documenting the injury by photography, magnetic resonance imaging (MRI) can localize and document soft-tissue masses and defects.

Timing of Soft-Tissue Repair

Ideally, the wound is treated definitively in the first few hours after injury. When definitive treatment is delayed however soft-tissue repair can safely be performed for as long as 24 hours after injury if the wound has been properly cleansed and dressed. The exceptions to this rule are animal bites and accidental tatoos, which should be treated soon after injury to reduce the likelihood of infection and tissue entrapment of foreign material.

Soft-Tissue Repair

The cheek is the area of the face most frequently lacerated. Deep structures of concern are the facial nerve, the parotid gland, and the parotid duct.

A. **Facial nerve injury.** Facial nerve injury should be diagnosed on the basis of physical examination and anatomic landmarks. Under ordinary circumstances, muscle paralysis on the involved side of the face indicates nerve injury. An uncooperative patient, an extensive soft-tissue injury, or extensive edema may make the physical examination inconclusive. A functional and cosmetic deformity results from an unrepaired proximal facial nerve laceration.

Most surgeons believe that division of branches of the facial nerve medial to the midpupillary line does not require repair. Branching cross-innervation is likely to reinnervate the appropriate muscle spontaneously. Lateral to the midpupillary line, nerve repair should be attempted to guide the advancing axons to the motor end-plate in the muscle.

B. **Parotid injury.** The parotid duct courses from the tragus of the ear to the midportion of the upper lip. It lies deep near the anterior border of the masseter muscle, emptying into the oral cavity adjacent to the first maxillary molar tooth (Fig. 21-1). It can be divided by a deep laceration posterior to the anterior border of the masseter muscle. Such lacerations also frequently damage the buccal branch of the facial nerve. When there is complete laceration of the parotid duct, end-to-end anastomosis over a small Silastic catheter can be performed. As an alternate procedure to maintain parotid function, the proximal cut end of the duct can be sutured to the oral mucosa.

When clear fluid is seen leaking from a wound in the parotid region, injury to the gland should be suspected. The gland itself need not be sutured. Salivary fistula is a common complication after skin repair of an underlying glandular laceration. The fistula usually closes without further treatment in approximately 3 weeks.

C. **Eyelid injury**

▼ Injuries to thin eyelid skin may result in small avulsion flaps having questionable viability. However, these flaps usually survive if replaced anatomically. Divided muscle and tarsal plate should be identified and sutured separately with fine absorbable suture. Simple direct anatomic repair is the best approach. The tarsal plate is adherent to the conjunctiva and can be repaired with the conjunctiva. Lacerations of the thin orbital septum usually do not require a separate closure provided that the orbicularis oculi muscle is repaired.

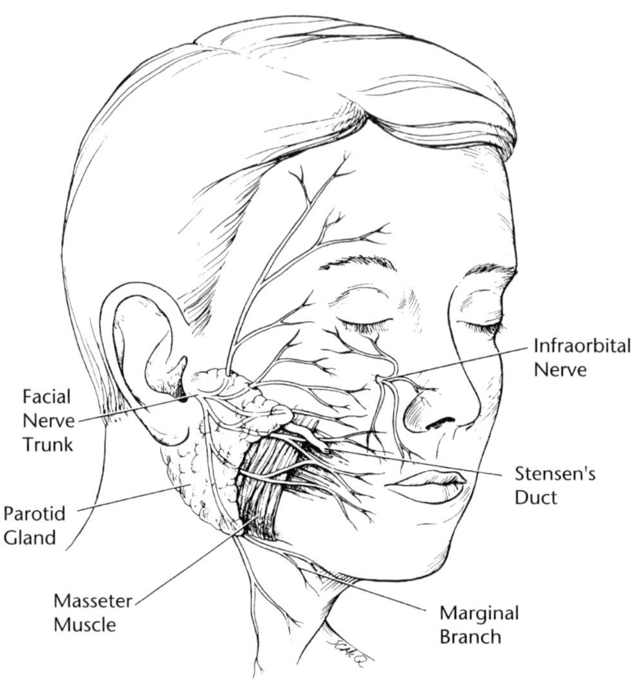

FIG. 21-1 *Soft-tissue anatomy of cheek showing relationships of facial nerve, parotid gland, parotid duct, and masseter muscle.*

▼ Lacerations of the lacrimal apparatus must be recognized and repaired to prevent postoperative epiphora and dacryocystitis. The divided lacrimal duct is cannulated with a heavy nylon suture and then reapproximated with fine absorbable sutures. After a week, the nylon stent is removed. Fine, soft polyethylene catheters can also be used for cannulation. When injury to the lacrimal system is severe, primary dacryorhinocystostomy should be considered.

FACIAL BONE FRACTURES

Diagnosis

The severity of soft-tissue destruction should not distract the physician from a complete examination of the facial skeleton. The initial x-ray film examination may not demonstrate facial fractures. As a result, the diagnosis of facial bone injuries may depend on the clinical evaluation alone.

Observation can disclose depressed frontal sinuses, a deviated nasal complex, a depressed zygoma, enophthalmos, an asymmetrical mandible, or a malaligned dental arch. Poor dental occlusion may be the first clue to mandibular or maxillary fracture. Diplopia may be the only positive finding associated with a fractured orbital floor.

Systematic bimanual palpation will help to avoid missing, less obvious fractures (Fig. 21-2A, B). Palpation of the bony parts can usually elicit tenderness and sometimes motion and crepitus at the fracture sites.

To simplify and systematize facial bone fracture diagnosis, the facial skeleton can be divided into three zones: upper, middle, and lower (Fig. 21-3).

Upper Third Facial Fractures

Fractures of the upper third of the face are less common than those of the lower two thirds because of the protection afforded by the nose, which serves as an energy-absorbing projecting part. Fractures of the frontal area usually involve the thinner bones of the frontal sinuses or the supraorbital ridges. Because of the close proximity to the brain, injuries in this area are more likely to be accompanied by greater morbidity and to be more life-threatening than any other facial fracture.

A. **Physical findings.** Positive physical findings usually appear in the ocular region because of extravasation of blood into the orbital area. Periorbital ecchymosis is observed in nearly all cases. Diplopia is inconstant; it is seen with depressed supraorbital fractures, but it is not commonly found with glabellar fractures. Nasal fractures and overlying lacerations of the forehead often are found in association with fractures of the upper third of the face.
B. **Treatment.** Treatment of facial fractures involves reduction of the bony fragments by either a direct or an indirect approach. The direct approach may be through the wound, a selected skin line, or a "gull wing" type

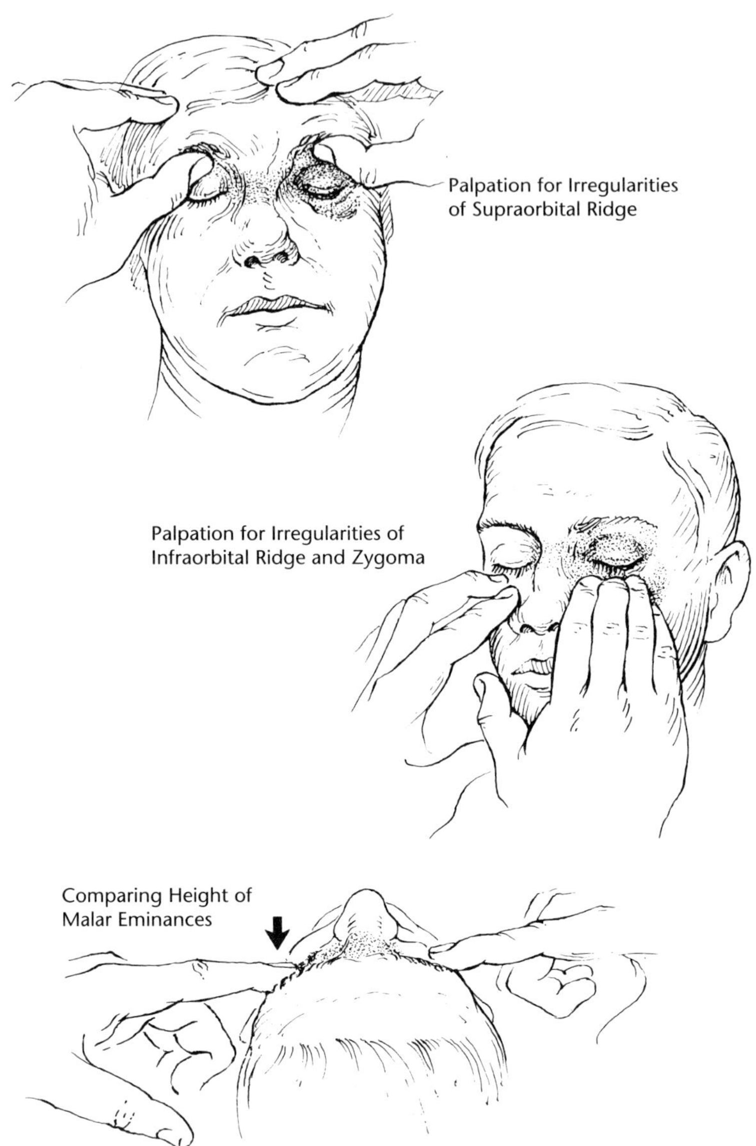

Fig. 21-2 A *Systematic bimanual palpation to aid in diagnosing facial fractures.*

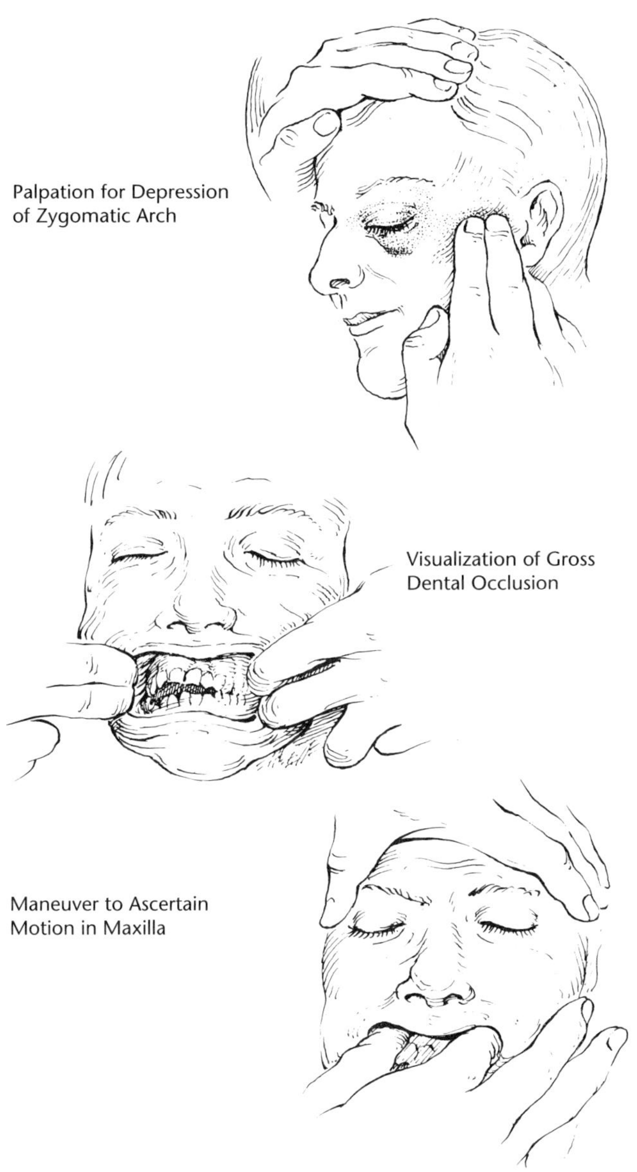

FIG. 21-2 B—***cont'd.***

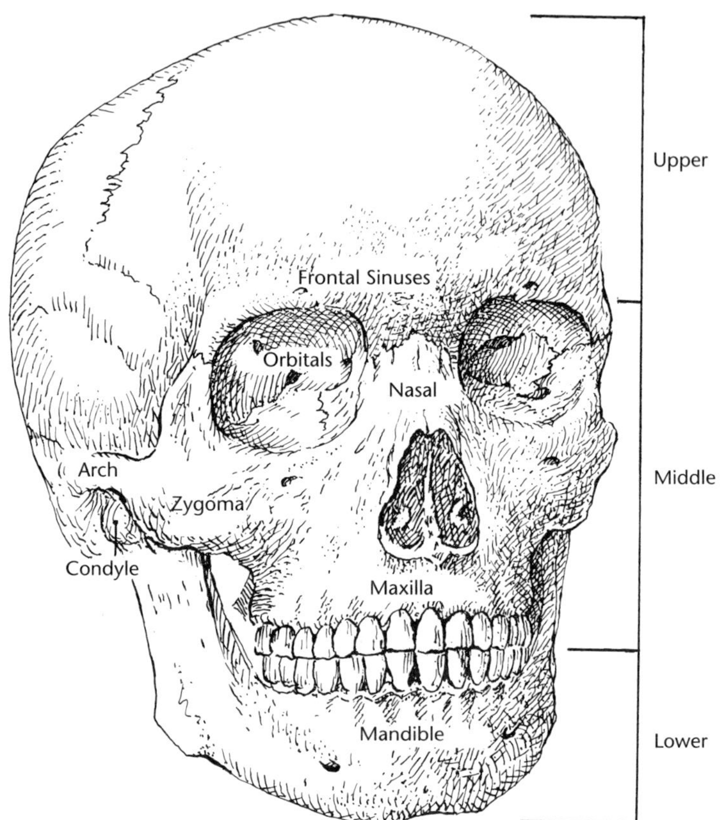

FIG. 21-3 *Area identification of facial bones.*

incision through the eyebrows. An excellent indirect approach to upper face fractures can be achieved through a coronal incision (Fig. 21-4 A-C). Appropriate débridement of avascular or pulped sinus mucosa, accurate replacement of soft tissue, and systemic antibiotic therapy should accompany the bony reduction. Some surgeons advocate removal of the comminuted bone fragments and extirpation of the sinus, but this bone loss results in gross deformities, requiring extensive secondary reconstructive procedures. Conversely, primary bony reconstruction as just described gives excellent functional and aesthetic results without complications.

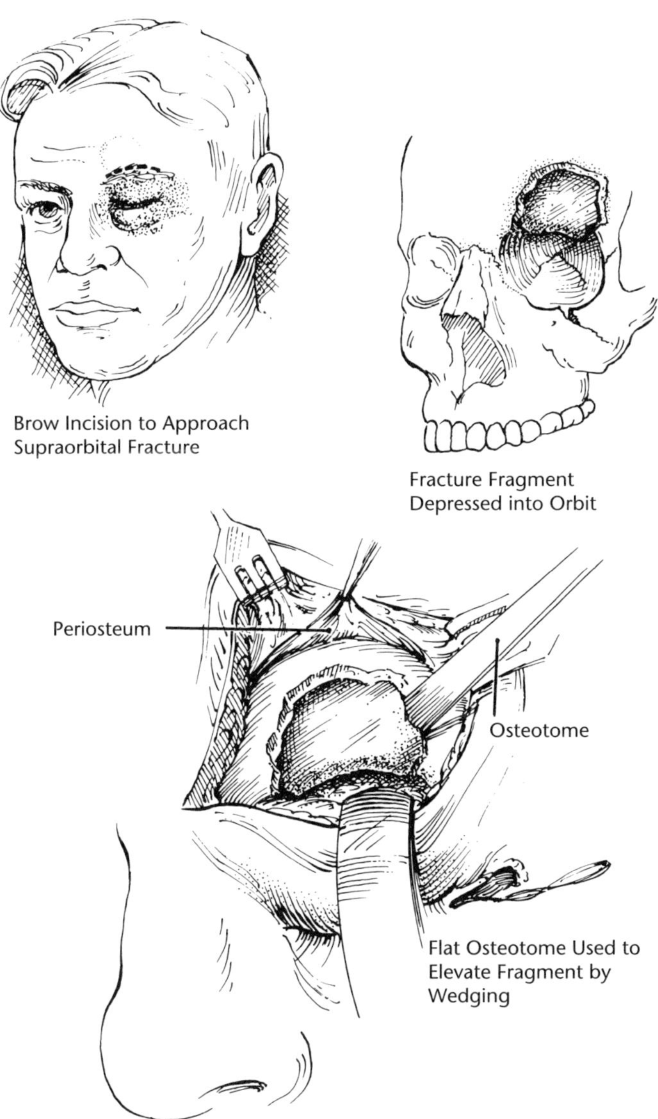

FIG. 21-4 *Surgical approach to reduction of segmental fracture of supraorbital rim.*

Middle Third Facial Fractures

Facial fractures of the middle third region often result from injury to unrestrained passengers within an automobile. They range from the nasal fracture, which is the simplest, to the maxillary fracture, which is the most complex of all facial fractures. Because of the prominence of the nasal complex and the thinness of the bones supporting it, nasal fractures are the most common of all facial fractures. Other fractures frequently seen in the middle third of the face involve the maxilla, the zygoma, the zygomatic arch, and the orbital bones.

A. Nasal fractures

- ▼ Diagnosis. Clinical findings are the most reliable means of making the diagnosis of a nasal fracture. Positive radiographic visualization is sometimes absent even when the nose shows gross traumatic deformity. A medical history of a nosebleed after injury, deviation of the nasal pyramid, and crepitus on palpation are the most helpful clinical findings. Sometimes, lateral and occlusal radiographic projections of the nasal bones will document these fractures precisely, but it is possible such films will not indicate them even with repeated attempts. The medical history of a previous fracture or nasal deviation is important because a healed displaced nasal fracture often cannot be reduced by the usual closed reduction techniques. Fracture-dislocation of the nasoseptal cartilages, diagnosed by symptoms and nasal speculum examination (Fig. 21-5) should be reduced at the time of nasal bone fracture reduction.
- ▼ Treatment. Unless the patient can be treated before the onset of edema, closed reduction should be delayed 5 to 7 days to allow for its resolution. Reduction can be delayed as long as 2 to 3 weeks if necessary. The need for reduction can best be determined after the edema has resorbed. Undisplaced nasal fractures require no manipulation.

Anesthesia of the nose is accomplished by insertion of intranasal packs soaked in a 5% cocaine solution accompanied by an external block using 2% lidocaine

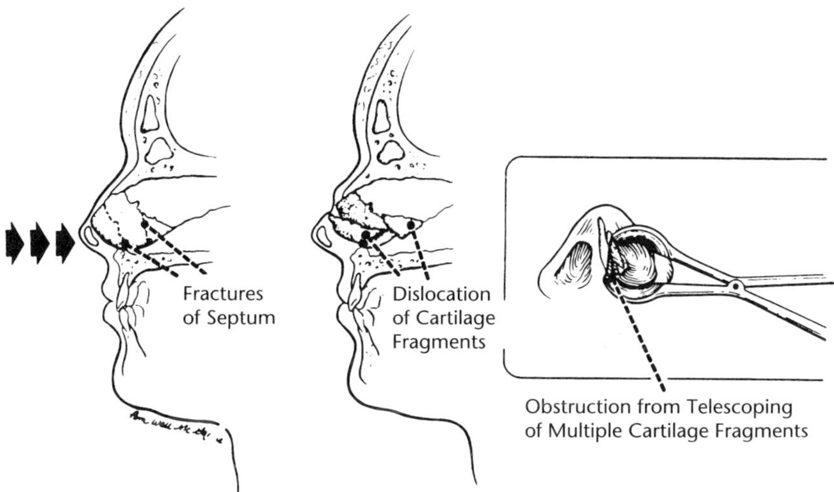

FIG. 21-5 *Fracture-dislocation of nasoseptal cartilages, visualized by nasal speculum examination.*

with epinephrine (Fig. 21-6 A, B). After the nose has been anesthetized, disimpaction and reduction of the nasal bone fragments are done with three nasal reduction instruments (Fig. 21-7). Reduction of the fracture is followed by immobilization of the fragments with a plaster splint for 1 week.

Although a severely displaced nasal fracture may be reducible by closed techniques for several months, a minimally displaced fracture will often become fixed by fibrous union within 3 to 4 weeks. Efforts to correct the deformity after such healing often requires open reduction and osteotomies.

B. **Maxillary fractures.** The mechanism of injury in maxillary fractures is usually a direct impact to the midface as in an automobile or motorcycle accident. In 1901 the French surgeon Le Fort described three common lines of fracture of the maxilla based on weak points of the midface (Fig. 21-8). Clinically, however, maxillary fractures are often a modification or combination of these classic fracture lines. Combinations of such fractures have given rise to the term "panafacial fractures."

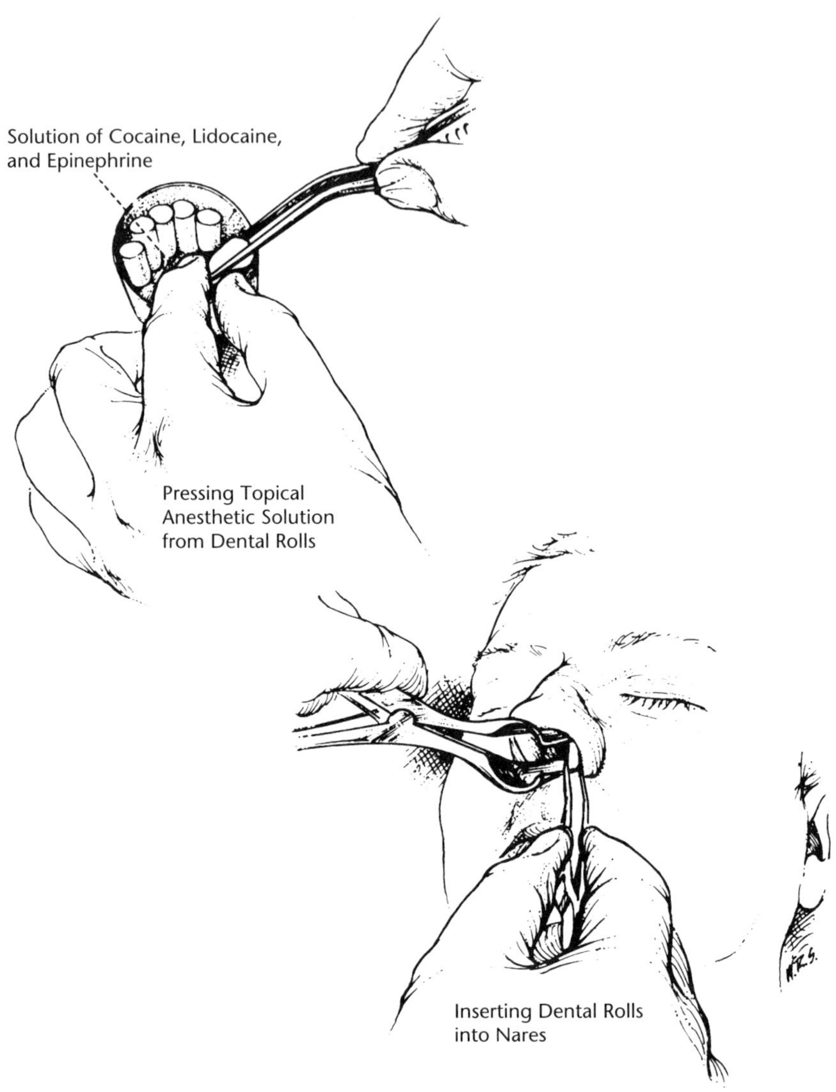

Fig. 21-6 A *Achieving local anesthesia of nose:* ***A,*** *Anesthetizing mucous membranes with a 5% cocaine solution.*

- Transverse maxillary fracture (Le Fort I). This fracture can be associated with a blow to the upper lip. The detached portion is often a single segment composed of the alveolar process, the palate, and the pterygoid process. Inspection of the dental arches usually dem-

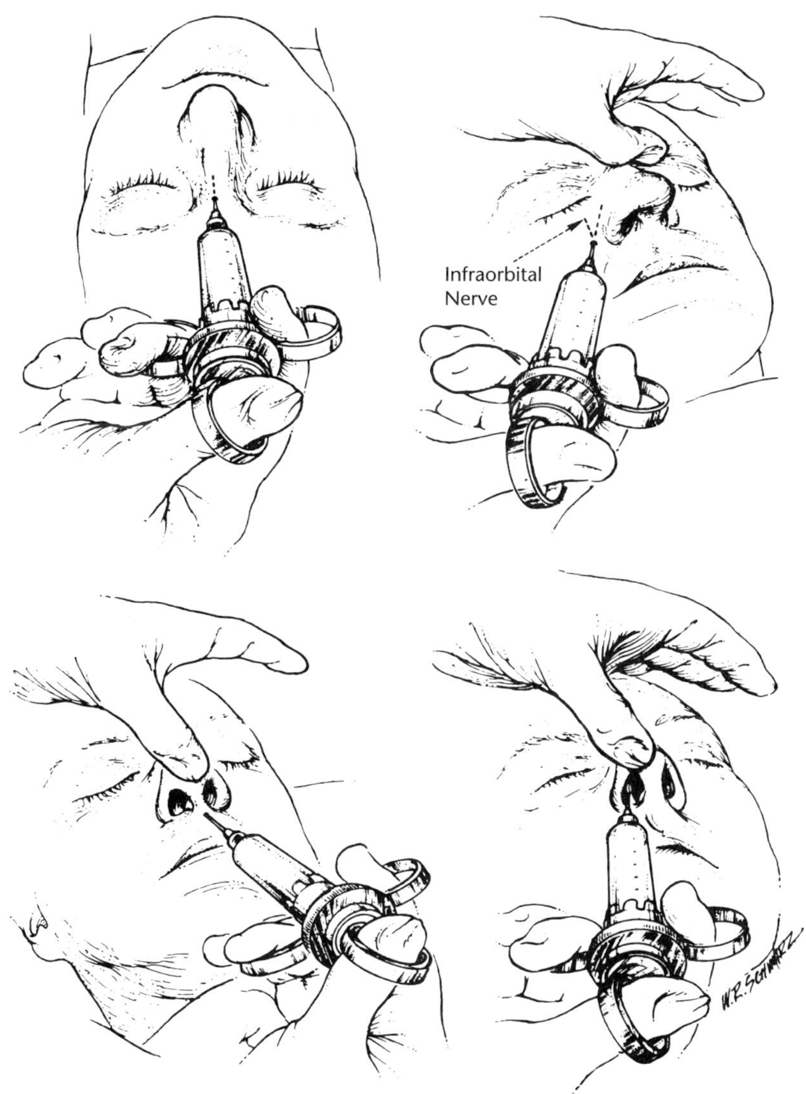

FIG. 21-6 B **B,** *Technique for achieving external nasal block with 2% solution of xylocaine and epinephrine.*

onstrates an open bite with superior displacement of the maxillary incisors. With this fracture, grasping the upper teeth may detect motion of the entire upper dental arch and palate. An isolated alveolar ridge fracture also may permit motion of the upper dental arch.

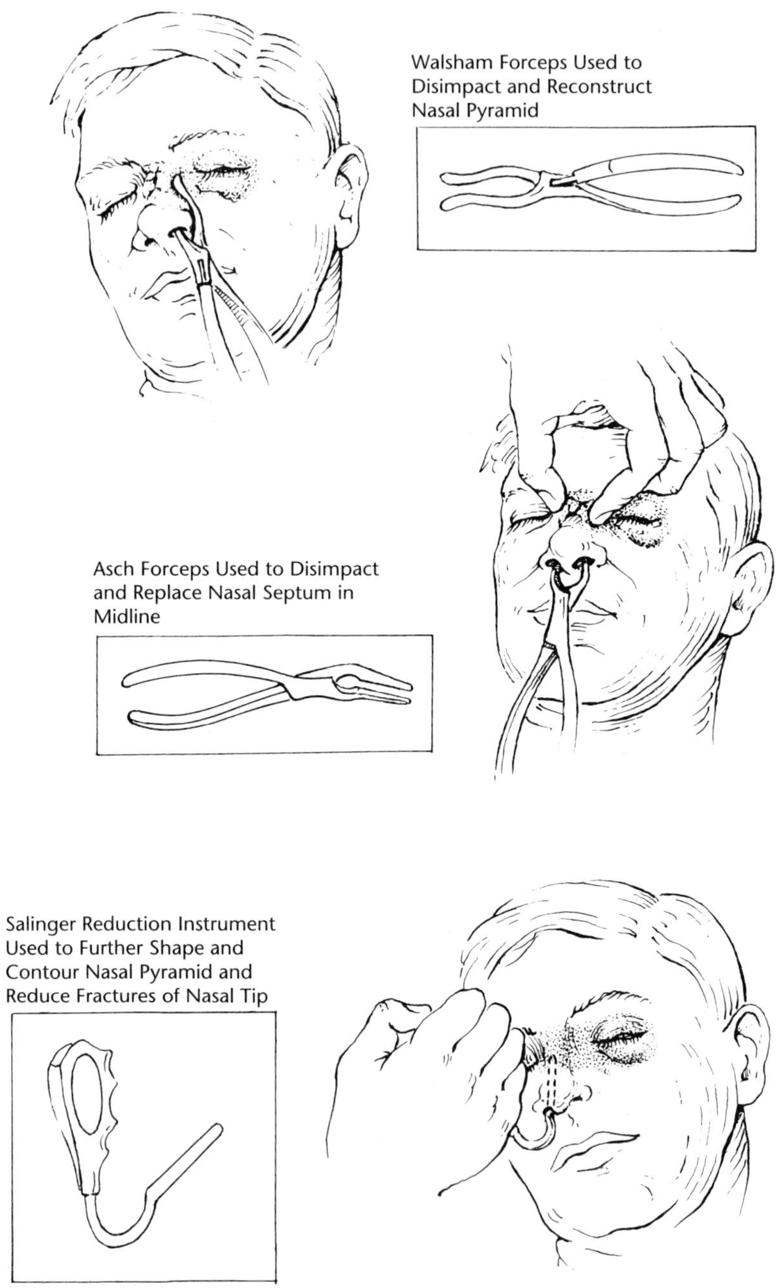

Fig. 21-7 *Technique for accomplishing closed reduction of nasal fracture with three nasal reduction instruments.*

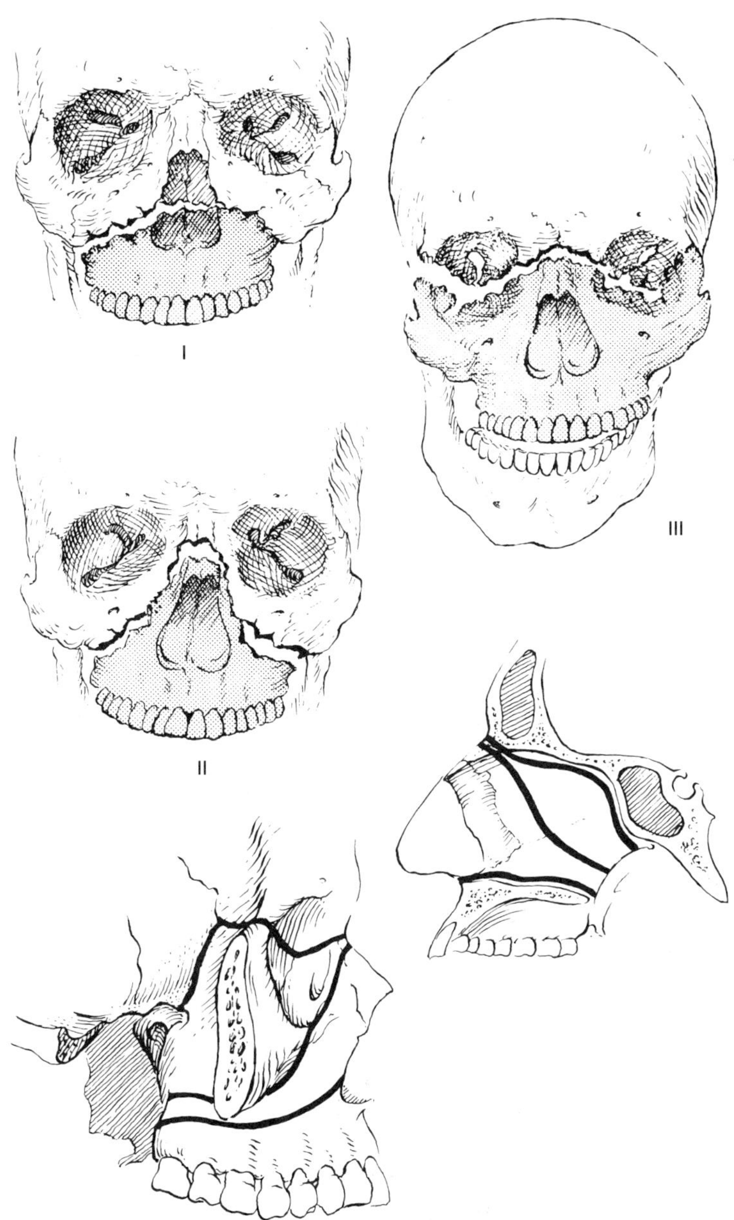

FIG. 21-8 *Le Fort classification of maxillary fractures.*

Treatment of a transverse maxillary fracture consists of reduction and immobilization. The reduction and immobilization usually are accomplished best by miniplates and screws (Fig. 21-9) or by intermaxillary fixation with arch bars and suspension from the lateral orbital rims. In some cases however interosseous wire fixation at the fracture site combined with intermaxillary fixation may be sufficient for stabilization.

- Pyramidal fracture (Le Fort II). An impact higher on the midface may result in a fracture that passes

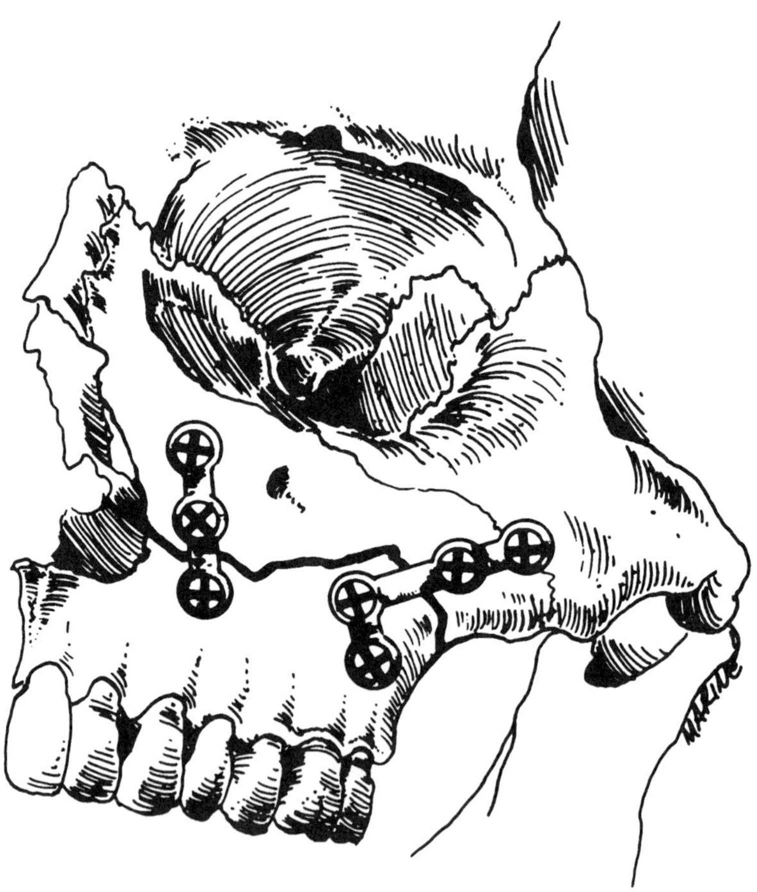

Fig. 21-9 *Use of miniplates and screws for stabilization of Le Fort I maxillary fracture.*

from the alveolus posteriorly along the nasal processes of the maxillary bone, across the root of the nose, and posteriorly through the lacrimal bones, the floor of the orbit, and the pterygoid process. The isolated maxillary fragment is pyramid-shaped. Unless the blow has impacted the maxilla posteriorly or superiorly, grasping the upper teeth and rocking the segment back and forth can detect motion at the medial portion of the orbital floors. Reduction and immobilization of this fracture can be accomplished with miniplates and screws or with wire suspension from the frontal bone or zygoma (Fig. 21-10). This fracture is unstable because of its tendency to become displaced posteriorly. Direct wiring at the infraorbital rim may add to the stability of the repair. Comminution sometimes is found at these points however and makes interosseous wiring difficult. Autogenous bone grafts spanning the fracture site are sometimes useful in the reduction and immobilization of these fractures.

- ▼ Craniofacial disjunction (Le Fort III). Powerful forces delivered to the maxilla may completely separate the facial bone structures from the base of the skull. The only remaining attachment of the face to the skull is soft tissue. This injury is more severe than the pyramidal fractures because the fractures extend transversely across the nasal bridge, both posterior orbital walls, the lateral orbital rims, and the zygomatic arch, separating the face from the cranium. A patient with this facial fracture often has an associated intracranial injury.

Treatment consists of reduction and immobilization of the fracture similar to those used in the Le Fort II fracture with the addition of interosseous plates and screws or wiring at the zygomaticofrontal suture to provide greater immobilization. Here also bone plates or autogenous bone grafts spanning the fracture sites may enhance both reduction and immobilization of the fractures. Cerebrospinal fluid rhinorrhea is not a contraindication to operative reduction of this fracture. In some instances, reduction will stop the rhinorrhea. The deformity that results from in

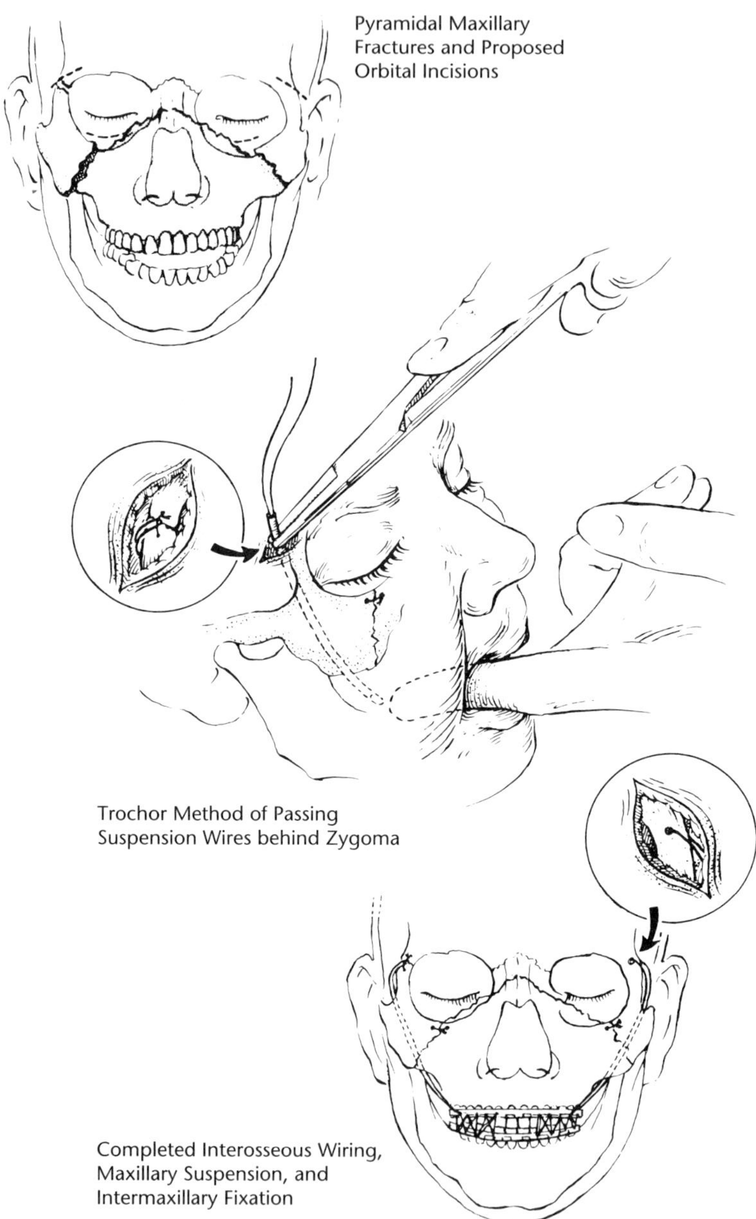

Fig. 21-10 *Technique for wire suspension of displaced maxillary fractures from lateral orbital rim.*

inadequate treatment of a severe maxillary fracture is a flattened, elongated, or depressed midface.

▼ Zygomatic fractures. The zygoma has two components: the malar eminence and the zygomatic arch. Fractures may occur in either segment separately or in both, but isolated arch fractures are less common. The most common fracture of the zygoma involves depression of the malar eminence. This type of fracture was once thought to consist of three parts—thus the use of the terms "tripod fracture" and "trimalar fracture." The fracture sites are usually found at the zygomaticotemporal and zygomaticofrontal suture lines and at the infraorbital foramen. A fourth fracture site is also sometimes found where the zygoma tapers into the maxilla. The fractured zygoma may undergo varying degrees of rotation and depression, depending on the mechanism of injury. Treatment usually requires open reduction and miniplate and screw fixation or internal interosseous fixation at two of the three fracture sites. The inferior and lateral orbital rims are the sites fixed most commonly (Fig. 21-11, A-C). Occasionally, reduction and stability cannot be achieved until rigid fixation is accomplished also at the zygomaticomaxillary junction (Fig. 21-12). Failure to effect an anatomically stable reduction can result in a flattened and depressed malar eminence after the swelling has resorbed.

C. **Orbital fractures.** The bones making up the orbital walls include the zygoma, maxilla, frontal, sphenoid, and ethmoid. Any of these bones may be fractured in extensive midface fractures. Commonly, however, an orbital floor fracture, involving the thin maxillary portion, accompanies a depressed zygoma fracture. Rarely does an isolated fracture of the orbital floor leave the orbital rim intact. The usual mechanism of this injury is a blow to the globe that transmits the force posteriorly and inferiorly through the weakest point in the orbital walls, the paper-thin orbital floor. Because of this mechanism of injury, this fracture has been named a

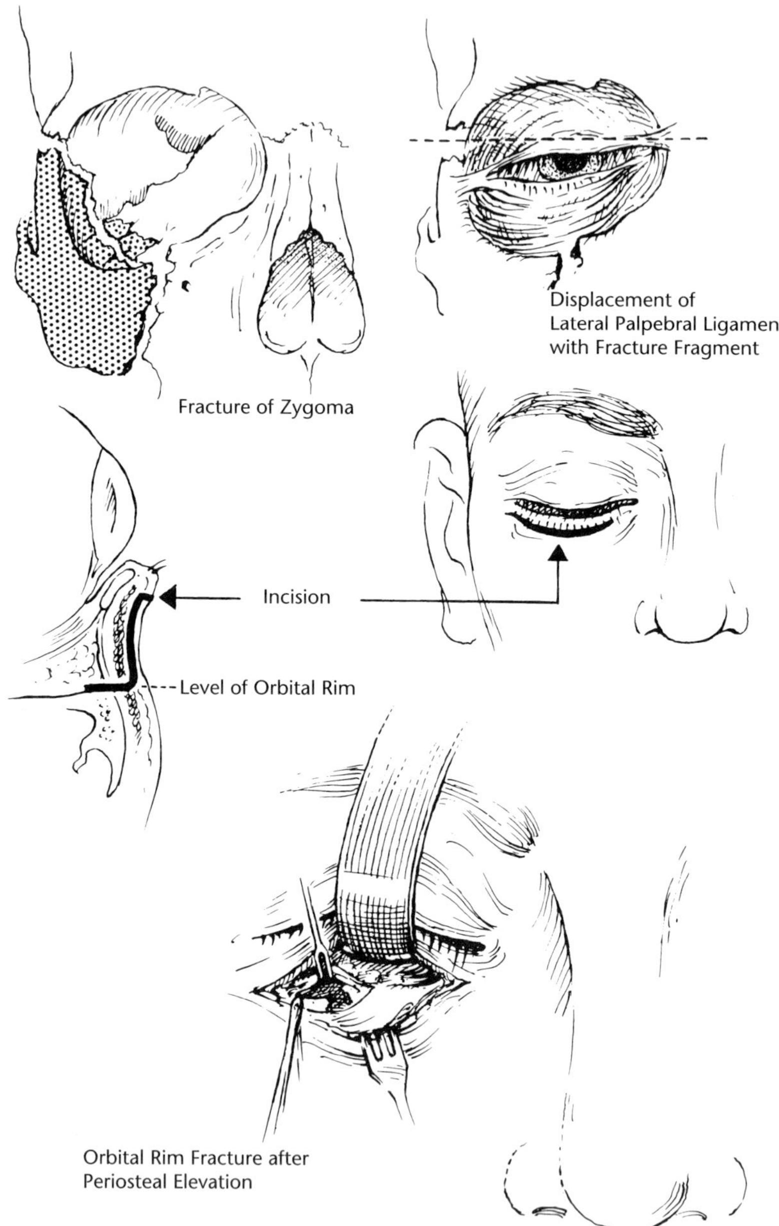

Fig. 21-11, A-C *Operative technique for open reduction and interosseous wire fixation of fractures of zygoma and orbital floor.*

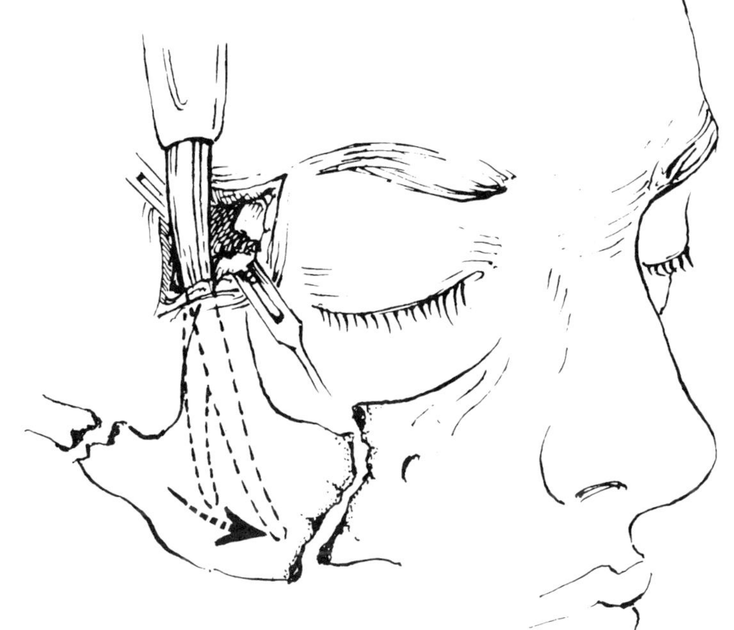

Elevation of Zygoma by Upward-Forward Force

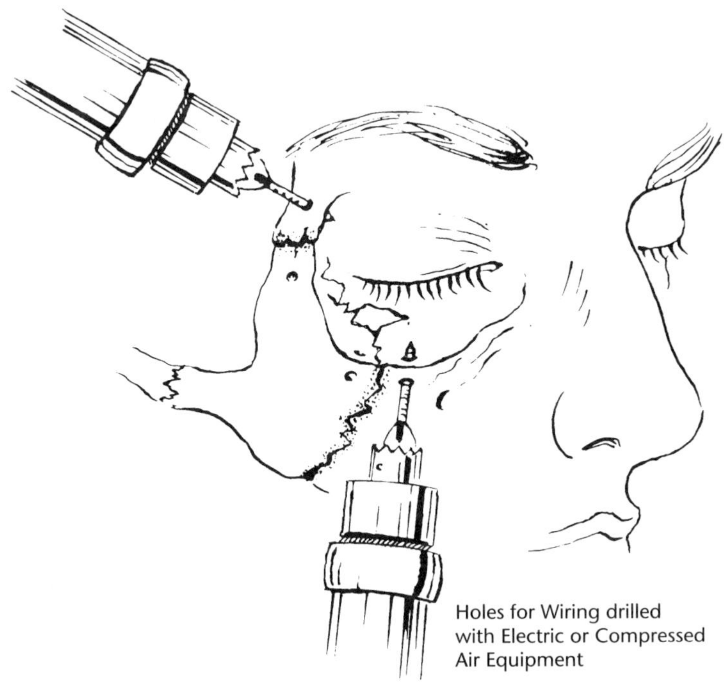

Fig. 21-11 B—*cont'd.*

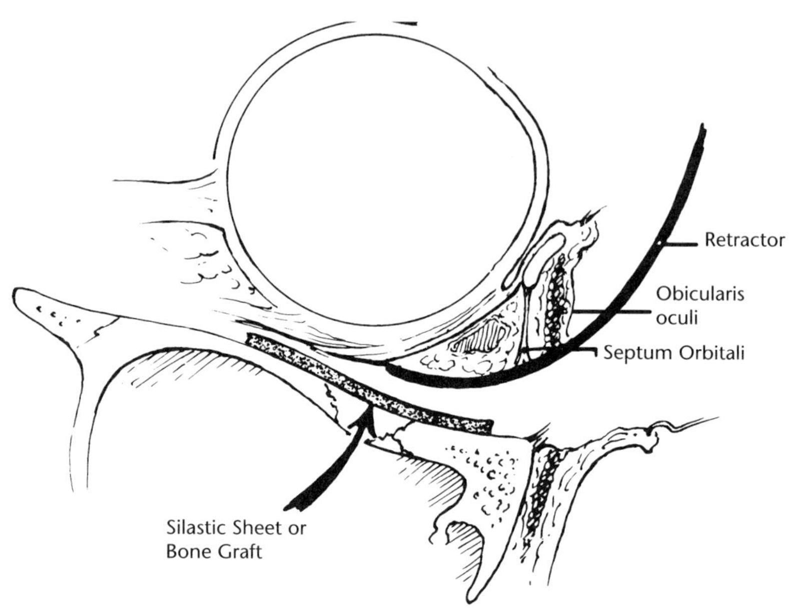

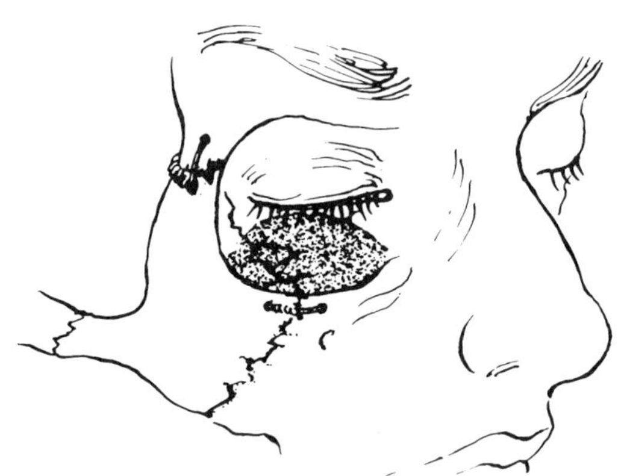

Silastic Sheet and Wiring in Place

Fig. 21-11 C–*cont'd.*

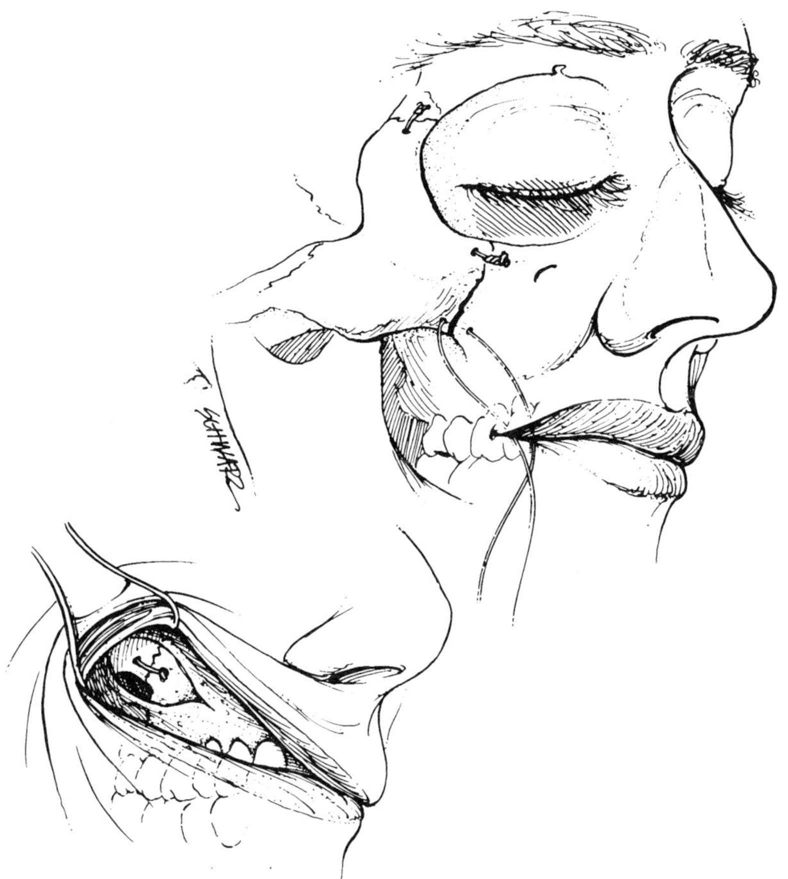

FIG. 21-12 *Interosseous wire fixation at zygomaticomaxillary junction to enhance stability of zygoma reduction.*

"blowout" fracture. Clinical findings may include diplopia, enophthalmos, and malfunction of the extraocular muscles. Entrapped periorbital fat and extraocular muscles may have to be freed from the fracture site. Often the floor is reinforced with a thin Silastic sheet or bone graft at the time of the reduction, as shown in Figure 21-13.

Some physicians advocate waiting for resolution of the swelling and hematoma so that the permanency of the

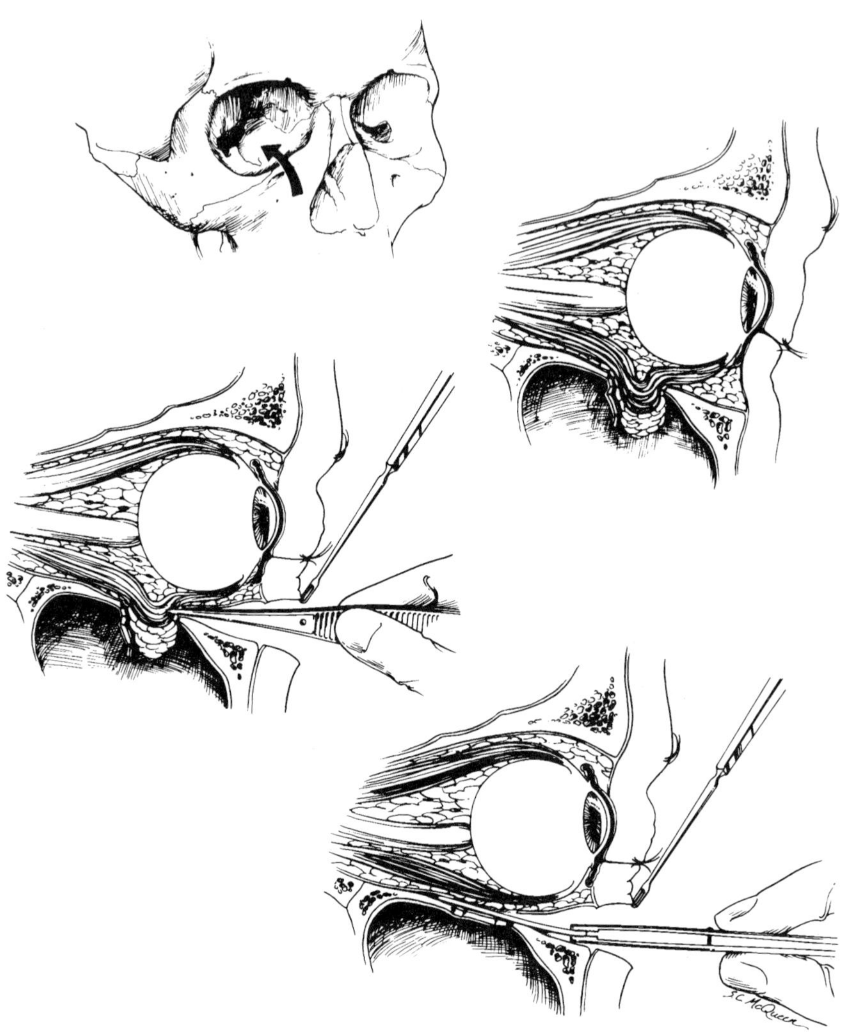

Fig. 21-13 *Technique for treatment of "blowout" fracture of orbital floor with herniation and entrapment of extraocular muscles and periorbital fat. Final drawing shows placement of thin bone graft or silicone sheet beneath orbital floor periosteum.*

enophthalmos, diplopia, and muscle entrapment can be evaluated more adequately. Experience has shown however that the presence of posttraumatic induration and fibrosis often precludes an acceptable functional and aesthetic result when treatment is delayed.

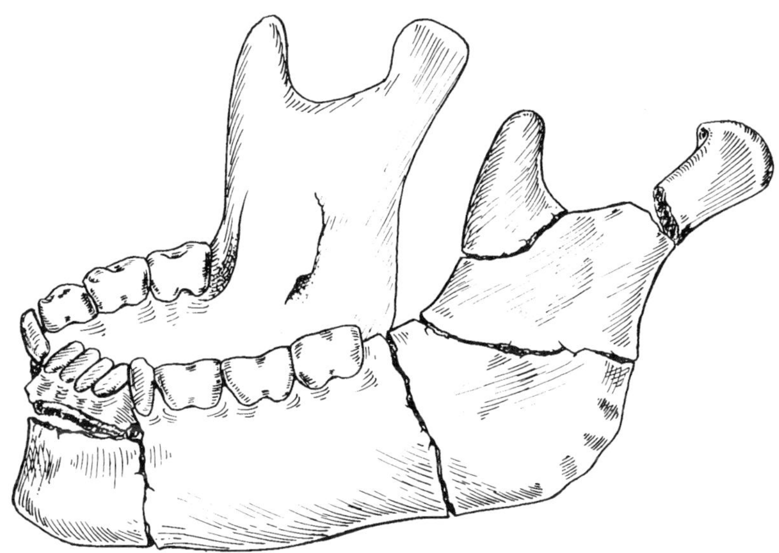

FIG. 21-14 *Common sites of mandibular fractures.*

Lower Third Facial Fractures (Mandibular Fractures)

Among facial fractures, those involving the mandible rank third in frequency behind those of the nose and zygoma. Patients with mandibular fracture, in contrast to other facial bone fractures, sometimes experience pain because of muscular distraction of the fragments. The fracture sites frequently are predictable on the basis of the mechanism of injury (Fig. 21-14).

Treatment of a fractured mandible is dependent on the location of the fracture, the angle of the fracture line, and the amount of displacement. The directions of muscular pull around the mandible are shown in Figure 21-15. A fracture line at the mandibular angle, which is angulated anteroinferiorly from above and behind, would tend to be impacted into a favorable position because of the action of the masseter and internal pterygoid muscles inserting on the lower border of the mandible at the angle. Conversely, the muscle pull on a fracture line angulated in the opposite direction would draw the fragments farther apart.

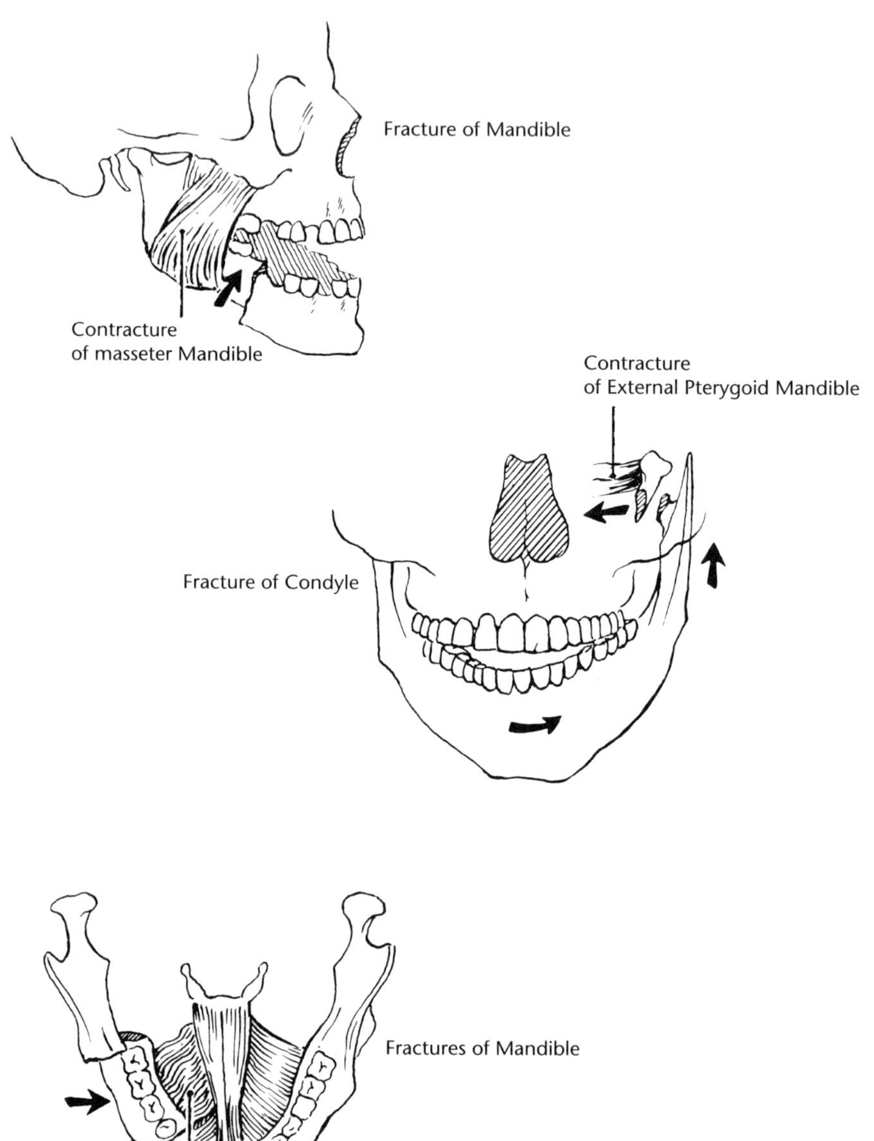

FIG. 21-15 *Muscles that tend to distract mandibular fracture fragments.*

A nondisplaced unilateral mandibular fracture can usually be treated by intermaxillary fixation with the teeth held in occlusion by arch bars or Blair-Ivy loops (Figs. 21-16, 21-17). A fracture that is unstable because it is markedly displaced, has an unfavorable angle, or is bilateral usually will require open reduction and interosseous fixation by wire or various types of metal bone plates and screws (Fig. 21-18). Either a cutaneous or intraoral incision can be used for access to these fractures. Stabilization by intraoral splinting, percutaneous Kirschner wires, or external traction devices has been used in various circumstances, but the indications for these methods are limited.

Facial Fractures in Children

In general, the mechanism of injury, the diagnosis, and the management of facial bone fractures in children do not differ greatly from those in the adult; however, a few differences do exist. Incompletely developed sinuses, mixed dentition, and lack of patient cooperation make interpretation of facial bone x-ray films in children more difficult.

Because of greater resiliency in the facial bones of children, greenstick fractures are more common than completely displaced fractures. Because bony union may occur early in children, fractures should be reduced in the first week after injury.

Subcondylar fractures in children, especially when bilateral, may involve epiphyseal growth centers and cause growth disturbance. As with adults, closed treatment is the preferred method of management even in instances of a medially displaced condyle. Intermaxillary fixation is more difficult in children because of the instability of deciduous teeth. This instability occasionally precludes using the teeth to maintain occlusion and indicates use of intraoral acrylic splints.

AUTOGENOUS BONE GRAFTS

Despite timely and skillful reduction, postoperative deformities occasionally cannot be avoided. They may result from severe comminution or displacement that cannot be

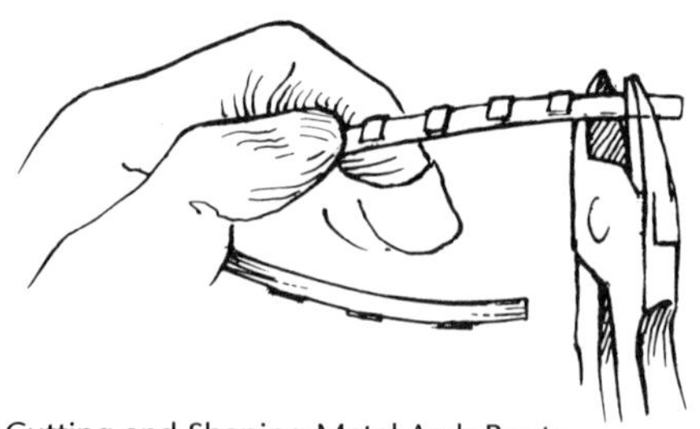

Cutting and Shaping Metal Arch Bar to Fit Dental Arch

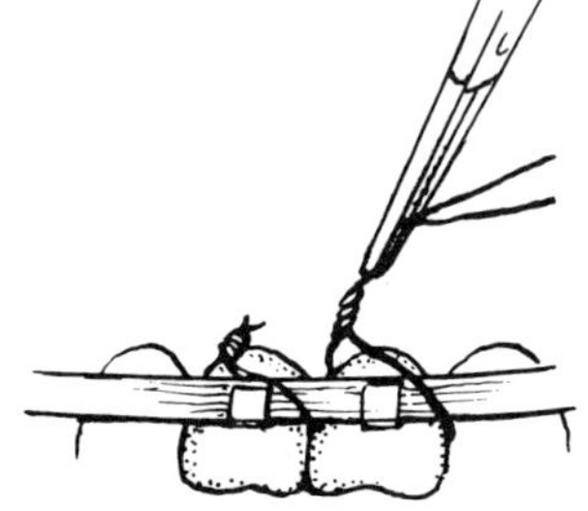

Simple Ligation of Arch Bar to Teeth with Wire

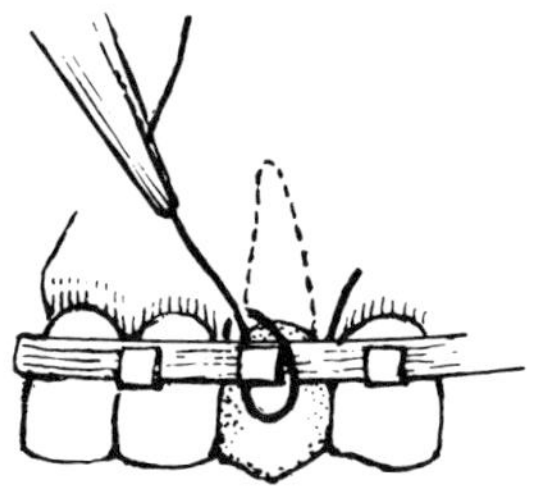

Special Technique for Fixation to Canine Tooth

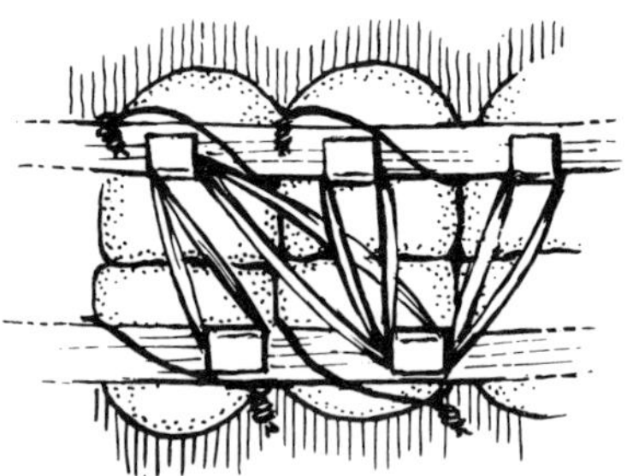

Intermaxillary Fixation with Dental Elastics

Fig. 21-16 *Formation and application of dental arch bars for intermaxillary fixation.*

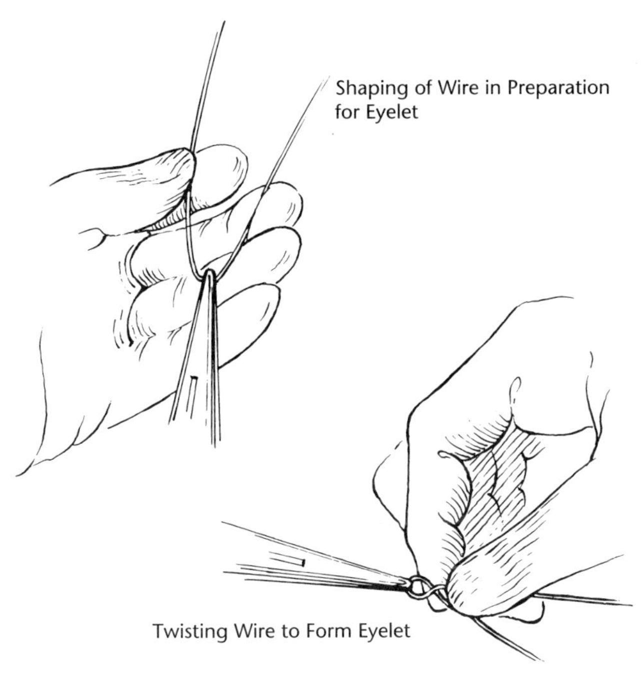

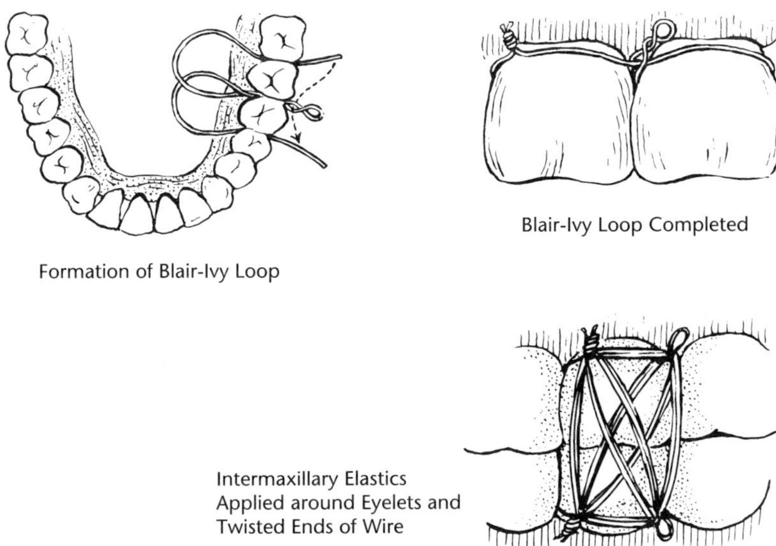

Fig. 21-17 *Formation and application of Blair-Ivy loops for intermaxillary fixation.*

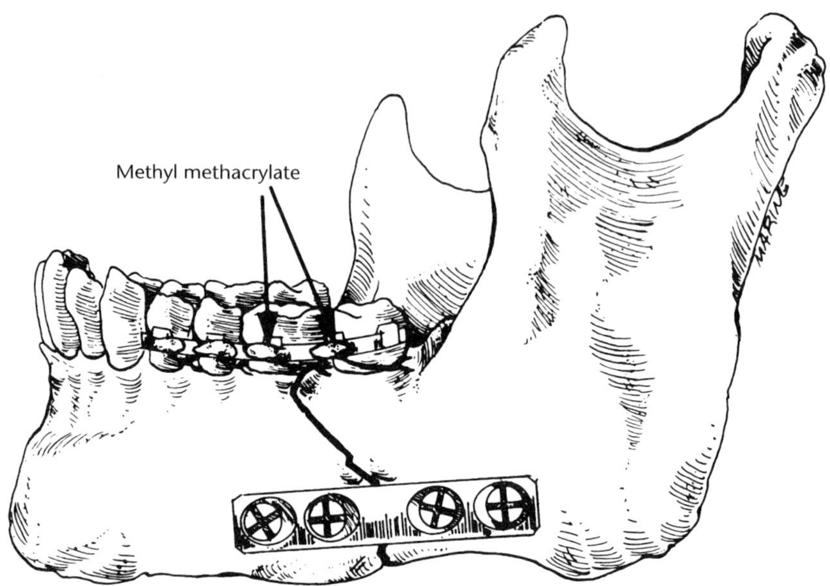

Fig. 21-18 *Rigid fixation of mandible with lower border compression plate and screws. Arch bar fixed to teeth adjacent to mandibular fracture made rigid by application of methylmethacrylate over ligating wires.*

adequately corrected. Reconstruction of these defects with many different materials has been described; the most physiologic graft material however is autogenous bone.

Donor Sites

Bone grafts for facial reconstruction usually are taken from rib, iliac crest, tibia, or calvarium (Fig. 21-19), depending on the specific requirements at the recipient site. All four areas contain cortical bone. Large amounts of cancellous bone can be obtained from the iliac crest and the tibia.

Grafting of Recipient Areas

Recipient areas requiring structural support must be grafted with cortical bone. When large defects must be spanned, split-rib grafts are usually the most suitable. Smaller defects can easily be filled with iliac or calvarial bone grafts cut to the needed shape.

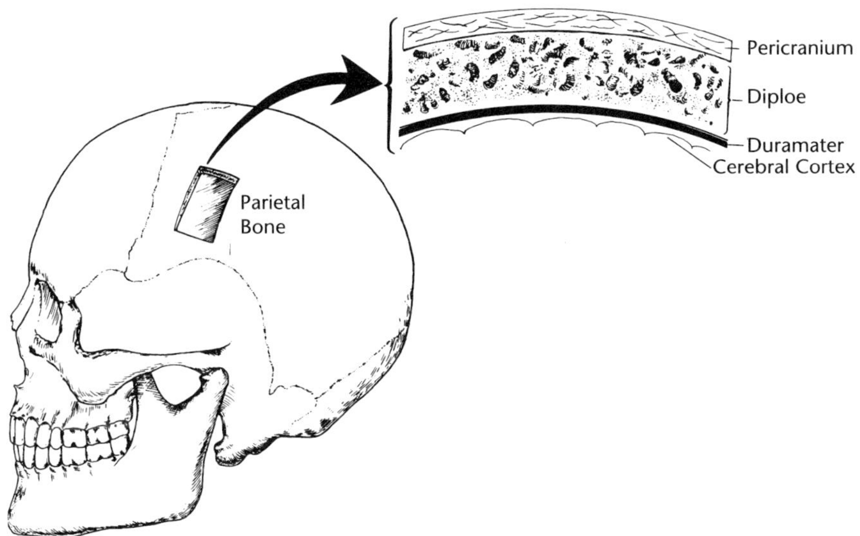

Fig. 21-19 *Calvarial bone graft taken from parietal bone.*

Disadvantages

The disadvantage of cancellous bone is its lack of structural strength and the unpredictable resorption that may take place. The healing that occurs after bone grafting is one of continuing resorption and new bone formation. Adding chips of porous cancellous bone may increase the volume of a viable bone graft. Areas of the facial structure most amenable to bone grafting include the nose, mandible, forehead, and orbital rims.

ALLOPLASTIC MATERIAL

As new compounds are developed, alloplastic materials are being implanted with increasing frequency. Silicone rubber, methylmethacrylate and hydroxyapatite are currently the most commonly used. Each has its own advantages.

Silicone Rubber

Silicone rubber can be custom prefabricated to fit the existing defect. It is inert, having essentially no antigenic potential. It is however a foreign body and has a higher incidence of extrusion than do autogenous bone or cartilage grafts.

Methylmethacrylate and Hydroxyapatite

Methylmethacrylate is a cold-curing acrylic that has the advantage, as does hydroxyapatite, of being molded in situ. These alloplastic materials are most applicable for reconstruction of the glabellar, supraorbital, and infraorbital areas.

FURTHER READINGS

Baker SP, Schultz RC: Recurrent problems in emergency room management of maxillofacial injuries, *Clin Plast Surg* 2:65, 1975.

Le Fort R: Experiemental study of fractures of the jaw, *Plast Reconstr Surg* 50:600, 1972.

Schultz RC: Facial injuries from automobile accidents: a study of 400 consecutive cases, *Plast Reconstr Surg* 40:415, 1967.

Schultz RC: One thousand consecutive cases of major facial injury, *Rev Surg* 27:394, 1970.

Schultz RC: The changing character and management of soft tissue windshield injuries, *J Trauma* 12:1, 1972.

Schultz RC: Frontal sinus and supraorbital fractures from vehicular accidents, *Clin Plast Surg* 2:93, 1975.

Schultz RC: *Facial Injuries,* ed 2, Chicago, 1988, Year Book Medical.

Schultz RC, DeVillers YT: Nasal fractures, *J Trauma* 15:319, 1975.

CHAPTER 22

Cleft Lip and Palate

D. RALPH MILLARD, JR., AND BERNARD M. BARRETT, JR.

Although the exact etiology of cleft lip and palate is unknown, Richard Stark and Joshua Kaplan demonstrated in 1973 that insufficient mesoderm migration into the lip and nasal floor is the basic cause of cleft formation. During the fourth to seventh weeks of intrauterine life, development of the primary palate occurs, including the medial upper lip, premaxilla, and structures anterior to the incisive foramen. The secondary palate develops from the seventh to twelfth weeks of intrauterine life, forming the hard and soft palate. When sufficient mesenchyme fails to migrate into a specific area, a cleft is established. Cleft lip and palate occur together in approximately 1:1300 live births. Cleft lip occurs in 1:1000 live births; cleft palate occurs in 1:2500 live births.

INITIAL CONSULTATION

Timing of Surgery

Anxious parents often encourage the plastic surgeon to operate immediately on the infant's cleft deformity (Fig. 22-1). It should be explained to the parents that newborns have better cardiovascular-pulmonary adjustment, nutritional status, and ability to combat infection after 1 month of age. The carefully planned design of treatment is explained to the parents. Another aspect of the cleft syndrome, otitis media, is treated at the same time. The otolaryngologist performs bilateral myringotomy and insertion of ear tubes during one of the surgical procedures.

Counseling Parents

Parents, who frequently experience unwarranted guilt, should be reassured that nothing could have been done during the pregnancy to prevent cleft lip formation and that

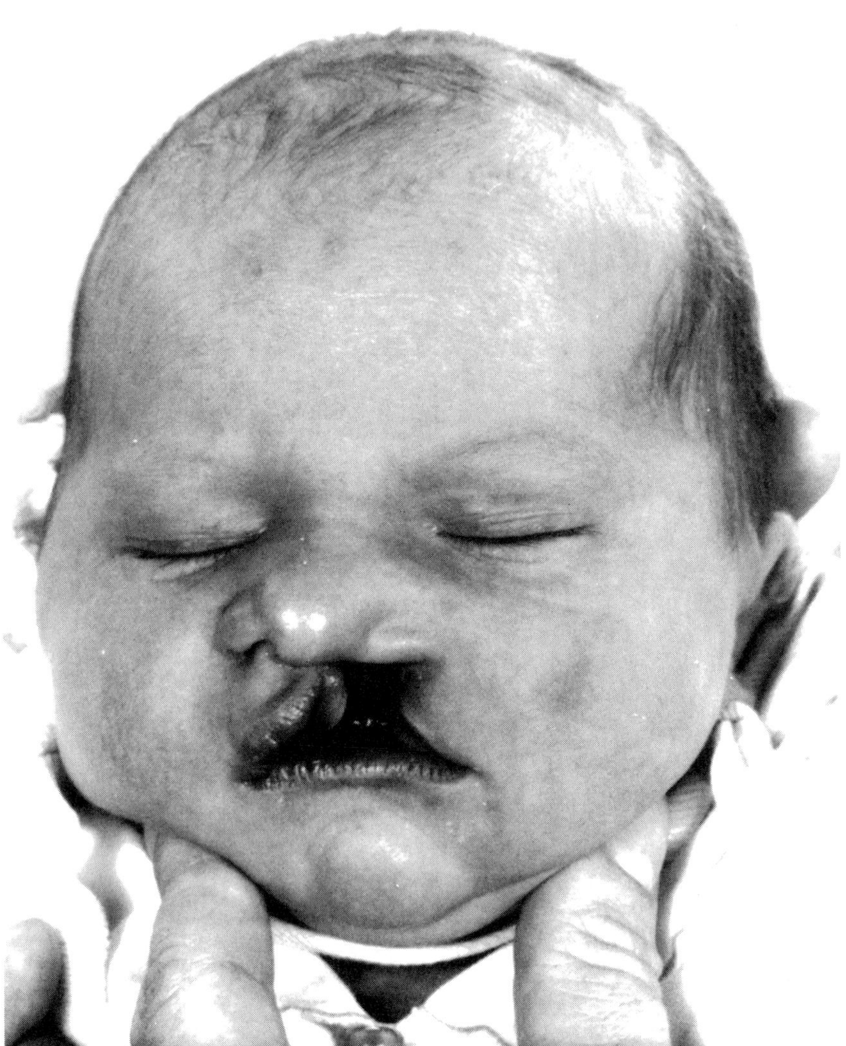

FIG. 22-1 *Complete unilateral cleft of lip and palate at 4 days of age.*

nothing was done that should not have been done. It should be explained that, although there is a hereditary factory, it is only partly to blame because the ratio of cleft to normal births in the United States is approximately 1:750. Parents with one or more children with clefts can have a normal infant, while normal parents with an uninvolved family history can have an infant with a cleft.

Geneticist Clarke Fraser has studied various cleft situations and established the following percentages for cleft lip (CL) and cleft palate (CP) occurrences:

- If both parents are unaffected and they have an affected child, the probability that their next infant will have the same condition is 4% in CL and CP and 2% in CP if they have no affected relatives.
- If unaffected parents have two affected children, the probability that their next infant will have the same condition is 9% in CL and CP and 1% in CP.
- If one of the parents is affected and they have no affected children, the probability that the next infant will be affected is 4% in CL and CP and 6% in CP.
- If one of the parents is affected and they have an affected child, the probability that their next infant will be affected is 17% in CL and CP and 15% in CP.
- If both parents are affected, the risk of the infant being affected is approximately 60%.

The more severe the patient's defect, the higher the recurrence risk is in subsequent children. It is recommended that persons with clefts not marry others with cleft deformities.

PREOPERATIVE CARE

Feeding

Feeding is the only special treatment for most affected children before surgery. A cleft in the lip or palate decreases the infant's sucking ability, making breast-feeding improbable and bottle feeding difficult. Formula is given by compression through a 50-ml syringe with a 3-cm rubber tube extension (Fig. 22-2). The infant is supported with the head in the upright position, and the catheter is slipped over the tongue, giving formula as the infant is able to take it. After the parents and infant are used to this feeding routine, they are allowed to go home from the hospital to increase the infant's weight before surgery. Other special feeding devices are available, including a commercially available bifid cleft palate nipple (made by Dow Corning) for infants with absent or minimal sucking reflex. For severely malnourished infants, forced feeding can be provided through a nasogastric tube.

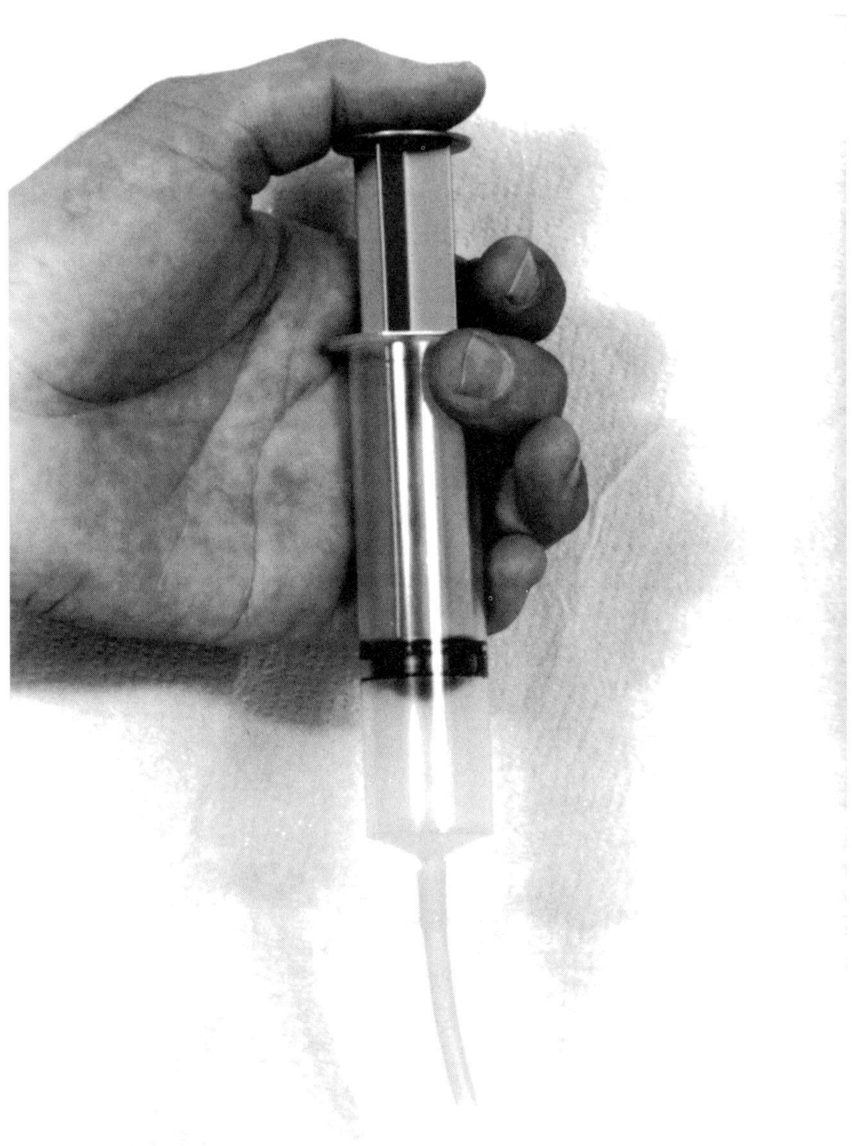

FIG. 22-2 *Syringe with rubber tube extension to aid in feeding infants with clefts of palate.*

Presurgical Orthodontics in Complete Unilateral Clefts

For children with complete clefts and alveolar distortion, the coordination of dental and surgical treatment has improved the preparation for surgery. What was once done crudely with pressure appliances and lip adhesion has been developed into an accurate procedure of presurgical orthodontics. It focuses the parent's attention and the immediate treatment on aligning the alveolar segments so that a balanced platform is created to support the lip and nose.

Latham created an orthopedic appliance custom made on the infant's plaster cast of the palate. Accurately fitting methylmethocrylate bases are formed on each palate segment. They are connected by a metal transverse strut posteriorly with a pivot at each end to allow movement. A 25-mm activating screw is embedded into the posterior part of the methacrylate polymer for the noncleft side near the midline (Fig. 22-3). The appliance is fixed to the maxillary segments by two wire pins on each side with the palate bone medial to the tooth follicles. Turning the screw pushes the cleft maxilla forward and places an opposite force to pull back on the unrotated noncleft segment. This appliance is applied under

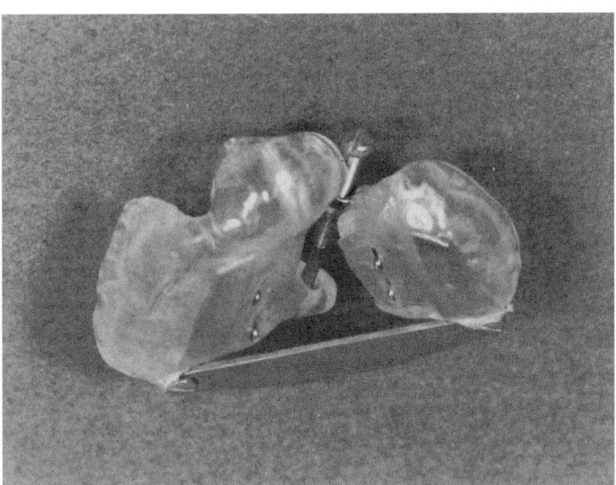

FIG. 22-3 *Latham expansion appliance to be pinned onto maxillary segments. Each turn of screw brings segments into better alignment.*

sedation as an outpatient, and the parents are taught to keep the mouth and appliance clean and turn the screw one twist each day (Fig. 22-4). This will move the segments into alignment and within 2 to 4 mm apart in 2 to 4 weeks. Once this has been accomplished, the appliance is removed and the irritated mucosa is allowed to heal for 2 to 3 days.

Presurgical Orthodontics in the Complete Bilateral Cleft

Repositioning the protruded premaxillary segment requires use of a continuous tractional force to pull on an attachment to the premaxillary bones. A pin-retained maxillary expansion appliance is used (Fig. 22-5). Double wire pins are passed through the stem of the premaxillary bones behind the incisor tooth follicles and in front of the premaxillary-vomeral suture. An orthodontic elastic chain is passed from

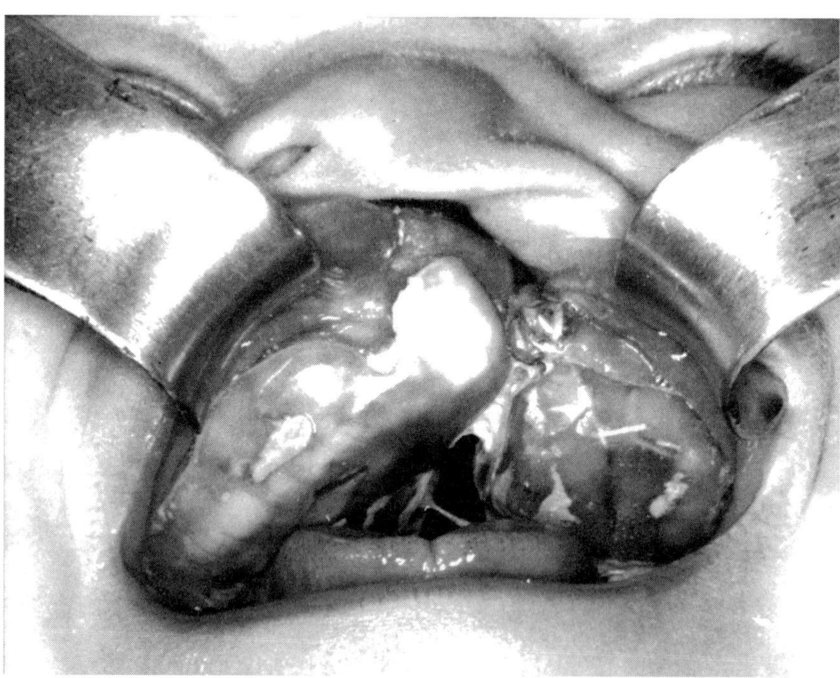

Fig. 22-4 *Appliance has been pinned onto maxillary segments. Parents taught how to turn screw.*

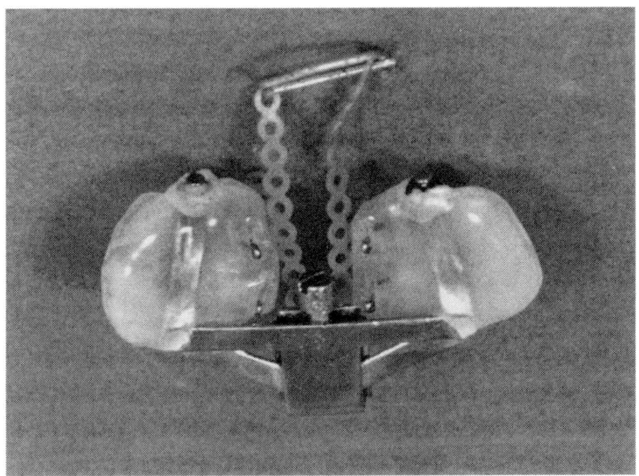

FIG. 22-5 *Latham expansion appliance with elastic chain and two pins for attachment to vomer provide retraction of premaxilla.*

the double premaxillary pins back around rollers on the expansion appliance and then forward to retaining hooks. The traction force on the chain is set at a continuous 2 ounces on each side. The parents are taught how to tighten the chain (Fig. 22-6). The forces set up bring the premaxilla back without septal deflection and spread the maxillary segments to accept the premaxilla. Slight undercorrections are ideal. The appliance is removed 2 to 3 days before surgery to allow the irritated mucosa to heal.

General Requirements

Ideally the infant should be healthy and gaining weight before the initial surgery is performed. A unilateral periosteoplasty and lip adhesion does not usually cause great blood loss, but in a bilateral case, it can be a problem. Use of local anesthesia with 1:200,000 adrenalin injected into the mucoperiosteum along the cleft can reduce the bleeding. Great care with hemostasis should be exerted. As the periosteoplasty and lip adhesion are carried out as soon as the segments are in alignment and the surgery is less extensive, the rule of 10 can be used with moderate license:

- Weight: Approximately 10 pounds
- Hemoglobin: 10 g

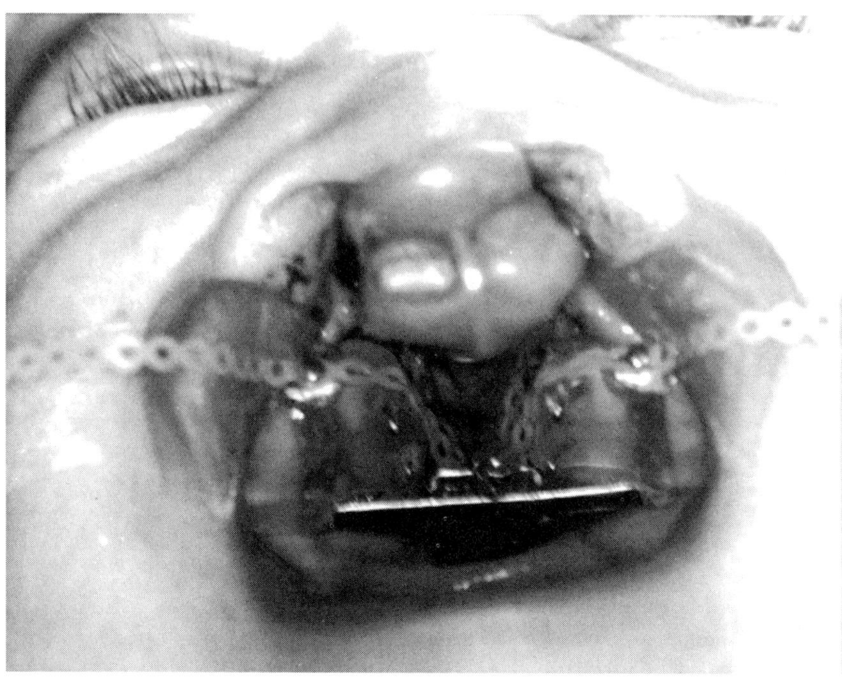

Fig. 22-6 *Appliance pinned into position and elastic chain used to retract premaxilla.*

- White blood cell count: Less than 10,000
- Age: Can be less than 10 weeks

The child should be trained to sleep on the back so that the healing lip will not come in contact with the bed in the postoperative period.

OPERATIVE CARE

Complete photographic records and a well-thought operative plan are essential before the surgeon enters the operating room (OR).

Anesthesia

General endotracheal anesthesia is required for primary cleft lip and palate surgery in children.

Positioning

Correct positioning of the child is important for the plastic surgeon, who sits at the head of the operating table. Head extension must be maximal for cleft palate surgery. The entire body is raised with a thick foam mat or folded blanket, allowing the head to drop back, hyperextended, into a soft stockinette head support. Not only does this position provide good exposure but it also allows blood to flow away from the larynx and toward the nasopharynx allowing it to be removed by suction.

Operative Procedure

▼ An orogastric catheter should be passed to empty the stomach of gas and secretions, and it should be removed before preparation of the surgical field.

▼ Before cleft lip closure, a posterior pharyngeal pack is placed deep into the pharynx around the endotracheal tube (Fig. 22-7). This along with a single piece of plastic tape placed externally around the tube and low down on

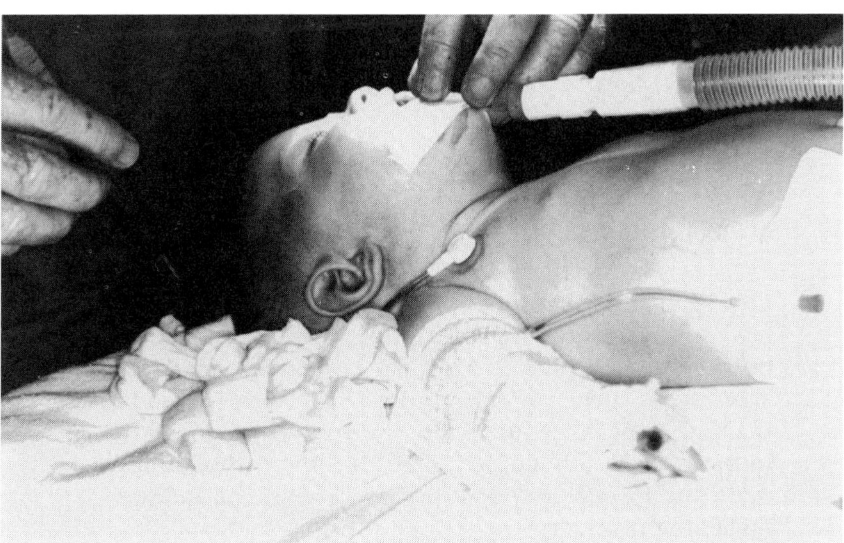

FIG. 22-7 *Patient anesthetized with tube taped in position and anesthetist ready to stabilize tube further with a pharyngeal pack.*

the chin keeps the endotrachael tube in place. The Millard-Dingman mouth gag allows the surgeon easy access to the field during cleft palate surgery, while stabilizing the endotrachael tube without using a pharyngeal pack.

- ▼ To avert eye injury, an ocular lubricant is placed in the eyes, and the upper eyes are splinted shut with tape (Fig. 22-8).
- ▼ Pulse, respiration, blood pressure, temperature, and electrocardiogram (ECG) are monitored at all times. A warming blanket is used to prevent hypothermia.
- ▼ Blood loss determination is made by a calibrated catchment trap in the suction line and by weighing sponges. Blood loss rarely exceeds 10% of the estimated circulating volume; however, properly crossmatched and screened blood should be available but used only if absolutely necessary.
- ▼ While the patient is still under anesthesia, by using an operating microscope, the otolaryngologist performs myringotomy, suction of accumulated fluid, and insertion of tubes when indicated (Figs. 22-9, 22-10).
- ▼ On completion of the surgical repair, the pharynx is carefully suctioned under direct vision, and extubation is carried out with the patient in the surgical plane of anesthesia.
- ▼ Instead of an oral airway, which is avoided to minimize trauma to the surgical field, a tongue stitch is used to maintain an adequate airway until reflexes return (Fig. 22-11). The patient is placed in the lateral position.
- ▼ If oxygen administration is necessary before the patient has regained protective reflexes, the tongue is pulled out by the stitch, which is then passed through the mask aperture, and the mask is connected to oxygen. Gentle traction may be required on the tongue stitch in the immediate postoperative period to remind the child to open the mouth and breathe. As soon as the infant is breaching normally, the tongue suture is removed.
- ▼ Infants with respiratory distress are placed in a unit with warm vaporization and increased oxygenation.

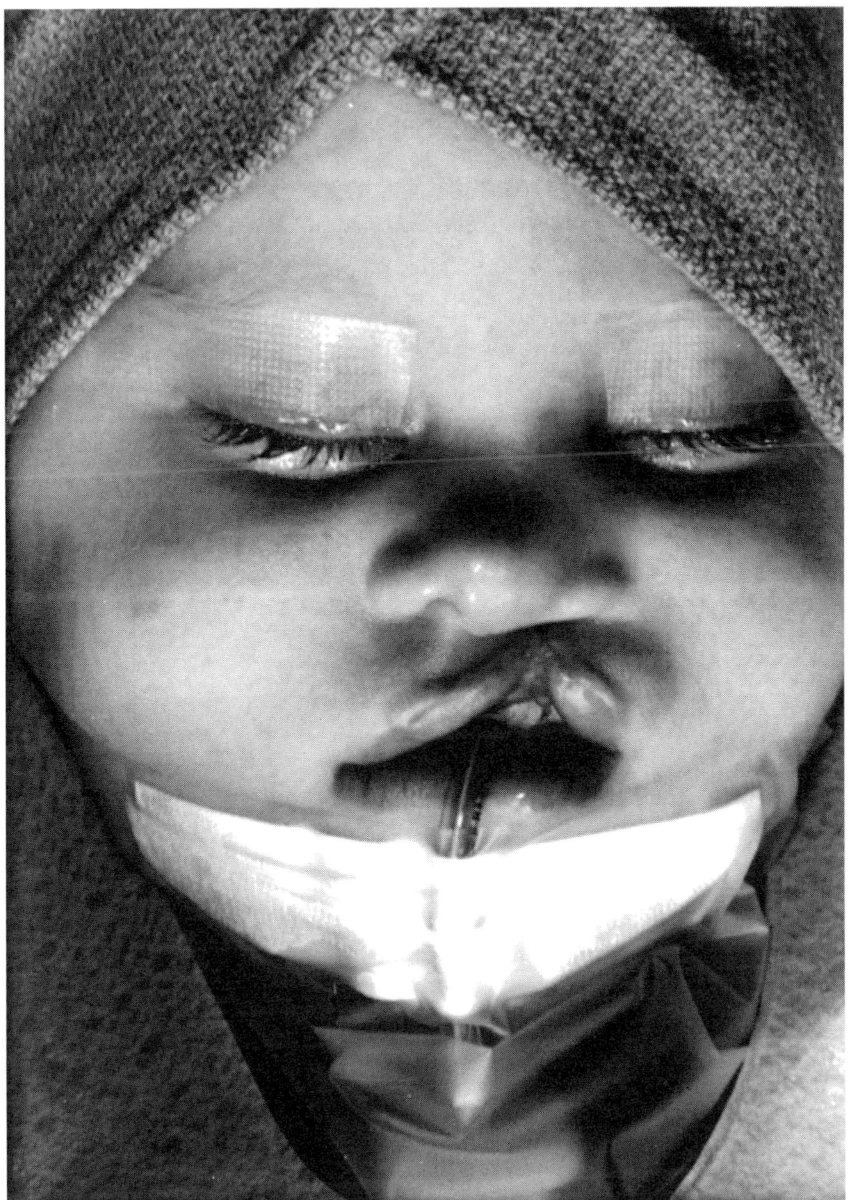

Fig. 22-8 *Periosteoplasty and lip adhesion has been carried out so patient is ready for rotation-advancement of lip and nasal correction. Endotrachael tube in position and taped. Upper eyelids have been splinted with paper tape after ocular lubricant placed in eyes.*

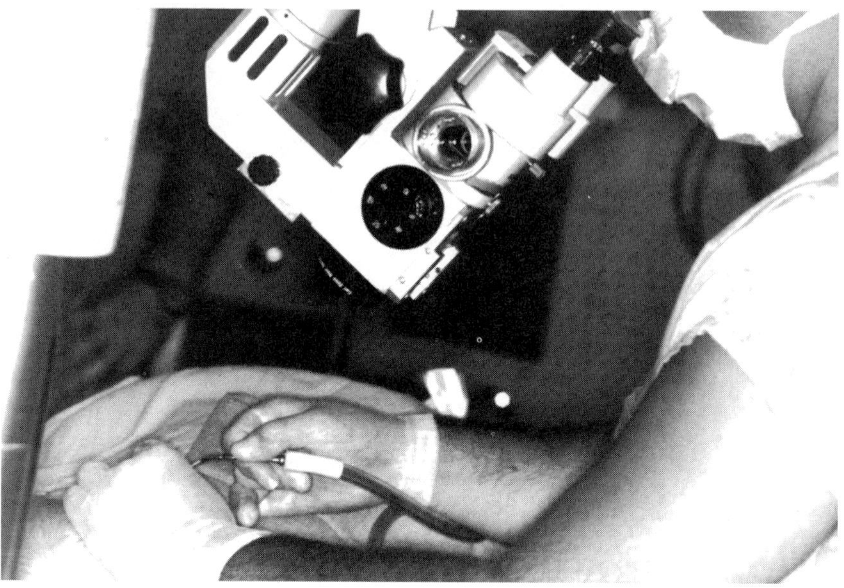

FIG. 22-9 *Otolaryntologist using microscope for myringotomy.*

SPECIFIC PROCEDURES

Periosteoplasty and Lip Adhesion

Once the segments have been aligned and the patient's general health is good, the mucoperiosteum, abnormally lining the alveolar and anterior hard palate cleft, can be incised and elevated out of the cleft to be joined across the cleft on the nasal and oral sides. This creates a periosteal tunnel from bone edge to bone edge across the cleft into which first a clot will form followed by a bony bridge. Teeth will eventually move into this bone. At the time of periosteoplasty, a simple lip adhesion dresses the area without constrictive tension. No special postoperative care is required except removal of a few skin sutures at 4 days postoperatively. The parents are warned to prevent the infant from striking the newly joined lip.

Definitive Lip and Nose Surgery

Alignment of the maxillary segments and their union by periosteoplasty should have a 3- to 4-month healing period. Then the definitive lip surgery is carried out. In the unilat-

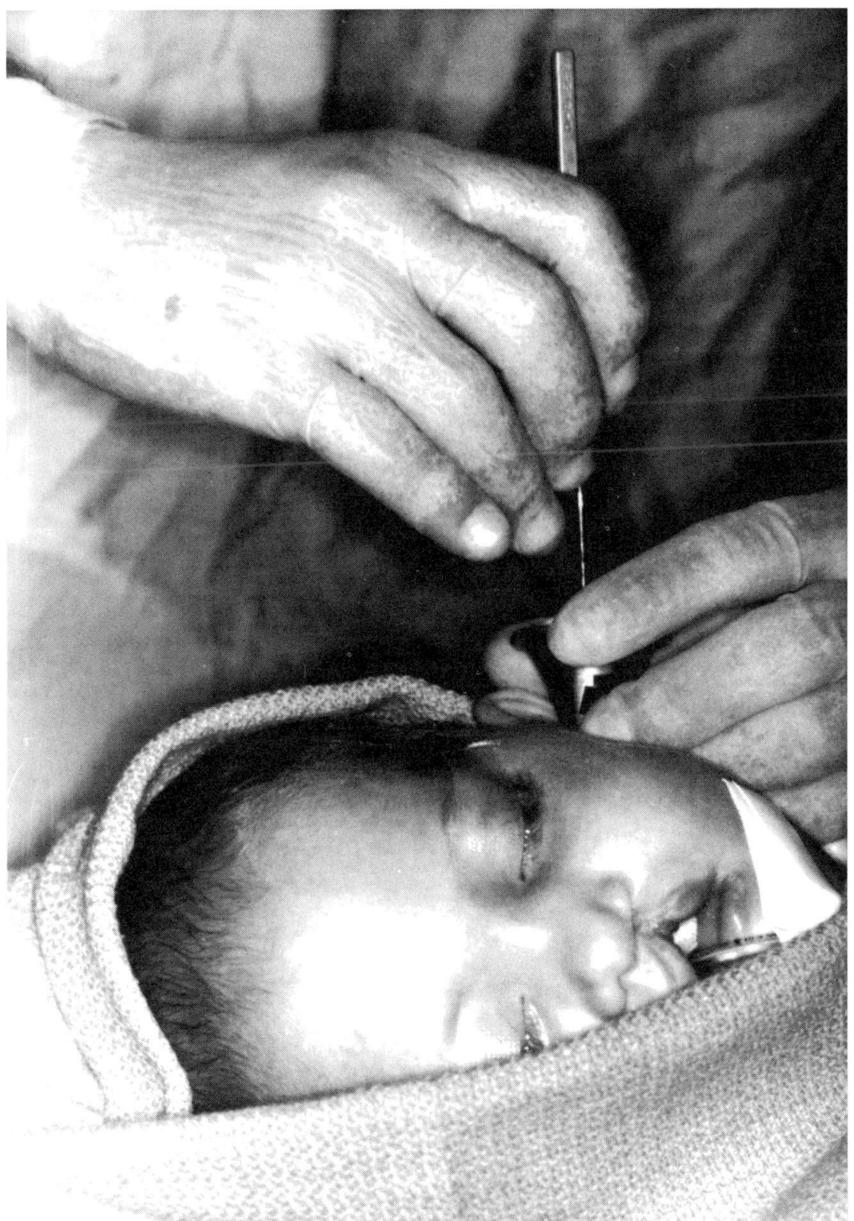

FIG. 22-10 *After myringotomy, polyethylene tubes inserted.*

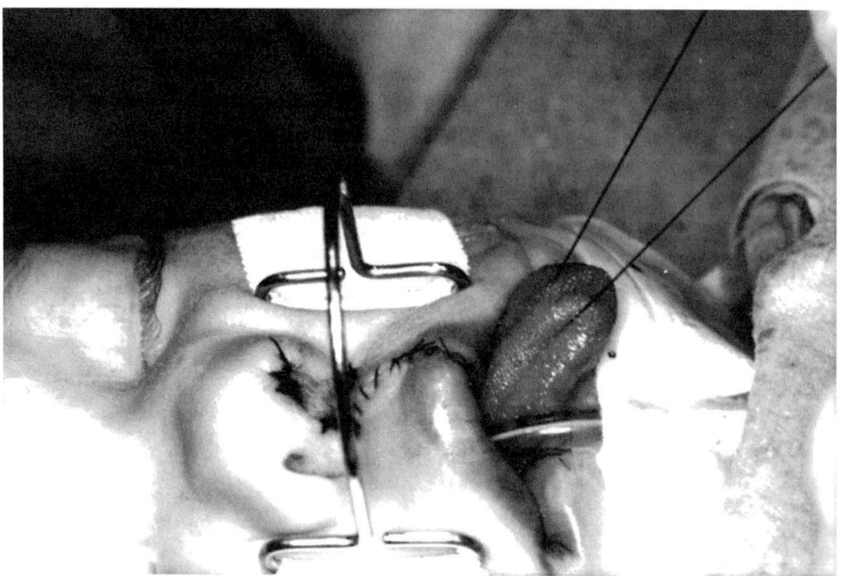

FIG. 22-11 *Safety stitch placed in tongue for retraction during immediate postoperative phase.*

eral cleft, rotation-advancement will position elements best, and alar cartilage positioning will correct the nose. In the bilateral cleft the width of the prolabium determines when the forked flap is taken. If the prolabium is wide, a forked flap can be banked at the time of bilateral lip closure. If the problem is too small, an adhesion can be used to stretch it wide enough to supply a forked flap later for columella lengthening.

Palate Closure

As the alveolar and anterior hard palate cleft is closed early, the remaining hard and soft palate cleft is closed at 18 months of age.

POSTOPERATIVE CARE

Suture Line

- ▼ The infant should lie with the face up at all times.
- ▼ Sutures in the lip and nose are covered with antibiotic ointment (Cortisporin) to avoid the wounds being bathed with nasal discharge.

- A Logan bow is placed across the operated lip, with tension centrally on the cheeks (Fig. 22-12). Although some surgeons do not use the Logan bow, both authors feel that it relaxes the surgical site and counteracts the harmful effects of crying and laughing on the suture line, thus insuring superior healing.
- Aside from the Logan bow, the wound is otherwise left open to facilitate treatment of the suture line. Constant cleansing of the sutures with hydrogen peroxide should be avoided because this is painful and irritates the sutures. The nurse should instead keep the sutures covered with antibiotic ointment, applying it 3 times a day, after feedings. Antibiotic ointment protects the stitch holes from nasal drainage, prevents crusting and keeps the sutures soft, for easy removal on the fourth day after surgery. Antibiotic ointment is continued 24 hours after suture removal until the suture holes are sealed.

Laboratory

The hemoglobin level should be checked the first day after surgery to make sure that whatever blood loss occurred during surgery is tolerated. Blood transfusion will be necessary for a severely low red blood cell level (See Chapter 7.). Iron drops (Fer-In-Sol) can be given for treatment of moderately low hemoglobin levels.

Sedation

Sedation with sodium pentobarbital elixir (Nembutal). To prevent excessive crying, 1 mg/kg is ordered because crying causes unwanted tension on the corrected lip.

Splints

Arm restraints, made by placing tongue blades side by side between two pieces of 4-inch adhesive tape, are applied to the elbows to prevent the patient from inserting a finger into the mouth and separating the incision. These restraints are wrapped around the child's elbow in the OR and pinned to the pajamas to prevent displacement (Fig. 22-13). Plaster of Paris elbow splints also can be used for difficult-to-control children.

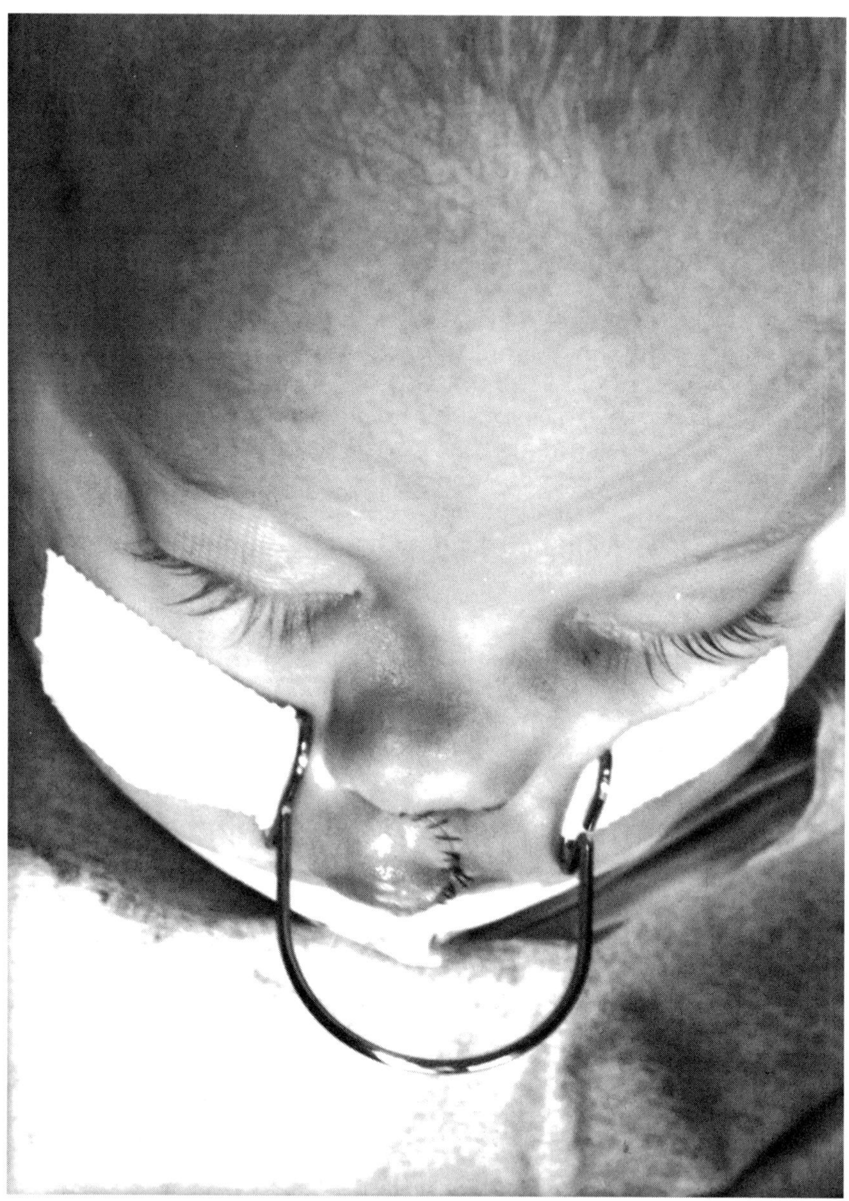

FIG. 22-12 *Logan bow placed to reduce tension on sutured lip.*

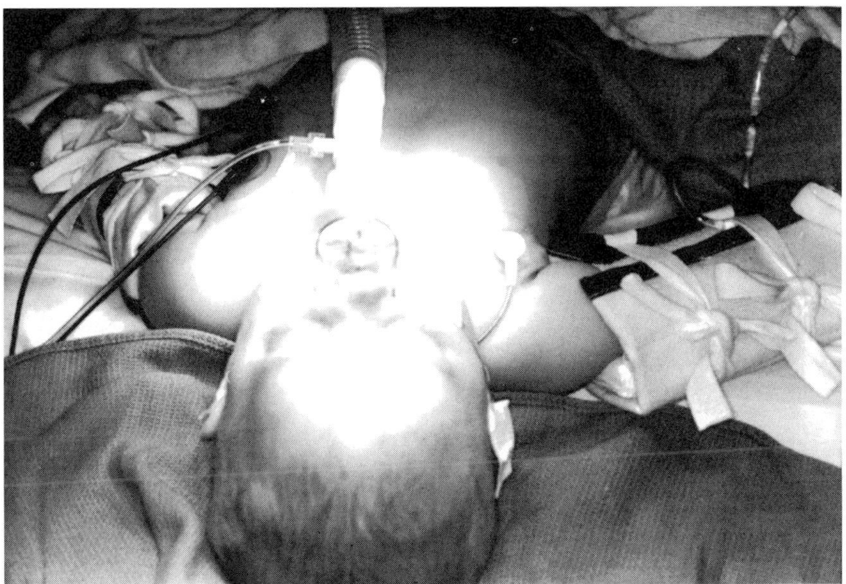

FIG. 22-13 *After operation and while infant sleeps, arm restraints placed on the elbows.*

Removing Sutures

Suture removal is one of the more difficult procedures in postoperative lip care. Some surgeons resort to general anesthesia to accomplish this. Instead, both authors recommend feeding the infant on the fourth postoperative day and giving medication equal to the preoperative order. One hour later, the side of the bed is quietly let down and sutures are removed with fine, smooth forceps and small, sharp scissors while the infant is asleep (Fig. 22-14).

Feeding after Surgery

After lip correction, the infant is fed best by a method that does not require sucking, which is the same routine used preoperatively. The child is held upright as a rubber catheter attached to a 50-ml Asepto syringe is slipped past the healing lip and over the tongue. Nourishment is provided by squeezing the bulb or pushing the syringe at a rate the patient can easily tolerate. Clear liquids are safe as soon as the infant is fully reactive. Regular formula can be started 12 hours

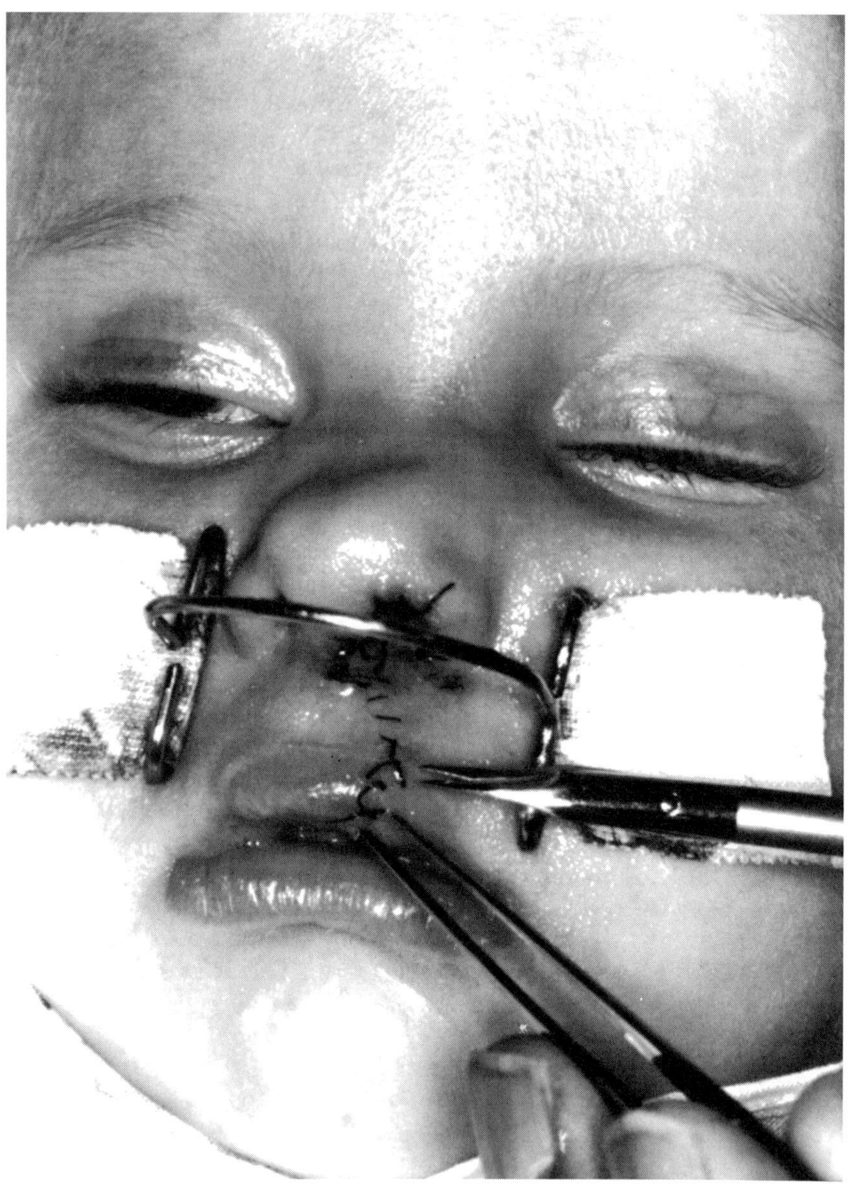

Fig. 22-14 *Infant has been sedated so that sutures can be removed on fourth postoperative day.*

postoperatively. Bottle feedings are allowed 1 month after lip surgery, unless there is also a cleft of the palate; the syringe technique should be continued until 1 month after palate surgery. Each feeding should be finished by passing water through the Asepto tube to clean the palate suture line. Antibiotics are now used routinely but can be instituted only if the lip shows inflammation or there is an elevated temperature that cannot be attributed to low fluid intake.

Discharge from Hospital

Usually the patient can leave the hospital as soon as fluids are well taken. The patient should have elbow restraints and a Logan bow in place (Fig. 22-15). The parents should be taught again to feed the child with the syringe and should feel confident in doing this before taking the infant home. Both the Logan bow and elbow restraints can be removed 2 weeks after surgery. Wounds are allowed to heal in the lip without massage. Banked fork flaps will settle into the nostril floor of the bilateral cleft lip patient and must be kept clean until they are needed to lift the nasal tip.

SECONDARY PROCEDURES

When a minor lip revision is needed, it can be done 6 months postoperatively or at the time of any additional surgery, such as a palate or nose procedure. Because the cleft lip and palate patient is evaluated by a prosthodontist, orthodontist, pedodontist, otolaryngologist, speech therapist, and even a psychiatrist, any of these professionals may recommend additional treatment procedures.

Tonsils and Adenoids

The need for bulky tissue in the posterior pharyngeal area to aid in velopharyngeal closure enjoins restraint in removal of the adenoids in a cleft palate patient. However, chronic nasal discharge, recurrent otitis media, and partial respiratory obstruction are accepted indications for tonsillectomy and adenoidectomy. Hearing improves in approximately three fourths of cleft palate patients after tonsillectomy and adenoidectomy. Some surgeons therefore recommend partial adenoidectomy to treat otitis media and to preserve speech by removing only the lateral adenoid tissue under direct

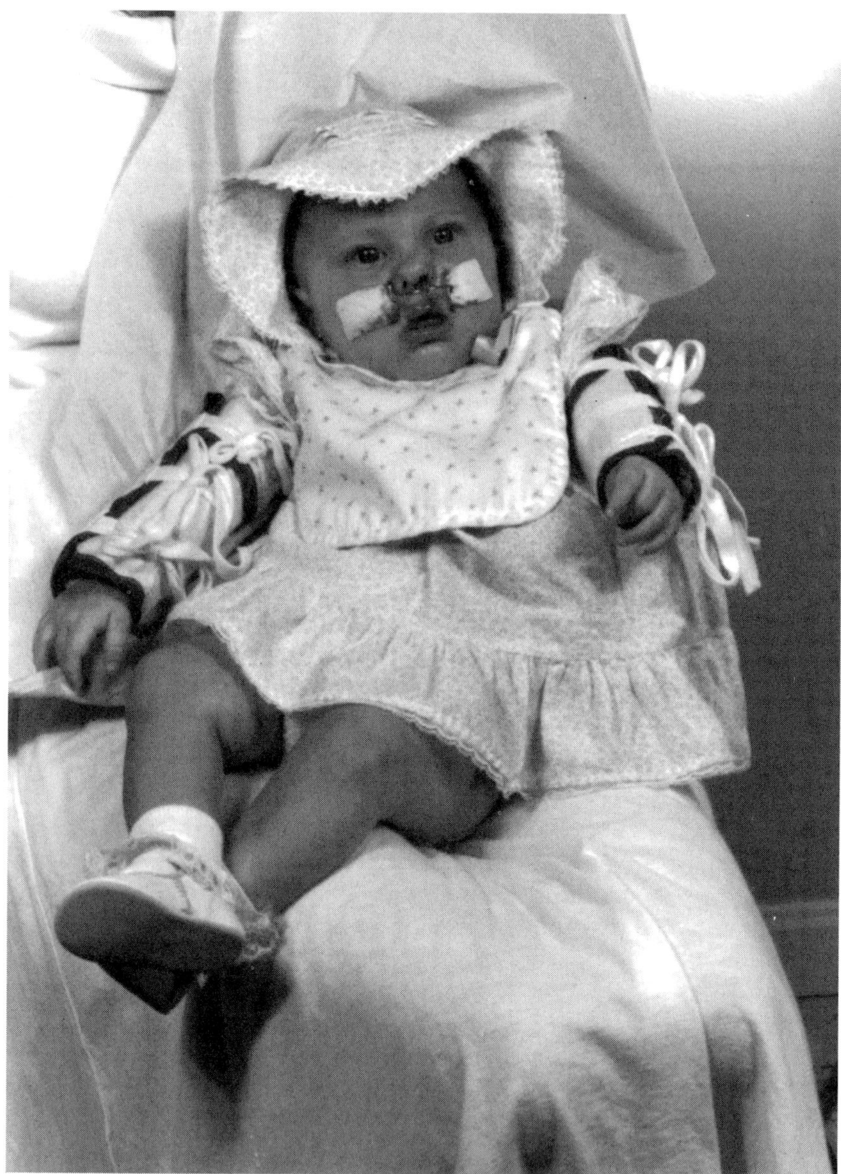

FIG. 22-15 *Patient ready to go home. Logan bow and arm restraint in position so that patient will do least amount of harm to healing lip and nose.*

vision. In removing tonsils, care must be taken by the surgeon to preserve the anterior and posterior pillars and thus reduce postoperative scarring.

Ears

Cleft palate children have a high incidence of fluid in the middle ear. Hearing loss is increased if middle ear fluid is ignored. Early evacuation under the microscope, myringotomy, suction of fluid, and insertion of tubes (plus repeated examinations and reinsertion of tubes) are essential patient care procedures to aid in hearing and speech. As craniofacial growth occurs, improved ear tubal function results in an adequately treated patient.

Secondary Palate Procedures

The care of a patient undergoing a secondary cleft palate procedure, such as a pharyngeal flap is similar to that required for any other operation in this region.

Rhinoplasty

Although the alar cartilage correction is carried out simultaneously with the definitive lip closure, further nasal procedures can be carried out at preschool age or when nasal growth is completed (i.e., age 16 in girls and age 17 in boys). Rhinoplasty patient care is discussed in Chapter 16.

FURTHER READING

Millard DR Jr, Latham RA: Improved primary surgical and dental treatment of clefts, *Plast Reconstr Surg,* 86: 856–871, 1990.

CHAPTER 23

Craniofacial Surgery

S. Anthony Wolfe and Terri L. Hill

Patients with major craniofacial abnormalities come to the surgeon with acquired or congenital conditions that may involved the cranium, the orbital cavities, the maxilla, and the mandible. Correction of their deformities may require complex surgical procedures on any or all of these structures simultaneously.

The length and magnitude of the operation, the frequent need for use of the transcranial surgical route, and the requirement for bone grafts taken from many areas of the body (e.g., ilium, rib, tibia, skull) are all factors that make these types of abnormalities one of the few areas in reconstructive plastic surgery wherein operative and postoperative mortality looms as a real threat even in the best of hands, just as it does in major general surgical or cardiothoracic procedures. Such surgery therefore should not be undertaken lightly. Besides having a thorough background in plastic surgery, the craniofacial surgeon should have received advanced training in this specific area of surgery.

The craniofacial field of plastic surgery owes its beginning and much of its continuing development to Paul Tessier of Paris, who has also devoted much time and energy in helping to establish a number of craniofacial surgical teams in the United States. This chapter borrows heavily from his methods and general approach.

PREOPERATIVE PLANNING

Patient Selection

The most important decisions are usually the ones made preoperatively, that is, the careful and meticulous assessment of the patient and the deformity and the planning of the operative procedures. One must always remember that some patients are not surgical candidates. Severely retarded patients although they may have a correctable craniofacial deformity, should not undergo surgery unless correction of the deformity will result in a definite functional improvement. The risks of surgery and the probability of postoperative complications in severely retarded patients are considerably greater than in individuals of normal intelligence, who comprise the vast bulk of patients with craniofacial deformities.

Team Approach

Although much or all of the surgical procedure is usually performed by the craniofacial surgeon, close collaboration with other members of the team, such as the orthodontist, neurosurgeon, anesthesiologist, ophthalmologist, pediatric "syndromologist," and others, is essential to the successful outcome of the operative procedure.

Alloplastic Materials

Sir Harold Gillies performed the first Le Fort III osteotomy in 1954, but he considered the procedure a failure because of the almost complete late relapse of the advanced midface. In the mid-1960s Tessier showed that the advancement could be maintained if fresh autogenous bone grafts were interposed between the two sides of the osteotomy. Although an occasional situation may be found for the use of alloplastic materials such as methyl methacrylate, polymeric silicone (Silastic), or Proplast in reconstructive surgery of the face, they should not be used in primary craniofacial surgical procedures. The almost unanimous opinion of surgeons in major medical centers performing this type of surgery is that alloplastic substances should not be used in procedures in which there is exposure of osteotomy areas to the mouth, sinus cavities, and nasal passages.

The use of alloplastic materials and heterologous freeze-dried bone or cartilage grafts is restricted to late contouring procedures that are confined to limited areas. An example of this use might be the filling of the temporal depression that occurs in a patient with Möbius' syndrome after the temporal muscles have been used for facial animation. The transient postoperative pain experienced in bone graft donor sites after most such procedures should not influence the surgeon to try using alloplastic material.

PATIENT PREPARATION

Psychologic Preparation

A thorough explanation of the proposed operative procedure to patients and their families does much to relieve anxiety and help them through the operative and postoperative periods. It is often useful to have the surgeon explain the procedure in the preoperative period to patients and their families on several different occasions and also to have the nurse-clinician member of the team spend time reviewing the same material, using somewhat different terminology. It is no help and is often a hindrance to have patients or their families ask questions of the floor nurse in the hospital, who may have little or no familiarity with this type of surgery. Answers to the following questions should be supplied to all patients:

- Will surgeon eyes be covered after surgery?
- How long can they expect to have visual disturbance (e.g., diplopia)?
- What tubes can they expect to have?
- Where will the tubes come from, and where will they go?
- Why are the tubes there, and how long can they be expected to remain?
- If the teeth are to be wired together in intermaxillary fixation, how are patients going to manage to feed themselves after the surgery? (Families of patients should be instructed to purchase a Water-Pik or similar irrigation device to help patients maintain a clean mouth.)
- Where can patients expect to have pain after the surgery and how long might it continue? (Surprisingly, the head itself is generally pain free after most of these major craniofacial procedures, and the pain that is usually experienced is from the bone graft donor areas (e.g., hip, rib, or tibia). It is advisable therefore to use the cranium itself as a source of bone graft material whenever possible.)

SURGICAL PREPARATION

Antibiotics

Antibiotics are started preoperatively in patients who are having bone grafting and the surgeon is using a transcranial approach. (We use high doses of penicillin in nonallergic patients, together with antistaphylococcal agents). Penicillin, when it is used, is given in an IV dose of 1 million units every 4 hours, adjusted as needed for children. The dosage for cephalothin (Keflin) is 1 to 2 g IV every 8 hours. In patients with penicillin and cephalosporin allergies, vancomycin 500 mg to 1 g IV every 6 hours is used. Antibiotics are continued for the first 5 days after surgery. In some cases in which there has been extensive swelling, antibiotics may need to be continued longer.

Shaving

Shaving of hair is done only to the extent required to make the coronal incision. Often no hair need be shaved at all. Although contrary to the training of some neurosurgeons, if the occipital hair can be spared, it will provide some protection against occipital pressure sores that can occur during lengthy procedures.

Positioning

Other bony prominences (e.g. elbows and heels) are padded with cotton before lengthy procedures.

Temperature

Temperature regulation should be provided for, particularly in infants, by a rectal temperature probe and a standard surgical heating blanket.

Endotracheal Tubes

Oral endotracheal tubes should be wired to a tooth or the mandible with a circummandibular wire. Nasal tubes should be sutured to the septum. There is nothing more disconcerting than having an endotracheal tube become displaced during one of the procedures. Armored endotracheal tubes are of considerable help because they do not kink as readily as other tubes (Figs. 23-1, 23-2, 23-3).

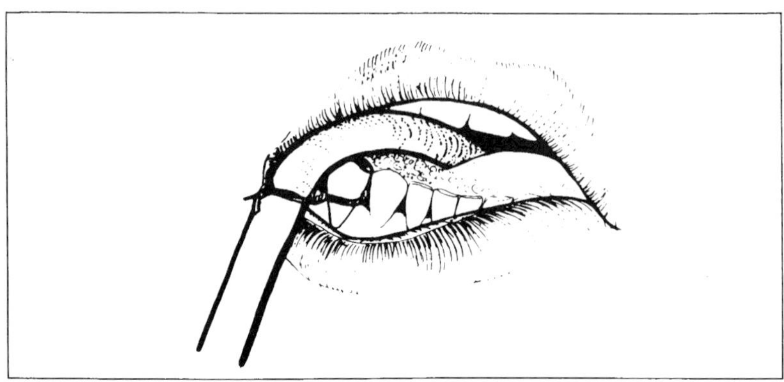

Fig. 23-1 *Fixation of oral endotracheal tube is done by ligating a tooth, usually the canine, and wiring tube firmly in place so it does not slip during surgery.*

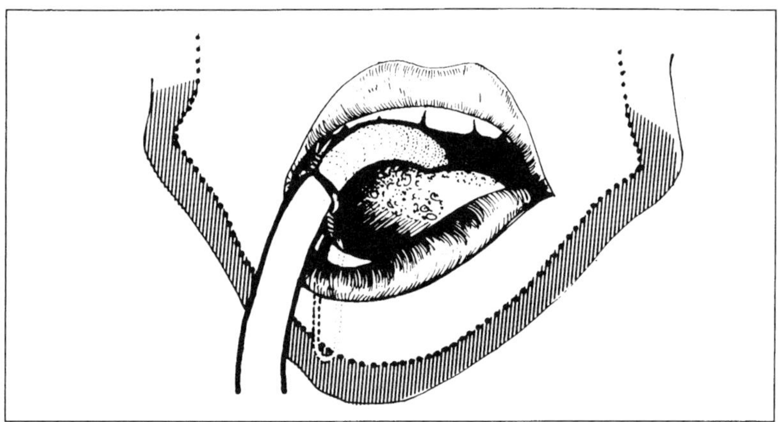

Fig. 23-2 *If patient is edentulous or a child, a circummandibular wire can be used to fix oral tube.*

Eyelid Closure and Scalp Clips

Eyelid closure is maintained by Steri-strips or temporary tarsorrhaphy sutures. Raney or Children's scalp clips are placed along the edges of coronal incisions to minimize incisional bleeding, and preliminary infiltration is performed with a 1:500,000 epinephrine-hyaluronidase solution before incisions are made. There is no benefit in using lidocaine (Xylocaine) under general anesthesia.

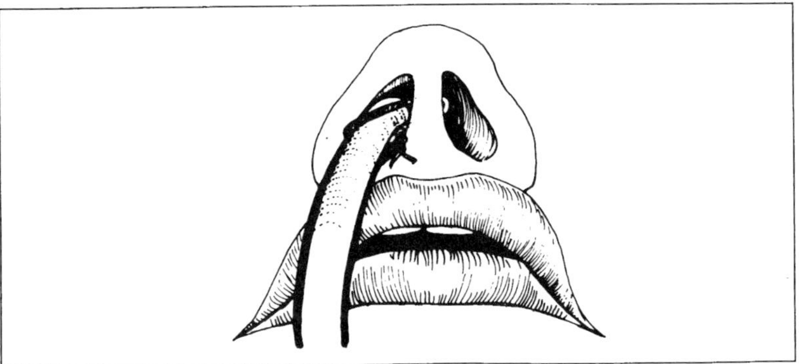

FIG. 23-3 *If nasal intubation is used, a heavy silk suture generally is taken through nasal septum to fix tube in desired position.*

Skin Preparation

Thorough skin preparation for 10 minutes (with Betadine or pHisoHex) and preparation of the nasal and oral cavities, in particular, is important.

INTRAOPERATIVE PROCEDURE

- Lengthy procedures in which blood loss is anticipated require direct arterial and central venous monitoring and installation of a Foley catheter. It is usually unnecessary to use translumbar cerebrospinal fluid drainage when the transcranial approach is used because adequate decompression of the brain often can be obtained by the use of hyperventilation, IV Mannitol, and furosemide (Lasix), 20 to 40 to 80 mg. In the rare case in which the brain is still tense after the use of Mannitol and furosemide combined with hyperventilation, a ventricular puncture can be performed.
- Care must be taken not to manipulate or traumatize the brain during the transcranial procedure. After the neurosurgeon has completed the dissection of the anterior cranial base in a procedure to correct hypertelorism, the upper orbital osteotomies should be performed. It is good to replace the skull flap with several wires during the rest of the procedure so that the assistant's hands or

instruments do not make contact with the brain. The amount of cerebral edema that occurs postoperatively is directly related to the trauma sustained by the brain.

- Because most infections develop where hematomas are present, dead spaces are avoided whenever possible. A large catheter is used as a passive drain in each temporal space. Suction is not used with the drainage because it is undesirable to stress the recently closed nasal mucous membranes. Compressive dressings as discussed later are used for 2 to 4 days after these procedures.
- Hip or rib bone donor sites are drained only if there is a large amount of oozing. If a drain is required for the hip or rib donor site, a standard Hemovac is used. With the increasing use of cranial bone grafts, hip and rib donor sites have become infrequent.

POSTOPERATIVE CARE

- For patients who have had intracranial procedures, the major concern of the postoperative period is the possible development of subdural or epidural hematomas or cerebral edema. A computerized axial tomography (CAT) scan or magnetic resonance imaging (MRI) can differentiate between the various causes of intracranial pressure.
- The usual steroid dosage is 8 to 10 mg of IV decadron, generally given only once, at the end of the operative procedure. Steroids may be given however for the first few days after surgery in tapering doses to postpone—not prevent—postoperative edema.
- Use of intermittent positive-pressure breathing devices without endotracheal intubation with an inflated cuffed tube is contraindicated after almost all craniofacial procedures. There may be a tenuous mucosal closure in the nasal cavity next to a bone graft or the anterior cranial base. Increased intranasal pressure is dangerous in this situation.
- Dressings are of vital importance and should be applied carefully, beginning with a film of antibiotic ointment over sutures, then a covering of petroleum jelly gauze, and then a thick layer of cotton to prevent pressure over

bony prominences (e.g., forehead, orbital rims). When pressure dressings cover the eyes, tarsorrhaphy sutures should be used to prevent eye opening and irritation by the dressings. The orbital cavity should be adequately drained. Sufficient drainage of the orbital cavity is obtained with catheters brought out through the temporal region if a coronal incision is used. If osteotomies are done through the floor of the orbit, drainage into the maxillary sinus will be adequate. More danger exists in placing pressure dressings on the eyes of a patient who has had a blepharoplasty than exists in one who has had a Le Fort III osteotomy or has had a correction of hypertelorism. For example, if a hematoma develops in the blepharoplasty patient, it has no room to expand and vision may be threatened.

- If possible, the patient should be kept in a semisitting position in bed to minimize facial swelling postoperatively. A portable car seat can be used for infants.
- If intermaxillary fixation has been used, cleansing of the mouth with water should begin immediately postoperatively. Gentle toothbrushing with a small toothbrush or use of a Water-Pik can begin after a few days, even with intraoral sutures in place. The lips should be kept lubricated with petroleum jelly to prevent crusting and drying in a patient who is unable to lick the lips.
- Skin sutures that are exposed are kept scrupulously free of crusts with hydrogen peroxide and saline. Thin films of antibiotic ointment are applied. When dressings are removed from the eyes, iced saline compresses are applied; this may not hasten the disappearance of swelling but is of considerable comfort to the patient. Chemosis (extrusion of edematous conjuctiva) is unsightly but generally disappears within a few days if the conjunctiva is kept moist with iced saline compresses.
- Patients are moved to a chair and ambulated as soon as possible, notwithstanding pain from bone graft donor sites. These patients, like cardiac surgical patients, are subject to the "intensive care unit syndrome" in which the constant noise, difficulty in sleeping, lack of difference between day and night, and a number of other factors frequently result in confusion and disorientation.

The sooner the patient can be out of bed and into a chair or can be ambulated, the better. In most cases, this means placing the patient into a chair on the day after surgery.

OUTCOME

If the surgical procedure has been properly planned, carefully executed, and care taken in the postoperative period, results obtained in the craniofacial surgical patient should be dramatic and gratifying.

CHAPTER 24

Head and Neck Cancer

STÉPHANE CORRIVEAU AND WILLIAM P. MAGEE, JR.

Head and neck carcinomas are responsible for approximately 5% of the total number of cancer patients today. Despite recent trends indicating a decrease in the use of tobacco and alcohol in the adult population of the United States, because of the delayed appearance of these tumors, one can still expect to see and treat many patients of both sexes afflicted with head and neck cancer in the next 20 years. For physicians to be comfortable with treatment of head and neck tumors they should be able to project a suitable plan encompassing the usual preoperative and postoperative requirements of these patients.

Fortunate patients will have the lesion discovered as a small, asymptomatic growth either by an observant member of the medical or dental profession or by the patients themselves. When the patient comes to the plastic and reconstructive surgeon with a suspicious entity, the patient has usually already experienced considerable fear. That fear might have caused some delay in between the lesion discovery and the patient's appearance in the office. Therefore one of the first things the physician should do is to spend the time necessary to separate fact from fiction in the patient's mind and to establish rapport, which will be important in the physician-patient relationship that will be developed. The next step is to confirm the diagnosis and establish the clinical staging of tumors, nodes, metastases (TNM); if the clinical suspicions prove to be correct these should be the priorities.

DIAGNOSIS

The suspicious lesion should be biopsied to establish its histologic nature as soon as possible. When the diagnosis of carcinoma is confirmed, planning for preoperative care and operative treatment should begin. Surgical treatment techniques vary according to the type and location of the head and neck tumor and are not included in this book. Differences of opinion (e.g., surgery versus radiation) and confusion may exist about whether, when, and how to treat specific cases. A few basic principles presented here hold relatively true in all patients and once these are understood, one should have a better comprehension of head and neck cancer patient care.

Basal Cell Carcinoma

Basal cell carcinomas are the most common tumor in humans. They come in a variety of shapes and forms, but usually these are less aggressive tumors than squamous cell carcinomas.

A. **Etiology.** The most common underlying cause of basal cell cancer is the ultraviolet B rays (UVB) from sunlight. Blond-haired, blue-eyed persons of fair complexion whose ancestors are from northern regions of Europe have skin not intended genetically to be constantly exposed to the sun and are therefore susceptible to this type of cancer. The most effective treatment for these individuals is prophylaxis, that is, staying out of sunlight and protecting skin with sunscreening agents as much as possible. This includes winter and cloudy days for persons who are at high risk (e.g., outdoor workers, fishers).

B. **Growth patterns.** Complete local excision is usually effective as treatment of basal cell carcinoma. These grow by local extension, rarely metastasizing. Once these tumors are detected, they should be adequately excised, and microscopic evaluation of the specimen should be done to make sure that the tumor has been removed completely. A small subgroup of these tumors with a high degree (75% or more) of irregularity in the peripheral palisade at the border of the tumor, or absence of small lymphocytes at the tumor base, or ulceration, have a more aggressive behavior and must be treated aggressively because of higher recurrence rates. Neglected or incompletely treated tumors can progress silently and create major reconstructive problems. Sometimes they can even kill the patient by direct invasion of vital structures. Although technical solutions vary with the extent and the location of the tumor, their common denominator is that all of the tumor must be excised or irradiated, regardless of its location.

Squamous Cell Carcinoma

The great majority of significant carcinomas in the head and neck regions are squamous cell carcinomas. Contrary to basal cells carcinoma, squamous cells metastasize to lymph nodes in a high percentage of cases. Approximately 34% of patients with floor of the mouth squamous cell carcinoma and a clinically negative neck will have positive nodes during elective neck dissections.

A. **Etiology.** These cancers can occur externally on the facial skin, frequently resulting from sun exposure. Alcohol and tobacco are also known to be etiologic agents in head and neck tumors.
B. **Cell differentiation.** Lesions generally advance from a well-differentiated state into a more undifferentiated state as development of the tumor progresses farther into the mouth. This progression of undifferentiation is probably not related to the local anatomic site as much as it is related to the larger size, which deeper lesions develop before clinically detectable. Generally the farther back the lesion is on the oral pharynx, the more serious is the problem.
C. **Tumor metastases.** As is true of all tumors, lesions that are diagnosed early and are well differentiated entail the best patient survival rates. Lesions that have grown and are detected later in the course of their development are usually poorly differentiated and entail the worst survival rates. Metastatic lesions often are present in this latter group at the time of their initial discovery. The treatment of head and neck cancer is based on a principle similar to that in skin cancer; that is, one should remove sufficient tissue to obtain adequate margins. Because these lesions commonly metastasize to the node-bearing areas, *en bloc*

lymph node resection is usually required for adequate treatment.

PRINCIPLES OF RECONSTRUCTION

A description of the reconstructive techniques available to plastic and reconstructive surgeons for the head and neck area is not relevant to this chapter. Nevertheless, the following principles apply:

- After the tumor is totally excised, a variety of reconstructive techniques can be used, depending on the extent of the extirpative endeavor. These reconstructive modalities range from primary closure of the wound (when possible) to the use of skin grafts, local flaps, distant flaps (fasciocutaneous or myocutaneous), and the use of free tissue transfers when the defect requires it.
- The extirpative surgeon should not base the size of the tumor resection on what the surgeon is comfortable in reconstructing but rather on what is necessary for complete resection. To resect less than the total would in many cases lead to inadequate margins and further difficulties with the tumor in the future. The extirpative surgeon, therefore must either feel comfortable with reconstructive techniques or have on the team another surgeon skilled in cancer reconstruction.
- Occasionally, the surgeon is confronted with a tumor that extends far beyond what was initially suspected. Efforts should be made to complete the tumor excision at the first setting. Chemosurgeons using Mohs' technique have proved many times that patients tolerate well an open wound with an appropriate dressing. Consequently the surgeon faced with a massive resection and inadequate preparation (i.e., few or no assistant surgeons, few operating personnel, little time, few blood products) should complete only the extirpative part of the procedure to have the opportunity of preparing for a second procedure and to explain the situation to the patient and family. Acceptance by the patient and family of the cosmetic or functional defect, of both the tumor and the reconstruction is much better, if complete information is given and consent is obtained preoperatively.

PREOPERATIVE EVALUATION

The problems that arise in the care of head and neck cancer patients usually can be attributed to the general health of the patient, the tumor size and its stage of development, or the extent of treatment that is necessary in the attempt to eliminate the disease.

Oropharyngeal and Upper Respiratory Tracts

An important part of the preoperative evaluation is a thorough examination of the entire oropharyngeal and upper respiratory tracts. An indirect laryngoscopy should be done in the office. To obtain a more complete evaluation, a direct laryngoscopy can be performed under anesthesia before surgery. In approximately 10% of all patients with oral cancers, a second primary lesion will be found at some time during the life of that patient. This second tumor may well have been present at the time of the discovery of the initial lesion because the same insulting agents were in contact with the entire oral mucosa and respiratory tract.

Alcohol and Tobacco

Because a large number of patients with oropharyngeal cancer have a significant history of excessive drinking and smoking, the initial planning should include the patient's clear understanding of these adverse conditions. Plans should be made for their elimination and reversal. Surgeons must assume that the poor habits and disease states of head and neck patients have negatively affected their general health. Surgeons must be prepared to treat all of the potential problems associated with heavy drinking, smoking, and malnutrition, including prolonged bleeding time, decreased respiratory functions, and delirium tremens. High doses of multivitamins, including vitamins B, E, C, and zinc (Z-Bec) are recommended, with addition of vitamin K (Mephyton) to promote wound healing and blood clotting. Careful assessment of hepatic function before vitamin and nutritional therapy is mandatory to determine the extent of liver damage present and its potential reversibility. Evaluation and treatment of clotting factors preoperatively ensures that blood coagulability will be adequate during surgery.

A. **Evaluation of respiratory function.** Heavy smoking causes a significant decrease in respiratory function. Complete evaluation of the patient's pulmonary functions, with spirometer and blood gas measurements, should be performed when any doubt exists about the respiratory reserve. This evaluation can begin with a simple clinical test (e.g., ability of patient to blow out a match held 1 foot away) and can advance to considerably more scientific evaluations as needed. Respiratory function can be improved before surgery with intermittent positive-pressure breathing therapy, nebulization, blowing exercises, and the cessation of cigarette smoking. Cessation of smoking for as little as 24 hours before surgery will significantly decrease carboxyhemoglobin levels and increase the oxygen delivery to tissues by shifting the oxyhemoglobin dissociation curve to the right. If smoking is actually stopped for a longer period of time, the patient will experience a massive increase in sputum production after 10 to 14 days, which is due to the accumulation of mucus and the renewed activity of the remaining cilia in the tracheobronchial tree. One must remember that 7% of all patients with moderate to severe lung disease die within 9 weeks after general anesthesia. Optimizing medical therapy of patients at risk should reduce this mortality rate.

B. **Evaluation of hepatic function.** The surgeon also must be concerned about the possibility of esophageal varices or other gastric anomalies secondary to liver disease, such as peptic ulceration, gastritis, or esophagitis. The presence of a dull contracted liver, large hemorrhoids, spider angioma, and gynecomastia should alert the physician to the possibility of liver cirrhosis and all associated conditions. Nasogastric tubes inadvertently placed against exposed blood vessels in the course of the surgical treatment could easily be the nidus of a significant upper gastrointestinal bleeding episode when any of these conditions exist. If halogenated inhalational agents (halothane enflurane, isoflurane) are considered for use during the general anesthesia, any history of hepatitis (chemical or infectious) should be carefully elicited and alternatives sought.

Nutritional Status

Head and neck tumor patients may have clinically significant nutritional deficiencies not only from alcohol abuse and decreased appetite but also because of the discomfort that they experience in eating, drinking, and swallowing while the disease progresses. Complete evaluation of the patient's nutritional status and recommendations and treatment by someone well versed in nutrition are important so that the patient will be in positive nitrogen balance before and after surgery. Special diets, carbohydrate or protein supplements, and even total parenteral nutrition (TPN) may be required before and after surgery.

Personal and Oral Hygiene

Heavy drinkers have a tendency not only toward poor nutrition but also toward laxity in personal and oral hygiene. Because any surgery performed in the mouth can alter its physiologic properties, careful attention must be given to the patient's oral hygiene status. Lack of normal tongue mobility in head and neck tumor patients decreases the cleansing action that the tongue provides. Removal or irradiation of salivary glands can also lead to a drier and less clean environment. Xerostomia and dental carries often increase when radiation therapy is included as one of the modalities of treatment. Significant problems of gingival and periodontal abscesses can often be present because periodontal disease is not uncommon in this group. A thorough evaluation by a periodontist well versed in the care of the cancer patient and treatment of these dental problems, with either incision and drainage or extraction and antibiotics is mandatory before head and neck surgery. An oral hygiene program should be instituted before surgery.

Acquired Immunodeficiency Syndrome and Hepatitis

The incidence of acquired immunodeficiency syndrome (AIDS) in patients with head and neck cancer is not known to be increased as compared with the general population. The incidence of hepatitis A has been shown to increase among people who abuse alcohol. Also patients with liver disease, are likely to have received multiple transfusions during previous hemorrhagic episodes, which makes them at risk for blood-transmitted diseases. Consequently, the physician should order a hepatitis screen and human immunodeficiency virus (HIV) ELISA or Western Blot tests in the appropriate patient.

Social Considerations

The social situation in which some of these patients find themselves can either contribute to or detract from their complete medical progress. If patients live by themselves or are alienated from their family to any extent, it may be necessary to have a social worker closely involved with the supportive team in planning for nursing home or intermediate care facility placement to foster recovery after hospital discharge.

HOSPITAL ADMISSION

On admission, the usual preoperative x-ray examinations and blood studies are obtained. Any extra studies that may be necessary because of medical problems that a patient might have, such as heart disease, liver dysfunction, or diabetes, are ordered and carefully evaluated before surgery. If the patient does not have a family physician or internist, a consultant may be brought into the case so that a thorough evaluation becomes part of the medical record. Any signs or symptoms suggestive of distant metastasis are evaluated preoperatively with the indicated x-ray films or scans. The surgeon must remember that the TNM staging is done by clinical evaluation only; the presence of enlarged nodes on computerized tomography (CT scan) or magnetic resonance imaging (MRI) does not alter the stage. At this time, CT scanning is as accurate for nodal evaluation as MRI.

INTRAOPERATIVE CARE

Preparation for Procedure

- ▼ All areas that will be operated on for extirpation and that may be used for reconstruction should be prepared and draped at the outset so that time is not wasted during surgery.

- A variety of modalities are available for reconstruction after the extirpative procedure has been completed; these should be well thought out by the surgeon before the extirpation. This is important not only for proper planning of incisions but also for correct positioning of the patient on the operating table. If possible, the surgeon must avoid having to reposition the patient in between the extirpative and the reconstructive portion of the operation; this not only invariably requires a significant time delay but also exposes the patient to risks of contamination, hypothermia, and increased anesthesia time.
- Because of the length of some procedures, special attention has to be placed on prevention of pressure sores; gel or foam cushions can be used judiciously to good effect. Pressure and traction injury to the brachial plexus are particularly disturbing because they always relate to the intraoperative positioning. One can often trace them back to a "quick" position change in the middle of the procedure without removal of the sterile drapes and appropriate verification of the patient's new position.
- The use of heating blankets, fluid warmers, and hot humidified gauzes will help to prevent intraoperative hypothermia.
- Urinary catheter drainage is standard because many patients experience bladder atony after prolonged anesthesia.

Tracheostomy

For any significant resections of the tongue, oropharynx, or mandible, it is wise to initially perform a tracheostomy—not because of the now rare possibility of tracheal damage from the low-pressure endotracheal tubes but because tracheostomy (1) liberates the operative field; (2) allows easier postoperative pulmonary care; (3) reduces dead space in the respiratory circuit, facilitating the weaning of the respirator in patients with marginal respiratory reserve; (4) prevents the possibility of damage to a complex reconstruction from traction or pressure from the oral or nasal endotracheal tube; and (5) is not associated with maxillary sinusitis, as are nasal tubes. Tracheostomy can be done with the patient under local anesthesia with some sedation before the initiation of general anesthesia; or, if oral intubation is easily performed, the tracheostomy may be done with the patient under general anesthesia after intubation and before beginning the formal tumor resection.

Pressure Monitoring

When the patient's condition or the anticipated length of the procedure warrant it, a central venous line and an arterial line should be established at the beginning of the operation. These lines allow complete pressure monitoring during the procedure and are extremely valuable during the postoperative phase, when the patient is in the intensive care unit.

A. **Central venous catheter.** An antebrachial or subclavian approach is recommended for the central venous catheter, so that the line stays well away from the area of resection. If the insertion of the subclavian line is difficult, an immediate upright chest x-ray examination is recommended, because the patient will be under positive-pressure ventilation during the procedure and consequently will be at high risk for tension pneumothorax.
B. **Arterial line.** The arterial line usually can be obtained by a percutaneous stick in the wrist. When necessary, a small cutdown can readily be performed. An Allen test to determine patency of both the radial and ulnar arterial systems should be done before insertion of the line. The patient makes a tight fist to express blood from the skin of the palm and fingers. Digital compression on either the radial or the ulnar artery is exerted by the physician. If blood fails to return to the palm and fingers on opening the hand, obstruction is present in the artery that has not been compressed.

A pulmonary artery catheter (PA line) for monitoring is usually not indicated for head and neck surgery cases. Despite the fact that the complexity of the procedures might require extended operative time, the total blood loss is usually small. Consequently, unless specifically indicated by the previous cardiac history of a patient, we do not recommend the routine use of PA lines.

Resection and Reconstruction

The effectiveness of radical neck dissection is well documented and has been proved for years. The size of the lesion, its location, and the degree of metastatic involvement, all determine the extent of the resection. In the 1950s surgeons first attempted to improve the quality of life of head and neck cancer patients by using skin grafts to reconstruct the lost tissues. Although skin grafts proved beneficial in some smaller defects in which the floor of the mouth was not disturbed, results remained far from satisfying. Monumental advancements in head and neck cancer reconstruction were made by Bakamjian with the use of the *deltopectoral flap* and by McGregor with the use of the *forehead flap* in rebuilding difficult composite defects. These flaps required multiple-stage surgery but were a significant improvement over the skin grafts, even though their donor defects were noticeable. More recently the *trapezius myocutaneous flap,* the *pectoralis major myocutaneous flap* and its extended skin paddle, and the *latissimus myocutaneous flap* have all contributed significant refinements to intraoral cancer reconstruction. In the last 15 years the use of free tissue transfers has revolutionized the head and neck reconstruction possibilities. Muscle bulk, vascularized bone, and soft-tissue coverage can be brought together or can be used as independent elements of a complex reconstruction.

These new reconstructive modalities have significantly improved not only the lifestyle of patients but also their chances of survival, because more aggressive tumor resections can now be done with the advanced methods of reconstruction available. Patients who have had irradiation therapy and still have residual tumor present can now be operated on with less trepidation, because these newer reconstructive techniques bring fresh skin, muscle, bone, and blood supply from nonirradiated donor areas.

Intravenous Fluorescein Testing of Flap Viability

For patients who have had previous irradiation, there is a good reason to question the vascularity of the local flaps, because radiation produces periarteritis and fibrosis, which in turn lead to reactive ischemia of the treated areas. The use of distant transposition flaps for reconstruction may also present questions about their vascularity and their viability. Intravenous (IV) fluorescein is routinely used to document flap viability during operations. With the use of an ultraviolet light, fluorescence can be noted after the fluorescein has been injected. When this fluorescence is not observed, the surgeon should be cautious about using the nonfluorescent portion of the flap and, if at all possible, eliminate this ischemic portion from the reconstruction.

A. **Dosage.** An initial dose of 1 ml is recommended at least 10 minutes before 10 to 20 ml diagnostic dose to recognize potential allergic reactions.
B. **Effectiveness in reducing postoperative complications.** Since performing this fluorescein test, the complication rate with flap nonviability has decreased dramatically, because necrosis of skin flaps is almost always due to lack of vascularity. Before fluorescein testing, necrosis was not usually seen until 2 to 5 days postoperatively. With fluorescein, the surgeon is able to determine flap viability intraoperatively and essentially eliminate this postoperative complication. False-negative tests rarely occur (e.g., flap that is alive looks avascular); they are usually due to systemic shock or hypothermia.

Free Flap Monitoring

Fluorescein cannot be used to determine survival of a free flap. Early pedicle thrombosis, often only venous initially, is the primary problem causing free flap failure. Occasionally, one can use fluorescein before a transfer to demonstrate, after isolating a pedicle, that the vascular territory desired is, in fact, what was dissected. Early detection of free flap failure remains a goal to be achieved by investigators worldwide. Detection of the thrombotic problem before the transferred tissue has suffered any ischemic damage would be ideal. Current techniques using laser Doppler, traditional Doppler, and photoplethysmograph have their proponents and detractors. Careful bedside examination of the flap by an experienced surgeon remains the standard against which any diagnostic device must now be compared. The use of temperature probes is not recommended, because these devices are not sensitive enough to determine anastomotic failure before tissue damage has occurred. Tissue pH monitoring however is a possible physiologic monitoring method under development.

POSTOPERATIVE MANAGEMENT

The procedures and techniques used in the operating room (OR) dictate the recovery of the patient. This is particularly true in the case of head and neck surgery in which large neck flaps are elevated for access to the neck dissection.

General Aspects of Intensive Care

Patients who have undergone significant extirpative or reconstructive head and neck procedures are usually admitted to the intensive care unit (ICU) after surgery.

A. **General care.** Vital signs are continuously monitored and intake and output carefully recorded.
   - ▼ Any special needs of the patient, such as aseptic tracheostomy suction, are met.
   - ▼ In major reconstructions, respiratory support is usually continued for the first postoperative night, because delayed circulation of fat-soluble anesthetic gases might prevent sustained respiratory efforts, especially in a patient with marginal liver function.
   - ▼ A chest x-ray examination is performed with a portable postoperative unit to check for possible pulmonary infiltrates or pneumothorax.
   - ▼ Blood counts are monitored so that an adequate red blood cell (RBC) level is maintained.
   - ▼ Acceptable white blood cell (WBC) counts are controlled by appropriate respiratory, urinary, and wound therapy, including use of systemic antibiotics.

B. **Positioning of patients.** Positioning of the patient may be critical, especially if free-tissue transfer was performed.

Head elevation to 30° to 45° is essential to decrease swelling. A pillow should not be used because the neck angulation might reduce an already diminished venous return if one of the jugular veins has been sacrificed. Adequate vascular pedicle length must be placed intraoperatively to prevent kinking of the venous return on bony prominences (i.e., the angle of the jaw), once the postoperative swelling has set in at 24 to 48 hours. We discourage the use of any ribbons or string around the neck (e.g., tracheostomy tape, face mask elastic) because pressure from them could cause flap failure if applied at a critical location. What might appear appropriately loose when leaving the OR might be too tight after a couple of hours of swelling.

C. **Nutrition.** Patients unable to receive oral nourishment may receive high-caloric liquid tube feedings through an oral gastric-jejunal tube or alternatively through gastrostomy-jejunostomy tubes. Even when the recovery period is prolonged and weight loss pronounced, the gastrointestinal (GI) route is the preferred method. Total parenteral nutrition (TPN) should be reserved for cases where the gut cannot be of use or will not tolerate the osmotic load of the tube feedings. Even then, as soon as the GI tract can resume normal function, TPN should be discontinued in favor of tube feedings. This is not only because of the costs involved in TPN but also because of the rate of sepsis and associated complications.

D. **Removal of urinary catheter.** The urinary drainage catheter should be removed as soon as the patient can be confidently expected to use bedside containers.

E. **Ambulation and discharge.** Early ambulation—the morning after surgery or as soon thereafter as possible—is encouraged. The patient is discharged from the ICU as soon as the postoperative progress allows it, usually 1 to 5 days after surgery, to a section of the hospital where the nursing personnel are familiar and comfortable with postoperative head and neck patient care.

Drainage

Adequate drainage is essential under all flaps, especially in head and neck surgery. Numerous large and small blood vessels are encountered and severed during neck dissection. When the patient awakens and there is an increase in positive pressure with coughing and stress, any of these small vessels can easily open, producing a significant hematoma. Adequately placed close suction drainage in the neck usually will handle this situation, and such drains have been shown not to increase the rate of infections. The surgeon should use as many suction drains as are necessary to hold down the skin flaps adequately. Bring these drains out through separate stab incisions in the skin, so that surgical incisions are not stressed. In free-flap surgery, place a drain in proximity but not in contact to the anastomosis. Beware of loops in the trajectory of the drain, because they may cause bleeding at the anastomotic site when they are removed. If a collection of blood accumulates under the flap despite these drains, bring the patient immediately back to the OR for evacuation of the hematoma and suture ligation of the open vessel or repair of the anastomosis (see "Hematomas and Seromas" later in the chapter).

Wound Care

Postoperative care of the surgical incisions is a relatively simple matter. Antibacterial ointment (e.g., Neosporin) is used on the suture line only to make encrusted blood easy to remove. No specific dressing is placed on the wound, so that the skin flaps may be observed by the physicians and the nursing personnel at all times. In an irradiated neck, the skin sutures are left in place for a longer period (2 weeks) than in the nonirradiated neck (1 week). Intraoral reconstructions should be kept clean and the suture lines unstressed. The use of a hand-held tonsil-tip suction helps keep patients happy and their mouths clean by removing excess saliva and intraoral drainage, because most of them have swallowing difficulty secondary to the tracheostomy and the tongue swelling. A gentler regimen or oral cleaning every 2 hours with mouthwash or 0.12% chlorhexidine (Peridex) tends to decrease the bacterial count, and accordingly, diminish the smell originating from the oral flora. Aggressive mouth care tends to increase the compassion demonstrated to the patient by the medical personnel.

Respiratory Care

Aggressive respiratory support is often necessary to decrease the incidence of postoperative atelectasis and infiltrates.

Incentive spirometry is usually effective in mobilizing secretions. Warm humidified oxygen therapy when indicated will usually suffice to prevent desiccation of the mucous membranes and secretions, but occasionally a mucolytic agent is helpful. *N*-acetylcysteine (Mucomyst) is effective in a vaporizer, but because of its bronchospastic potential it should be used preceded or mixed with an inhaled beta-adrenergic agonist (e.g., metaproterenol, isoetharine).

Corticosteroids

No consensus exists on the use of corticosteroids intraoperatively and postoperatively to decrease the massive swelling that sometimes accompanies head and neck surgery. Physicians who use dexamethasone routinely are convinced of its effectiveness. Unfortunately, no consistent scientific data can support their claim. Consequently, we cannot recommend the routine use of steroid for the prevention of edema in the head and neck area.

Anticoagulant and Antiplatelet Agents

The use of heparin, aspirin, and low molecular weight dextran (LMD) during free-tissue transfers varies from surgeon to surgeon. Patients with a medical history of ulcers and esophageal bleeds who need treatment with systemic anticoagulants should be treated with heparin at a lower dose. Most commonly, low-dose heparin (300 IU/hr IV) is used at a rate not affecting either the prothrombin or the partial thromboplastin times (PT-PTT). Heparin has a short half-life and can be reversed by protamine sulfate IV if a life-threatening GI bleeding episode starts. Aspirin has an irreversible effect on platelets which have a 10-day half-life, and the effect of LMD is also irreversible.

MANAGEMENT OF POSTOPERATIVE COMPLICATIONS

Hematomas and Seromas

As previously mentioned, a hematoma collection unresolved by adequate drainage should be evacuated in the OR. Seromas, which usually occur between the third and fifth postoperative day after the drains have been removed, can be an annoying complication. When seromas occur, they are almost always treated by sequential aspiration with a 19-gauge needle and a syringe for 1 to 3 weeks. Chylous fluid also can collect under the neck flap, owing to unrecognized cutting of some of the major lymphatic channels during surgery. This is usually a self-contained problem, and it will resolve itself in 1 to 3 weeks. Sequential aspiration may also be necessary for removal of chylous fluid during this time.

Infection

It is well understood that the oral and nasal pharynx, with a variety of bacteria always present, have significant contamination potential. For this reason, all head and neck cancer patients are begun on prophylactic broad-spectrum antibiotics, a first generation cephalosporin (cefazolin 1g IV), or clindamycin 600 mg IV the evening before surgery. Antibiotic therapy is continued for 1 to 2 weeks postoperatively, depending upon the overall progress of the patient. Significant periodontal disease and cavity formation in the teeth increase the amount of bacteria present within the mouth. Proper preoperative attention to intraoral hygiene is therefore essential.

When infection becomes a problem postoperatively, it is almost always due either to the presence of necrotic tissue or to a breakdown in the oral closure. To prevent a breakdown in the oral closure, horizontal mattress sutures are used to properly evert the edges of the wound. Mucous membranes are difficult to evert with a simple running suture or simple interrupted suture, because the mucosal edges have a tendency to invert. This is especially true when one is trying to bring dissimilar tissues into approximation (e.g., the skin of a flap and the mucous membranes). Delay in primary wound healing is believed to be one of the prime factors in infection and fistula formation. The choice of antibiotics for treatment of postoperative infections should be guided by specific sensitivity cultures. It is better to open a suture line to drain accumulated fluids and let it heal secondarily than to lose a flap completely.

Nerve Deficits

A postoperative complication of which all patients should be warned is loss of sensory or motor nerve function because of surgical resection. All of the superficial nerves, such as the greater auricular, posterior occipital, and transverse cervical branches, are removed during the neck dissection. For this reason, areas of the head and neck supplied by these nerves will be anesthetic. Likewise, when portions of the body of the mandible are removed that contain the inferior alveolar nerve, the ipsilateral half of the lower lip becomes anesthetic.

The surgeon should exercise caution and concern for mouth motor functions supplied by the marginal mandibular nerve, because this nerve is intimately associated with the upper part of the neck dissection and the submandibular triangle. In neck dissection, nerve simulators should be used to isolate, protect, and preserve the marginal mandibular nerve whenever possible. If it has to be sacrificed because of tumor involvement, the surgeon should try to replace the mandibular nerve with a nerve graft by using the operating microscope for anastomosis. Following this same philosophy, the surgeon should always try to preserve the spinal accessory, phrenic, or recurrent laryngeal nerves, unless it is directly involved with tumor. When the spinal accessory nerve is resected because of its tumor involvement, the surgeon should attempt reconstruction.

The anesthesiologist must be notified in advance of the surgeon's intention to use nerve stimulation so that a long-acting muscle relaxant will not be used. Nerve stimulators can be used as early as 20 minutes after intubation with a short-acting muscle relaxant.

Once a muscle is denervated it will atrophy rapidly. Transcutaneous electrical stimulators can be used to preserve muscle bulk and function while waiting for the neural regeneration to travel the distance between the microneural coaptation site to the end plate of the muscle.

Delayed Hemorrhage

Significant hemorrhage is known to occur late after extensive extirpation head and neck cancer. The possibility of catastrophic bleeding is always worrisome, especially in the neck after irradiation. Postoperative hemorrhage is often associated with an oral cutaneous fistula in which inadequate protection of the carotid system leads to its being bathed in saliva. Well-established methods of neck reconstruction have helped considerably with this problem. A surgeon can cover the entire neck dissection with muscle by using the pectoralis major flap. This flap provides superb protective coverage of the neck contents with well-vascularized distant tissue. Especially when irradiation has been used in treatment of the tumor, this new, nonirradiated musculature is important for protection of the neck contents. After using the pectoralis major muscle flap in more than 50 cases, half of which were irradiated necks, we have encountered no significant problems with bleeding or wound healing.

Aspiration

Aspiration can be a problem in patients in whom significant amounts of the base of the tongue or the oral pharynx have been compromised, either by the extirpative surgery or by the concomitant swelling and paralysis. This is due to the inability of the respiratory tree to protect itself by its normal physiologic mechanisms. When this occurs, extreme care must be taken in feeding these patients, many of whom will go to temporary tube feeding, either by a gastrostomy or jejunostomy. A nasogastric feeding tube is routinely used for the first 5 to 7 days after head and neck surgery, so that adequate nutritional support can be provided during the immediate postoperative period. Time usually helps this situation through the resolution of edema and wound healing.

Osteoradionecrosis

Osteoradionecrosis can be a problem in patients who have received preoperative or postoperative radiation therapy. In postoperative care of head and neck cancer patients, one must remain cognizant of this possible complication and be well prepared to treat it.

A. **Symptoms, signs, and contributing factors.** Pain is a dramatic symptom in patients with osteoradionecrosis, and wound breakdown over the necrotic bone is common. Osteoradionecrosis can occur relatively early or after a number of years postoperatively. Often it is preceded by a minor surgical procedure such as the extraction of a tooth, which allows entry of bacteria into the poorly vascularized bone bed.

B. **Treatment.** Treatment of this condition requires extensive débridement of the involved bone and adequate coverage of the remaining bone with a viable flap. When dealing with a badly scarred bed that failed previous reconstructive efforts with bone graft as is common for the mandible, a free-vascularized bone transfer has provided reliability and flexibility.

Delirium Tremens

With any alcoholic patient, delirium tremens (DTs) can be a serious complication, especially in the immediate postoperative phase. When full blown, it is associated with an amazing 50% mortality rate. When possible, it is wise to have patients under close observation and free of alcohol for at least 1 week before surgery.

A. **Clinical signs and differential diagnosis.** In the postoperative phase, DTs must be suspected, but not assumed, when a patient becomes confused, disoriented, or combative. Hypoxemia can cause a similar clinical state, and the assumption must not be rashly made that a patient has DTs. Sequential chest x-ray examinations and blood gases are ordered at intervals to differentiate the diagnosis and ensure that the respiratory tract is functioning appropriately.

B. **Treatment.** When blood gases are normal and the diagnosis of DTs is made, a variety of medications, IV benzodiazepine, in small increments (Diazepam 2 to 5 mg) is helpful. Constant reorientation to time and location by the nursing staff and low-level light for 24 hours a day will decrease the severity of hallucinations and will help to reassure the usually distressed patient. Careful immobilization is mandatory to protect the recent reconstruction, and aggressive pulmonary toilet by respiratory therapists is mandatory if and when the patient becomes unable to cooperate. IV alcohol administration is one of the more effective means of bringing DTs under quick control; it should be considered early in the course of the disease.

Orocutaneous Fistulae

One of the most distressing sights a surgeon can see is saliva escaping from the reconstructed oral cavity and reaching the skin of the neck, often bathing bone grafts along the way. Although nonvascularized bone grafts might not survive such an insult, well-débrided bone will. The majority of these fistulae will close spontaneously if devascularized bone is débrided and given the appropriate time.

Frye's Syndrome (Auriculotemporal Syndrome)

This syndrome is a condition in which gustatory sweating occurs. This is due to aberrant regeneration of the auriculotemporal fibers to the skin flaps overlying a parotidectomy dissection. This condition has been associated with excessively thin skin flaps. The diagnosis is confirmed by the minor iodine test for starch. A tympanic neurectomy may be necessary for severe cases. Interposing the deep temporalis fascia has been tried in the past. More commonly, local skin excision is sufficient, because the involved skin area is small in most cases.

Depression

Being given a chance to beat cancer might not be enough for the patient who has to live sometimes with a less than perfect reconstruction. Many of these patients have poor family support systems and are subject to thoughts of suicide when confronted with what is sometimes disfiguring surgery. Psychiatric evaluation and psychologic support through body image clinics or group therapy should be organized as soon as depression appears to be a problem for the patient.

OUTCOME

Head and neck cancer patients usually do well after surgery if all the necessary precautions have been taken preoperatively, operatively, and postoperatively. They usually can resume useful lives. The advances in the reconstruction of large head and neck defects secondary to cancer that have been made possible by increased knowledge and use of skin, muscle, and bone transfers have made this type of surgery a rewarding experience for those surgeons involved in resection and reconstruction. However, additional modifications and refinements in surgical technique and patient care are necessary so that plastic surgeons can continue to improve outcomes and help these patients to resume satisfactory lives.

CHAPTER 25

Breast Augmentation and Capsular Contractures

James L. Baker, Jr.

Augmentation mammaplasty has been one of the most sought after cosmetic operations in the United States. Conservative estimates place the number of breast augmentations done annually in excess of 100,000 patients. Approximately 2 million women have had breast augmentation using silicone prostheses.

In 1992 the Food and Drug Administration (FDA) banned the use of silicone gel prostheses for cosmetic augmentation mammaplasty. Currently, there is a 5-year study that has been proposed by the FDA, which will involve 1,000 patients in an attempt to answer questions raised by that governmental agency in early 1992. These involve the rupture rate of the prostheses and their questionable link to autoimmune disease. Currently, saline inflatable implants are the only prostheses available for cosmetic augmentation mammaplasty. It should be noted that the saline inflatable implant has to date not been approved by the FDA (in addition to approximately 300,000 other nonapproved medical devices) but is coming up for review in 1998.

Although augmentation mammaplasty has recently undergone criticism, we must remember that the majority of patients have not experienced adverse effects. The strong, positive psychologic benefits to the women who suffer from poor body image because of breast hypoplasia must be considered. Breast augmentation remains one of the safest and most requested aesthetic procedures and is one of the most gratifying cosmetic operations performed, yielding instant alteration of body image for the patient. For surgeons to repeatedly produce an aesthetically pleasing breast and a satisfied patient, they must have a complete understanding of the psychosexual dynamics of the female desire for increased breast size.

PSYCHOSEXUAL DYNAMICS

From the earliest of times, the breast has been the symbol of womanhood. Kinsey reported in 1984 that an American man found the sight of a female breast a greater sexual stimulus than that of the female genitalia. The size and shape of the breasts are extremely important to a woman in her perception of her body and in her concept of self. Although cultural and biologic pressures encourage women to seek breast augmentation, previous studies have reported that the personal symbolism of the breast is the most important stimulus to the women seeking surgical correction.

In 1973 I reported a psychiatric study of patients undergoing breast augmentation. The study was designed to evaluate the motivational factors and the psychiatric prognostic indicators for patient selection. In this study, the average woman requesting breast augmentation was an educated, upper middle-class mother of two children who was in her early 30s. She had considered augmentation for many years. Feelings of inadequacy had developed early in puberty, when she compared her own breast development with that of her peers. The feelings of inadequacy became deeply rooted and had an effect on her interpersonal relationships. She usually decided to undergo surgery after discussing it with a friend who had undergone a satisfactory breast augmentation. The study also showed that these patients rejected using a padded brassiere to give the illusion of adequate breast size, no matter how natural it may feel or appear. Use of padding further enhanced their feeling of inadequacy and was considered a deceptive maneuver. For an artificial device to be effective, it must be implanted beneath the skin, so that it may become incorporated into the patient's body image.

In the early postoperative period, the patient spends much time in front of the mirror admiring her new body image and feeling her breasts. This is the psychologic mechanism by which the patient incorporates the implant into her own body image. Postoperative evaluation of breast augmentation has shown that patients experience a marked increase in self-esteem, adequacy, and self-confidence. There is frequently an increase in the quality and quantity of sexual relations. Apparently this is secondary to a release of sexual inhibitions caused by previous feelings of inadequacy as a result of small breasts.

PATIENT SELECTION

In evaluating the psychologic acceptability of a patient for augmentation, the following three key questions must be asked; the answers to these questions are excellent indicators as to which prospective patients will be satisfied and have a positive response to their changed body image:

- Why do you want your breasts enlarged?
- What size would you like to be?
- If you have had a pregnancy, did your breasts enlarge, and if so, what was your reaction to this change?

The typical positive prognostic responses to Question 1 are (1) "I dislike wearing a padded bra," (2) "I have always felt inferior or inadequate about my small breasts," and (3) "I used to have good breasts before I had children; they just seem to get smaller with each child." These responses usually indicate a stable, realistic woman who will be pleased by breast enlargement.

The responses to Question 2 regarding new breast size indicate whether the desires are realistic. It is not realistic to take a small framed, thin woman with a triple A cup size and turn her breasts into double Ds without making her look grotesque. The typical correct patient response to Question 2 is "I don't want to be too big, just normal, and in proportion to the rest of my body."

Question 3, regarding breast enlargement with pregnancy, may be the best indicator for evaluating the prospective augmentation patient. If breast enlargement during pregnancy produced positive feelings for the patient, breast prostheses should have a similar effect. Conversely, if the patient was displeased with breast enlargement during pregnancy, there is a high probability that surgically enlarging the breasts will produce similar adverse feelings. In essence, pregnancy provides a temporary breast augmentation. If the patient was unhappy then, it is naive to expect her to be pleased with permanent enlargement from surgical augmentation. A typical positive response to this question is "That was the only good part of the pregnancy; I tried to breastfeed forever to keep them large. I loved it."

PREOPERATIVE EVALUATION

Physical Examination of Breasts

The office nurse prepares the patient for examination and remains present during the examination and taking of photographs. The patient's clothing is removed to the waist. The examination is begun from behind the patient to evaluate her spinal alignment. Scoliosis in varying degrees is a common finding and often will cause asymmetry of the breasts or nipple alignment and rotation of one side of the anterior thoracic wall, which can appear as a breast asymmetry. Any discrepancies that produce asymmetry must be pointed out to the patient, because most patients are unaware of these anomalies. Any anomalies noted are marked on the body sheet and pointed out to the patient in the mirror (Fig. 25-1).

The breasts lie on the thoracic wall similar to a building resting on its foundation, projecting off this bony foundation. Any alteration in the thoracic wall will produce projection alterations of the breasts. A patient may believe this will be corrected by breast augmentation. When the ribs slant or lateralize with a prominent sternum, a patient will never have a tight cleavage and must be made aware of this before surgery. The implant will produce fullness beneath the breasts in the position in which they are lying on the chest wall. It does not alter the direction in which the breasts or nipples project. The nipple distance is measured from the sternal notch and noted on the body sheet.

A. **Symmetry.** If the breast volumes are not symmetrical one should plan to use different fill volumes or different

ANATOMIC FORM

NAME ____

DATE ____

Breast and Chest Circumference

Inframammary Chest Circumference

ABD Circumference

Hip Circumference

1. Have you or any family member had breast pathology, such as cysts, tumors, infection or cancer?

____

2. What is your bra size now?__________ Desired size?__________

3. Is nipple stimulation important in your sex life?

____

FIG. **25-1** **A,** *Example of body sheet for noting anatomic breast anomalies.*

ANATOMIC FORM

NAME ____

DATE ____

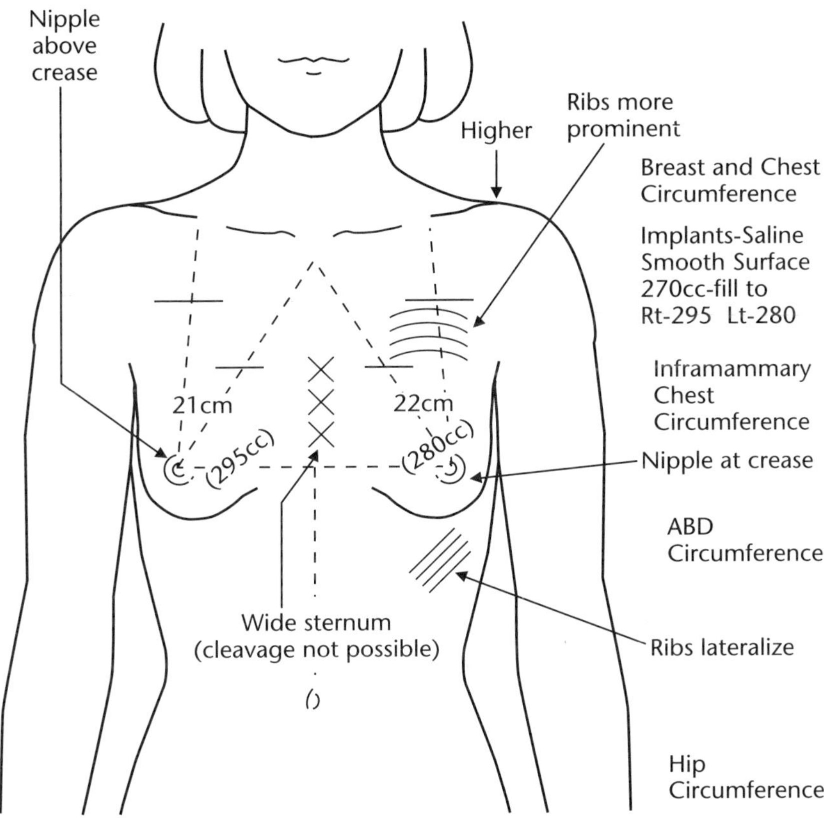

1. Have you or any family member had breast pathology, such as cysts, tumors, infection or cancer?

   Mother: benign cysts

2. What is your bra size now? *34-A* Desired size? *34-C*

3. Is nipple stimulation important in your sex life?

   Yes (but patient NOT orgasmic from nipple stimulation alone)

FIG. 25-1—***cont'd.*** **B,** *Example of body sheet with surgeon's notes entered.*

size implants to minimize the discrepancy. The patient is warned during the examination that symmetry should be greatly improved, but that perfect symmetry is impossible to attain.

B. **Presence of ptosis.** Ptosis of any great degree is not improved by augmentation and can be accentuated. If the nipple is far below the inframammary crease, mastopexy with or without simultaneous augmentation is recommended. When the nipple is at the crease or marginal to the crease, the patient is warned that the nipple will not be moved up on the chest wall by augmentation unless a superior areolar ellipse is excised. Some degree of ptosis will still be present and may even be increased postoperatively. The patient is discouraged from going without a brassiere after surgery because this will produce greater loss of elasticity and further ptosis. If the patient is willing to accept the limitation produced by her degree of ptosis, augmentation is performed with the warning that further mastopexy may be necessary as progressive loss of elasticity and further descent of the breasts occurs.

The nipples are measured down from the sternal notch. Any difference in position is pointed out to the patient. Augmentation will not appreciably change the nipple alignment unless a periareolar ellipse is removed. Many patients assume that augmentation will produce perfect symmetry, exact nipple alignment, and lovely cleavage. Unless the anatomic prerequisites are present preoperatively, this will not be evident postoperatively. If the patient is aware of the limitations of her anatomy and of the surgical procedure and she accepts these limitations, she will be pleased with the postoperative result. Unrealistic expectations are the most common cause of patient dissatisfaction after surgery.

C. **Breast palpation.** Bilateral palpation is performed, and the nipples are examined for any abnormal discharge. If any questions of breast pathologic disorders are present, bilateral mammography is performed preoperatively. If biopsy is indicated, it may be performed at the time of augmentation.

Decision on Implant Size

Implant size is decided upon, and a note is made on the chart. The patient's expectations are evaluated, and volumes are discussed with the patient. Templates are available showing base diameter and sizes, and the implant base may be related to these templates to aid the surgeon in choosing the right implant. If the base diameter of an implant is too large for the base of the breast and chest wall, an abnormally full appearance will occur, with convexity in the upper poles caused by attempting to squeeze too large an implant into too small a space. A general rule of thumb is that approximately 100 to 125 cc of volume will produce a one cup size change postoperatively. When different volumes are necessary for improving breast symmetry, the different fill volumes are marked on the body diagram to avert confusion in the operating room (OR). Implant sizes are marked on the patient's breasts with gentian violet in the OR to avoid a mistake by placing an incorrect volume implant on the wrong side.

Preoperative Photographs

Photographs with a solid background are taken of all patients undergoing surgery. Standard frontal, right and left lateral, and oblique views should be taken from neck to waist. The arms should be at the side unless a thoracic or breast anomaly is present, in which case views may be taken with arms overhead as well. The same distance from camera to subject should always be used so that preoperative and postoperative photographs can be compared accurately.

Preoperative Mammography

See Chapter 29.

INFORMED CONSENT

After discussion of the following points, a written informed consent form is always obtained preoperatively (Fig. 25-2).

Discussion of Possible Complications

The possible complications are fully discussed. Any physical anomalies observed during the examination that may affect

INFORMED CONSENT TO OPERATION

Patient:______________________________
Date:________________________________ Time:____________

I hereby authorize Dr. James L.Baker, Jr., and/or associates to perform the following procedures on myself:

____

____

____

1. I recognize that during the course of the operation unforeseen conditions may necessitate additional or different procedures than those set forth above. I therefore further authorize and request that the above-named surgeon, the assistants, or the designees perform such procedures as are, in professional judgement, necessary and desirable, including but not limited to procedures involving pathology and radiology. The authority granted under this paragraph shall extend to remedying conditions that are not known to the above doctors at the time the operation is commenced.

2. I consent to the administration of local anesthesia to be applied by or under the direction and supervision of the above doctors, with the exception of

____
(None or a particular one)

3. I recognize that when general anesthesia is used it presents additional risks over which the above doctors have no control, and I agree to discuss the risks of general anesthesia with the anesthesiologist before surgery is performed.

4. I am aware that the practice of medicine and surgery is not an exact science, and I acknowledge that no guarantees have been made to me as to the results of the operation or procedure.

5. I consent to be photographed before, during, and after the treatment; these photographs shall be the property of the above doctors and may be published in scientific journals and/or shown for scientific reasons.

6. I agree to keep the above doctors informed of any change of address so that they can notify me of any late findings, and I agree to cooperate with the above doctors in my care after surgery until completely discharged.

7. I am not known to be allergic to anything except the following:________

____

____

Fig. 25-2 *Example of informed consent forms for patient undergoing augmentation mammaplasty.*

PREOPERATIVE INSTRUCTIONS
OFFICE SURGERY

1. **DO NOT TAKE ANY ASPIRIN OR ASPIRIN-CONTAINING PRODUCTS (BUFFERIN, ANACIN, EXCEDRIN, ETC.) FOR 2 WEEKS BEFORE OR AFTER SURGERY**. Aspirin interferes with normal blood clotting. If needed, you may take **Tylenol.** If you have any doubts about a product, check with your pharmacist.
2. Have your lab work completed **7 to 10 days** before your surgery date. We must receive the results in our office before your surgery date.
3. Fill in the **DATE** on each of your prescriptions the day you have them filled, before going into the pharmacy. Do this **1 week** before surgery. Begin taking medications **as the labels direct.** The pain pills are for after surgery, should you need them. Bring medications with you to the clinic.
4. **DO NOT** take the antibiotic the day of surgery; bring it with you to the clinic to be administered after surgery when you have eaten.
5. **NO FOOD OR DRINK SHOULD BE TAKEN AFTER MIDNIGHT THE DAY OF SURGERY.**
6. Remove nail polish from and trim your **left index** fingernail to normal length so the pulse monitor can be applied to this finger.
7. If you wear contact lenses, bring something to put them in because they **must** be removed before surgery.
8. A responsible adult **must** remain with you from the time you return to your room after surgery until you are discharged from our clinic. You must be driven home and have someone stay with you for at least the first **24 hours** after leaving the clinic.
9. **SMALL CHILDREN ARE NOT ALLOWED IN THE CLINIC.**
10. Please call the office several days before your surgery to reconfirm and inform us of any changes in your address or phone number.
11. **FACELIFTS AND ABDOMINAL LIPECTOMIES:** You must **STOP SMOKING** for at least **2 weeks before** and **2 weeks after** your surgery. **Two days** before surgery start taking **50 mg zinc, 3 times** a day for **1 month,** because it aids in healing.
12. **FACE, NECK, AND EAR SURGERY:** For **3 days** before surgery, wash face, neck, ears with an antibacterial soap such as **Dial** or **Betadine** (available without a prescription from your pharmacy). The night before surgery, remove all makeup and wash your face, neck, and ears with the soap. The morning of surgery, wash your face, neck, ears, and hair thoroughly with the antibacterial soap. **DO NOT** use any makeup or creams after cleansing. **DO NOT** use any hair conditioners, gels, sprays, or mousses on your hair after washing it.
13. **BREAST SURGERY:** For **3 days** before surgery, wash breasts and under arms with an antibacterial soap such as **Dial** or **Betadine** (available without a prescription from your pharmacy). Wash with the soap the night before surgery and again on the morning of the surgery. **DO NOT** use deodorants or powders on the day of surgery. **DO NOT** wear perfume. Wear comfortable, loose fitting clothes, especially a blouse that is easy to slip on and off that buttons down the front. Wear flat heeled shoes. Do not wear a pull-on sweater or tight fitting pants.

Fig. 25-2—*cont'd.*

matory response, and formation of silicone granulomas. If a rupture does occur, additional surgery may be required to remove the gel implants and the gel contents.

Research indicates that the material implanted in the body does not cause malignancy in human subjects.

There is a possibility that the body may not tolerate these implants, making it necessary to remove the implants. This occurs in a small percentage of cases.

A cyst may form in the area adjacent to the implants, causing fluid accumulation that may require drainage by needle or removal of the implants.

No guarantee has been given as to size and shape of the breasts. Good results are experienced but not guaranteed.

In some patients, the margin of the implants can be felt.

Postoperative bleeding may occur around the implant requiring a second operation for its removal.

After being exposed to cold temperatures (i.e., swimming in cold water), the breast may feel cooler than surrounding body tissues.

Pregnancy is not recommended for at least 6 months after the surgery.

Change in Nipple Sensation
It has been reported in medical literature that some patients undergoing breast surgery may experience either complete numbness, diminished nipple sensation, or hypersensitivity. These changes may be temporary or permanent.

Connective Tissue Disorder
A possible association between implanted silicone and connective-tissue disorders (i.e., adjuvant disease) has been referred to in some medical literature.

Scarring
Although your surgeon will make every attempt to minimize the scarring that results from breast surgery occasionally a raised, thickened scar may occur.

Gel Breed
Small microscopic droplets of silicone gel may leak or bleed through the silicone shell of a breast implant. The long-term effects of silicone gel in the body are unknown.

Breast implants may interfere with postoperative mammography. Before having a mammogram procedure performed, you should inform the radiologist of the presence of mammary implants.

Fig. 25-2—***cont'd.***

Although every effort has been made to produce a reliable long lasting silicone implant, we cannot guarantee that this implant will last a lifetime. Implants may simply wear out or break because of external trauma—stress forces. It is understood that breakage can occur at any time after surgery, and surgery may be required to remove or replace the implant.

Saline Inflatable Implants
Saline inflatable implants are medical grade silicone shells filled with saline (salt water). These implants are subjected to all of the above complications other than any silicone gel bleed or complications resulting from silicone gel. As it was explained to you, saline implants can develop a leak through the shell wall or the valve mechanism by which they are filled, which results in deflation and necessitates reoperation for insertion of a new implant. Whenever a saline inflatable implant is used, the patient must accept the deflation risk as a distinct possibility and that one or both implants may have to be replaced during their lifetime as a result of deflation.

Textured-Surface Silicone Implants
The texturing of the implant surface was developed to diminish the incidence of capsular contracture (hardness) following breast augmentation with a silicone implant. As a result of the bonding of the capsule membrane that walls off the implant from the body (i.e., a thin layer of scar membrane), this could result in a rippling effect along the edges, especially in the inner edge along the sternal border. This is most commonly seen in extremely thin women with a low fat content in the subcutaneous layer of the skin.

Patient Acknowledgement
I have read the above information and understand it. I realize that all of these problems cannot be completely eliminated by even the best medical technology and surgical care, and I accept these conditions and limitations.

Witness	Signature	Date

FIG. 25-2—*cont'd.*

the final result are stressed to the patient and noted in her chart. The relatively more frequent complications of postoperative bleeding, infection, unattractive scars, loss of nipple sensation, and firmness of the breasts (i.e., capsular contracture) are explained in detail. The treatment of each complication is explained. It is explained that (1) hematomas usually require surgery for correction; (2) if infection occurs, it could necessitate removal of the prosthesis for several weeks to

14. **OTHER AREAS OF SURGERY:** For **3 days** before surgery, wash with an antibacterial soap such as **Dial** or **Betadine** (available without a prescription from your pharmacy). Wash with the soap the night before surgery and again on the morning of surgery. **DO NOT** apply underarm deodorants, powders, perfume, or lotions the day of surgery.
15. If you have any questions about any of these instructions, please call our office for assistance.

Do not be concerned if your temperature elevates 1 to 2° for a few days after surgery. This is normal.

NOTES TO REMEMBER

Your surgery is scheduled for:____________________at o'clock

Please arrive in the clinic at:_________________o'clock

Your prepayment for surgery is due by:

READ ALL INSTRUCTIONS THAT WE HAVE GIVEN YOU

Do NOT Forget:

- To have your lab work done 7 to 10 days before surgery
- To have you prescriptions filled, take as directed, and bring with you on the day of surgery
- To have your prepayment for surgery in 2 weeks before surgery

- Please have NO alcohol 24 hours before lab work and surgery
- Please DO NOT take any ASPIRIN or ASPIRIN COMPOUNDS for at least 2 weeks before and after surgery. You may take Tylenol or any acetaminophen compound in its place.
- It is required that a responsible adult stay with you from the time you return from the recovery area until you are discharged from our clinic by the doctor.
- We will provide all meals and beverages for the patient; however, while we will be happy to provide beverages for the person staying with you, arrangements for meals must be made. If you have any special dietary requirements, please discuss them with us before surgery.
- On day of your surgery go directly to our surgical suite located on the first floor of the building. The sign on the door reads "Surgical Suite."
- Please call us with any questions that you have. We are here to help you.

Thank You

Fig. 25-2—***cont'd.***

months; (3) revision of an unattractive scar may be necessary, but not always successful; and (4) alteration in sensation on one or both sides, which can include the nipple areolar complex or skin of the breast, occurs in 15% of patients undergoing this procedure, on a permanent basis. This can be total or partial numbness or a slight loss in sensation. Even removing the implant will not alter this condition. Numbness or loss of sensation is considered permanent when it is present 1 year or longer; if firmness occurs, it may require surgical or nonsurgical treatment, which is not always successful. Pregnancy is discouraged for the first 6 months postoperatively. This allows the breast to adjust over the prosthesis and the incisions to heal before the breasts are subjected to the stresses of engorgement during pregnancy.

Discussion of Textured Surface Implants versus Nontextured-Surface Implants

The saline inflatable prostheses, which include the textured and nontextured-surface implants, are shown to the patient. It is explained that a textured-surface prosthesis has a lower reported contracture rate currently than a smooth-surfaced implant; however, it has its own inherent possible complications. Because the implant surface bonds to the posterior wall of the breast, in a very thin patient when placed suprapectorally, a ripping effect can occur in the upper inner quadrant from the internal mammary vessels that supply the gland at this point. Because the smooth-surfaced implant glides beneath the breast tissue, this phenomenon has not been encountered. To avoid this problem, subpectoral placement of the prostheses should be discussed. I show a photograph of a patient with the rippling effect to prospective patients and a photograph of a patient with a subpectoral placement of the implants, because this placement usually produces a more convex upper pole of the breast. If the patient desires suprapectoral placement of the implants and I feel the rippling effect is a probability, I will recommend a smooth-surfaced implant to avoid this complication.

Discussion of Deflation

The patient is warned that saline implants may deflate at a later date. Deflation is usually a slow process with a slight softening of the breast tissue originally noted, then a gradual diminution in volume. There can however be a rapid deflation, and the patient should be aware that this phenomenon can occur at any point in time. The implant manufacturers estimate deflation rates at approximately 2% in the lifetime of the implant, however this may not mean the lifetime of the patient. It must be assumed that there will be a 100% deflation rate if the patient lives long enough. The surgeon should explain that exchange of a deflated saline implant is a simple procedure that can be performed with the patient under local anesthesia on an outpatient basis with minimal inconvenience to the patient. Normally the manufacturer will provide a prosthesis free of charge, and if I have done the primary surgery, I do not charge the patient to replace a ruptured implant.

Discussion of Anesthesia

Unless otherwise indicated for medical reasons, the augmentation procedure is usually performed on an outpatient basis. General or local anesthesia is offered to the patient.

PREOPERATIVE PREPARATION

Patient Instructions

Patients are informed by the surgical secretary of the routine to follow before the surgery. All instructions, both preoperative and postoperative, are given to the patient on printed forms. One should not rely on the memory of an apprehensive patient or family member to recall all of the instructions that a surgeon wishes to be followed (Figs. 25-3, 25-4).

A. **Cleansing of surgical area.** Instructions for cleansing surgical areas are also given to the patient in writing. I recommend that the patient wash the skin of her chest wall, breast, and axillae with povidone iodine (Betadine) skin cleanser or an antibacterial soap (Dial) daily for 1 week before surgery. Scrubbing reduces skin bacteria and gets the patient used to handling her breasts, which she will massage frequently postoperatively if smooth surfaced implants are used.

B. **Prohibited medications.** All surgical patients are warned against taking aspirin for 2 weeks before and 2 weeks after the operation because of its potent anticoagulant effect. Preoperative laboratory studies are ob-

James L. Baker, Jr., M.D., P.A.
400 West Morse Blvd., Suite 203
Winter Park, Florida 32789

PLEASE DO NOT WEAR OR BRING ANY VALUABLES TO THIS FACILITY.

I FULLY UNDERSTAND THAT THIS FACILITY WILL NOT BE RESPONSIBLE OR LIABLE FOR ANY LOSS OF VALUABLES.

____
Patient

____________________ ____________________
Date Witness

FIG. 25-3 *Example of preoperative instructions for patient undergoing outpatient plastic surgery.*

tained, including complete blood count (CBC), bleeding time, sequential multiple analyzerwitt computer (SMAC) and urinalysis. Any abnormalities are investigated, and any questionable medical problems are referred to the appropriate physician for definitive treatment before surgery.

C. **Clothing.** Loose-fitting clothing that is easy to slip on after surgery is recommended. Low-heeled slip-on shoes should be worn, because many patients experience equilibrium disturbances from the preoperative and intraoperative sedation.

D. **Driving.** As a result of the effects of the sedation and postoperative analgesics, no driving of a vehicle is allowed for several days. The patient must plan accordingly.

E. **Foods.** Ingestion of solid food or milk products is not allowed on the day of surgery. If the patient is taking a routine medication, such as an antihypertensive, she should take this medication with a small amount of water on the day of surgery.

INTRAOPERATIVE CARE

A board-certified physician-anesthesiologist is used for all patients undergoing surgical procedures. At the patient's

PREOPERATIVE INSTRUCTIONS
OFFICE SURGERY

1. **DO NOT TAKE ANY ASPIRIN OR ASPIRIN-CONTAINING PRODUCTS (BUFFERIN, ANACIN, EXCEDRIN, ETC.) FOR 2 WEEKS BEFORE OR AFTER SURGERY**. Aspirin interferes with normal blood clotting. If needed, you may take **Tylenol.** If you have any doubts about a product, check with your pharmacist.
2. Have your lab work completed **7 to 10 days** before your surgery date. We must receive the results in our office before your surgery date.
3. Fill in the **DATE** on each of your prescriptions the day you have them filled, before going into the pharmacy. Do this **1 week** before surgery. Begin taking medications **as the labels direct.** The pain pills are for after surgery, should you need them. Bring medications with you to the clinic.
4. **DO NOT** take the antibiotic the day of surgery; bring it with you to the clinic to be administered after surgery when you have eaten.
5. **NO FOOD OR DRINK SHOULD BE TAKEN AFTER MIDNIGHT THE DAY OF SURGERY.**
6. Remove nail polish from and trim your **left index** fingernail to normal length so the pulse monitor can be applied to this finger.
7. If you wear contact lenses, bring something to put them in because they **must** be removed before surgery.
8. A responsible adult **must** remain with you from the time you return to your room after surgery until you are discharged from our clinic. You must be driven home and have someone stay with you for at least the first **24 hours** after leaving the clinic.
9. **SMALL CHILDREN ARE NOT ALLOWED IN THE CLINIC.**
10. Please call the office several days before your surgery to reconfirm and inform us of any changes in your address or phone number.
11. **FACELIFTS AND ABDOMINAL LIPECTOMIES:** You must **STOP SMOKING** for at least **2 weeks before** and **2 weeks after** your surgery. **Two days** before surgery start taking **50 mg zinc, 3 times** a day for **1 month,** because it aids in healing.
12. **FACE, NECK, AND EAR SURGERY:** For **3 days** before surgery, wash face, neck, ears with an antibacterial soap such as **Dial** or **Betadine** (available without a prescription from your pharmacy). The night before surgery, remove all makeup and wash your face, neck, and ears with the soap. The morning of surgery, wash your face, neck, ears, and hair thoroughly with the antibacterial soap. **DO NOT** use any makeup or creams after cleansing. **DO NOT** use any hair conditioners, gels, sprays, or mousses on your hair after washing it.
13. **BREAST SURGERY:** For **3 days** before surgery, wash breasts and under arms with an antibacterial soap such as **Dial** or **Betadine** (available without a prescription from your pharmacy). Wash with the soap the night before surgery and again on the morning of the surgery. **DO NOT** use deodorants or powders on the day of surgery. **DO NOT** wear perfume. Wear comfortable, loose fitting clothes, especially a blouse that is easy to slip on and off that buttons down the front. Wear flat heeled shoes. Do not wear a pull-on sweater or tight fitting pants.

FIG. **25-3—*cont'd.***

14. **OTHER AREAS OF SURGERY:** For **3 days** before surgery, wash with an antibacterial soap such as **Dial** or **Betadine** (available without a prescription from your pharmacy). Wash with the soap the night before surgery and again on the morning of surgery. **DO NOT** apply underarm deodorants, powders, perfume, or lotions the day of surgery.
15. If you have any questions about any of these instructions, please call our office for assistance.

Do not be concerned if your temperature elevates 1 to 2° for a few days after surgery. This is normal.

NOTES TO REMEMBER

Your surgery is scheduled for:__________________at o'clock

Please arrive in the clinic at:______________o'clock

Your prepayment for surgery is due by:

READ ALL INSTRUCTIONS THAT WE HAVE GIVEN YOU

Do NOT Forget:

- To have your lab work done 7 to 10 days before surgery
- To have you prescriptions filled, take as directed, and bring with you on the day of surgery
- To have your prepayment for surgery in 2 weeks before surgery

- Please have NO alcohol 24 hours before lab work and surgery
- Please DO NOT take any ASPIRIN or ASPIRIN COMPOUNDS for at least 2 weeks before and after surgery. You may take Tylenol or any acetaminophen compound in its place.
- It is required that a responsible adult stay with you from the time you return from the recovery area until you are discharged from our clinic by the doctor.
- We will provide all meals and beverages for the patient; however, while we will be happy to provide beverages for the person staying with you, arrangements for meals must be made. If you have any special dietary requirements, please discuss them with us before surgery.
- On day of your surgery go directly to our surgical suite located on the first floor of the building. The sign on the door reads "Surgical Suite."
- Please call us with any questions that you have. We are here to help you.

Thank You

Fig. 25-3—***cont'd.***

**AUGMENTATION MAMMAPLASTY
(BREAST ENLARGEMENT)**

POSTOPERATIVE INSTRUCTIONS

THE FOLLOWING INSTRUCTION SHOULD BE READ CAREFULLY BY YOU AND THE PERSON OR PERSONS WHO WILL BE CARING FOR YOU DURING THE FIRST 48 HOURS FOLLOWING SURGERY.

* Upon arriving home, go to bed immediately.

* For the first **3 days,** sleep on your back with your head elevated on two pillows.

* **DO NOT TAKE ASPIRIN OR ASPIRIN-CONTAINING PRODUCTS (BUFFERIN, ANACIN, EXCEDRIN, ETC.).** Aspirin interferes with normal blood clotting. If needed, you may take **Tylenol.** If you have any doubts about a product, check with your pharmacist. Take pain pills ONLY AS NECESSARY for discomforts as directed. **TAKE ANTIBIOTIC AS DIRECTED.**

* A surgical brassiere will be furnished at the time of surgery. Do not worry if it does not fit properly. Your breasts should be supported at all times, including the times you are sleeping, for **1 week.** Do not wear a brassiere with metal wires or stays for **6 weeks.** You may sleep without a brassiere in **1 week,** but wear it throughout the day for an additional week. You may also try to sleep on your abdomen at **1 week** postoperatively.

* Arm movements should be kept to an absolute minimum during the first **48 hours.** No heavy lifting, pushing, or driving a car. After **2 weeks,** you will be able to resume normal activities with the exception of golf, tennis, swimming, etc. These activities may be resumed in **3 weeks.**

* You may eat whatever you like, feed yourself, comb your hair, and brush your teeth. Care should be taken when dressing and undressing.

* After the **third day,** the brassiere may be removed, and you may bathe or shower. The tapes overlying the incision should remain in place; pat them dry.

* If there are any questions or doubts, please call our office at **644-5242.**

* You will be called on the first postoperative day by my staff.

Fig. **25-4** *Example of postoperative instructions for patient undergoing augmentation mammaplasty.*

request, the anesthetic may be IV sedation administered by the anesthesiologist with local anesthesia or standard general anesthesia.

Preparation of Chest Wall and Local Anesthesia

After sedation or induction of the patient by the anesthesiologist, the patient's chest wall is prepared with Betadine, and local anesthesia is accomplished with 100 cc of 0.25% lidocaine and 1:400,000 epinephrine infiltrated with a 20-gauge spinal needle connected to a Pitkin syringe. This relatively large-bore needle will not bend or deflect and enter the thorax if a rib is encountered, as is possible with a flexible 25-gauge spinal needle. It is important to keep the needle at a right angle to the ribs to avoid entering an intracostal space and producing iatrogenic pheumothorax.

Markings

The implant sizes are marked on the patient's breast with gentian violet. A 4-cm incision is marked 1 cm above the inframammary crease bilaterally. The patient is again prepared with Betadine and then draped.

Operative Technique

The incision is opened and a subcutaneous flap 1.5 cm is made and is dissected inferiorly down to the chest wall.

- ▼ Dissection is then turned cephalad, and the pocket is developed over the pectoralis fascia (or under the pectoralis muscle, according to the desires of the patient). I use an inframammary approach in almost every patient.
- ▼ After developing the pocket, it is irrigated with Betadine solution, and 25 cc of 0.25% bupivacaine with adrenalin is infiltrated into the muscle and soft tissues to reduce postoperative discomfort.
- ▼ The saline inflatable implant of the desired size, is inflated outside the body, checked for leaks, dipped in Betadine, inserted into the pocket, and positioned.
- ▼ The flap is reapproximated with a running 3-0 Surgilon suture, and the skin is closed with a running intracuticular 4-0 Vicryl suture with Steri-strip reinforcement.
- ▼ A standard brassiere is used as a final dressing.

▼ The patient is then sent to the recovery room and is discharged when she feels well enough to return home.

POSTOPERATIVE CARE

Activity Restrictions

Upper arm motion, which causes movement of the pectoralis major muscle, is discouraged for 48 to 72 hours. The patient then may begin driving a vehicle, but should limit heavy lifting or pushing for the first 2 weeks. At the end of 2 weeks, she may begin aerobics, walking, jogging, bicycling, and at the end of 4 weeks she may begin upper body weight lifting.

Medications

Systemic antibiotics, which are started 1 to 2 days preoperatively, are continued for 1 week postoperatively. Oral analgesics are prescribed for comfort.

Vitamin E

Alpha-tocopherol (vitamin E) is an effective antiinflammatory agent. Its effect is similar to that of corticosteroids in reducing inflammatory response. Patients are encouraged to take the synthetic form of vitamin E 1,000 IU orally, twice a day. It is recommended that they continue on this dosage indefinitely because it is also effective in reducing fibrocystic diseases of the breast.

Return Office Visits

A. **Third to fourth postoperative day.** The patient is rechecked between the third and fourth postoperative day. The Steri-strips are changed, and the patient is then instructed to remove the Steri-strips in approximately 1 week. She is encouraged to minimize strenuous activities in the first 2 weeks and to follow the adage, "If it doesn't hurt, do it." The patient may go without a brassiere at the end of 2 to 4 weeks. She is encouraged to sleep in a brassiere for the first postoperative week.

B. **Two to three months postoperative.** The patient returns at 2 to 3 months for examination, and postoperative photographs are taken. She is given her preoperative photographs at this time. The patient should be encouraged to return annually thereafter.

POSTOPERATIVE COMPLICATIONS

Early Complications

A. **Hematoma.** The most common early postoperative complication is hematoma. This usually occurs within the first 48 to 72 hours postoperatively. All patients are warned preoperatively to notify the office of any rapid enlargement of the breast or excessive or undue pain, particularly pain not relieved by oral narcotics. Bilateral hematoma, although possible, is extremely rare. Moderate to large hematomas are surgically evacuated in the OR. Small accumulations can be left to reabsorb, if they are not causing any discomfort to the patient.

B. **Minor wound separation or suture reaction.** This is an uncommon finding. When encountered, it usually occurs within the first 2 weeks after surgery. Separated wounds usually can be resutured, or Steri-strips can be applied without any adverse reaction.

C. **Postoperative infection.** The usual treatment for a postoperative infection is removal of the prosthesis for several weeks or months. When there is no evidence of residual infection, reimplantation may be performed.

D. **Ptosis of implant.** This condition can occur when the subcutaneous flap has not been reapproximated to the proper fascial plane or steroids have pooled inferiorly, causing a resorption of the subcutaneous fat, which allows the prosthesis to settle. This condition can be corrected by resuturing the subcutaneous flap or having the patient wear a brassiere with underwires for extended periods. Occasionally the pocket has been made inadequately through a periareolar or transaxillary approach, causing asymmetry of the inframammary crease.

E. **Mondor's disease.** This disease is an idiopathic phlebitis affecting the large subcutaneous veins normally coursing along the rectus abdominus muscles and is encountered in approximately 1% of breast patients. It appears as a tender band near the inframammary crease and is a benign, self-limiting condition. No specific treatment is necessary. The patient should be reassured.

F. **Alteration of nipple sensation.** Although in most cases changes in nipple sensation is a temporary condition lasting 6 to 12 months, it is permanent in approximately 15% of all patients undergoing this procedure. As long as the patient is aware preoperatively that there can be permanent sensory loss, she should not be upset should it occur. Paresthesias are much more common and usually disappear by the sixth postoperative month.

G. **Leakage of inflatable prostheses.** This complication is a distinct possibility. The patient should have been told of this possibility preoperatively and should have been made aware that if it occurred, it is a relatively simple procedure to exchange the deflating prosthesis for a new one.

Late Complication: Capsular Contracture

Capsular contracture after breast augmentation usually occurs between 6 and 12 months. Although the exact cause of capsular contracture remains obscure, it is in essence a basic wound-healing phenomenon common to all wounds. It appears to be more host related than implant related. Although multiple etiologic factors have been implicated, it appears that the myofibroblast probably initiates the process of wound and capsular contracture. As the capsule wall is laid down around the prosthesis, the myofibroblast causes the collagen bundles to be pulled together and decreases the surface area of scar membrane around the implant, thus compressing the prosthesis.

A. **Prophylaxis of capsular contracture.** Prevention of capsular contracture is more desirable than treatment, both to patient and surgeon alike. The effectiveness of steroids, either in the pocket at the time of implantation or within the prosthesis itself, is controversial and their use has led to numerous complications as a side effect. *The use of any drug or substance within an inflatable prosthesis should be discouraged. The manufacturer voids the warranty on its product if anything other than sterile saline is used to fill the implant.* Vitamin E is effective in diminishing capsular contracture, because of its antiinflammatory and steroidlike effect, and use is encouraged for all of my patients.

B. **Breast massage.** Many surgeons encourage their patients to massage the breasts daily. It is believed that by moving the implant inside the pocket, it will produce a "bursalike effect", keeping the capsule walls stretched. Squeezing and pressing on the breast appears to be as effective as 5- and 10-minute involved massage programs, which some people prefer. If the textured-surface prosthesis is used, massage is not indicated because the implant surface and capsule wall unite.

C. **Treatment of capsular contracture**

- Medical. Research has shown that the myofibroblast population is highest in younger contracted capsular tissue. The pharmacologic effect of drugs, such as papaverine hydrochloride, can cause a relaxation of the myofibroblast, and thus reverse the contracture procedure. This drug will be most effective when given early at the onset of contracture. It is less effective in long-standing capsular contracture. At the first sign of capsular contracture, a time-release papaverine hydrochloride capsule (Pavabid) 150 mg is given twice a day. It is recommended that patients continue the drug's use until softening of the capsule occurs, which will normally be within 3 to 6 months. Patients will continue massage during administration of this drug (including patients with textured surface prostheses). If no results have been obtained in 6 months, the drug is discontinued. The side effect of orthostatic hypertension is discussed with the patient, and she is warned not to mix alcohol with the drug because of its synergistic effect on blood vessel dilatation.
- Nonsurgical squeeze closed capsulotomy. The technique of compression around the prosthesis, building a force great enough to cause a fracture in the capsular wall, has proved highly successful in a majority of patients. The technique should be performed with the discomfort of the patient in mind, and the patient should be aware that damage to the prosthesis can result in this procedure. In the case of

CLOSED CAPSULOTOMY CONSENT

Patient:____

Date:________________________ Time:__________________

1. I hereby authorize Dr. James L. Baker, Jr., and/or his associates to perform a procedure to attempt to rupture the scar capsules surrounding my breast implants by squeezing the breasts, known as closed capsulotomy, on myself.
2. The procedure listed in Paragraph 1 has been explained to me by the doctor and/or nurse, and I completely understand the nature and consequences of the procedure. The following points have been made specifically clear:
   A. There is a possibility that a blood clot may form in the area adjacent to the implants that might require surgical correction, which may have to be performed while I am under general anesthesia.
   B. The procedure is not always successful, and bizarre shape of the breast can occur, which could necessitate surgery for correction.
   C. Recurrence of the contracture (hard breast) can occur even if the capsulotomy is successful.
   D. Breakage of the implant can occur, which would necessitate surgical correction.
   E. Thinning of an area of the tissue over the prosthesis may occur, which could necessitate surgical correction or removal of the implant.
   F. If surgery is necessary following the capsulotomy, it may be necessary to make an incision in an area other than where the previous scar is located.
   G. Surgical fees would be charged if surgery should become necessary as a result of this procedure.
   H. No guarantee has been given as to the expected result.
3. I am aware that the practice of medicine and surgery is not an exact science, and I acknowledge that no guarantees have been made to me as to the results of the operation or procedure.
4. I agree to keep the doctor informed of any changes of address so he can notify me of any late findings, and I agree to cooperate with the doctor in my care after surgery until completely discharged.
5. I have read the above consent and fully understand the same and do authorize the doctor to perform this procedure on me.
6. I am not known to be allergic to anything except: (List)

____

__________________ __________________
(Witness) (Patient)

Fig. 25-5 *Example of informed consent form for patient undergoing closed capsulotomy.*

a saline inflatable implant, this compression could cause deflation of the prosthesis, resulting in a need for replacement. It has the advantage of no cost to the patient and no time loss from work or other duties; also, it is without surgical risk (unless a complication occurs that would necessitate surgical intervention). The procedure is simple to perform in the office and usually causes only slight discomfort to the patient. Sedation or other means of diminishing pain response should not be administered. The patient's discomfort should be the surgeon's guide. A special consent form (Fig. 25-5) is reviewed with the patient before the procedure is performed. Hematoma that requires surgical intervention can occur from the closed capsulotomy. Incomplete rupture of the capsule wall can cause bizarre shapes caused by herniation of the prosthesis through the weakened defect in the capsule wall. This condition could require later surgical correction.

▼ Surgical capsulotomy. Surgical capsulotomy is recommended when the medical or nonsurgical treatment is ineffective or when frequent recurrences have developed within 6 months to 1 year of repeated closed capsulotomies. The technique may involve capsulectomy or simple capsulotomy. General anesthesia is usually preferred, because it is difficult to obtain adequate analgesia with local anesthetic infiltrated into the scar tissue. Normally a new prosthesis is used after the procedure. After the operation, the same postoperative regimen is continued as with primary augmentation.

FURTHER READINGS

Baker JL Jr: Augmentation mammoplasty. In Owsley Q Jr, Peterson RA, editors: *Symposium on aesthetic surgery of the breast,* vol 18 (Scottsdale, Ariz, 1975), St Louis, 1978, Mosby, pp 256-263.

Baker JL Jr: Augmentation mammoplasty. In Grabb WC, Smith JW, editors: *Plastic surgery,* ed 3, Boston, 1979, Little, Brown, pp 719-736.

Baker JL Jr: The effectiveness of alpha-tocopherol (Vitamin E) in reducing the incidence of spherical contracture around breast implants, *Plast Reconstr Surg* 65:696 1981.

Baker JL Jr: Augmentation mammoplasty: a personal approach. In Marsh L editor: *Current therapy in plastic and reconstructive surgery, trunk, and extremities,* Toronto, 1989, Decker, pp 1-9.

Baker JL Jr, Donis R: Genesis and management of the hard augmented breast. In Habal M, editor: *Advances in plastic and reconstructive surgery,* vol 6, Chicago, 1989, Mosby.

Baker JL Jr: In Lars V, editor: *How they do it: procedures in plastic and reconstructive surgery,* Boston, 1990, Little, Brown, p 203.

Baker JL Jr: Augmentation mammoplasty. In Peck G, editor: *Complications and problems in aesthetic plastic surgery,* New York, 1991, Gower Medical.

Baker JL Jr, Penn JG: Augmentation mammoplasty. In Goldwyn RM, editor: *The unfavorable result in plastic surgery, avoidance and treatment,* ed 2, Boston, 1984, Little, Brown, pp 719-733.

Baker JL Jr, Bartels RJ, Douglas WM: Closed compression technique for rupturing a contracted capsule around a breast implant, *Plast Reconstr* Surg 58:137, 1976.

Baker JL Jr, Chandler ML, LeVier RR: Occurrence and activity of myofibroblasts in human capsular contracture tissue surrounding mammary implants, *Plast Reconstr Surg* 68:905, 1981.

Baker JL Jr, Kolin IS, Bartlett ES: The psychosexual dynamics of patients undergoing mammary augmentation, *Plast Reconstr Surg* 53:652, 1974.

Baker JL Jr, LeVier RR, Speilvogel DE: Positive identification of silicone in human mammary capsular tissue, *Plast Reconstr Surg* 69:56, 1982.

Baker JL Jr, Mara JE, Linville J: Diagnosis and treatment of masses in the augmented breast, *Rocky Mountain Med J* 74:255, 1978.

Little GA, Baker JL Jr: Results of closed compression capsulotomy for treatment of contracted breast implant capsules, *Plast Reconstr Surg* 65:30, 1980.

CHAPTER 26

Reduction Mammaplasty

PAUL K. MCKISSOCK

In mammaplasty, like in most plastic surgical procedures, good preoperative and postoperative care will not salvage the results of poor craftsmanship during surgery. But patients and civil courts alike are generally more forgiving of errors of surgical technique than of negligence in the overall care of the patient. The care of the reduction mammaplasty patient embodies the same principles of patient care common to all major pedicle flap operations done with the patient under general anesthesia, including observation of proper blood replacement, wound drainage, early ambulation, flap design, preoperative assessment, and intraoperative and postoperative care. Because reduction mammaplasty is a quasi-cosmetic procedure that is performed upon paired cancer-prone organs of considerable sexual importance to the patient and involves several skin flaps, it should not be undertaken without a careful determination by the physician of the benefit to the patient. If the physician decides that reduction mammaplasty is indicated, the preoperative, intraoperative, and postoperative phases of patient care must adhere to certain basic principles and procedural steps.

INITIAL VISIT: PATIENT SCREENING AND INTERVIEWING

The first consultation should include (1) a general assessment of the nature and scope of the problem by the surgeon and the suitability of the patient for the operation, and (2) information to the patient covering as thoroughly as possible all aspects of the surgery, including its drawbacks, so that she can determine intelligently whether to proceed. The most efficient use of the consultation time will result if the patient is examined first and if the patient's medical history is taken subsequently.

Initial Examination

The physical examination is limited to the breasts. The surgeon should take special note of the following characteristics:

- Breast size and weight compared with the patient's stated symptoms of discomfort; in borderline cases, the presence of grooves on the shoulders caused by brassiere straps will lend credibility to the patient's complaints of discomfort
- Degree of ptosis, as determined by the relationship of the nipple to the submammary fold level transposed to the anterior surface of the breast
- Asymmetry in breast size, nipple size and location, and submammary fold level
- Overall length of the proposed nipple-bearing flap (distance from the submammary fold to the upper rim of the new areolar window
- Character of the parenchyma (fatty, densely fibrous stroma, or cystic)
- Presence of old surgical scars, especially in the vicinity of any planned flaps
- Presence of any inflammatory conditions, such as areolar hidradenitis or pustules

On completion of this brief physical examination, the surgeon should have a clear understanding of the patient's problem, her suitability for surgery, and any special problems that might arise in her particular case.

Consultation

The initial consultation should include the following items:

- A statement from the surgeon to the patient concerning her need for the surgery and whether there are any special risks in her case, such as an increased risk of vascular problems, a suspected prolonged healing time, or the need for a free nipple graft
- A period of time to let the patient talk and describe her symptoms and her motives in seeking the surgery; common symptoms include back, shoulder, and breast discomfort

- A statement from the surgeon reassuring the patient that the operation will alleviate most, if not all, of her principal concerns, such as the inability to participate in sports, fit easily into clothing, and enjoy unrestricted activities
- An honest and comprehensive description of the principal drawbacks inherent in the operation. The four drawbacks listed below can be expected to occur, at least to some degree, in 100% of patients and the patient deserves to be informed of them. It is a rare patient who will be dissuaded from surgery by this candid disclosure of the operation's negative side.

  - Scars. A graphic description of the expected scar pattern, either by diagrams or photographs, is appropriate and will be appreciated by the patient. If photographs of previous patients are used, it is important to select the pictures carefully so that they do not influence the patient by the quality of the result they depict. It would be wise to illustrate both good-quality scarring and hypertrophic scarring in patients that the surgeon believes represent an average result in terms of contour and symmetry. Even above-average results usually have imperfections. The surgeon should expose these and take this opportunity to inform the patient that some imperfections in contour and symmetry are usual.
  - Alterations in nipple-areolar sensibility. Regardless of the technique used, the resection of substantial amounts of the parenchyma should be expected to jeopardize the normal innervation of the nipple-areolar complex. The effect often will not be the same between the two breasts and during the months and years after the operation, sensibility often will improve. All of this should be discussed with the patient, and perhaps followed-up by the statement that the degree of this effect cannot be predicted in any given case. It would also be wise to inform the patient that total and permanent denervation of one or both nipples, although not usual, is a possibility.
  - Interference with lactation. In patients who are distinctly unable to bear children by reason of age or

sterilization procedures, interference with lactation as a possible adverse result of reduction mammaplasty need not be discussed beyond a mere mention. With all other patients, this result should be stressed, regardless of the patient's stated plans regarding future pregnancies or her desire to breastfeed. This is particularly true in the case of the young, unmarried, nulliparous woman whose negative perception concerning the values of breastfeeding may be conditioned by immaturity, and thus is subject to change. Although some originators of breast reduction techniques make claims of noninterference with lactability, it is unwise to promise anything in this regard to a woman with childbearing potential. A properly informed patient is one who understands that her surgery might inhibit or defunctionalize lactation.

- Late shape change. Although future loss of breast shape is not a drawback to the surgery, the prudent surgeon will begin at this point to condition the patient to accept the undesirable gradual loss over time of the classic breast shape she hopes to achieve immediately postoperatively.

GENERAL PREOPERATIVE PROCEDURES

Blood Transfusion

The thorough surgeon will include a statement concerning the need for blood replacement in the first description of the operation. Except for the occasional procedure involving minor glandular reduction, all reduction mammaplasty operations should be performed in a setting in which blood transfusion is available.

A. **Autologous versus homologous transfusion.** Autologous transfusion may be more difficult for patients living at great distances from the hospital, because of the need for extra hospital laboratory visits before surgery; however it should be offered and encouraged. Because exposure to homologous blood is thereby decreased, autologous transfusion has a high patient acceptance as well as being medically desirable (See Chapter 7.).

B. **Procedure.** Usually, only 1 unit of blood (500 ml) is necessary, and this may be drawn 7 to 10 days before surgery. When autologous transfusion is impractical, 1 or 2 units of homologous blood should be available for transfusion at the time of surgery. In either case, blood should be transfused only if the patient's condition justifies its use. This will be necessary in less than 25% of cases if dilute solutions of epinephrine are injected into the parenchyma during surgery and the electric cutting current is used for resection.

Although the risk factors associated with the use of autologous blood are significantly less than with homologous blood, the risks of clerical error are essentially the same, and the physician should be aware that serious and sometimes fatal transfusion reactions can occur with autologous blood. The use of autologous blood as replacement therapy should be no different from the use of homologous blood.

Preoperative Mammography

A. **Current use of mammography as screening procedure.** The value of the routine use of mammography as a screening procedure for the general population has developed widespread acceptance in recent years. With the advent of film mammography, the doses for mammographic procedures are low, and radiation risks are not considered significant at this time even with yearly examinations beginning at the age of 35. The National Cancer Institute (NCI) and the American College of Surgeons (ACS) both recommend a routine baseline mammogram from ages 34 to 40, with a mammography yearly or every 2 years thereafter until age 50 and then yearly after 50. In fact, if there is a strong family medical history of breast cancer in either a mother or sister, a baseline mammogram may be recommended before 35 years of age.

Although the NCI does not make any statement regarding the place of mammography as a routine preoperative study in association with operations such as mammaplasty, it does recognize that there may be a place for single-study mammography as a baseline test. NCI also does not recommend withholding mammography from a patient of any age group if both she and her physician deem it to be in her best interest. This may be the pertinent area of recommendation for the mammaplasty patient.

B. **Purposes of mammographic studies in mammaplasty.** The NCI indicates there are two purposes in obtaining a mammogram: (1) to rule out an undetectable early cancer in a preoperative mammaplasty patient, and (2) to establish a baseline study for later comparison. In accordance with these NCI recommendations, the plastic surgeon may be justified in obtaining at least a preoperative mammograph in all reduction mammaplasty patients (especially those more than 35 years of age), and another mammogram 9 to 12 months postoperatively.

IMMEDIATE PREOPERATIVE VISIT: MARKING PROCEDURE

Aside from the usual routine of the prehospitalization office visit (e.g., preoperative physical examination, review of relevant laboratory or x-ray studies and photographs), the most important thing to accomplish during this visit is the breast pattern marking, assuming the visit is scheduled for the day immediately preceding surgery. This visit provides the ideal time and setting to perform this important planning step. The surgeon who postpones the marking procedure until a more convenient time will, more often than not, never find the time and will be confronted the next morning with an unmarked patient already on the operating table and sedated, if not already anesthetized. Under those circumstances, the surgeon has provided the worst possible setting in which to plan the operation.

Ideally the patient should be seated fully upright and not sedated. The surgeon should be comfortably seated facing the patient and should not be rushed. A felt tip marking pen will provide a mark that can be erased with alcohol if necessary, yet when left on overnight, the ink will seat itself into the skin sufficiently to survive a surgical preparation the next morning. The steps of the marking procedure are summarized in Fig. 26-1.

INTRAOPERATIVE PROCEDURES

With the possible exception of cases of minimal glandular resection, all patients undergoing reduction mammaplasty should be operated on in a hospital where general anesthesia and blood transfusion facilities are available. At least 1 unit (500 ml) of whole blood, preferably autologous, should be readily available.

Patient Positioning

The patient is positioned supine and flat on the operating table with both arms abducted 80° from the side. Many surgeons prefer to elevate the head of the operating table as much as 20°. If this is done, it would be wise to apply support hose or leg wraps to counteract the effects of dependent venous stasis. It is important that the surgeon not be deluded into believing that 20° of elevation will eliminate the distortion of recumbency enough to allow artistic decisions that will be as accurate as when the patient is fully erect.

Surgical Preparation of Patient

The surgeon should remain in the operating room (OR) during surgical preparation of the patient to ensure that the dye markings are not being erased. In most cases, if the markings have been applied 12 hours or more earlier, they will not be erased by the preparation. If it appears that some erasure is occurring, the preparation should be stopped, and the markings scratched with a needle or scalpel point. The surgical preparation should extend from umbilicus to jugular notch, and laterally to the midhumerus, including the entire axilla. The drapes should be applied so that both breasts are exposed. A bulk of absorbent sterile sponges stuffed down into the axilla and along the posterolateral thorax will help to keep the patient's back from becoming blood stained.

(*Text continues on p. 426.*)

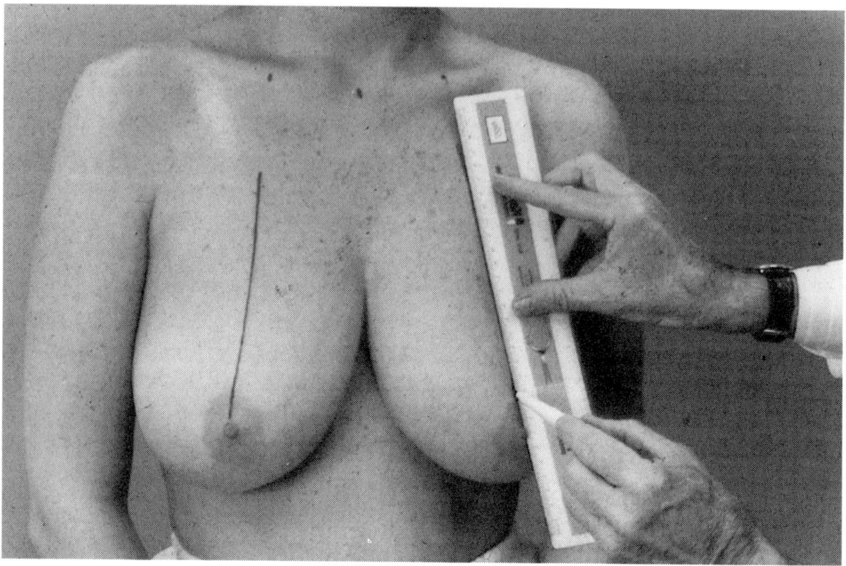

Fig. 26-1 *Marking procedure for reduction mammaplasty.* **A,** *Breast meridians drawn.*

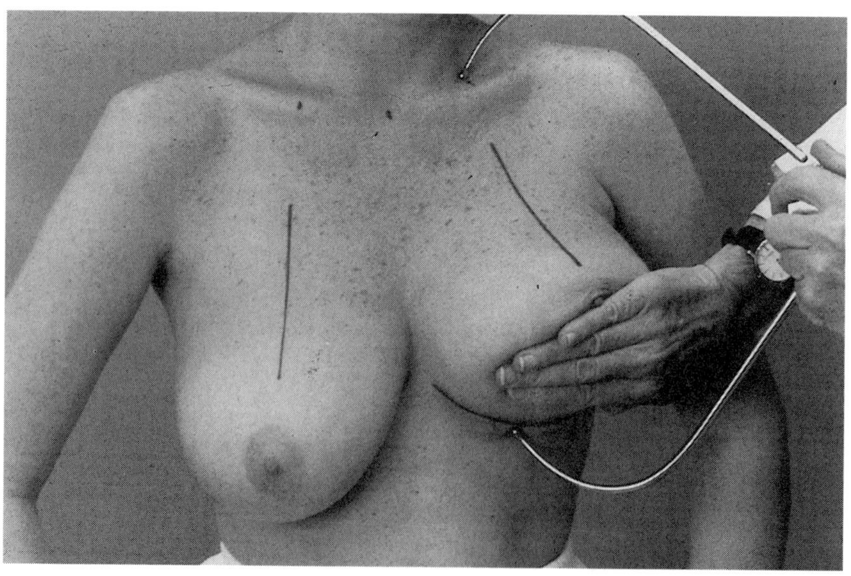

Fig. 26-1 **B,** *Measuring inframmary fold level by caliper.*

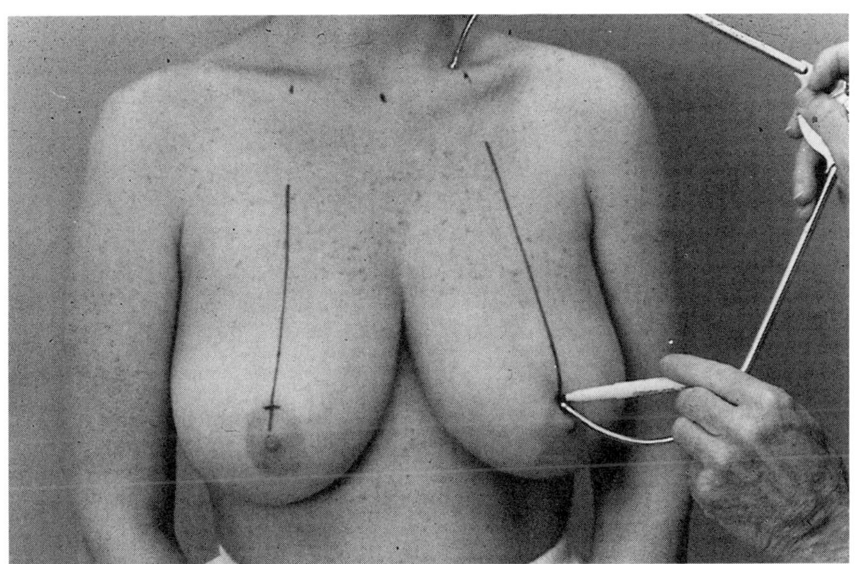

FIG. 26-1 **C,** *Transposing inframammary level to front of breast.*

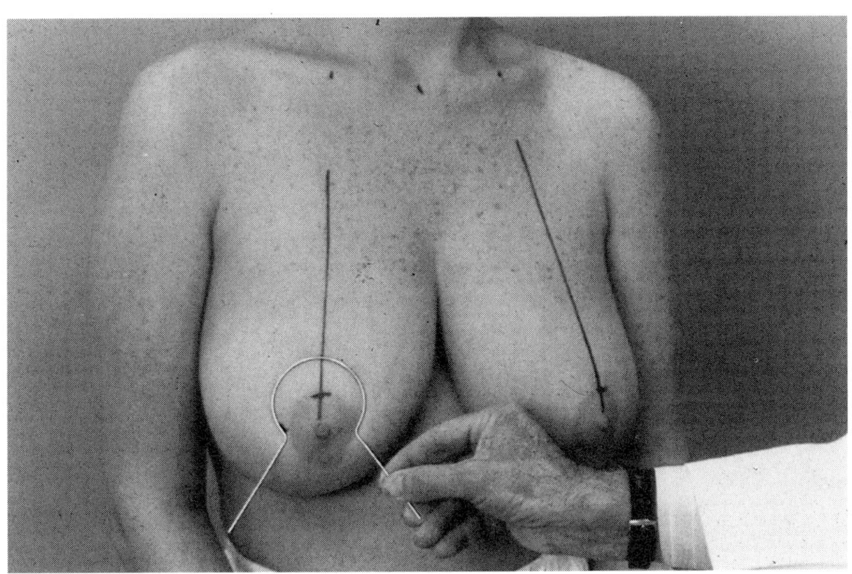

FIG. 26-1 **D,** *Centering keyhold pattern around new nipple site.*

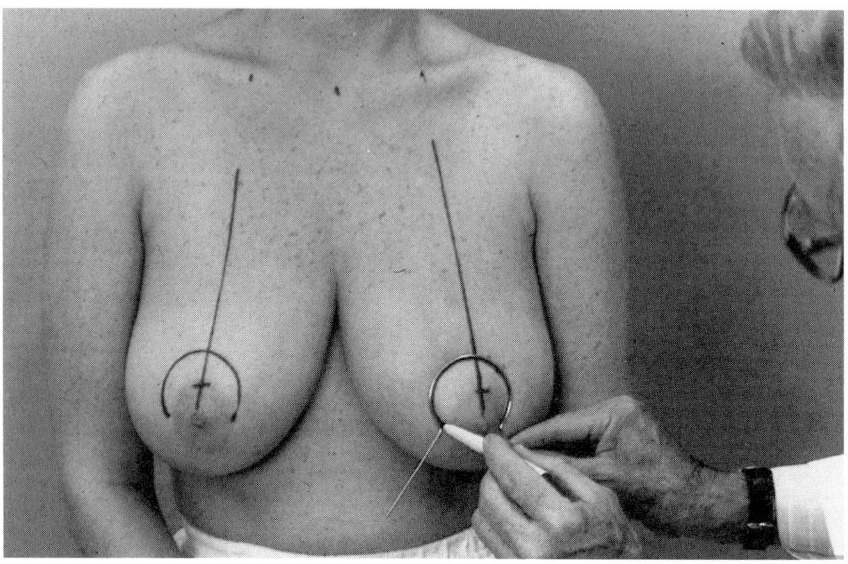

Fig. 26-1 **E,** *Areolar circles drawn.*

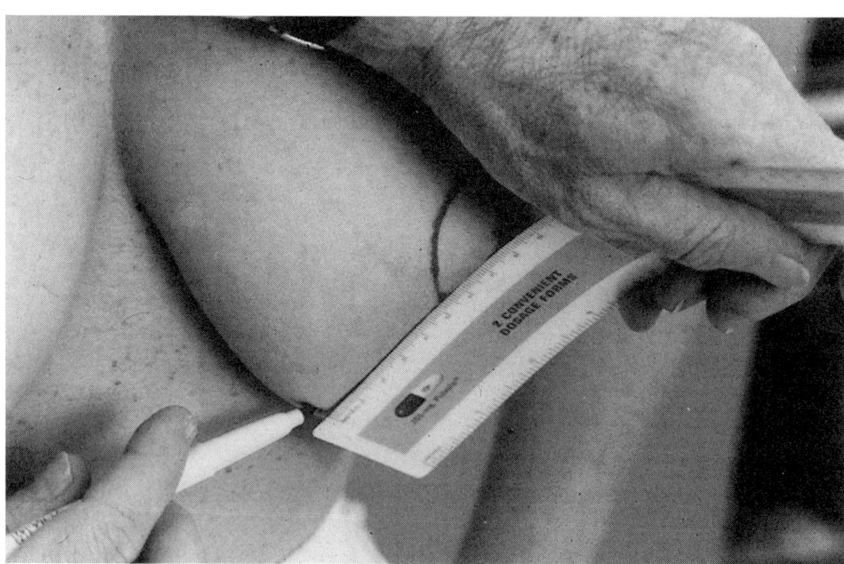

Fig. 26-1 **F,** *Measuring down oblique limb 5.5 cm.*

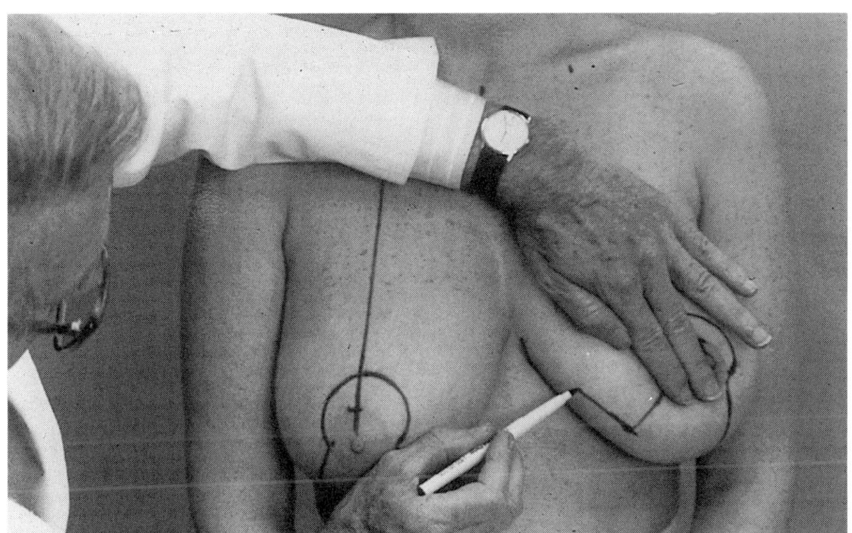

FIG. 26-1 **G,** *Completing medial pattern.*

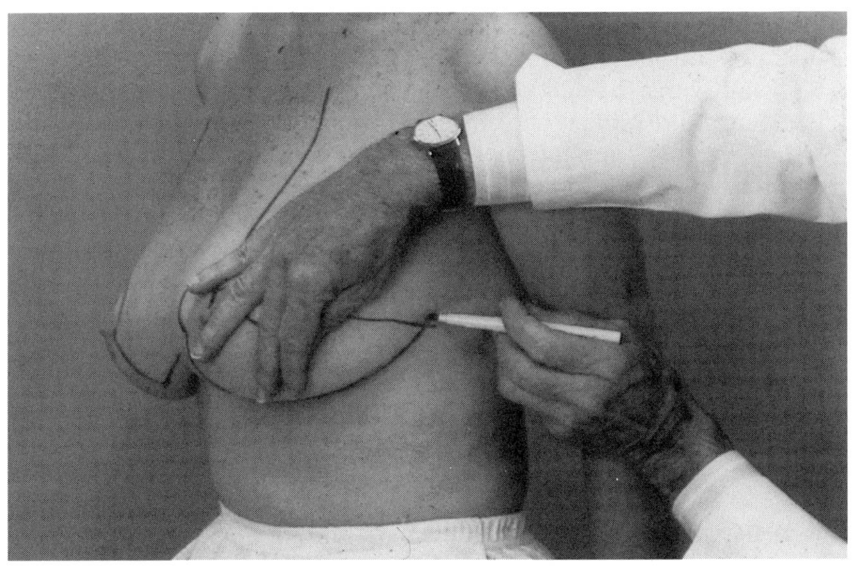

FIG. 26-1 **H,** *Completing lateral pattern.*

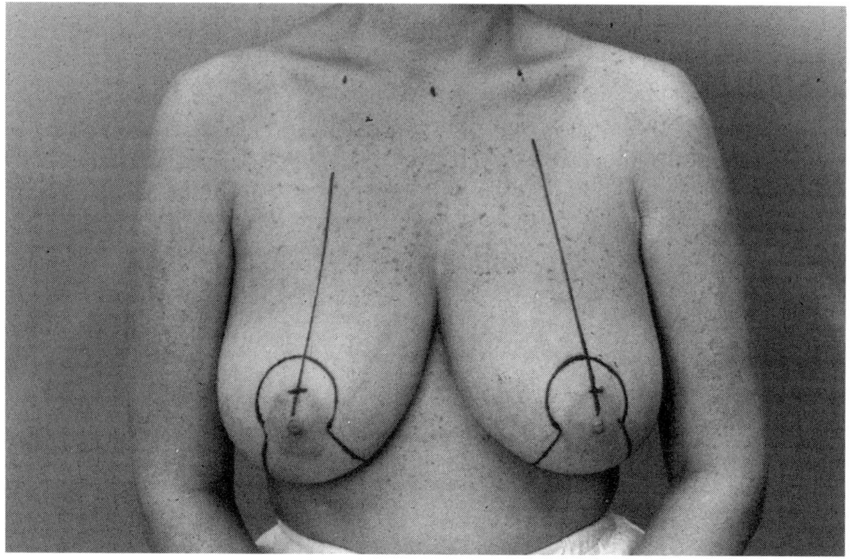

FIG. 26-1 **I,** *Patterns complete.*

Operative Technique

With the approval of the anesthesiologist, the first breast to be operated on should be infiltrated with 20 ml of 0.5% lidocaine with a 1:200,000 dilution of epinephrine to decrease bleeding. To maximize the effect, yet minimize the exposure to epinephrine, the surgeon should exercise some thought in administering these injections. The parenchyma should be infiltrated only along planes of intended parenchymal incisions, not indiscriminately throughout the entire gland. This, combined with the use of the electric cutting current, will minimize blood loss during the resection. The bleeding encountered during the parenchymal resection can usually be controlled entirely by electrocoagulation, with a suture ligature required only rarely. To help the surgeon achieve symmetry, the circulating nurse should weigh the resected breast specimens on an accurate scale in the OR.

Closure

It is usually preferable to complete the closure of the first breast before beginning the second. If autologous blood has been prepared, it may be given at the end of the resection of the second side. In all techniques using a keyhole-type pattern of skin resection, it is wise to perform the closure of the submammary wound from the medial and lateral ends, toward the middle. This will avoid "dog ear" formation at the ends, and any discrepancy in the lengths of the wound edges to be approximated can be adjusted at midbreast at the site of the vertical scar. The upper wound edge should always be longer than the lower, if the keyhole pattern is initially designed to be as narrow as possible.

A. **Drainage.** In any operation, such as reduction mammaplasty, which leaves a large, freshly resected surface area, it is an acceptable surgical technique to provide drainage for a short period of time. A 0.5-inch Penrose drain should be installed across the full width of the breast and led out the extreme lateral end of the submammary wound. It should be sutured in place at the exit point or its end should be protected from retraction by a safety pin. An untied "waiting" suture should be placed through the wound edges separated by the drain to close the drain site defect after removal of the drain. In most cases, the drain may be removed after 24 hours.

B. **Sutures.** The type of suture material to be used for closure varies with the preference of the surgeon but involves some buried absorbable suture material for approximation of the skin flaps and a direct suturing of the dermal edges. The contour of the breast does not lend itself to the use of Steri-strips as the primary agent for skin edge approximation. They are however useful as a reinforcement. There is no need for the suturing of the buried nipple-bearing flap to its surrounding tissues, and the use of such a suture is contraindicated. In general, it is wise to keep the use of buried absorbable suture to a minimum. The most important point concerning the suture closure of the skin is the avoidance of suture marks. The skin of the breast is particularly susceptible to the formation of unsightly stitch marks from any suture that penetrates the skin. The use of subcuticular suturing of all skin edges, either by removable nylon or Prolene, or even an absorbable synthetic suture material to be left in place, is worth the slight extra effort and time involved in subcuticular suturing.

Dressings

The dressings usually are applied while the patient is still asleep. A grease-impregnated antibiotic gauze is applied in strips over all suture lines. A bulk of absorbent dressings is placed over the two drain sites, and the remainder of the dressing consists of a wraparound of two rolls of Kerlix to hold everything together and provide breast support without compression. A metal arm board dusted with baby powder can be placed beneath the patient's back and used to elevate her sufficiently to apply the wraparound dressing; it then can be withdrawn like a shoehorn. To provide some breast support, the dressing should crisscross the chest and surround the neck. The dressing should not be applied tightly. The key to a proper dressing is simplicity. There is no need for a bulky dressing with absorbent pads over the suture lines, engulfing the breasts. This simply adds to the compression of the wraparound dressing. Furthermore, a complex dressing by its very nature discourages frequent changing.

POSTOPERATIVE CARE

Immediate Postoperative Period

Immediate postoperative orders need not be elaborate but should include the following items:

- Early ambulation with nurse assistance
- Reinforcement of the dressing over the drainage sites as needed
- Appropriate diet as desired by the patient
- Pain medication: meperidine (Demerol) up to 100 mg every 3 to 4 hours as needed
- Antinausea agent: prochlorperazine (Compazine), 10 mg intramuscularly (IM) every 3 to 4 hours
- Supplemental iron by mouth: ferrous sulfate 250 mg daily
- Hemoglobin and hematocrit determination the next morning

Four-Hour Check

Within 4 to 6 hours after the end of the operation, it is wise for the surgeon to check the patient to assess the vascular status of the nipple-areola and the skin flaps and to evaluate the breasts for the presence of a hematoma. The surgeon should not rely on the opinion of the floor nurse obtained by a telephone call. This examination can be done quickly and usually does not require removal of the dressings. If a simple dressing has been applied, the areola and the tips of the skin flaps can be inspected by simply retracting the dressings.

A. **Routine postoperative care.** If the 4-hour check reveals all to be well, an uneventful course can be expected. From this point, the patient's hospital care consists of the following routine procedures:

    - Dressings should be changed daily, leaving only the Xeroform gauze as long as it adheres to the wound.
    - The Penrose drain (when utilized) may be removed on the morning of the first postoperative day, and the waiting suture may be tied down to close the site defect.
    - Prophylactic antibiotics, although not contraindicated, are not believed to be necessary in routine cases. A transient temperature elevation on the first postoperative night is common, but the patient should be afebrile by the morning of the second postoperative day.

B. **Management of complications**

    - Hematoma. If both breasts are soft and appear the same size and the pain is symmetrical, a hematoma is unlikely. However, if there is the slightest question, the entire dressing should be removed. If examination reveals a hematoma, plans should be made immediately for return of the patient to the OR for evacuation. This usually will require a second general anesthesia.
    - Vascular insufficiency. If examination reveals an impending vascular insufficiency of either the areola or the skin flaps that was not evident before closure, and if the surgeon perceives the breast to be excessively compressed by the closure and aggravated by the forming edema, then at this point, the breast should be decompressed.

- Decompression. Decompression can be done, without returning to the OR and without any anesthesia, by cutting some of the sutures of the submammary wound or the vertical wound, or both, after first strapping the flaps with adhesive tape. This procedure will usually allow a few hours reprieve before the surgeon has to decide on the need for more aggressive treatment. If decompression is followed by prompt improvement of areolar perfusion, the patient can be kept in this state for several days until the resolution of edema can allow a secondary closure or a temporary skin graft closure.
- Reoperation. If areolar perfusion does not appear to improve on decompression, the surgeon must suspect a basic vascular insufficiency of the nipple-bearing flap and must be prepared to return the patient to the OR and convert the operation to a free-nipple graft procedure. An intravenous (IV) fluorescein study may be helpful at this point to aid in making the decision to operate and shorten the period of procrastination. Under the best of circumstances, the areola is not intensely fluorescent because of its pigmentation; however, spicules of fluorescence scattered throughout the areola can be considered a positive viability test and sufficient reason for further observation.

▼ Areolar cyanosis. An areola that remains mildly cyanotic for several days postoperatively, without the degree of cyanosis substantially changing, will usually not result in a total loss of the nipple and areola. Occasionally, this will eventually result in a partial loss of the areola in the form of a fading of 3 to 4 mm of the areola edge (circumferentially) around its periphery. This entire process may take as long as 4 to 6 weeks to be completed. In most cases in which this degree of vascular insufficiency has occurred, some fat necrosis can be expected. In fact, some amount of fat can be expected in many cases in which extensive resections have been performed, whether or not the blood supply to the nipple has been compromised. Fat necrosis commonly manifests itself as spontaneous drainage from one of the suture lines of a copious amount of oily, purulent-appearing liquid or sometimes as an area of low-grade localized erythema and tenderness, suggestive of an underlying abscess. Characteristically, these signs of fat necrosis will appear some time after discharge from the hospital. Treatment includes establishment of adequate drainage, saline irrigation, and appropriate oral antibiotics (Keflex, 250 to 500 mg 4 times a day).

Discharge from Hospital

The patient may be discharged from the hospital on the first or second postoperative day if she is afebrile and otherwise feels so inclined. The pathologist's report should be examined, and the patient should be informed before discharge of the absence or presence of malignancy in the specimen.

A. **Wound dressing for discharge.** A light wraparound dressing held in place by a brassiere will eliminate the need for a dressing that loops around the neck and will provide enough support for comfort.
B. **Medications.** Discharge medications can be limited to an oral pain reliever such as acetaminophen (Tylenol) with codeine (30 mg) and supplemental iron.
C. **Patient instructions on discharge**
    - ▼ The patient should be instructed to wear a well-fitting brassiere that immobilizes the breasts day and night for 4 to 6 weeks.
    - ▼ She should be told that she may shower 1 week after surgery if a subcuticular suture has been placed or immediately after suture removal if conventional suturing has been done.
    - ▼ She should be instructed not to lie directly upon the breasts for 6 to 8 weeks after surgery to avoid unnecessary stress on scars.
    - ▼ Arm and shoulder motion after surgery is not believed to be harmful to the breasts, and a reasonable instruction in this regard is simply to direct the patient to keep within the limitations of her discomfort.

Follow-up After Discharge

The patient should be seen in the office 1 week after discharge from the hospital, and any remaining sutures should be removed at that time. The frequency of follow-up visits beyond this point will be dictated by the presence and nature of complications. In routine cases presenting no unusual treatment problems, it is wise to follow-up each patient quarterly for at least 1 year. This will be mainly for the edification of the surgeon, not only to evaluate the final quality of the work but also to determine the need for minor surgical revisions. The surgical revision of hypertrophic scars and the elimination of "dog ears" will comprise the majority of secondary revisions needed. These should not be considered earlier than 6 months after surgery and ideally should not be considered for 1 year. Although nothing can be done to restore lost sensibility to the areola, a year-long record of the status of nipple-areolar sensibility, observed in comparison to its importance to the patient, will enlighten the surgeon.

CHAPTER 27

Breast Reconstruction After Mastectomy

John Bostwick III and Benjamin H. Johnson III

The breast is the most salient sign of womanhood. It is no wonder that operations on the breast evoke feelings of fear in the patient. Many women feel the loss of a breast represents the utmost mutilation. As has been shown by Halsted, Haagenson, and many others, when cancer is present, a cancer operation with local ablation should be performed. For many years the standard Halsted radical mastectomy, which sacrifices the pectoral muscles, was the operation chosen most often. It has been shown more recently that a modified radical mastectomy, leaving the pectoral muscles intact, has an identical patient survival rate. Choice of the ablative procedure is best made by the educated operating surgeon and is not the purpose of this discussion. Breast amputation offers the best chance for cure, but it is usually psychologically damaging and may result in physical discomfort as well.

Breast reconstruction has changed dramatically with the advent of the silicone implant, tissue expander, and the musculocutaneous flap. The latissimus dorsi musculocutaneous unit and the transverse rectus abdominus island flap (TRAM) provide the means for a one-stage reconstruction. We present an approach to the care of the patient who seeks breast reconstruction and care for the opposite breast with regard to symmetry and reduced risk of development of malignancy. Preoperative evaluation, intraoperative consideration, postoperative care, and possible complications are discussed.

PREOPERATIVE EVALUATION

Medical History and Age

Breast cancer is primarily a disease of middle-aged women. In the United States 190,000 new cases of breast cancer are diagnosed and treated yearly. Nine percent of women will develop breast cancer; of these, 15% are less than 40 years of age. No one is refused breast reconstruction because of age. Patients less than 60 years are more likely to seek reconstruction. Any medically stable patient seen in consultation, after thorough preoperative evaluation by an internist, oncologist, and general surgeon, is given every consideration.

Family History

Simple mastectomy, total mastectomy, or subcutaneous mastectomy is often offered by the general surgeon to those at high risk of developing carcinoma; that is, these patients have a strong family history of this disease. One of these procedures is often considered in the contralateral breast in patients who have had a previous cancer operation.

Pathologic Grade, Clinical Staging, and Timing of Reconstructive Procedure

The presence or absence of axillary nodal metastasis has been demonstrated to correlate with survival. No patient is refused consideration for breast reconstruction on the basis of the clinical stage if she can be shown to be free of distant and local disease.

A patient would be considered eligible 6 weeks after radical or modified radical mastectomy, assuming no adjuvant therapy is planned. If radiation or chemotherapy is undertaken postoperatively, a 6-week waiting period is recommended after cessation of this treatment. Immediate reconstruction is offered to stage I patients. Any method may be used. Immediate, synchronous reconstruction is desirable after prophylactic mastectomy.

Type of Procedure Performed by Oncologic Breast Surgeon

If possible, preoperative consultation between the reconstructive and oncologic surgeons is desirable for planning of incision. An oblique or transverse incision is preferable for reconstruction. If the patient is seen only postoperatively, the procedure should be discussed with the referring surgeon with regard to pectoral muscle integrity and the status of the thoracodorsal nerve and vessels. If this consultation is not feasible, the initial surgical report should be reviewed by the reconstructive surgeon.

Preoperative Discussion with Patient

The patient is included as much as possible in the preoperative planning. She is informed of the possible surgical risks, including those of bleeding, infection, and anesthesia. The possibility of seroma and its treatment are also discussed. A breast reconstruction information brochure can be useful to the patient.

The patient is encouraged to discuss what she dislikes about her appearance and what physical dysfunctions she is experiencing. Her preferred types of dress also are reviewed for incision orientation. Because symmetry is so critical, any needed modification of the opposite breast also must be discussed.

A. **Patient medical history.** A thorough medical history is taken with attention particularly to the following items:
   - ▼ Medications taken by the patient such as aspirin and antiinflammatory drugs, which should be stopped 2 weeks before surgery
   - ▼ Family history of breast cancer. (Consideration should be given to the opposite breast for prophylactic mastectomy.)
   - ▼ Surgical history and abdominal incision

Physical Examination and Tests

Before breast reconstruction, the patient should be thoroughly examined by an internist or oncologist and cleared for general anesthesia. Particular attention should be directed to the following areas:

- ▼ Search for metastatic disease, including the tests indicated:

- Chest x-ray examination
- Liver function tests and clotting studies
- Bone scan (not recommended routinely unless bone pain or back pain is elicited from the medical history or physical examination)

▼ Local conditions. Tightness of skin, orientation of incision, and presence of skingrafts are noted.

▼ Axilla. Aside from possible adenopathy, the amount of scarring and presence of tight bands in the axilla are noted. This is important in operative planning of the approach to the axillary vein and brachial plexus, especially after radical mastectomy, and if a free flap is being considered.

▼ Arm edema. Both arms are measured and compared for edema. There is some evidence clinically of improvement of edema after a latissimus dorsi flap procedure. Liposuction can reduce upper arm fullness.

▼ Pectoral muscles. Infraclavicular defects are noted. The muscles may be tested by having the patient abduct the arm against resistance. Even though a modified radical mastectomy was performed, the muscle may have been denervated and may now be atrophic because of division of the pectoral nerves.

▼ Latissimus dorsi muscle. It is important to test the latissimus dorsi muscle by instructing the patient to place the hands on the hips and press down. Any winging of the scapula is noted. Both tests are indicative of the integrity of the thoracodorsal and long thoracic nerves and the adjacent vascular pedicles.

▼ Contralateral breast. The other breast and axilla are thoroughly examined for signs of malignancy, masses, or fibrocystic disease. A mammogram is recommended. If the remaining breast is not to be removed, attention and planning toward symmetry is most important (i.e., consideration of mastopexy, augmentation, and nipple-areolar complex).

Preoperative Mammography.

See Chapter 29.

OPERATIVE PLANNING

Indications for Flap

- Absent pectoralis muscle
- Tight skin
- Thin skin
- Previous irradiation
- Skingraft
- Size of opposite breast, ptosis

Orientation of Skin Island Donor Site

Usually, if the patient has had a modified radical or radical mastectomy, skin is needed. The amount of tissue to be transferred depends on the presence or absence of the pectoral muscles.

A. **Absent pectoralis muscle because of radical mastectomy.** The orientation of the skin-island donor site should be transverse or oblique. The patient should be examined and marked with her brassiere in place, so that the alignment of the donor incision leaves the resultant scar on the back beneath the brassiere. This orientation also necessitates placing the patient in the lateral decubitus position for the operation. The use of the entire latissimus muscle is necessary to ensure filling of the infraclavicular and anterior axillary fold defects. To ensure primary closure of the donor defect, the skin island should be no greater than 8 to 9 cm in width, depending somewhat on the patient's body habitus, amount of fat, and laxity of skin. The skin length runs from the posterior axillary line to the spine (Fig. 27-1).

B. **Pectoralis muscles remain but patient has thin or irradiated skin, tight skin, or skin graft.** A skin island may be planned parallel to the anterior axillary line. Patient preference is considered, but if this incision is used, the patient may remain supine during the procedure. She also may wear low-backed dresses, bathing suits, and other revealing clothing without exposure of the resultant scar from the donor defect.

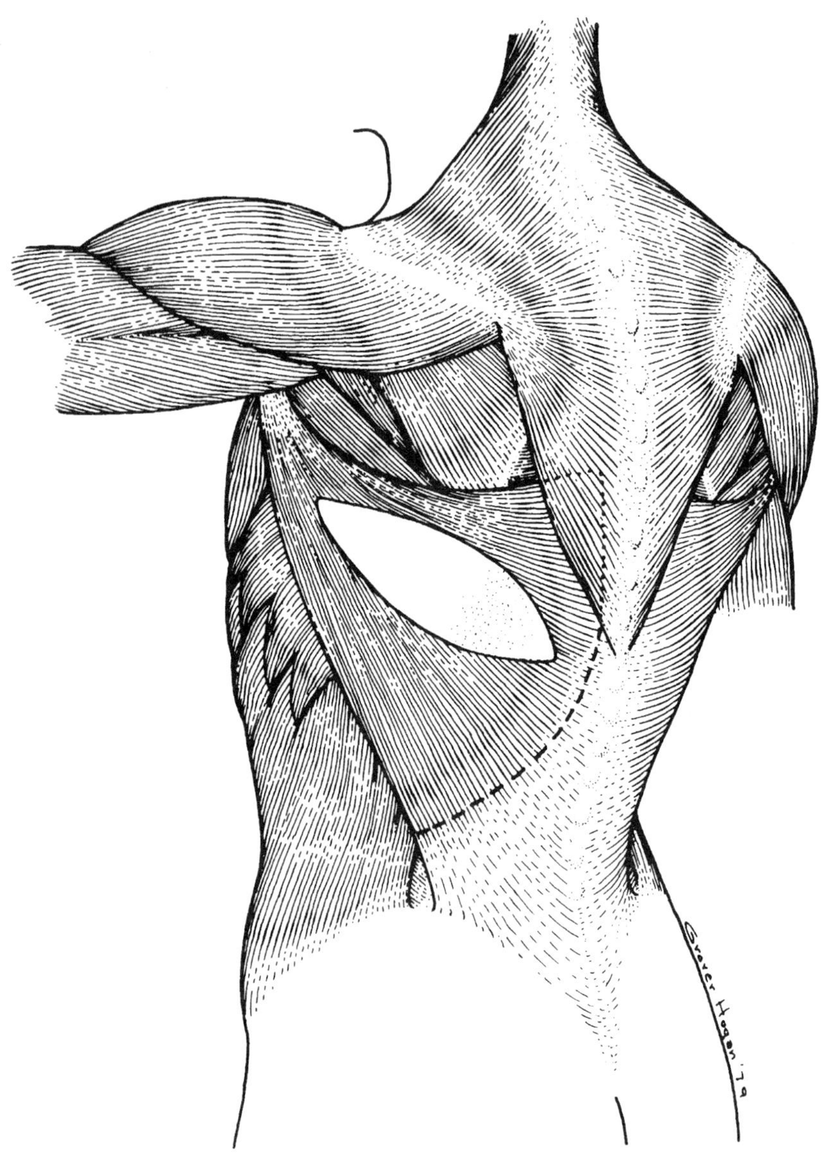

Fig. 27-1 *Skin island placement.*

Contralateral Breast and Breast Symmetry

To ensure breast symmetry, the proper procedure is selected. Whether this be mastopexy, augmentation mammaplasty, or total mastectomy, the inframammary line is marked on the opposite breast and corresponding ipsilateral inframammary line. The placement of the nipple-areolar complex is usually determined intraoperatively.

PREOPERATIVE ORDERS

Aside from the routine orders, the following procedures are carried out:

- Hibiclens or Betadine scrub 1 week before surgery
- Typing and cross-matching for 2 units of whole blood. When feasible, autotransfusion is recommended (See Chapter 7.). (Autologous blood donation: 2 units for unilateral; 3 to 4 units for bilateral)
- Designing the operation and drawing to be done the day before surgery to allow sufficient time
- Clear liquid diet 24 hours before surgery; fleet enema on day of surgery
- Intravenous (IV) fluids beginning night before surgery
- Solu-Medrol 250 mg IV at midnight and 6 AM day of surgery
- Foley catheter

OPERATIVE MANAGEMENT

- Warming blanket, heated IV fluids, and blood
- Solu-Medrol 500 mg IV intraoperatively
- IV antibiotics: cephalosporin
- Replenish fluid loss

OPERATIVE PROCEDURE

It is preferable for the reconstructive surgeon to be present before the ablative breast procedure to discuss the selection of the incision with the general surgeon.

Nonflap Reconstruction

This technique is usually used after a total mastectomy. To achieve symmetry, the procedure is done with the patient in the semisitting position. In reconstruction, we use the submuscular position for the implant. If the reconstruction is a delayed surgery, the previous incision is opened secondarily. Dissection of the submuscular plane is continued down to the previously marked inframammary line. The inframammary line is sutured to the fascia.

Latissimus Dorsi Musculocutaneous Flap

A. Incision

- ▼ A transverse back incision is indicated if a large amount of muscle is needed (or if the patient prefers this incision). The patient is placed on the operating table in the lateral decubitus position. The upper arm is placed in a supporting device similar to that used for thoracotomy incisions. Care must be taken to pad this arm sufficiently to protect against nerve damage from pressure during the procedure.
- ▼ If the vertical incision is chosen, the patient may lie supine, with folded sheets placed beneath the shoulder and flank to provide some tilt.
- ▼ Both the donor incision site and mastectomy wound should then be prepared and draped so that simultaneous dissection can be undertaken. The dissection of the latissimus dorsi muscle itself has been adequately described elsewhere. (Fig. 27-2).
- ▼ At the site of the mastectomy, if the orientation of the closure is transverse or oblique, the scar is removed and the skin island is inserted. If a radical mastectomy was done and muscle is needed to fill the infraclavicular area, the skin island is oriented low on the muscle. If a vertical mastectomy scar is present, a new incision is made transversely or obliquely to receive the skin island.

B. Closure of donor defect

- ▼ A Jackson-Pratt drain is placed in the depths of the donor site and exited through a separate stab wound.

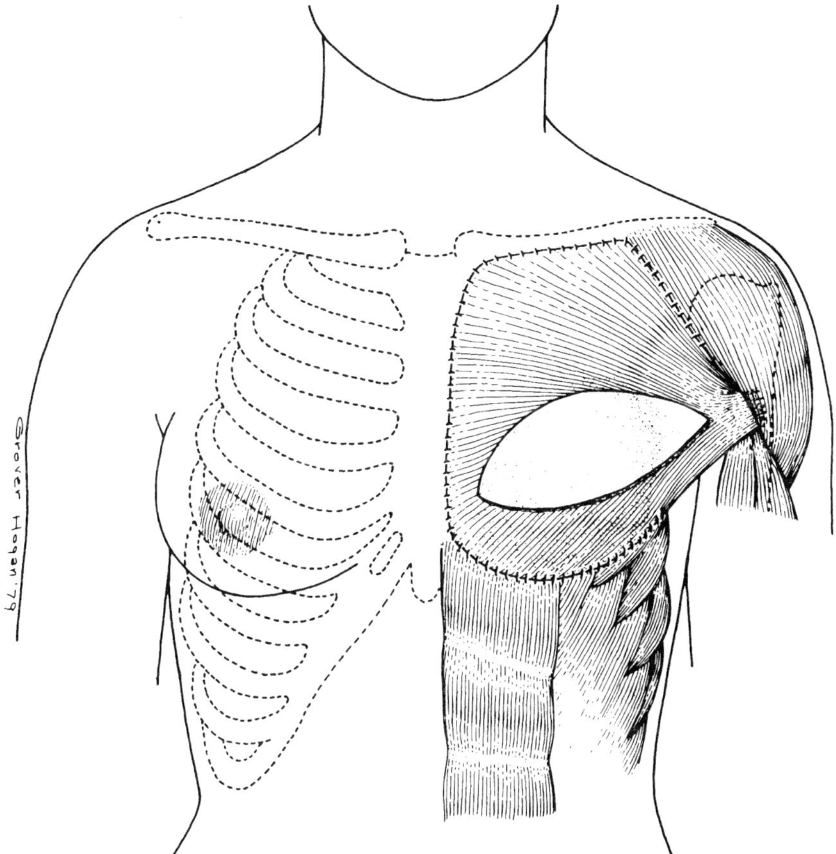

FIG. 27-2 *Transposed muscle in position and transfer of divided insertion of latissimus dorsi muscle, with transfer to previous insertion of pectoralis major muscle higher on humerus.*

- ▼ The wound edges are at first approximated with skin staples for good alignment. There is usually some tension on the wound edges.
- ▼ The donor defect is then closed in layers by using 00 Vicryl in the deeper tissues and interrupted and running intracuticular 000 Proline in the skin, after which the staples are removed.

Breast Reconstruction

- ▼ If the patient was positioned in the lateral decubitus position, she is now turned to the supine position. The anterior chest wound is covered with a sterile towel before repositioning. The patient is reprepared an draped.

- If a bilateral reconstruction is planned, the patient is placed prone at first; the latissimus dorsi dissection is completed; then she is turned supine.
- The tunnel for passage of the muscle must be ample, usually three finger-breadths' wide, so as not to compromise blood flow to the flap.
- If the pectoralis major muscle is present, it is dissected free of its attachments to the chest wall. The dissection is carried inferiorly to the insertion of the muscle, corresponding to the inframammary line, as determined previously. The latissimus dorsi muscle is then sutured to the inferior portion of the pectoralis major, thus creating a pocket to receive the implant. Absorbable suture is used (e.g., Vicryl, Dexon).
- If the pectoralis major muscle is absent, the inferior portion of the transposed latissimus dorsei muscle, which is now superior on the chest wall, is sutured to the clavicle and high on the shoulder to recreate the anterior axillary line and infraclavicular fossa.
- An implant of appropriate size is placed in the pocket beneath the muscle. The skin island is then approximated to the wound edges in two layers. An intercuticlar 000 Prolene is used in the skin.

Transverse Rectus Abdominus Island Flap

Since the advent of the TRAM in the early 1980s by Hartrampf, many variations and refinements have been introduced, but their explanation is beyond the scope of this chapter. Choices of the type of flaps include unipedicle, contralateral, bipedicle, free TRAM, or other free flap, depending on the patient's anatomy, opposite breast, amount of abdominal tissue and abdominal scars, general physical condition, age, and smoking history. In the obese (25% more than ideal body weight) or the very thin patient, other options for reconstruction are often a better choice. Other risk factors must be considered, such as diabetes, vascular disease, and smoking. As always, the patient must be included in the decision. The patient's working history and psychologic factors must also be considered. This includes determining if the patient is able to accept the time involved in healing and the presence of a large abdominal scar.

Nipple-Areola Complex

Currenty the nipple can be constructed from existing tissue on the reconstructed breast or by a sharing technique.

A. **Local tissue.** Either a winged flap placed superiorly as described by Hartrampf or the skate flap used by Little is used, with the former giving the best projection. Either is best suited for a TRAM flap or a latissimus flap. These methods are done in the office approximately 6 weeks postoperatively, usually requiring no anesthesia. The areola is tattooed. Tattooing gives a better color match and avoids a painful groin scar.
B. **Contralateral nipple shaving.** This is a viable alternative, especially in the tissue overlying a prosthesis like in tissue expander reconstruction.
C. **Skin graft.** If a skin graft areola is preferred, a "dog ear" from a TRAM flap abdominal closure is often used.

POSTOPERATIVE MANAGEMENT

Aside from routine postoperative care, the patient should be managed as follows:

- ▼ Particular attention paid to pulmonary care—provides incentive to use spirometer
- ▼ Patient-controlled analgesics (PCA); pump extremely useful 24 to 48 hours postoperatively
- ▼ Antibiotics for 48 hours
- ▼ Ambulation first postoperative day
- ▼ Removal of Foley catheter first postoperative day
- ▼ Clear liquids given first postoperative day and advance
- ▼ Removal of Jackson-Pratt drains postoperative day 2 to 3 from chest, 3 to 4 from abdomen, when drainage is less than 20 ml in 8 hours
- ▼ Patient discharged 5 to 7 days postoperatively

COMPLICATIONS

Bleeding

Transfusion is rarely required except with TRAM flap; unilateral TRAM requires 2 units; bilateral TRAM requires 3 to 4 units. Blood should be administered intraoperatively or soon postoperatively. Attempt should be made to keep hemoglobin in the normal range.

Skin Necrosis and Partial Flap Loss

This complication should be prevented with careful patient selection and correct surgical technique. Flap viability should be monitored. If there is evidence of vascular compromise, usually venous congestion, early consideration should be given to exploration for twisting or other pedicle compromise.

Fat Necrosis

This often occurs as a late side effect. Areas should be recorded and followed-up, because they may be confused with tumor recurrence. Good communication between surgeon and patient is essential.

Seroma

Obese patients have a higher incidence of this complication. The condition usually responds to needle aspiration, often multiple. Elastic garments may be preventive.

Contour Irregularities

Patients should wait 2 to 3 months for edema to subside and muscle to atrophy. These irregularities are often treated with liposuction.

Ventral Hernia

Now incidence of this complication is less than 5%. Care must be taken not to take fascia below the line and close the fascia to the pubis. If a postoperative hernia is present, it usually must be repaired, often with mesh.

POSTOPERATIVE MAMMOGRAPHY

See Chapter 29.

FURTHER READINGS

Bostwick J III: *Plastic and reconstructive breast surgery,* St Louis, 1990, Quality Medical.

Hartrampf CR: *Transverse abdominal island flap technique for breast reconstruction after mastectomy,* Baltimore, 1984 University Park.

Hartrampf CR: *Clin Plast Surg* 15:703, 1988.

Little JW III: Nipple-areola reconstruction, *Clin Plast Surg* 11:351, 1988.

CHAPTER 28

Nipple-Areola Reconstruction

SCOTT L. SPEAR AND HOWARD HEPPE

Nipple-areola reconstruction has become an integral part of breast reconstruction. No matter how symmetric a reconstructed breast mound appears, an aesthetic result will remain elusive until the nipple-areolar complex has been reconstructed. Advances in nipple reconstruction now provide a means to create adequate and stable projection. In addition, tattoo has revolutionized areolar reconstruction by eliminating the morbidity of specialized skin graft donor sites, while providing an improved method of attaining areolar color match. The following discussion will emphasize the important goals in preoperative evaluation, operative planning, execution, and postoperative care of the various forms of the skate flap and tattoo.

DISCUSSION WITH PATIENT

The decision to pursue nipple-areola reconstruction should begin before breast reconstruction.

Operative Procedure

At this time the patient should be made aware that the optimal aesthetic result will require two, or possibly more, operative procedures. The initial procedure should focus on reconstructing the breast mound, with subsequent procedures necessary to modify the shape and to reconstruct the nipple-areolar complex. It should be emphasized that nipple-areola reconstruction is minimally inconvenient to the patient, at times only requiring an office procedure with local anesthetic.

Tattoos

The benefits of tattoo should also be explained to the patient. Tattoo has allowed surgeons to eliminate the morbidity of specialized skin graft donor sites, such as the paralabial tissue, while providing improved control over the final color match. More than one procedure may be required to achieve the desired color match, and this should be mentioned to the patient.

PREOPERATIVE EVALUATION

Symmetry

Before planning a nipple-areola reconstruction, the surgeon must assess the current status of the breast reconstruction with regard to size and symmetry. Positioning of the nipple is dependent on the position of the contralateral nipple and the convexity of the reconstructed breast mound. Therefore the reconstructed breast must be close to its final shape to avoid malposition of the nipple-areolar complex. In addition, if a contralateral mastopexy or reduction is required, these procedures should be performed before nipple-areola reconstruction can take place. Once the major revisions have been performed on the reconstructed or the contralateral breast or both, a symmetric position can be determined for the nipple-areolar complex.

If nipple reconstruction has already taken place, but the position is not optimal (the usual error is too lateral and superior), a corrective procedure must be planned. The easiest way to camouflage this problem is to tattoo the areola in the correct position, with the nipple eccentrically placed. However, if the misalignment is too great, nipple transposition will be necessary and can be obtained with techniques such as V-Y plasty. In severe cases of nipple ectopia, a new nipple reconstruction is required, followed by simple excision of the ectopic nipple. The ease of this latter step is another virtue of this low effort, low morbidity methodology.

Timing

Nipple reconstruction is usually performed no sooner than 2 to 3 months after the breast reconstruction. This allows time for the reconstructed breast to reach its final shape. Areola reconstruction by tattoo then follows 2 to 3 months later, allowing scar hyperemia to resolve, and thus avoiding difficulty in determining color match. This delay also allows the surgeon an opportunity to fine-tune the breast one last time, including scar revisions, size and shape adjustments, and nipple refinements.

Skin Graft

The original "skate" flap (Fig. 28-1) called for a large circular skin graft, usually harvested from the paralabial area as a source for the pigmented areola. Creating an incision in the paralabial area was the cause of significant patient morbidity and dissatisfaction. With the advent of tattoo, the skin graft was required only to close the donor defect for the skate flap, relying on tattoo for simulation of the areola. Currently, a modified skate flap is performed by not deepithelializing the area above the wings of the skate flap as originally described. The requirement for a skin graft is then reduced to only a small horseshoe-shaped defect, a size that can be harvested as a 2- by 1-cm ellipse based on the lateral aspect of the mastectomy incision, or other scar, eliminating the need for a new incision. Even this small skin graft can be eliminated, in the appropriate patient, by using the newer, abbreviated skate flap, which allows primary closure of the donor site.

Nipple Projection

As with any surgical procedure, the skate flap has undergone several refinements while experience was gained with its execution. The greatest improvement allowed elimination of the skin graft when only minimal to modest nipple projection was required. In this modification, the skate flap leaves three V-shaped defects that can all be closed primarily, with areolar tattoo to follow at a later date. However, if the contralateral nipple projection is significant, a standard skate flap may be required, with concomitant skin graft. Alternatively, nipple sharing may be an option in patients with true unilateral nipple hypertrophy.

TECHNIQUE OF NIPPLE RECONSTRUCTION USING MODIFIED SKATE FLAP

The new nipple position is determined by measuring the distance from the clavicle and sternum to the nipple on the contralateral side and then duplicating these measurements on the reconstructed site. This position can then be modified

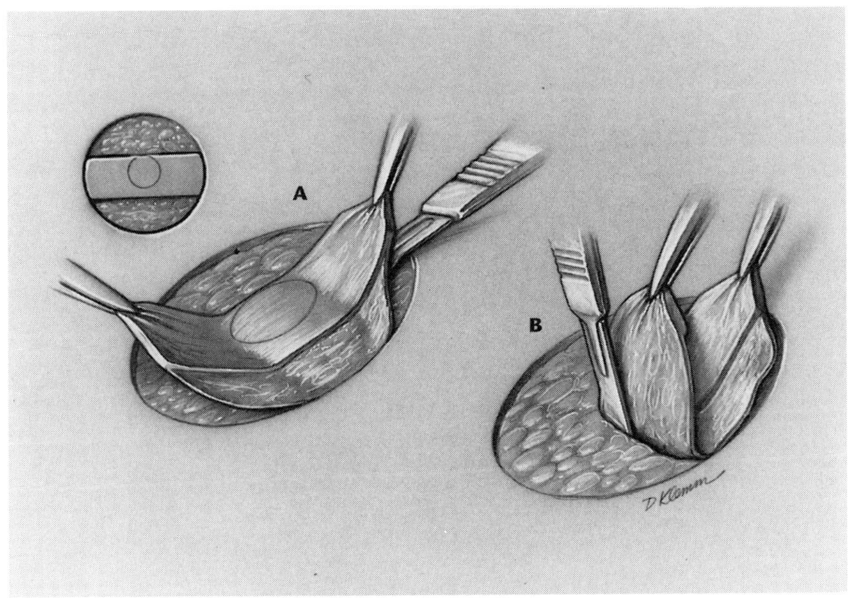

FIG. 28-1. *Original skate flap.* **A,** *Flap markings with area outside tangents deepithelialized and wing elevation at deep dermal level.* **B,** *Plane of dissection changing from horizontal to vertical to create central wedge.*

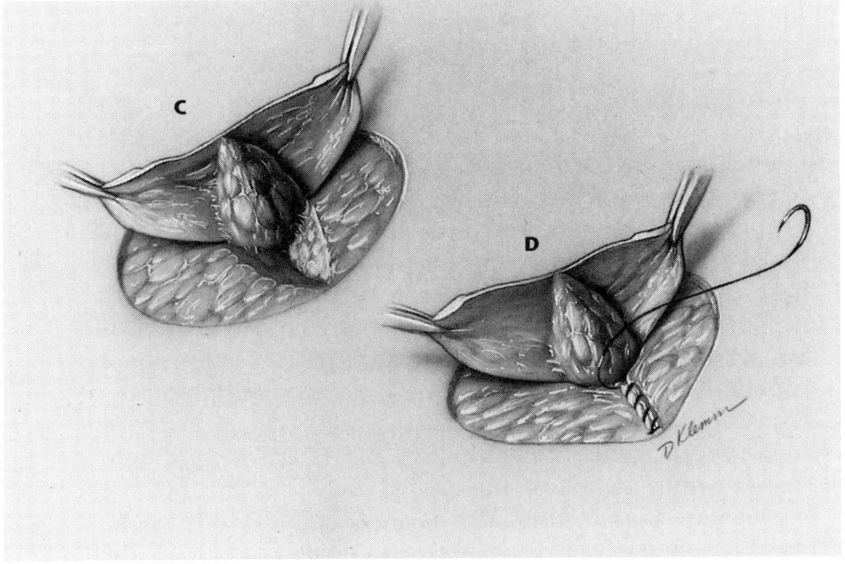

FIG. 28-1 **C,** *Skate flap elevated, with central wedge defect remaining.* **D,** *Closure of central defect with a running 5.0 Vicryl suture.*

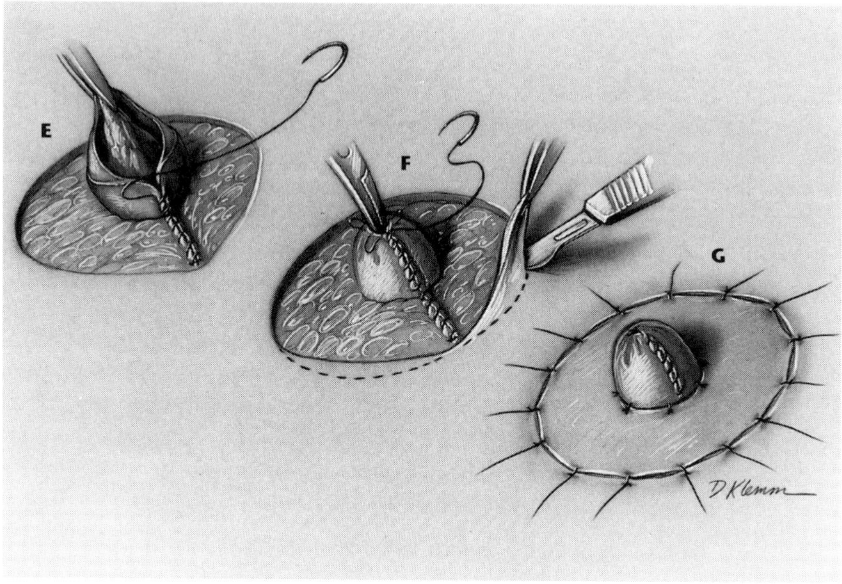

FIG. 28-1 **E,** *Running vicryl suture continues up epithelial portion of nipple column.* **F,** *Vicryl suture continues around epithelial margin as a purse string to invaginate dermal and subcutaneous components. In addition, revision of skin margin is performed to maintain circular border.* **G,** *Completed nipple with skin graft and tie-over sutures in place.*

somewhat, depending on the shape of the reconstructed breast. An areolar circle is then drawn with an additional inner concentric circle corresponding to the diameter of the nipple. The modified skate flap (Fig. 28-2) is designed with a central wedge of skin and subcutaneous tissue flanked by partial thickness wings. The central wedge is outlined by dropping two curvilinear arcs from either side of the inner (nipple) circle to a point on the outer (areolar) circle. If these arcs started at the 3- and 9-o'clock positions on the inner (nipple) circle and extended to the 6-o'clock position on the larger (areolar) circle, then the wings are designed by drawing a tangent to the inner circle at the 12-o'clock position. This tangent extends to the areola circle and outlines the base of the wings. Another line is drawn parallel to the base, two-thirds of the way down the central wedge, creating the upper border of the wings. Flap elevation then begins at the lateral aspect of the wings. These are dissected just above the

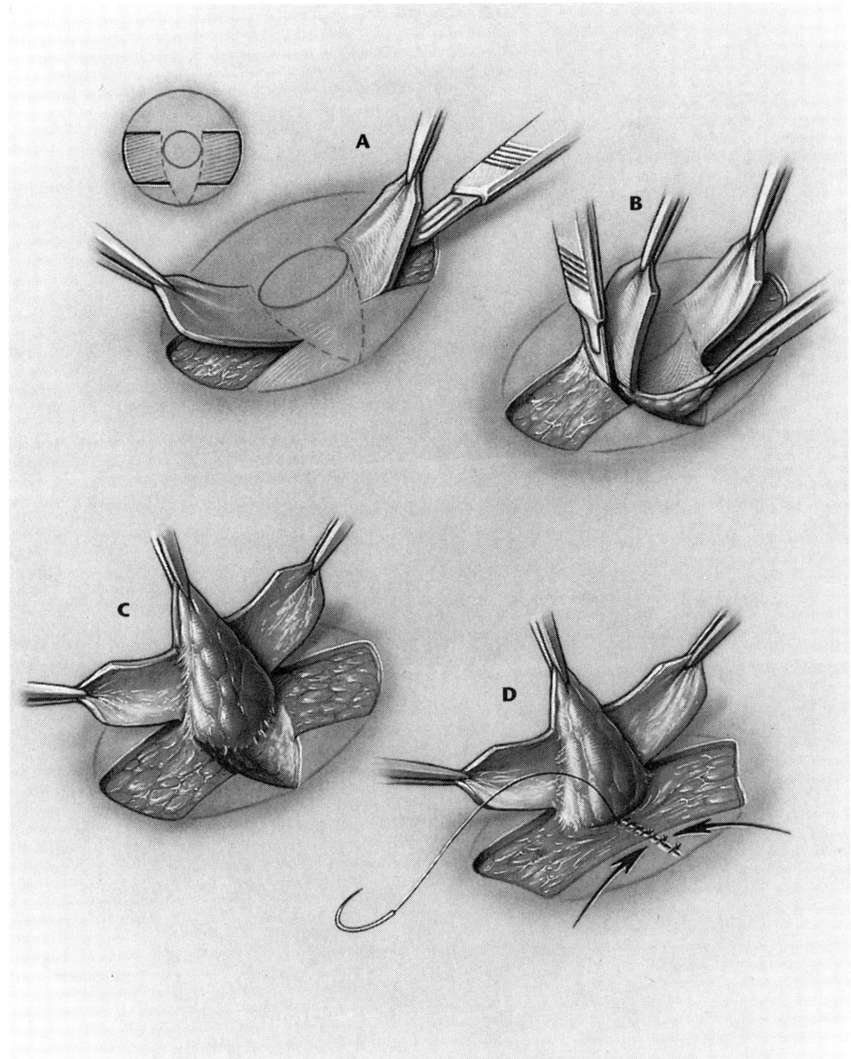

FIG. 28-2 *Modifed skate flap.* **A,** *Flap markings, with wing elevation at deep dermal level up to dotted line.* **B,** *Dissection changing from horizontal to vertical at dotted line to develop central wedge.* **C,** *All aspects of modified skate flap elevated.* **D,** *Closure of central wedge defect with running 5.0 Vicryl.*

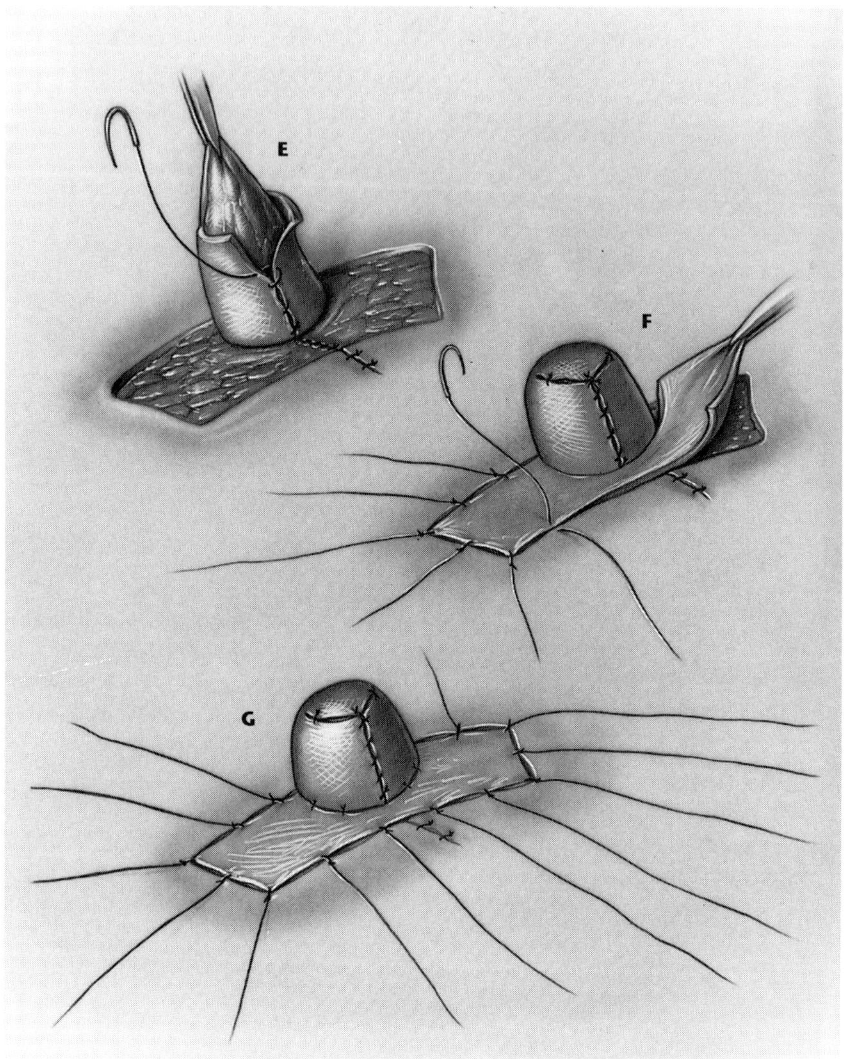

FIG. 28-2 **E,** *Closure of wings around central wedge as continuation of running stitch.* **F,** *Placement of skin graft.* **G,** *Completed skate flap with tie-over sutures in place.*

subcutaneous fat, deep within the dermis, to the lateral border of the central wedge, at which point the dissection goes deep. The central wedge carries subcutaneous tissue, and occasionally muscle or even implant capsule, to provide a dual blood supply to the flap from the dermis and the deep tissues. After the flap is raised, the central wedge defect is closed primarily, and this suture is continued up the nipple column, suturing the wings together, around the subcutaneous and other tissues of the central wedge. A skin graft of suitable size is then sutured in place at the donor site.

Abbreviated Skate Flap

To eliminate the need for a skin graft, the lateral wings are designed similar to the central wedge. When elevating the wings in this method, though, the level of dissection is full-thickness skin just below the dermis, not necessarily including any subcutaneous tissue. This allows both the lateral and central wedge defect to be closed primarily, obviating the need for a skin graft. Closure begins with a 5-0 Vicryl intradermally to approximate the central and lateral defects. The skin is further approximated with an interrupted 5-0 chromic. The central Vicryl then continues up the nipple column to suture the lateral wings around the central tissue.

DRESSING AND POSTOPERATIVE CARE

The skin graft, when it is included, is covered with a greasy dressing, and the nipple is protected with the cut base of a plastic syringe barrel or other such protector. Wet cotton is wrapped around the syringe barrel to facilitate the use of a tie-over dressing. This dressing remains in place for 4 days, when it is removed, and the area is redressed with a greasy dressing, which is changed daily by the patient. At the end of the first week, the dressing is discontinued, and the patient is allowed to bathe completely. In the case of nipple reconstruction with a skin graft, postoperative care is even easier. In the operating room a greasy dressing with nipple protector is held in place with tape. After the operation, there are no restrictions on bathing at any time, because there is no skin graft to be protected.

TECHNIQUE OF AREOLAR TATTOO

After determining the desired location of the areola, the patient is placed in the supine position. Local anesthetic with epinephrine is injected to reduce bleeding, which would complicate the determination of color match. The appropriate pigment is chosen by swabbing the pigment next to the normal areola. Mixing of the pigments may be necessary to obtain the best color match, but pure colors are preferred because of the difficulty and inaccuracy of mixing. Once the color has been selected, the pigment may be swabbed into the marked areola circle or the needle may be dipped into the pigment. The tattoo device is held like a pencil at an approximate 60° angle, and tattooing is performed with a side-to-side retreating motion. The tattooist must avoid advancing or carelessly pushing the device away, because this may tear the skin. The power setting should be set to allow easy dermal penetration but not to the point of causing abrasion of the skin. Progress is determined by removing excess pigment with alcohol swabs and then continuing the process until the desired color is reached.

The tattoo procedure takes approximately 15 to 20 minutes for each nipple-areola complex. At completion the color will appear considerably darker than the normal side because of the mixing of blood with the pigment. The entire area is covered with a greasy dressing for 7 to 10 days, and the patient is not allowed to fully bathe during that time. If an eschar develops, this usually indicates that an area was overtreated or abraded. Unfortunately, when the eschar sloughs, so does most of the pigment. Fortunately, a second, more gentle tattoo will usually be effective at a later date.

The early dark shade of the areola will fade rapidly during the first several weeks, but the final color will not be achieved for 2 to 3 months. Additional tattooing procedures can be performed at any time to optimize the result.

FURTHER READINGS

Adams WM: Labial transplant for correction of loss of the nipple, *Plast Reconstr Surg* 4:295, 1949.

Allison AS, Howorth MG Jr.: Carcinoma in a nipple preserved for heterotropic auto-implantation, *N Engl J Med* 298:1132, 1978.

Andersen JA, Pallesen RM: Spread to the nipple and areola in carcinoma of the breast, *Ann Surg* 189:367, 1979.

Becker H: The use of intradermal tattoo to enhance the final result of nipple areola reconstruction, *Plast Reconstr Surg* 77:673, 1986.

Broadbent RR, Woolf RH, Metz PS: Restoring the mammary areola by a skin graft from the upper inner thigh, *Br J Plast Surg* 30:220, 1977.

Cohen IK, Ward J: Pinwheel nipple-areolar reconstruction, *Plast Reconstr Surg* 77:995, 1986.

Hartrampf CR, Culbertson J: A dermal fat flap for nipple reconstruction, *Plast Reconstr Surg* 73:982, 1984.

Little JW, Munasifi T, McCulloch DT: One-stage reconstruction of a projecting nipple: the quadrapod flap, *Plast Reconstr Surg* 72:422, 1983.

Little JW: Nipple-areola reconstruction, *Clin Plast Surg* 11:351, 1984.

Millard DR: Nipple and areolar reconstruction by split graft from the normal side, *Plast Reconstr Surg* 77:676, 1986.

Quinn RH, Barlow JF: Involvement of the nipple and areola by carcinoma of the breast, *Arch Surg* 116:1139, 1981.

Schwartz AW: Reconstruction of the nipple and areola, *Br J Plast Surg* 29:230, 1976.

Spear SL, Convit R, Little JW: Intradermal tattoo as an adjunct to nipple-areolar reconstruction, *Plast Reconstr Surg* 83:907, 1989.

Wexler MR, O'Neal RN: Areola sharing to reconstruct the absent nipple, *Plast Reconstr Surg* 51:176, 1973.

Wellisch DK, Schain W, Noone RB: The pyschological contribution of nipple addition in breast reconstruction, *Plast Reconstr Surg* 80:699, 1987.

CHAPTER 29

Mammography in Aesthetic and Reconstructive Breast Surgery

F. Parker Gregg

Primary breast carcinoma currently affects one woman out of every nine in the United States at some time in her life. Incidence of breast carcinoma begins to increase at approximately 35 years of age, with the greatest incidence at more than 50 years of age. The best evaluation of the breast for breast cancer remains for the physician to use a combination of good mammography and thorough breast physical examination.

Mammography for detection of breast carcinoma uses ionizing radiation to create images. In recent years, fear of breast cancer caused by radiation exposure has received great publicity, recognizing the breast as a radiosensitive organ. The value of mammography nonetheless remains evident, despite this fear, based on relative risk-benefit considerations. An asymptomatic woman might have a two-view bilateral mammogram annually for 35 years before she approaches a threshold accumulation of radiation doses that would cause concern.

Mammography conducted alone, without physical examination, has been shown to detect clinically occult breast cancer in community hospital settings in 2.3% to 38% of cancers detected. It also detected 41.6% of cancers found in 275,000 women during the Breast Cancer Detection Demonstration Project that was jointly sponsored by the National Cancer Institute and the American Cancer Society.

INDICATIONS FOR SCREENING MAMMOGRAPHY

The American College of Radiology has suggested the following indications for screening mammography:

- ▼ Patient should be asymptomatic woman at least 40 years of age
- ▼ Initiation of screening mammography at younger age may be considered with a patient at high risk for breast cancer
- ▼ Mammography screening should be done every 1 to 2 years between 40 and 49 years of age and at same interval if screening begun at younger age
- ▼ Mammography screening should be done annually after 50 years of age

MAMMOGRAPHY IN AESTHETIC PLASTIC SURGERY OF BREAST

Preoperative Period

The surgeon should determine from the patient considering cosmetic breast surgery if a recent mammography has been performed. If so, a review of mammography images and their interpretation is prudent to reinforce the physical examination findings and to exclude an occult lesion. If the patient has not had a recent mammography, consider discussing screening mammography with patients in high risk categories and appropriate age groups.

Postoperative Period

Following breast augmentation or reduction, conducting a mammography earlier than 9 to 12 months postoperatively is not necessary, but the physician should consider returning to using interval examinations based on age groups and relative risk factors as before.

MAMMOGRAPHY IN BREAST RECONSTRUCTION AFTER MASTECTOMY

Preoperative Period

The plastic surgeon should perform a preoperative review of any recent breast images and interpretations obtained before breast biopsy or mastectomy. This review is useful to confirm the site and the extent of the noted disease for record and to exclude an undetected coincident primary breast mass in the contralateral "normal" breast.

Postoperative Period

Follow-up mammography screening based on age groups and relative risk factors may resume. The physician should allow for a time interval for resolution of postoperative tissue changes in order to obtain an adequate baseline mammography (approximately 9 to 12 months postoperatively).

CHAPTER 30

Tissue Expansion

Louis C. Argenta

Tissue expansion is a mechanical process that facilitates standard movement of tissue flaps by significantly increasing their surface area and by creating an augmented blood supply that increases the safety of flap movement. The success of tissue expansion presupposes a thorough knowledge of standard flap techniques. In addition, it requires technical facility and patience to mechanically manipulate tissue in a safe and predetermined way. There is a definite learning curve in tissue expansion that increases not only the safety of the procedure but also the scope of patients to which it may be applied. The limitations of the applications of this technique and the underlying pathophysiologic conditions are still being elucidated.

INDICATIONS FOR TISSUE EXPANSION

Tissue expansion allows for the generation of specific tissues of appropriate color, texture, and hair-bearing qualities that may be necessary for reconstruction of specific defects. It allows an increase in surface area, thus increasing the potential size of a flap, which can then be turned for coverage of a given defect and for closure of the "donor defect." During normal expansion, nerve integrity is preserved so that a flap of relatively normal sensitivity can be created. By inducing an increased blood supply by a process similar to delay, the safety of a random or extended axial flap can be significantly increased. If overlying muscle is expanded during the process of tissue expansion, a functional motor unit can be created for specific needs, such as in the brow.

CONTRAINDICATIONS TO TISSUE EXPANSION

The tissue expansion process requires a competent, compliant patient who is willing to return to the clinic for multiple visits for safe expansion.

- A patient who is mentally incompetent, uncooperative, or who has excessive expectations will not benefit from this procedure.
- Tissue that has received significant amounts of irradiation can be expanded slowly but at significant increased risk and compromise to a late overall cosmetic result.
- Placement of a tissue expander adjacent to a lymphangioma or vascular malformations results in significant seroma formation with a risk of secondary infection.
- Expansion adjacent to an existing malignancy is not recommended because its influence on the neoplasm is not yet defined. Extirpation of such lesions is best performed before undertaking expansion.
- Ongoing adjacent infection is a relative contraindication, because this risks the prothesis to infection and exposure. A distant incision for implant placement away from the site of infection may be helpful in such a patient.

PATIENT EDUCATION

A compliant patient is essential to a successful tissue expansion. A long-term relationship is required between the patient and physician. Frank discussion of the proposed procedure, including an explanation to the patient concerning the duration of the procedure and the amount of discomfort and deformity that may result during expansion, is necessary. Because significant deformity can occur during expansion, allowing patients to see other patients with an expander in place or permitting them to see photographs of examples in other patients can be extremely useful. The risk and potential complications, including infection, extrusion, and deflation should also be explained preoperatively. With proper education, the majority of patients, once realizing the benefits of this procedure, will become compliant and allow the procedure to be completed. The deformity that occurs during expansion, particularly in the head and neck, is well tolerated by an informed, mature patient or by a child who is appropriately supported by understanding parents. Explanation of potential alternatives with their complications, risk, and benefits is also helpful in helping the patient to make a more meaningful decision.

FLAP DESIGN

General Considerations

The specific design regained for any flap to cover a given defect is dictated by the preexisting nature of the size and location of the defect and surrounding tissues, the potential systematic limitations, and the surgical expertise of the surgeon. A thorough knowledge of the basic flaps, whether random, axial, myocutaneous, or free, that can be applied to a given situation is necessary. Tissue expansion is a "graduate-level" flap exercise that should be preceded by a meaningful residency in plastic and reconstruction surgery. The specific modifications of tissue expansion in any anatomic area of the body will be outlined at a later time.

Donor Site

The majority of complications in tissue expansion are caused by inadequate planning and improper selection of a donor site for the flap. In general, when evaluating and selecting a donor site, considerations should be given to the following recommendations:

- Avoid areas of previous trauma and scars.
- Select an area of adequate size (one that allows generation of sufficient tissue to safely and aesthetically cover the recipient area).
- Consider the donor site's hair-bearing qualities, not only at the time of the procedure but also its potential for later hair growth, particularly in children. At attempt to develop a flap that fits into an aesthetic unit, particularly on the face, minimizes later abnormal scars and secondary surgery.
- On the arms, legs, and trunk, consider whether the ability to dress and undress and to sleep, sit, and ambulate is excessively compromised.

- Carefully plan and design incisions for placing the implant so that they do not later compromise potentially necessary cuts to make the flap fit into an ideal location. In general, use one edge of the flap, either advanced or rotated, as the incision site through which the implant is placed.

IMPLANT SELECTION

A large number of standard designs and custom shapes are available to the plastic surgeon. Differential expansion prostheses facilitate advancement of flaps around curved surfaces, such as the scalp. The size and shape of the implant should be selected on the basis of the implant size that best fits the donor area and shape. The actual volume of the implant is less important than its base size, because most prostheses will hold 3 to 4 times the manufacturer's recommended volume. An implant of adequate size to cover all or as much as possible of the donor site, should be used. Excessively large prostheses, especially on the trunk and neck, may cause problems because of their sheer weight and dependent movement of fluid during normal daily activities. Although implants are available holding in excess of 600 cc, multiple implants are usually better when large volumes are necessary, particularly in children. Specific implants for breast reconstruction are discussed later under that heading. Textured expanders have been quite helpful in breast reconstruction although their use elsewhere in the body is probably less useful.

INFLATION VALVES

Valves for inflation of the prostheses either can be at a distant site and connected to the prosthesis through a fill tube or can be integrated into the prostheses. Integrated valves have the advantage of not requiring more dissection, but they may be more difficult to find and offer a slightly higher risk of inadvertent perforation of the implant. Integrated valves are most frequently used in breast reconstruction. Prostheses with distant reservoirs are best used in children, particularly in the head and neck areas. Placing the inflation reservoir to exit from the skin to avoid percutaneous puncture with each injection has been largely abandoned by most surgeons, because the risk of infection is significantly higher.

PLACEMENT OF THE EXPANDER

The individual requirements for placement of soft-tissue expanders will be discussed under regional placement.

Anesthesia and Perioperative Medication

Prostheses can be placed with the patient either under general anesthesia or under local anesthesia. Children are best treated under general anesthesia as used in dissections of the neck, face, and scalp in adults. Systemic perioperative antibiotics (e.g., cephalosporin) are usually given, but long-term antibiotics are usually avoided.

Incision and Dissection

The incision for placement of the expander must be carefully planned so that it does not compromise alternatives in flap reconstruction. Usually one margin of the defect, adjacent to the flap to be rotated, is the ideal site for the incision. Ideal incisions for placement of the prostheses avoid tension on the incision line. Usually incisions are placed in such a position that they are not dependent to the prostheses when the patient is standing, sitting, or lying down.

The base size of the expander dictates the size of the dissection necessary. An excessively large space is developed so that it adequately accommodates the prosthesis. Several centimeters are allowed between the margin of the implant and the suture line. If a prosthesis abuts the incision, the risk of exposure is significantly higher.

Procedure for Distant Reservoir

If a distant reservoir is used, a separate tunnel of sufficient size is created with scissors or a hemostat into the subcutaneous space to ensure that the reservoir will not retract. The tubing is shortened to an appropriate length. It is important that a minimal excess remains to minimize erosion. The tubing must also be in such a position that it cannot come into contact with the suture line. The ends of the tubing are then secured to an adapter and tied in place with permanent suture if an internal adapter is used. Recently developed external adapters do not require sutures.

It is important to note that when shortening and reanastomosing the tubing, instruments should not be used to hold the tubing. Hemostats and forceps produce structural weaknesses that may rupture when fluid is placed into the prosthesis.

Drains

Drains are infrequently used and should not be used as an alternative to good hemostasis. One significant exception however is the placement of expanders in immediate breast reconstruction where drains in the excision site are always used until drainage stops.

Wound Closure

The wound is closed in multiple layers using absorbable sutures and permanent monofilament. I prefer to leave the sutures in as long as possible during expansion. If the expander is properly positioned, this will not create tension sufficient to result in would disruption.

INFLATION

Inflation Procedures

Limited amounts of saline can be placed in the implant at the time of surgery to fill dead space. Excessive tension should not be placed on the overlying tissue until the wound has had a significant opportunity to heal. Inflation is usually begun 7 to 10 days after the implant has been placed. Normal saline is used; preservatives in the saline do not have a significant effect. Although some physicians have advocated intraluminal antibiotics, the use of dimethyl sulfoxide (DMSO) to facilitate expansion or the use of local anesthetics to decrease discomfort is not routinely recommended.

A. **Use of distant reservoirs.** When distant reservoirs are used, the following procedures are employed:
   - ▼ The valve site is sterilized with Betadine, and then, using sterile gloves, the physician holds the reser-

voir between two fingers and inserts a 23-gauge "butterfly" intravenous needle to puncture the reservoir. (Butterfly needles with silicone tubing allow the patient some movement and are not as hostile as a straight needle.) If there is any question of whether the physician is in the appropriate place in the reservoir, watching for back flow into the tubing of the butterfly is helpful.

- ▼ Injection is then begun and fluid is placed into the prosthesis until the overlying skin becomes tense. Skin color, capillary refill, and patient discomfort are important criteria that should be monitored. Pressure-monitoring devices are not a substitute for clinical judgment. It must be remembered that expansion is an aesthetic refinement, and nothing should be done to compromise or jeopardize the overlying skin that will ultimately impair the final result. Patience in an expansion is critical. With children, it is helpful to allow them to decide when enough fluid has been placed and discomfort becomes significant.
- ▼ The patient is then observed in the office for approximately 15 minutes. If discomfort or excessive blanching persists, fluid can be withdrawn from the prosthesis.

B. **Use of integrated valves.** When integrated valves are used, they can either be palpated in the subcutaneous tissue, or magnetic devices can be used to locate the inflation reservoir. It is important to use metal detectors in at least two directions so that the exact position of the valve can be marked out on the skin before puncture.

Problems with Inflation

With both types of implant, it is possible to miss the reservoir, resulting in difficulty in injecting saline. Unnecessary force should not be used. If the physician observes no back flow of saline then the needle is not in the proper position for injection. The needle should be withdrawn and a second attempt made. If the second attempt fails, particularly if any fluid has been injected into the reservoir, further attempts should be abandoned for approximately 5 to 7 days.

SPECIFIC SITES FOR RECONSTRUCTION OR EXPANSION

Scalp Reconstruction

The aim of scalp reconstruction by expansion is to expand as much of the remaining scalp as possible so that hair follicles will be evenly distributed after flap creation, thus obtaining a homogeneous final distribution. Usually, it is best to defer expansion in neonates and infants until some cranial suture ossification has occurred when they are 2 years old. However, many such children have been successfully expanded much earlier in life in urgent cases. If expansion is attempted before 2 years, frequent small-volume inflations are best to avoid excessive pressure on the skull.

In correction of scalp defects, multiple expanders are usually necessary around the defect area. Multiple expanders are helpful in avoiding excessive tension in one area and minimizing poor distribution of follicles during expansion. Expanders are best placed beneath the galea frontalis to minimize the risk of exposure. Croissant-shaped expanders or rectangular expanders without reinforced backing are helpful.

Distant reservoirs are usually used either with the reservoir external to the skin or, more preferably, on the top of most cranial aspects of the scalp. If a nevus is present, the valve is placed under it, because sensation is usually diminished in this area. Valves should not be placed under skin grafts or scars.

Some discomfort usually occurs early in the course of expansion, but as expansion proceeds, the galea stretches and expansion is easier. Discomfort is usually treated with mild analgesics. At the second procedure, the capsule is incised when necessary with an electrocautery to allow movement of the expanded scalp in all directions. Care is taken not to damage follicles or major blood vessels with the electrocautery. Minor "dog ears" are ignored because most of these redistribute spontaneously.

Forehead Reconstruction

The forehead can be expanded to create adequate tissue for defects of the forehead and adjacent scalp. The total non–hair-bearing forehead can be increased or decreased by approximately 20% by expanding and mobilizing adjacent scalp or forehead without making the change obvious. Expanders of any appropriate size or shape, usually without reinforced backing, are best. Expanders are selected on the basis of their covering as much surface area of the remaining forehead and adjacent scalp as it is reasonably possible. Some discomfort is always encountered in expanding the forehead; frequent, slow small-volume expansion can minimize this. The critical factor in reconstructing the forehead is to obtain a final symmetric alignment of the brows and a relatively normal hairline, even if this requires discarding some of the expanded forehead. Fixation of the brows to underlying periosteum minimizes later distortion. An attempt to preserve the frontal branch of the facial nerve is always made in the placement of the prosthesis and during the flap advancement.

Nose Reconstruction

To reconstruct the nose, large rectangular expanders encompassing the entire forehead are placed through an incision in the scalp. This allows generation of adequate tissue for both the nose and the primary closure of the forehead. Expanders in excess of 400 cc are usually necessary. Expansion can usually be performed in 4 weeks, thus minimizing excess capsule formation.

At the time of development of the flap, a template is used to outline the shape, allowing a slight excess of tissue for reconstruction of the nose. The flap is then dissected with the expander in place. The capsule is taken with the flap until the supraorbital region is reached. Dissection is carried subperiosteally into the orbit. This technique minimizes risk to the supraorbital vessels and allows the arch of rotation to be in the orbit rather than in the forehead. The flap is appropriately thinned by excising excess capsule and subcutaneous tissue and is draped over an appropriate infrastructure of cranial bone and ear cartilage. Flaps placed over an inadequate infrastructure are doomed to long-term failure. Subcuticular long-term sutures are used to close the donor defect. The flap is divided and inset 2 weeks later.

Face Reconstruction

Defects of facial soft tissue in almost any location can be covered by tissue expansion of appropriate donor areas in the face and neck. Consideration of hair growth pattern at the time of expansion is critical in planning flaps, particularly in children, where there is the potential for later hair growth. Flaps should be planned to be of sufficient size and shape, so that the final suture lines ultimately lie in the normal position of the nasolabial fold and across the inferior orbital margins.

Thin expanders without reinforced backing are best suited with distant reservoirs for expansion of the face. Excessively large protheses in the face and neck are uncomfortable and prone to erosion. Expansion prostheses are best placed into the subcutaneous space through a face-lift type of incision or through incisions adjacent to facial defects. Inferomedial-based flaps are most frequently used based on branches of the facial arteries.

The neck in the preplatysmal space can also be expanded and advanced up into the face for correction of lower facial defects (See following section.). When neck flaps are brought into the face, they must be sutured to a relatively secure stable area, avoiding tension on the lower lip and its subsequent distortion. Permanent buried sutures placed lateral to the commissures are helpful for this purpose.

Neck Expansion

The neck expands rapidly with little difficulty in the majority of patients. Usually, one nonreinforced rectangular expander is used on each side of the midline. Excessively large expanders can become dependent in the neck and can result in thinning of tissue and in erosion. Expansion above the platysma facilitates flap rotation. As long as I have performed expansion judiciously, I have encountered no significant compromise of underlying respiratory or circulatory systems. Expansion in an older person, where atherosclerotic carotid plaque may be present, should be performed more carefully.

In the neck, it is usually best to move tissue from side-to-side rather than in a cephalocaudad direction. Planning where suture lines and hair will ultimately lie is important.

Extremities Expansion

Defects of the extremities are best covered by using expanders placed radially to the defect. Multiple expanders can assist in facilitating the wearing of clothes and in expediting safe expansion. When expanders are placed in a longitudinal fashion on the extremities, considerable difficulty can be encountered in obtaining and mobilizing adequate amounts of tissue for large defects. Nerves, such as the dorsal cutaneous nerves of the arm and the sural nerve in the leg, should be avoided, because they are more prone to trauma, and contact can result in significant neurologic complications.

There is a significant complication rate when expansion below the knee is attempted, and patients must be carefully selected. When isolated injuries have occurred, such as skin tumor or localized burns, expansion has been successful. When extensive degloving injuries or bony exposure has occurred, the lymphatics and vascularity are greatly compromised and the risk of implant infection and exposure is significant. Such patients are best treated with free flaps. Expansion of the palms and planter foot is extremely difficult and painful.

Trunk Expansion

Multiple large expanders can be placed around defects of the trunk. It is usually best to place expanders radially to the defect rather than axially. However, because of the size of implant that can be placed and the tissue tolerance to rapid expansion, this is less of a problem in the trunk than it is in the extremities. Care must be taken to ensure that expanders are placed and expanded in such a manner that the patient can lie down and sleep in at least one position. The patient must also be able to sit, so expanders in the buttocks must be judiciously placed. Expansion of local muscles, such as the pectoralis major, latissimus dorsi, and rectus abdominis, can be accomplished to develop expanded myocutaneous flaps to cover large defects.

Breast Expansion

Asymmetries in the development of the breasts, such as Poland's syndrome or unilateral hypoplasias, can be treated early in puberty once asymmetry has become significant. A small incision in the axilla or under the hypoplastic breast is used to place a round tissue expander with or without a distant reservoir. The tunnel is then created down to the appropriate level on the chest wall, preferably behind the pectoralis muscle. If the pectoralis is not present, like in Poland's syndrome, the prosthesis is placed subcutaneously as deep as possible. A Becker type of implant or a textured implant with a self-contained valve is the most frequently used. Textured expanders develop a better inframammary fold. The prosthesis is then gradually expanded over time as the opposite breast develops. In a patient aged 18 or 19 who has fully developed, the expander is replaced with a permanent implant, and the latissimus dorsi is transferred if necessary.

A. **Expansion in immediate breast reconstruction.** In carefully selected patients, an expander can be placed at the time of mastectomy for immediate breast reconstruction. Once the entire resection has been performed by the general surgeon, an incision is made in the pectoralis muscle and an entirely submuscular plane is created beneath the pectoralis major and the serratus anterior. The dissection is as extensive as necessary to properly locate an adequately sized prosthesis whose base size is symmetrical with the opposite breast. Textured prostheses with self- contained valves create a better inframammary fold and displace less than the usual prosthesis. The Becker permanent implant is also useful in avoiding secondary procedures in approximately 50% of patients. If the Becker implant with the distant reservoir is used, the valve is placed in the subcutaneous plane in the axilla away from the brassiere. It is critical to use suction drains in the axilla and to continue the patient's use of antibiotics as long as axillary drainage is present.

The implant is then expanded at a rate that is tolerable to the patient. Overexpansion of the implant by 200 to 400 cc for 3 to 4 months followed by partial deflation helps create ptosis at the second procedure. Reconstruction of the inframammary fold in the second procedure has been defined well elsewhere.

B. **Delayed secondary breast reconstruction after mastectomy.** Round expanders with a base size equal to the opposite breast base are used. Prostheses with either self-contained or distant reservoirs are useful. The textured implants expand more rapidly with less force, migrate less, and create a better inframammary fold, and they are the prosthesis of choice at this time. The Becker implant is useful in decreasing the need for a second procedure.

- ▼ Placement of implant. The lateral portion of the mastectomy wound is used for access to the subpectoral space. The implant is placed beneath the pectoralis muscle, but extensive dissection beneath the serratus anterior is not necessary in a patient with adequate subcutaneous fat. If the patient is particularly thin, it is best to place the implant beneath the serratus anterior.
- ▼ Expansion of implant. The implant is expanded at an adequate rate that is also comfortable for the patient. Patients who have received radiation treatments should be expanded with frequent small-volume expansion to avoid damage to overlying skin. Depending on the amount of ptosis in the opposite breast, the reconstructured breast is overexpanded by 200 to 400 ml for 3 to 4 months. The implant is then partially deflated to create ptosis. Expanders that are not planned to "permanent" are then exchanged in a second procedure for a permanent implant.
- ▼ Second procedure for possible removal. If malposition of the mound or a poorly defined inframammary fold has been created, a second procedure is performed in which the expander is removed and a permanent textured or high-projection implant is placed. The inframmary fold can be recreated at

this time. A nipple-areolar reconstruction is usually deferred for 2 to 3 months until mound position has stabilized.

EXPANSION OF FULL-THICKNESS GRAFT

In some patients, it may be difficult to generate local flaps, particularly in the periorbital and perioral areas. By expanding tissue as close as possible to the recipient area, a full-thickness graft with most of the characteristics of the recipient area can be generated. With respect to the face, the neck or upper chest in the paraclavicular area is ideal.

- A round or rectangular prosthesis is placed adjacent to but not directly over the clavicle and expanded for approximately 4 weeks.
- The potential recipient site is then excised, and a template is used to outline the exact size of the area.
- A full-thickness graft, approximately 20% larger than the recipient area is then outlined over the expander. The tissue is harvested with the expander in place.
- Once the graft has been harvested, it is extensively defatted down to the dermis, using scissors.
- The donor site is closed primarily after removal of the expander.
- The full-thickness graft is sutured in place and then totally immobilized with a tie-over dressing left in place for 3 to 5 days.

Absolute hemostasis is required in the recipient area to accept the graft. In patients where bleeding may be a problem, it is best to excise the recipient area and cover it with dressings for 24 hours before placing the full-thickness graft. Full-thickness grafts 5 to 6 cm in diameter are easily generated by the above technique.

EXPANSION OF FREE FLAP

The standard free flaps described in the literature can be significantly increased in size by preexpanding them with a tissue expander. Free flaps, almost twice as large as standard free flaps, can be generated by expansion.

- The axial vessel is carefully identified by using Doppler ultrasound.
- A large expander is then placed under the standard territory of the flap, avoiding damage to the axial vessel.
- In some patients where a musculocutaneous flap is desired, the expanders are placed beneath the muscle, expanding both the muscle and the overlying skin.
- It is important to keep the expander away from the artery and vein to be anastomosed, because some fibrosis will occur, which may make the anastomosis more difficult.

MANAGEMENT OF COMPLICATIONS

Complications are avoided by careful planning and meticulous surgical technique. There is a definite learning curve in the technique of tissue expansion, both in the scope of patients to which it may be applied and the finesse with which it can safely be performed. Most major institutions have reported an initial significant complication rate in the range of 25%, which rapidly decreased to less than 10% over 6 to 8 months.

Implant Failure

Deflation of implants is almost always total when any tear is made in the prosthesis. The use of needles greater than 23 gauge can cause damage to the inflation reservoir, which seals best when direct 90°-percutaneous perforations are made. When the reservoirs are incorporated with the prosthesis, meticulous care is required to ensure that the surgeon does not puncture the implant. Once deflation of the implant has occurred, the surgeon has only approximately 7 to 10 days to accomplish replacement. If one waits an excessive length of time, contraction of the overlying skin, development of seroma, and fibrosis in the capsule can occur. Replacement of prostheses is not an emergency procedure and should be done carefully under sterile conditions.

Infection

Infection of expansion implants, like any other prostheses, can be extremely subtle. The skin overlying noninfected tissue expanders is frequently somewhat erythematous but should not be warmer than usual or demonstrate *peau d'orange* changes.

A. **Prevention.** Meticulous sterile technique and careful hemostasis minimize risks of contamination during implant placement and inflation. All patients who receive implants should be given perioperative antibiotics, although I do not routinely continue antibiotics for a long time thereafter.

B. **Diagnosis.** Patients with implant infections frequently complain of malaise and discomfort, rather than acute pain. Monitoring of temperature, white blood cell count, sedimentation rate, and examination of the tissue overlying the prosthesis may be helpful.

C. **Treatment**

▼ Antibiotic therapy. A broad-spectrum antibiotic with particular emphasis toward staphylococcus may be tried if implant contamination is suspected. Long-term continuation of antibiotics for a questionably infected implant should be avoided. Implants, where external reservoirs are used, are almost always colonized, and the surgeon can note at the time of removal a thick and "beefy" capsular membrane, which is more prone to bleeding than the normal capsule.

▼ Removal of implant. Like all infections of prostheses, removal of the implant is required to clear the infection.

- If enough tissue has been generated by expansion to close the defect, the space within the capsule can be irrigated with Betadine and the flap advanced. Drains are placed under such flaps to remove seroma, and the wound is not closed excessively tightly. Revision of scars in such cases is frequently necessary.
- Cases such as breast reconstruction where a permanent implant is to be placed should be treated by removing the infected expander, allowing the space to clear the infection and then proceeding with expansion or implant placement several months later. I have witnessed the reinfection of permanent implants placed up to 3 months after removal of expanders infected with identical bacteria, despite the lack of clinical symptoms in the interval. Permanent implants placed into an area of infection are

almost doomed to infection extrusion or capsular contracture.

Implant Exposure

Implants can become exposed and later extrude. Radovan, early in the course of tissue expansion, recognized that because of the increased blood supply to this tissue, implant exposure does not necessarily mean that removal is required if a flap is to be generated. If exposure occurs late in the course of expansion, judicious frequent-fill expansion is continued until an adequate amount of tissue has been generated. The capsular space is then copiously lavaged and the flap turned. Obviously if a permanent implant or bone graft is to be placed under the expanded tissue, this regimen should not be carried out. In such patients, the expanders should be removed and the infection allowed to subside before reexpanding and placing a permanent implant.

Capsular Contracture

Rarely, capsular contracture can develop at a rate such that it becomes totally impossible to expand. Such patients are best treated with *open capsulotomy,* circumferentially cutting the capsule and then expanding at a more rapid rate. Usually, expansion twice a week, even if smaller volumes are tolerated, will help overcome this phenomenon.

Significant capsular contraction may occur during expansion for breast reconstruction. If this occurs, the risk of contracture around the permanent implant is significant. The capsule around the expander should be totally excised and meticulous hemostasis obtained. A textured silicone implant or polyurethane implant should be placed in such patients.

FURTHER READINGS

Adson MH, Anderson RD, Argenta LC: Scalp expansion in the treatment of male pattern baldness, *Plast Reconstr Surg* 79:906, 1987.

Antonyshyn O, Gruss J, Mackinnon S, Zucker R: Complications of soft tissue expansion, *Br J Plast Surg* 41:239, 1988.

Antonyshyn O, Gruss J, Mackinnon S, Zucker R: Tissue expansion in the head and neck, *Plast Reconstr Surg* 82:58, 1988.

Argenta LC: Controlled tissue expansion in reconstructive surgery, *Br J Plast Surg* 37:520, 1984.

Argenta LC: Reconstruction of the breast by tissue expansion, *Clin Plast Surg* 11:257, 1984.

Argenta LC, Austad ED, editors: Tissue expansion, *Clin Plast Surg* 14:435, 1985.

Argenta LC, Marks MW, Grabb WC: Selective use of serial expansion in breast reconstruction, *Ann Plast Surg* 11:188, 1983.

Argenta LC, Marks MW, Pasyk KA: Advances in tissue expansion, *Clin Plast Surg* 12:159, 1985.

Argenta LC, VanderKolk C, Friedman RJ, Marks M: Refinements in reconstruction of congenital breast deformities, *Plast Reconstr Surg* 76:73, 1985.

Argenta LC, Watanabe MJ, Grabb WC: The use of tissue expansion in head and neck reconstruction, *Ann Plast Surg* 11:31, 1983.

Bauer B: The role of tissue expansion in reconstruction of the ear, *Clin Plast Surg* 17:319, 1990.

Bauer B, Vicari F, Richard M: The role of tissue expansion in pediatric plastic surgery, *Clin Plast Surg* 17:101, 1990.

Becker H: Breast reconstruction using inflatable breast implant with detachable reservoir, *Plast Reconstr Surg* 73:678, 1984.

Cooper R, Brown D: Pretransfer and transfer expansion of a scalp flap, *J Reconstr Microsurg* 6:339, 1990.

DeHaan M, Hammond D, Mann R: Controlled tissue expansion of a groin flap for upper extremity reconstruction, *Plast Reconstr Surg* 86:979, 1986.

Forte V, Middleton WG, Briant TD: Expansion of myocutaneous flaps, *Arch Otolaryngo* 111:371, 1985.

Francis G, Jayarajah M: Bradycardia associated with insertion of inflation of tissue expanders under the scalp, *Acta Anaesth Scand* 35:366, 1991.

Gibney J: Use of a permanent tissue expander for breast reconstruction, *Plast Reconstr Surg* 84:607, 1989.

Gruss JS, MacKinnon SE: Soft tissue expanders in upper limb surgery, *J Hand Surg* 10A:749, 1985.

Hong C, Stark GB, Futrell JW: Elongation of axial blood vessels with a tissue expander, *Clin Plast Surg* 14:465, 1987.

Leighton WD et al: Experimental pretransfer expansion of free flap donor sites: I. flap viability and expansion characteristics, *Plast Reconstr Surg* 82:69, 1988.

Leonard AG, Small JO: Tissue expansion in the treatment of alopecia, *Br J Plast Surg* 39:42, 1986.

Manders EK, Graham WP III, Schenden MJ, Davis TS: Skin expansion to eliminate large scalp defects, *Ann Plast Surg* 12:305, 1985.

Manders EK, Schenden MJ, Furrey JA, Hetzler PT, Davis TS, Graham WP III: Soft-tissue expansion: concepts and complications, *Plast Reconstr Surg* 74:493, 1984.

Marks MW, Argenta LC, Thornton J: Burn management: the role of tissue expansion, *Clin Plast Surg,* 14:543, 1987.

Neale H, High R, Billmore D, Carey J, Smith D, Warden G: Complications of controlled tissue expansion in the pediatric burn patient, *Plast Reconstr Surg* 82:840, 1988.

Radovan C: Breast reconstruction after mastectomy using the temporary expander, *Plast Reconstr Surg* 69:195, 1982.

Radovan C: Tissue expansion for soft tissue reconstruction, *Plast Reconstr Surg* 74:482, 1984.

Tanine R, Miyasaka M: Reconstruction of microtia using tissue expansion, *Clin Plast Surg* 17:339, 1990.

Thornton J, Marks M, Izenberg P, Argenta LC: Expanded myocutaneous flaps: their clinical use, *Clin Plast Surg* 14:529, 1987.

Versaci A: Reconstruction of a pendulous breast utilizing a tissue expander, *Clin Plast Surg* 14:499, 1987.

CHAPTER 31

Excisional Body Contour Surgery

Frederick M. Grazer and W. Graham Wood

TYPES OF BODY CONTOUR SURGERY AND ITS EVOLUTION

There are two types of body contour surgery: suction-assisted lipectomy (SAL) and excisional, with or without SAL. Since the introduction of SAL, the factors governing patient selection have broadened remarkably. Not only has male body contour surgery emerged and increased in numbers, but the age spectrum for both male and female body contour surgery has also been greatly expanded to include much younger patients on one end of the spectrum and much older patients on the other. Genetically predisposed individuals of either sex are now considered appropriate candidates if they have significant contour deformity, including those in the preteen years. Modern anesthetic techniques using state-of-the-art monitoring equipment, such as pulse oximetry and endtidal carbon dioxide (E_T CO_2) assay, have allowed safe performance of body contour surgeries on much older patients. Many individuals in their seventh and eighth decade of life are now requesting surgery.

In prior years, many surgeons believed that there might be possible underlying psychologic problems in ectomorphic patients seeking correction of a minor body contour defect. Today, however, many ectomorphic and mesomorphic athletically inclined individuals are requesting minor refinements of their body contour defects. Today experienced body contour surgeons still must closely examine the motivations and expected goals of surgery based upon their experience, skill, and thorough understanding of the patient's desires. The astute surgeon should be able to advise the patient of the percentage of improvement that can be expected from a proposed procedure. On the basis of the patient's thorough understanding of the percentage of improvement that can be realistically expected, minor body contour defects may be corrected even though the percentage of improvement might be relatively small. The patient who is well informed by the body contour surgeon is gratified and appreciative of even small percentages of improvement.

There are numerous health enthusiasts who practice good dietary habits and indulge in extensive daily physical exercise programs but whose bodies are genetically oriented toward body contour defects. These types of deformities cannot be improved by either diet or physical exercise. Thus there are increasing numbers of ectomorphs and mildly affected mesomorphs that are requesting body contour refinement.

PATIENT SELECTION

Age of Patient

The ages of patients for SAL body contour surgery range from the preteen years to the eighth decade. Excisional body contour surgery with its commensurate scars should be reserved for patients who cannot expect a reasonable percentage of improvement by SAL alone. These patients' conditions may warrant trade-off of an improved body contour versus an incisional scar. The younger patient in the 20s or 30s with body contour deformity requiring excisional correction should understand that because the collagen content of their skin is greater than that of older individuals (more than 60), scar widening will be greater on them.

Motivation of Patient

No patient, regardless of how unrealistic the expectations may be, should be refused surgery, without the consulting surgeon taking the time to educate the patient as to why the requested surgery would not meet the the patient's expectations. Refusing surgery to patients without providing them with a concrete reason as to why it should not be performed only makes them more vulnerable to the next plastic surgeon's whims. This next surgeon may impose a surgical procedure upon these unsuspecting patients, who have now become susceptible because of the prior surgeon's refusal to perform the patients' surgery without supplying concrete reasons.

All patients requesting body contour improvement have been motivated by some reason. As long as patients are aware of their motivational stimuli and recognize and understand the total gamut of possible complications and the percentage of improvement that can be expected, these patients should then be considered as potential candidates for surgery.

In the past, recently divorced patients who are reentering the "marketplace" in search of a mate have been regarded with skepticism by the operating surgeon. It is still the plastic surgeon's prerogative to decline to perform surgery on any individual; however, it is that surgeon's responsibility to carefully evaluate the patient's motivations, without automatically labeling the patient as a poor candidate. The operating surgeon should be aware of the enlightened attitudes of our changing society and the motivational needs of the patient without being judgmental.

Medical History

Important aspects of the patient's medical history should always be investigated, including the following areas:

- Thorough review of symptoms
- Medical history
- Family medical history
- Surgical history, including prior aesthetic procedures
- History of coronary artery disease and diabetes and of family members who might have had malignant hyperthermia
- History of both over-the-counter and prescribed medications

Physical Examination and Diagnostic Tests

A thorough physical examination, including laboratory and diagnostic examinations (See Chapter 2.), should be done to rule out any medical or surgical problems that might cause detriment to the patient if the proposed surgery were performed.

PATIENT CONSULTATION

At the time of consultation the following actions should be taken:

- ▼ The patient should be fully informed of the placement of the incisions and what to expect in terms of bruising and the healing process.
- ▼ The patient should be informed of the probability or percentage of possible complications and the possible adverse effects if the surgery does not go as expected. By far the most frequent postoperative complication is an undesirable result. This may be caused not only from possible complications or their sequelae but also from poor physician-to-patient communication concerning the reasonable percentage of improvement that could be expected from the proposed surgery.
- ▼ The physician must be careful to examine the patient for umbilical hernias, inguinal hernias, abdominal wall hernias, and incisional hernias.

Informed Consent

For excisional body contour surgery, a significant number of complications are possible, including but not limited to wound infection, wound dehiscence, skin loss, hematoma, thrombophlebitis, pulmonary embolism, pulmonary fat emboli syndrome, fat necrosis, hypertrophic scars, keloids, and other formations of undesirable incision sites. With the use of appropriate autologous blood replacement, and fluid and electrolyte management intraoperatively, the true medical complications of pure SAL body contour surgery are few. In SAL alone, infection nerve injury and hematoma formation requiring drainage are rare. If the patient is properly treated preoperatively, intraoperatively, and postoperatively, pulmonary complications of grave significance are rare.

The most common postoperative complication is an undesirable result coming from inappropriate candidate selection or the inability of the operating surgeon to deliver the improvement predicted. The blame for an undesirable result with SAL body contour surgery can never be placed upon the patient. Almost always the failure of such an operation rests solely with the competency of the operating surgeon.

Although smoking is discouraged because of anesthetic morbidity, pure SAL without undermining and skin reduction usually can be done in tobacco users without fear of compromised circulation. In excisional body contour surgery, preoperative and postoperative smoking can produce catastrophic results. Such patients must be made aware of these probable anesthetic or circulatory complications should they use tobacco products.

The patient should also be given a list of all over-the-counter and prescription drugs that might prolong bleeding with the resulting complication of hematoma formation and the sequelae thereof.

Expenses of Surgery

At the time of consultation, the patient should be made aware of the surgeon's fee. The assistant surgeon's fee should be quoted when applicable. The patient should be aware of the operating room (OR) costs, anesthesia costs, expenses for postoperative medications, expenses for preoperative laboratory studies, and the possible additional expenses should a complication arise.

Unless operating surgeons have specific knowledge of the terms of a patient's insurance policy, they should not dismiss the patient's request for possible application for insurance coverage by stating that the proposed surgery would not meet the standards of the insurance company. In such a situation, the surgeon has a responsibility to give the patient a written diagnosis and the name of the proposed surgical procedure. Surgeons should explain that it is the patient's responsibility to inform the insurance company of the proposed operation in order to determine the probability of coverage. Today there are many high-end insurance policies that cover cosmetic procedures on the underwritten patient. The operating surgeon would be at fault for dismissing that possibility without having knowledge of the the patient's policy. However, whatever the terms of the policy may be, the operating surgeon has the option to accept or not accept insurance assignment on any proposed surgical procedure.

PREOPERATIVE PREPARATION

Autotransfusion

The replacement of blood should be considered on any operation where there is a probable blood loss of more than 1 unit. The economy and safety of autologous blood replacement is well established. Even though unit replacement for a unit lost is not necessary for the survivability of a patient, the postoperative recovery is greatly improved on patients who have a unit replaced for each unit lost. Not only do the patients look and feel better in the recovery room but they also return to their daily physical activities and their professional pursuits more rapidly than those patients who are not afforded autologous blood replacement. The ultimate decision for autologous blood replacement rests with the operating surgeon. Today many well-informed patients are requesting autologous blood replacement because of public awareness of its salutary effect.

Preoperative Education and Procedures

A. **Diet.** It is recommended that all patients be on a balanced diet and understand its necessity for optimum postoperative healing. A female patient should also be informed that the results of future pregnancy might impose deleterious effects on their prior breast reduction or abdominal surgery or both.

B. **Laboratory and diagnostic studies.** All preoperative laboratory and diagnostic studies should conform to the accepted practices of the medical community and should be ordered by the surgeon in concert with the physician anesthetist. All of these studies should be done, and the data should be analyzed in advance of the surgery, so that corrective action for any abnormality can be taken. The possibility of canceling surgery if there is an abnormality would be more appropriate if the decision were made earlier rather than if it were left until the "eleventh hour."

C. **Hygiene.** Good personal hygiene with daily total body showers is encouraged. Preoperative enemas should be ordered for thighplasty patients. Surgery that involves the undermining of a flap is contraindicated for patients who have used tobacco products within a 14-day period immediately before surgery. Such patients should be warned not to smoke for an additional 14-day period immediately after surgery. Preoperative shaving of hair-bearing areas is at the discretion of the operating surgeon. The required amount of autologous blood and fluid replacement will determine the need for an indwelling catheter for the duration of the surgery. This decision should always be made before the patient is prepared and draped.

D. **Skin cleansing and preparation.** Standard OR or surgery center policies for the operative skin cleansing and preparation should be followed closely. It is the responsibility of the operating surgeon to ensure that all appropriate areas have been sufficiently prepared before the surgical draping. It is particularly important that the patient's umbilicus be adequately cleansed and prepared before the beginning of surgery. The surgeon should drape the patient in a manner that ensures contamination is avoided during the surgical procedure.

E. **Skin marking and preoperative decisions.** It is now the expected standard of care for patients to be marked preoperatively in the upright position. Patients can also participate in the preoperative markings. They can use a different color marking pen to place marks in the areas where they desire a change. It is the surgeon's responsibility to inform the patient of inappropriate areas that they have marked. A preliminary premarking with the patient's participation can often eliminate false perceptions about what portions of the deformity can and cannot be corrected. All preexisting indentations and contour irregularities should be pointed out to the patient preoperatively. Preoperative decisions as to whether autologous fat grafting would be appropriate must be explained before surgery. If there is evidence that skin envelope problems would result from the removal of unwanted fat, this must be pointed out to the patient preoperatively. Decisions should then be made about limiting the amount of aspiration to prevent such occurrence or the necessity of skin reduction in addition to SAL. It is important to inform the patient that the only fat that is suctionable is between the skin and the muscle. Fat, particularly in the abdomen, that is intraabdominal (omentum and mesentery) cannot be removed by SAL.

F. **Equipment and supplies.** It is also the standard of care for a secondary backup SAL machine to be available in case the primary SAL machine should fail. It is recommended that the patient's preoperative photographs be available in the OR for convenient assessment by the operating surgeon. If the patient is to receive autologous blood, it is imperative that the surgery not begin until the surgeon receives definite assurance of its availability.

INTRAOPERATIVE CARE

General Care

Before the patients are anesthetized, anxiety-provoking conversation from the surgical team should be avoided. Adequate intravenous (IV) fluid volume replacement should generally follow the 3:1 rule. We use intraoperative corticosteroids IV and alcohol for prophylaxis and treatment of pulmonary fat emboli syndrome, although we believe the primary treatment of full-blown fat embolism syndrome is the use of large doses of corticosteroids. Intraoperative IV steroids and alcohol are routinely given to our patients; other surgeons choose not to use them. These consist of 500 mg of methylprednisolone sodium succinate (Solu-Medrol) or equivalent. Alcohol, 32 to 50 IV (5 mg dextrose and 5%

alcohol) are given during a 30-minute to 2 ½-hour period. With the alcohol protocol, anesthetic gases can be reduced. There may be the possibility of some mild hypotension during the immediate post-operative-recovery room phase.

Abdominoplasty

A. Preparation of patient and anesthesia

- The patient is marked in the upright position before surgery and is positioned in a supine position on the OR table.
- The patient is anesthetized by general endotracheal anesthesia and is prepared and draped in the normal manner. Care is taken to ensure that the umbilicus is properly prepared and that the patient does not have incisional hernias, abdominal hernias, or any umbilical hernias.
- Lidocaine 0.25% with epinephrine dilution 1:400,000 is injected into the area to be incised, or suctioned, or both at the discretion of the operating surgeon.

B. Operative procedure

- Flap elevation is done with electric current.
- In cases that have anterior abdominal wall weakness, plication of the rectus sheath is performed. A braided nonabsorbable suture of sufficient strength is used for the plication.
- The OR table may be flexed before suturing of the panniculus. Scarpa's fascia deep layer closure with the sutures of choice is at the discretion of the surgeon. Intracuticular closure with Vicryl sutures is used followed by placement of stainless steel staples or sutures. (Staples and sutures should be removed within 4 days of surgery to avoid epithelialization.)
- Last-minute suction contouring of any residual fullness where the upper flap joins with its lower counterpart and contouring of fullness in the lateral extensions of the incisions and dogears is accomplished by inserting the canula into the incision between two staples. Such last-minute suctioning of

the upper flap is performed after the final closure has been done.

- In the male patient, the surgeon must take extra care not to inadvertently injure the spermatic cord with its vas deferens and associated vessels. It is easy to contact these structures, particularly in male individuals with a large abdominal panniculus.

C. Thrombosis and embolism

- Risk factors. Age, obesity, smoking, and a medical history of previous phlebitis or pulmonary embolism all increase the incidence of deep vein thrombosis (DVT) in surgery patients. Use of oral contraceptives by women and the existence of varicose veins are additional risk factors.
- Prevention. Elastic stockings during and after abdominoplasty or alternating inflating-deflating antiembolism stockings may be used. Patients are encouraged to plantar-flex their feet and are mobilized the morning after surgery with the help of physiotherapy technicians.
- Management. If there are signs and symptoms of DVT or thromboembolism, a multidisciplinatory team composed of a vascular surgeon, a radiologic subspecialist, an internist, and a plastic surgeon must convene. Doppler ultrasound is a good diagnostic tool for DVT. First the clear-cut diagnosis or probability factors for DVT must be balanced against the risk factors of treatment, if the probability of DVT is uncertain.

D. Blood supply

- If the surgeon suspects that circulatory problems are developing on the abdominal flap during the operation, appropriate measures must be taken to make a determination as to the cause of the ischemia, and corrective measures must follow. Fluorescein analysis of the flap circulation may be helpful.
- If the umbilicus is relocated, that area is dressed with Xeroform gauze after it is exteriorized and

sutured into place. The dressing of choice is applied. Jackson-Pratt No. 7 drains are installed through a midline suprapubic stab incision and placed to the lateral extent in each side of the wound. An abdominal elastic binder is then applied.

▼ It is important for the surgeon to remember that excessive pressure on the abdominal flap from the binder may cause compromise of the circulation. Excessive pressure may also inhibit the excursions of the diaphragm and therefore could cause pulmonary problems.

▼ For the patient's comfort, the recovery room bed is flexed at the 45° position. Postsurgical bleeding is seldom encountered in abdominoplasty or abdominal wall reconstruction. Jackson-Pratt drains are usually left in for the first 24 to 48 hours. The patient is followed-up at appropriate intervals for the possible collection of serous fluid, which may necessitate aspiration at the discretion of the surgeon. If the duration of the surgery is to be more than 2 ½ hours, an indwelling catheter should be installed before beginning surgery. Another option is to do a straight catheterization at the end of the operation before the patient is extubated and moved to the recovery room. Orders may be written for straight catheterization if the patient has postoperative micturition problems, or an indwelling catheter may be left in for 24 hours.

E. **Hospital versus outpatient surgery.** Secondary to the increasing costs of hospitalization and because of more efficient outpatient surgery, more and more abdominoplasties with or without abdominal reconstruction are being performed on an outpatient basis. From a surgical standpoint, unless there are some unforeseen complications, most patients may have surgery on an outpatient basis. One technique that we have used to help pain-sensitive individuals is to inject 0.25% marcaine into the plication of the rectus abdominis muscle before the incision is closed. We find that this is helpful in reduction of the postoperative pain. Jackson-Pratt drain care must be taught to family members. The patient may be released after an uncomplicated recovery period to go home and be followed-up in the customary manner on an outpatient basis.

Thighplasty

A. Preoperative care

- ▼ Patients should be informed of possible complications of thighplasty, including but not limited to bleeding, skin loss, fat necrosis, asymmetry, deep vein thrombosis, pulmonary embolism, and the frequent need for secondary scar revision. Showing patients photographs of both poor and good results helps to properly inform them preoperatively.
- ▼ Restriction of activities such as the inability to sit for up to 10 days after surgery and the relative immobility after thigh surgery are explained.
- ▼ Patients are given a low-residue diet before surgery and receive a cleansing enema the night before surgery.

B. Operative procedure. The operative care of thighplasty patients is similar to that of abdominal patients.

Brachioplasty

A. General considerations. Because brachioplasty scars are usually not covered by clothing, patient selection is of great importance. Brachioplasty can be done as an outpatient procedure. Brachioplasty may be done at the same time as other procedures, such as abdominoplasty, thighplasty, or face-lift. Brachioplasty may also be performed in conjunction with breast reduction where the lateral thorax incision is extended into the brachioplasty incision.

B. Indications and contraindications. Flaccidity and wrinkling of the arm, which are usually seen in older individuals, comprise the major deformities that are amenable to surgical excision. The obese arm in which the skin is tense should not be considered for brachioplasty surgery; in this case, SAL alone would be the procedure of choice.

C. Intraoperative care

- ▼ Marking of the proposed incisions is performed with the patient standing with arms spread at a 90° angle.
- ▼ The patient is positioned on the operating table with bilateral arm boards.
- ▼ Sterile stockinette dressings are placed over the patient's hand and forearm so that the sterile arm is completely mobile during surgery. IV tubing is led out through a small opening in the stockinette, thus eliminating the need for an IV in the leg.
- ▼ The incision is placed between the medial epicondyle and the central axilla, so that the scar will lie in the most inconspicuous position.
- ▼ Resected arm specimens are weighed in the OR for comparison with those from the opposite side.

POSTOPERATIVE MANAGEMENT

Patient Information on Healing Process

- ▼ All body contour surgery patients must be instructed preoperatively and postoperatively on what to expect concerning bruising, bruise resolution, areas of induration, and induration resolution. They should be told that incision sites undergo color and consistency changes during the inflammatory period of healing. This knowledge helps the patient from being unduly anxious about the normal course of healing.
- ▼ All male patients who have abdominal SAL, body contour, or excisional body contour surgery, should be informed that they are not to be alarmed if swelling, bruising, and ecchymosis of the scrotum, testicles, and penis occurs.

Medical Staff's Observation and Care

- ▼ The medical personnel that will be removing sutures and following-up the patient at postoperative intervals must also know the unusual aspects and complications of healing, such as hematoma formation, seroma formation, signs of wound infection, signs of circulatory compromise, and signs of hypertrophic scarring. Serial injections of Triamcinolone acetonide (Kenalog 10) mixed with equal parts of lidocaine may speed the resolution of areas of induration, hardness, and hypertrophic scarring. Serial injections are sequenced appropriately so as not to cause fat atrophy. Stronger dilutions of more than 10 mg/mL should be avoided to prevent fat atrophy.

▼ Psychologic depression can often complicate the postoperative aesthetic surgery patient. The operating surgeon and other staff members must be alert for the signs and symptoms of postoperative depression. The operating surgeon has the responsibility of determining when postoperative depression cannot be treated by reassurance alone. The surgeon may decide to direct the patient to the appropriate health care specialist for psychologic treatment should the need arise.

Photographs

Because patients often forget how they looked preoperatively, we take preoperative and postoperative photographs. These comparative photographs can often alleviate the anxiety of the postoperative patient even before the ultimate period of time has transpired in which all swelling and induration would have resolved. If patients can identify a salutary change in the photographs, they will accept the inflammatory phase of healing with less apprehension.

Prophylactic Antibiotics

Cephalosporin antibiotics are used for 5 to 7 days postoperatively.

Patient Instructions upon Discharge

Patients are encouraged to resume normal activities as soon after surgery as pain and discomfort allow. If patients are smokers, they should have been warned preoperatively that they must not smoke 2 weeks before surgery, and they are also restricted from smoking for an additional 2 weeks after surgery. Patients and their families are again reminded of the "do's" and "dont's" of postoperative care before the patient is discharged from the outpatient facility.

FURTHER READINGS

Grazer FM: Abdominoplasty, *Plast Reconstr Surg* 51:617, 1973.

Grazer FM: Suction-assisted lipectomy, suction lipectomy, lipolysis, and lipexeresis, *Plast Reconstr Surg* 72:620, 1983.

Grazer FM: Unfavorable results in body contouring operations including psychological aspects. In Goldwyn RM, editor: *The unfavorable result in plastic surgery, avoidance and treatment,* ed 2, Boston, 1984, Little, Brown.

Grazer FM: Suction assisted lipectomy—its indications, contraindications, and complications. In Habal MB, editor: *Advances in plastic and reconstructive surgery,* vol 1, Chicago, 1984, Mosby.

Grazer FM, editor: Body contouring surgery, *Clin Plast Surg* 11:3, 1984.

Grazer FM: *Reflections on body imagery,* 1984, Uplift Productions.

Grazer FM: Lipexhairesis versus lipexeresis, *Plast Reconstr Surg* 77:857, 1986.

Grazer FM: Quantitative analysis of blood and fat in suction lipectomy aspirates, *Plast Reconstr Surg* 78:770, 1986.

Grazer FM, Davis TS: Body contouring and abdominal lipectomy. In Sohn SA, editor: *Fundamentals of aesthetic plastic surgery,* Baltimore, 1987, Williams & Wilkins.

Grazer FM, Goldwyn RM: Abdominoplasty assessed by survey, with emphasis on complications, *Plast Reconstr Surg* 59:513, 1977.

Grazer FM, Klingbeil JR: Abdominoplasty. In Courtiss E, editor: *Aesthetic surgery. Trouble: how to avoid it and how to treat it,* St Louis, 1978, Mosby, pp. 204-222.

Grazer FM, Klingbeil JR: *Body image: a surgical perspective,* St Louis, 1980, Mosby.

Grazer FM, Klingbeil JR: Pulmonary complications following abdominal lipectomy, *Plast Reconstr Surg* 71:814, 1983.

Grazer FM, Klingbeil JR, Mattiello M: Abdominoplasty. In Goldwyn, RM, editor: *Long term results in plastic and reconstructive surgery,* Boston, 1980, Little, Brown.

Grazer FM, Mathews WA: Fat embolism, *Plast Reconstr Surg* 79:671, 1987.

Kettunen R, Timisjarvi J, Saukko P et al: Influence of ethanol on systemic and pulmonary hemodynamics in anesthetized dogs, *Acta Physiol Scand* 118:209, 1983.

Mathews WA: Pulmonary complications following abdominal lipectomy *Plast Reconstr Surg* 71:816, 1983.

CHAPTER 32

Lipoplasty

RICHARD A. MLADICK

Lipoplasty evolved rapidly from its inception in 1977 by Dr. Gerard Illouz. It arrived on the American plastic surgery scene in 1982 and is now the most commonly performed cosmetic surgical procedure. When the proper technique is used by a trained plastic surgeon, lipoplasty is one of the safest procedures in plastic surgery. Nevertheless, errors and tragedies have been associated with this procedure when it has been performed by poorly qualified individuals or when individuals have deviated from a safe protocol. Safe lipoplasty requires an understanding of patient selection and examination, proper patient positioning, operative technique, and proper postoperative care.

After experience with more than 1,800 patients, I have had no serious complications. There have been no infections, hematomas, skin sloughs, or significant cosmetic problems. Minor dents and waves have occurred primarily in patients with poor quality skin with some preoperative dents and waves. I believe lipoplasty done with the proper technique can be one of the safest procedures in plastic surgery.

PATIENT SELECTION

The ideal candidate for lipoplasty is a healthy, young, average-size patient who is requesting correction of the typical bulges of the saddlebags, hips, lower abdomen, and knees. These areas respond well to lipoplasty and are the most common areas corrected in my practice. Other areas such as the inner thighs and lower legs (calves and ankles) require more skill and expertise on the part of the surgeon. The hardest areas in which to achieve a dramatic and beautiful result are the epigastric area and the buttocks. In those areas, the fat can be fibrous, and the skin may not contract well.

INITIAL CONSULTATION

Patient Interview

The initial consultation should address the following issues:

A. **Height and weight.** Obtain the patients' present height and weight and briefly review the range of their previous weight loss and weight gain. What is the most they have ever weighed, and what is the least they have weighed during their adult life? This range gives an indication of how much their skin has been stretched and loosened.

B. **General health and goals.** The patients' general health and their goals are carefully reviewed.

C. **Age of patient.** No age limitations are imposed for lipoplasty. The physiologic age of the patient is more important than the chronologic age, and I have successfully operated on teenagers and patients well into their 60s. In spite of this, common sense must prevail, and one must think twice about performing lipoplasty in patients more than 60 where the risk is higher and the benefits are few. The best results are obtained in patients in their 20s, 30s, and 40s, and the quality of the results decline as a patient reaches more than 50 years of age.

Physical Examination

A. **General approach and visualization of bulge(s).** The patient is examined totally undressed or in bikini pants while standing on a stepping stool, and the surgeon sits on a low sitting stool to visualize the bulges at eye level. The bulges are viewed from all angles. The overall appearance of the patient is one of the most important examinations. Does the patient have a definite bulge? The patient and the surgeon must agree on the exact location of the bulge to be corrected. It is helpful to point out the bulges while the patient looks into a large mirror. Photographs of the patient are helpful to discuss the posterior problem areas and their potential correction.

B. **Quality and quantity of skin.** I pay particular attention to the skin *elasticity* by noting the rebound to pinching. Skin elasticity is critical to the success of the lipoplasty procedure. Poor elasticity of the skin with slow rebound after pinching indicates it will be difficult to achieve good skin contraction. *Striae* and *overhang* are two other factors that work against a good result from lipoplasty alone. *Dimples* and *cellulite* changes in the skin are pointed out to the patient preoperatively, because they will usually not be improved by lipoplasty. I consider the triad of poor skin elasticity, striae, and overhang as contraindications to lipoplasty alone. The surgeon should pay particular attention to the saddlebag areas, the abdomen, and the inner thighs, because these areas create problems if the skin quality is poor.

C. **Quantity of fat.** After determining the quality and quantity of the skin, I evaluate the quantity of fat. The best test for measuring the quantity of fat is the simple *pinch test.* The pinch test will measure a certain number of inches in the areas to be corrected, and I explain to the patient that lipoplasty will reduce it to below 1 inch. If the patient does not have a pinch test of at least 1 inch, I am hesitant to recommend lipoplasty. Exceptions apply to the neck, cheeks, lower legs, or ankles, where the preoperative pinch test does not have to measure an inch. In those areas, one may achieve an improvement with a pinch test as little as ½ inch. I do not bother with tape measurements of the circumference of abdomens or thighs. Good preoperative and postoperative photographs document the improvement better and simpler than using tape measurements.

Estimate of Percentage of Correction

The consultation is concluded by giving an estimate of the probable percentage of correction. I rarely state a correction percentage of 100% but will often estimate a 90% or 95% correction in an ideal case. If the patient is not a good candidate for lipoplasty, I make it clear that I might achieve only a 30% improvement, and I note that figure in the patient's chart.

PREPARATION OF PATIENT

Good preoperative preparation of the patient is important for successful lipoplasty.

Preoperative Instructions

Patients are asked to discontinue the use of alcohol, aspirin, and tobacco and to take vitamins for at least 10 days before surgery. They are instructed to wash with a surgical soap beginning 3 days before surgery.

Preoperative Workup

On the day of the patient's routine medical history and physical, which is usually 7 to 10 days before surgery, photos are taken, and a complete blood count (CBC), urinalysis, Sequential Multiple Analyzer (SMA 18), and an electrocardiogram (ECG) (on patients 35 years and older) are obtained. No coagulation tests are done if there is a negative (normal) bleeding history. If there is any indication that patients have a prolonged bleeding time, then they are sent for a coagulation workup.

Preoperative Marking

Preoperative marking is done with the patient standing on a stepping stool while the surgeon sits. The markings are made in a topographic pattern with smaller concentric circles over the midpoint (highest) of the bulge and larger circles toward the periphery. The incisions, buttock crease, and preoperative depressions may also be marked. If the abdomen is to be suctioned, a final examination is made for possible weakened areas or hernias in the abdominal wall. A pinch test is done on all the areas to be treated to obtain the preoperative thickness for comparison with the final thickness after liposuction. The patient is placed in thromboembolus deterrent (TED) stockings unless the suctioning includes the calves and ankles.

INTRAOPERATIVE PROCEDURE

After premedication, the relaxed patient is wheeled on a stretcher to the operating room (OR).

Anesthesia

General anesthesia is used for all major trunk and extremity lipoplasty. Neuroleptics plus local block are used for face and neck liposuction and some larger touch-ups. Small touch-ups can be done easily under local anesthesia.

Intravenous Fluids and Intraoperative Monitoring

Ringer's lactate IV solution is started early to preload the patient, and all IV fluids are warmed. The patient is connected to all the monitoring equipment expected for any major surgical procedure (i.e., blood pressure, pulse rate, mean arterial pressure, temperature, pulse oximeter, end expiratory carbon dioxide pressure, ECG).

Positioning the Patient

There are two basic positions used for lipoplasty: prone or supine-supine lateral decubitus (SSLD). I advocate the SSLD position, and I have used it for 13 years for more than 2,000 patients. I have never used the prone position for lipoplasty. The SSLD position has many advantages. This position permits lipoplasty on all areas of the body without completely turning over the patient for repreparing and redraping. In the prone position, many commonly treated areas, such as the face, neck, abdomen, anterior inner thighs, and anterior knees are totally inaccessible. In the SSLD position, the patient may be prepared and draped entirely at one time for all areas. The SSLD position allows the head, neck, and shoulders to remain supine at all times for easy administration of anesthesia or for emergency resuscitation measures (Figs. 32-1, 32-2). There is also an advantage for the surgeon's schedule, because the SSLD position eliminates the extra time necessary to intubate patients, turn them prone on chest rolls, and carefully pad bony prominences. It should also be noted that an inherently greater risk is present in using general endotracheal anesthesia in the prone position than in using general anesthesia in the SSLD position.

Preparing the Patient

My staff has developed the following protocol for preparing the patient:

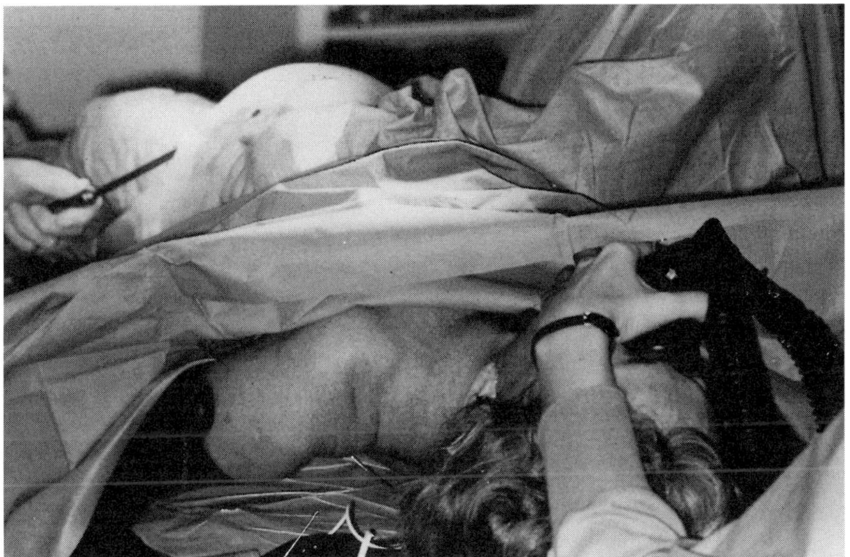

FIG. 32-1 *Patient's trunk is in lateral decubitus position while head and shoulders remain supine. This patient is receiving general anesthetic by mask for lipoplasty of saddlebags after first undergoing face-lift.*
(From *Clin Plast Surg,* April 16:252, 1989.)

- The patient is prepared while awake on the OR table. With the patient supine, the entire anterior and lateral surfaces of the trunk and extremities are prepared from the chest to below the knees or to the feet if the calves and ankles are to be done. Only the posterior surfaces remain unprepared initially.
- To prepare the posterior side, the patient lifts the buttocks and back off the table by bridging. While the patient's back is arched off the table (another nurse may help support the patient's back), the preparatory nurse thoroughly cleans the patient's entire back, buttock, and posterior thighs.
- After the posterior preparation of those areas is complete, a sterile sheet is passed under the patient, who then lowers the back and buttocks down onto the sterile sheet. The patient's legs are then lifted by the heels for preparation of the posterior lower thighs, knees, calves, and ankles.

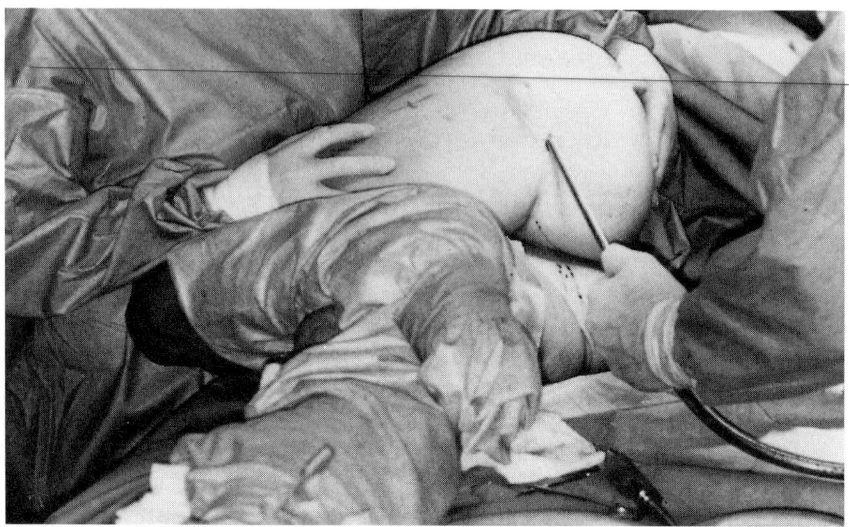

FIG. 32-2 *Access to saddlebag area is easy from buttock crease incision with head in supine position.*
(From *Clin Plast Surg,* April 16:252, 1989.)

- A sterile sheet is then placed over the lower half of the table to overlap with the previous sheet. Each leg is then covered with a sterile stockinette or sheet before it is lowered onto the table. Then the anterior chest draping is completed, a towel is placed over the perineum, and the patient is ready to be anesthetized.

An optional technique may be used but I do not recommend it. This is a technique where patients are prepared while they are standing and then are allowed to lie down on the OR table. This method goes against the established medical teaching that anything below the level of the OR table is considered unsterile. Even if the patient stands on a sterile sheet, it is not good technique to prepare all the way down to the calves and ankles because these areas are too close to the floor.

Preoperative Injection of Local Anesthesia

At one time there was some debate about whether it was better to perform lipoplasty by the "wet" technique, which is the preoperative injection of local anesthesia (lidocaine) with epinephrine or the "dry" technique, which is starting liposuction without preoperative injection. In repeated studies by different surgeons, the wet technique has conclusively shown a decrease of approximately 30% in blood loss. I have confirmed this with a computerized suction machine and always use the wet technique.

A. **Small resections.** For relatively small resections (less than 1500 ml) the basic wet technique of injecting 300 to 500 ml of anesthetic solution is satisfactory. An effective solution for injection is easily made by taking two 50 ml bottles of 0.5% lidocaine with 1:200,000 epinephrine and diluting that combination with 200 ml of saline. This provides a total of 300 ml of dilute lidocaine with epinephrine for injection, which provides excellent vasoconstriction and significant postoperative comfort. This volume can be increased to 1000 ml by adding more saline and can still have a good epinephrine effect.

B. **Large resections.** For large resections or for performing lipoplasty in multiple areas, a large volume of solution is injected through the *tumescent technique*. To use the tumescent technique, one ampule (1 mg of epinephrine) and one bottle of Ringer's lactate are mixed with one bottle of 1% lidocaine (Xylocaine). The amount of fat to be removed from each area is estimated and 2 times that volume of wetting solution is injected (e.g., for a patient who will have an estimated 1,800 to 2,000 ml removed, 3,600 or 4,000 ml are injected.). The tumescent technique has dramatically reduced the blood loss to a small fraction of the previous amount that resulted from the routine wet technique. The reduction in blood loss is so great that autotransfusions are rarely necessary. Whether this result is from the mechanical effect of the extreme increase in tissue turgor, the epinephrine effect, or both is unknown. The tumescent technique can also provide anesthesia, but I prefer to operate on all these patients under a general anesthetic agent.

There is some question about whether it is safe to use large quantities of lidocaine that are above the doses recommended by the package inserts. The pharmacologic studies that have been done on the blood serum levels of the lidocaine patients have all shown the level of lidocaine to be within the safe parameters. Surgeons must decide whether they are comfortable with using the large amounts of lidocaine that are recommended. The tumescent technique has an excellent track record, and no cases of lidocaine overdosage have been reported. The advantage is that patients wake up with considerable analgesia and comfort when lidocaine is used.

It is more effective to inject the solution before scrubbing and gowning. I use a 10-ml syringe and spinal needle to inject small amounts of local anesthetic. For larger volumes, the injection is done by the automatic filling syringe similar to the Pitkin type made by Byron. During the time the surgeon takes to scrub and gown, the wetting solution begins to produce good vasoconstriction from the epinephrine effect.

Technique

All lipoplasty patients who will have a significant volume of fat removed or will undergo a bilateral procedure are done with the *computer suction machine* (MD Engineering Company, 2536 Barrington Court, Hayward, CA 94545). This machine has been one of the greatest advances in lipoplasty and is invaluable for achieving safe and symmetrical results. The machine immediately analyzes the blood and fat components in the tissues removed. The computer screen accurately displays the total amount of blood and fat removed for each area and the overall totals. If a computer machine is not available, the circulating nurse carefully records the volume removed from each site.

The 4-mm round, Illouz, single-hole cannula is the main cannula used for the trunk and extremities. The 4-mm triple-hole accelerator cannula (Byron Manufacturing Company, 3280 E. Hemisphere Loop, Tucson, AZ 85706), which has three holes on the underside and no holes on the top, is also an excellent cannula to remove fat a little faster. The accelerator cannula is often used in larger liposuction cases but not always on the smaller, more delicate areas. It is helpful to have both a long cannula that is 12 to 14 inches and a short cannula that is approximately 6 inches.

The procedure for lipoplasty is conducted as follows:

- The operation starts by placing the patient into the supine lateral decubitus position. By using the ipsilateral flexed knee as a lever, the patient is turned at the waist to bring the hip and saddlebag area upward. I routinely start the saddlebag on one side, finish that area, and then do the hip roll on the same side. After finishing the hip roll and saddlebag on one side, the patient is turned at the waist in the opposite direction, and I move to the other side of the table to complete the opposite saddlebag and hip roll. Then I will do the abdomen, knees, and the inner thighs. I do the inner thighs last because it is the least sterile area; that is, the surgeon must grab the inner thigh skin near the perineum and buttocks to stabilize the area, causing a high risk of potential contamination.
- I always attempt to place the incisions in a hidden crease, (e.g., the buttock crease, or under the bikini area). The posterior buttock and the buttock crease incisions allow cross-tunneling of the saddlebag area, that is, suctioning from two different directions almost at right angles (Fig. 32-3). This gives a finer, more complete, smoother result. Cross-tunneling is also used for the abdomen and the lower legs. The one incision in the posterior buttock area is usually sufficient for the smaller hip roll bulge.
- The incisions are made with a No. 15 blade, and then a hemostat is used to penetrate through into the subcutaneous fat to permit easy insertion of the cannula. For trunk and extremities, I first insert the round No. 4 Illouz cannula to pretunnel the area. The technique of pretunneling means that the cannula is passed repeatedly without turning on the suction. The cannula is passed in the most superficial plane in which the surgeon desires to remove fat. This means the cannula is passed fairly close to the skin, usually 0.5 cm to 1 cm from the undersurface of the skin. Care is taken not to damage or

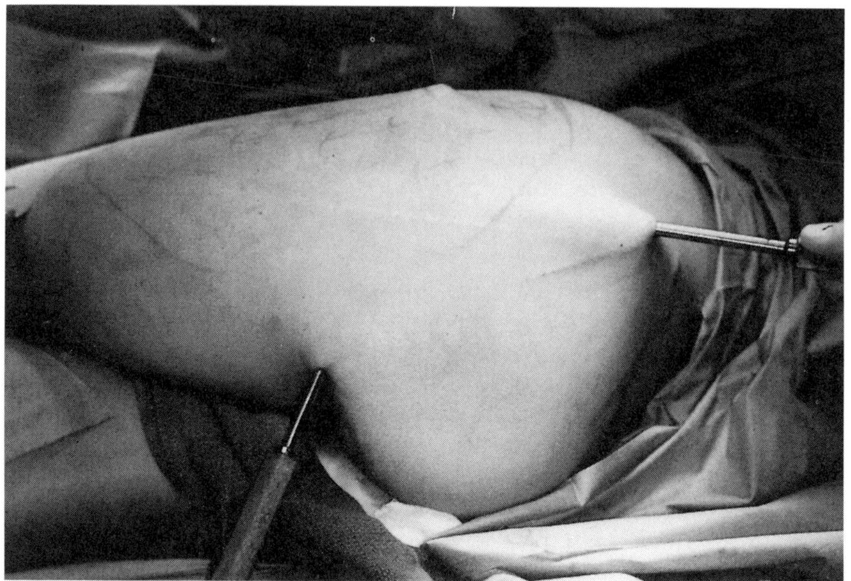

FIG. 32-3 *Two cannulas inserted to show right angle directions of tunnels used to suction saddlebag (lateral femoral area).*
(From *Clin Plast Surg,* April 16:253, 1989.)

enter into the firm subdermal fat. By passing the cannula without suction, the surgeon easily loosens up a pseudoplane at that superficial level. All fat to be removed will be suctioned below (i.e., from that level on down to the fascia). The surgeon starts pretunneling with short strokes as the cannula penetrates into fat and then moves to longer strokes. It is easier to pass the cannula accurately when there is no suction, because there is no force grabbing the cannula. When the suction is turned on, the cannula passes with more resistance and it requires more force, creating a condition that makes it easier to make a false or errant tunnel. The pseudoplane developed by pretunneling helps when the suction is turned on because the cannula tends to stay in the safe plane. I spend 2 to 3 minutes pretunneling the area to be treated.

▼ After the pretunneling is completed, the suction is turned on, and the surgeon passes the cannula in the same superficial level to begin the fat removal. The tip is always kept down and away from the undersurface of the skin to avoid damaging the subdermal layer.

- The suctioning procedure is two-handed. The hand not holding the cannula stabilizes the skin and palpates the cannula. I try to avoid totally obscuring the area with the stabilizing hand. I spread my fingers or keep the hand slightly to the side to allow visualization of the cannula under the skin.
- The surgeon passes the cannula with a sensitive but forceful touch. The technique should not be done with blind, crude thrusts. Lipoplasty is performed as a precise, sculpturing procedure. It is a three-dimensional procedure that requires all of the surgeon's senses to be tuned into the cannula, particularly, touch, visualization, and spatial placement in the subcutaneous plane. It is the surgeon's responsibility to always know the exact location of the cannula tip. The surgeon also pays attention to the fat coming out in the tube (to note the amount of blood) and also to the computer machine. As the tissue removed changes from mostly fat to blood, the surgeon knows that the end of the suctioning in that area is drawing near.
- How do surgeons know that they have completed treatment in an area? They check the amount of blood returning in the tubing and the computer totals. They note the feel of the cannula and whether it is soft and gives as it moves in fat or whether it feels gritty as when it rubs against fibrous bands or fascia. They constantly check the pinch and roll test of the area treated to measure the thickness of the remaining fat. They visualize the correction and compare it to the opposite side. Lifting the cannula up against the skin gives an indication of the uniform layer of fat left under the skin. Using all the above knowledge, they then decide when there is a satisfactory amount of fat removal.
- I emphasize that it is the surgeon's responsibility to *always* know where the tip of the cannula is located. There have been a few tragic penetrations of a cannula through the abdominal wall into the abdominal cavity.

In general, these cases have occurred in patients greater than 50 years. Often in older patients the abdominal wall is much thinner and more fragile than in the healthy, muscular abdominal wall of younger patients. Nevertheless, this kind of error should never happen and, if surgeons are paying attention by observation, by feel, and by carefully guarding the thrusts while they push the cannula, they should not have the problem of abdominal penetration.

- At the completion of the procedure when all areas appear to be suctioned adequately, a sterile towel rolls out the blood and serum from the suctioned area. Firm pressure on the towel while it rolls from the periphery toward the incision expels the blood, serum, and fat particles. It is not unusual after liposuction of the saddlebags or an abdomen to roll out 4 to 5 ml the first time, and then on the second or third roll the amount of drainage ceases.
- The same basic technique just described is used for all areas of the body. For the saddlebags, two incisions are used to allow cross-tunneling: one incision in the upper outer buttocks and the other in the buttock crease. For the abdomen, I prefer two incisions, each inside the upper outer portion of the pubic hair at the top of the escutcheon. These two incisions allow for excellent cross-tunneling of the abdomen. For the epigastric area, an additional single incision inside the umbilicus may be helpful.
- For the anterior inner thighs, I use the same incisions as I use for the abdomen. For the posterior inner thighs, I use the same buttock-crease incision used for the saddlebags. These incisions permit easy access to the entire inner thigh. The patient is supine with the thigh abducted for doing the anterior inner thigh. The thigh is flexed onto the chest into the knee-chest position for doing the posterior inner thigh.
- Lipoplasty for gynecomastia is performed through a small incision at the bottom of the areola. The cannula is passed like spokes of a wheel in all directions after which the incision is enlarged to facilitate sharp removal of the remaining subareolar fibrous parenchyma.

- ▼ The upper arms are reached through an incision placed on the medial aspect of the arm, usually by the elbow. It is preferable to have the arms abducted on an arm board with a sterile stockinette covering the hand and forearm to facilitate movement. Care and precaution are taken to avoid injury to the ulnar nerve when using the incision near the medial elbow. A midarm incision is also possible.
- ▼ Lipoplasty of the calves and ankles requires four incisions (Fig. 32-4). Two incisions are placed in the knee regions, one medial and one lateral, for tunneling downward with a 4-mm cannula. Two incisions are placed in the ankle region, one medial and one lateral, for tunneling upward with a 3-mm or 4-mm cannula. When the legs are placed in the "frog" position with the patient's trunk supine, the medial aspects of the calves and ankles may be reached to the anterior midline and to the posterior midline. For the lateral calf and ankles, the patient is turned to the supine lateral decubitus position and as the upper leg is rotated away from the surgeon, the lateral aspects of the calf and ankle are completely exposed from the anterior midline to the posterior midline to complete the circumferential treatment (Fig. 32-5).
- ▼ I have not used any drains in any of my lipoplasty patients (except in gynecomastia, which has a component of a sharp surgical resection of the fibrous breast tissue, and except in liposuction done with a face-lift). In any of the pure liposuction patients, rolling out the wounds from the periphery to the incision adequately drains off the blood, and I have not had a single hematoma in more than 1,800 patients. It is important to apply good compression to the area as soon as possible postoperatively. My staff places thromboembolic support stockings and compression garments on patients while they are still on the OR table.

POSTOPERATIVE CARE

Warming the Patient

The patient's body temperature is often lowered during lipoplasty; therefore, I warm the preparatory solutions and

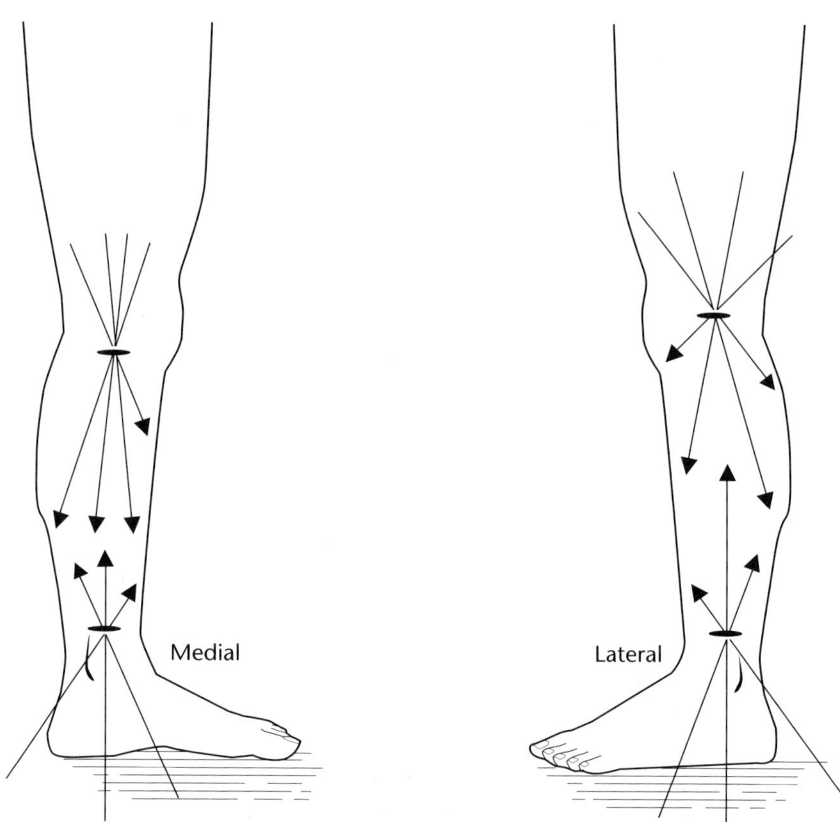

FIG. 32-4 *Four incisions used for circumferential lower leg suctioning. Two are placed on each midlateral ankle and knee, and two are placed on medial ankle and knee.*
(From *Clin Plast Surg,* April 16:251, 1989.)

the IV fluids. Postoperatively, I warm the patient with heat lamps or electric blankets.

Monitoring the Patient

Postoperative monitoring includes use of a pulse oximeter and the automated blood pressure and temperature machines.

Fluid Replacement

A. **After basic wet technique.** For safe postoperative care after the basic wet anesthesia technique, adequate fluid

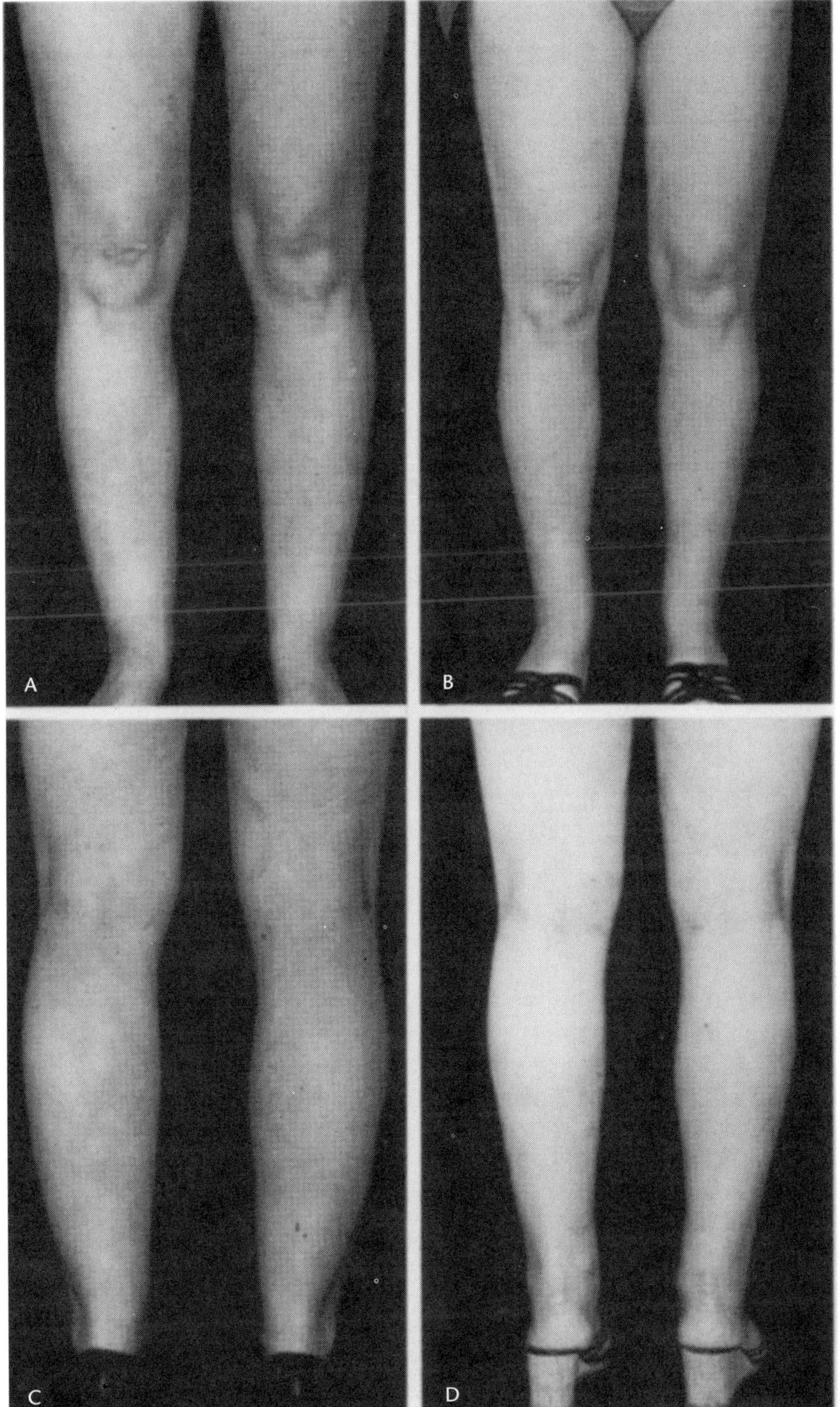

Fig. 32-5 *Patient, aged 37 years, with circumferential fat accumulations in lower legs.* **A,** *Preoperative view of moderately fat legs in young woman who desires circumferential removal of fat.* **B,** *Postoperative view of legs after 450 ml of fat were removed from each leg.* **C,** *Preoperative posterior view of legs.* **D,** *Postoperative posterior view.*
(From *Clin Plast* Surg, April 16:255, 1989.)

replacement with electrolytes or colloid or both is essential. I use the following formula for fluid replacement after lipoplasty: In resections up to 1,500 ml, I replace the volume of total fluids suctioned with at least 2 times that amount with Ringer's lactate. When the resection is more than 1,500 ml to 2,000 ml, I use the same amount or slightly more Ringer's lactate but will usually use 1 unit of hetastarch (Hespan) as a colloid replacement or 1 unit of an autotransfusion. For resections of more than 2,000 ml, I replace at least 2 times the volume of total fluids suctioned with Ringer's lactate and use 1 unit of an autotransfusion for every 500 ml over 2,000 ml.

B. **After tumescent technique.** For postoperative care after the tumescent technique, less IV fluid replacement is necessary. It may be assumed that half the fluid injected for the tumescent effect will be removed by suctioning, but the remaining fluid helps to decrease the IV fluid requirement. It is rare that these patients will need blood transfusions because many surgeons are removing volumes more than 3,000 ml with minimal drops in hematocrit percentage. Nevertheless, it behooves the surgeon to use all modalities—blood pressure, pulse rate, urine output, color, vasomotor stability, and postoperative hematocrit figures in evaluating the adequacy of fluid replacements.

Mobilization of Patient

Bicycle motion of the legs is started by the recovery room nurse, and patients are mobilized to the bathroom usually within the first 2 to 3 hours postoperatively.

Hemoglobin Check

In the larger liposuctions, a postoperative hemoglobin level check is done approximately 6 hours before the patient is discharged. Although it is recognized that not all fluids have equilibrated that soon postoperatively, my experience in a large number of patients indicates the 6-hour postoperative hemoglobin level check is a good guideline and is approximately within 1 gram of the postoperative hemoglobin check done at 24 to 48 hours.

Discharge

In the large liposuction procedures (more than 3,000 ml), I often keep the patients overnight. For resections less than 3,000 ml, I usually allow the patient to go home after I have observed them until late in the afternoon. Before discharge, they should be able to walk to the bathroom and void and not have any hypotensive problems.

Instructions to Patient upon Discharge

The patient is advised to rest for the next 24 hours except to get up for the bathroom, a drink of water, and food. By the second postoperative day, I prefer they begin some walking in the house or outside. After a smaller resection, patients can go back to work by the third or fourth postoperative day. By the end of the week, the patient should be walking at least ½ mile or more. After 10 days postoperatively, I allow my patients to return to any type of exercise they desire.

Follow-up Visits

The patients are checked 1 week postoperatively, and sutures are removed. It is normal to see significant bruising, swelling, and less than an optimum result. These conditions are carefully explained at that time, and reassurance is given that the result will improve and that the swelling and bruising will disappear. I then see the patient between 3 and 6 weeks later and then again at 3 to 6 months. Patients are advised to wait 6 months for touch-ups. Touch-ups are done in less than 5% of patients. For calves and ankle liposuction, all patients are instructed to use an intermittent or sequential compression machine for 2 months postoperatively.

CHAPTER 33

Hand Surgery

FRED B. KESSLER AND JEFFREY D. FRIEDMAN

Hand surgery requires a basic understanding of the principles of treating skin, tendon, vascular, nerve, joint, and bone disorders. The thorough mastery of hand anatomy and functional physiology are tantamount to successful treatment. We leave these details to the many hand surgical and anatomy texts. We will focus here on sound principles of preoperative, intraoperative, and postoperative patient care.

PREOPERATIVE CARE

Medical History

A complete medical history is essential to proper treatment. The following information, pertinent to the management of the upper extremity problem, should be obtained for all patients:

- What is the complaint, and what time did it begin?
- If an injury, what was its mechanism? Was the trauma blunt, sharp, or crushing?
- If the complaint is of pain, determine its location. What makes it worse and better; what is its character (e.g., sharp, dull, burning); how long does it last; from where does it radiate; and when does it predominantly occur? Certain hand problems have almost specific patterns of pain, and the more details of this complaint available, the better the chance of a proper diagnosis.
- If the pain occurs in the wrist, is there a pop or clunk sensation associated?
- If the complaint is of stiffness, inquire if this is a passive or active limited range of motion. This varies with

tendon entrapment, tendon injuries, and joint problems, and the detail helps delineate one from the other.

- What is the hand dominance of the patient? This is particularly important in evaluating a patient with a complaint of weakness.

Physical Examination

An appropriate physical examination should compliment the specific examination of the upper extremity. There are many monographs available on the details of upper extremity examination, and we strongly refer you to them. The techniques of observation, measurement, palpation, percussion, and even ausculation (Doppler) are useful as in any other part of the body. The examination should be systemized (e.g., skin, tendon, bone, joint, nerve, vascular). By using these standard techniques and examining the various systems, a routine for accurate assessment can be developed.

Patient observation should also include the following:

- Skin: Is it supple or tight?
- Scars: Do they restrict or not? Are they stable or not?
- Circulation: Use Allen's test, and observe capillary refill of nailbeds.
- Joints: Are they supple, stiff, or tight?
- Bones: Are they rotated or angulated?
- Tendons: Are they disrupted, adherent, or have tendinitis?
- Nerves: Observe motor and sensory nerve function.

It is essential to measure circumference (swelling), range of motion (extension, flexion, pronation, supination), deviation, angulation, grip, and pinch and to record this information. Use two-point sensibility (moving or static) as a recordable technique that will permit monitoring of the progression or improvement of peripheral nerve problems. Only through objective observation and documentation can the patient's course be accurately followed. All other techniques are not recordable or reliable means of examinations.

Diagnostic Tests

Medical history and physical examination make the diagnosis of a majority of problems occurring in the upper extremity readily possible. Adjuvant diagnostic testing is frequently used as needed for confirmation and documentation. In other situations, these are required to establish the diagnosis.

A. **Vascular testing**

- ▼ *Doppler examination* can be performed in the office or clinic. With it, the patency of the radial and ulnar arteries and the arches and digital branches can be evaluated.
- ▼ More sophisticated vascular tests can include *plethysmography,* with or without cold stress testing, to rule out vasospastic phenomena and *arteriography* to visualize vascular luminal compromises or disruptions and vascularized tumors.

B. **Electrodiagnostic testing of sensory and motor function.** This testing points out the absence of normal peripheral nerve function, the location or multiplicity of the problem, its severity, and the complication of peripheral neuropathy. We recommend liberal use of this technique in all suspected peripheral nerve problems, including carpal tunnel syndrome. Confirmation, documentation, and the knowledge of the presence of an associated peripheral neuropathy or a secondary more proximal compression problem is helpful in the management of these patients.

C. **Bone scans.** Bone scans are sensitive but nonspecific. We find them useful in evaluating problems with otherwise negative physical and x-ray examinations. A normal scan may be helpful in deciding that there are no pathologic changes present. Often the positive bone scan will require other tests in order to more specifically identify the pathology and make a diagnosis. It is often used in detecting early osteomyelitis, occult fractures, and reflux sympathetic dystrophy.

D. **X-ray examinations.** X-ray examinations should be taken in multiple views. Some fractures cannot be identified on posteroanterior and lateral views alone. Dislocations, dissociations, tumors, bone cysts, and calcifications are among the other entities that can be seen.

Stress views often assist in the identification of ligament disruptions, particularly at the scapholunate joint. Similar views of the opposite hand or wrist are frequently helpful in identifying pathologic changes. This is especially true in children, and we use this routinely with them.

E. **Tomograms.** Tomograms are helpful in identifying occult fractures, such as early scaphoid fractures. They can help appraise articular surfaces and the nonunion of fusions.

F. **Arthrograms.** Arthrograms are useful in identifying wrist joint ligament disruptions and triangular fibrocartilage tears. A three-phase study with intercarpal and radial ulnar joint injections followed several hours later by radiocarpal injection significantly increases the likelihood of identifying pathology. It is important to remember that not all perforations are traumatic and that the older the patient the more likely these changes are related to degenerative change.

G. **Computerized axial tomography scans.** These scans have limited value in the hand. Because they permit a sagittal view they are best to identify hook of the hamate fractures, radial ulnar dissociations, and pisiform-triquetrum arthritis.

H. **Magnetic resonance imaging.** These are relatively new in hand and wrist evaluation. Presently, some triangular fibrocartilage tears are identifiable, but the main value of magnetic resonance imaging (MRI) is in identifying early avascular necrosis of bone. MRIs are also helpful in evaluating articular surfaces and the extent of tumors. As experience is broadened and technique is refined, more intercarpal ligament problems will probably be evaluated with this noninvasive study as well as peripheral vascular ones with magnetic resonance angiogram.

I. **Other tests.** The patient's medical history should dictate the need for electrocardiograms (ECGs), chest x-ray examinations, coagulograms, blood sugars, and other tests.

Preoperative Medications

Preoperative management may require the addition of medications such as colchicine to prevent gout; steroid compliment dosages for patients taking them; and antibiotics such as in a patient with cardiac valvular disorder or before bone or joint surgery. There are pros and cons for the use of prophylactic antibiotics, but we do favor them in these cases and in patients with significant acute trauma. We usually give an intravenous (IV) loading dose of an antibiotic before tourniquet inflation. This is followed by 72 hours of a parenteral dose at appropriate intervals.

In other situations, medications may need to be deleted. These would include any medications that alter platelet adherence or have an anticoagulant effect. It is our opinion that this should not be done without the consultation of the prescribing physician.

Most hand infections involve *Staphylococcus* or *Streptococcus* organisms. Diabetic patients are prone to having mixed aerobic and anaerobic infections as a result of their poor microcirculation. Human bite infections are due to mixed organisms, but *Eikenella corrodens* is almost always present and requires pencillin. *Pasteurella multocida* is frequently encountered in cat bites and also requires pencillin. There are other specific combinations of injuries and types of infectious organisms, and one must be aware of these to start proper therapy.

Emergency Situations

Obviously, any patient with an acute injury should be evaluated and stabilized before proceeding with specific care for the extremity. "Life before limb" is a reliable adage to follow.

There are a few specific injuries requiring immediate surgical attention that merit special mention:

A. **High pressure injection injuries (e.g., injection of paint, cleaner, hydraulic fluid).** These injuries appear innocent on the surface but are associated with significant internal soft tissue injury. Patients with these injuries need immediate surgery with adequate exploration and débridement.
B. **Amputation.** If reattachment is indicated for an amputated part, it should be reattached as soon as possible.

Before surgery the stump should be treated as any other acute open wound. Further trauma to vascular or nerve stumps must be avoided while obtaining hemostasis. Shortening of these stumps may preclude the possibility of a satisfactory operation. The amputated part should survive for 6 hours at 4° C, and some reports indicate that parts without muscle last as long as 12 hours. Muscle does not tolerate even cold ischemia well, so the higher the level of amputation, the more the likelihood of ischemic necrotic changes occurring. The amputated part is most favorably protected by cleaning it of gross contamination, placing a moist dressing over the open wound, placing the part in a clean dry container, and placing the container in another one containing ice. Dry ice should be avoided because it freezes the tissue.

C. **Bleeding wounds.** Most bleeding wounds can be controlled by a combination of patient recumbency, bulky compression dressing, and elevation of the part. Laceration into an artery or severed sclerotic vessels may not respond to this. If need be, intermittent tourniquet use or ligation of the vessel can be performed. The rules of tourniquet use (mentioned later) should be followed. The surgeon should avoid blind probing of a wound to ligate a vessel. Adjacent nerves can be readily injured by such maneuvers.

INTRAOPERATIVE CARE

Each operation should be well planned by the surgeon. Mentally performing the operation before actually doing it while considering all contingencies and the management of them will ultimately make the operation go smoothly and efficiently with minimal waste of time and potential for mishap. This phase should also include planning of the sequence of the operation so that a sensible pattern is followed without one step negating the possibility of the next.

Wound Preparation

A. **Cleaning of wounds.** Acute wounds should be cleaned of all gross contamination (e.g., oil, grease, gravel) as soon as possible. There are many scrub preparations available to prepare a wound area. We do not recommend scrubbing the internal wound with these but only the skin up to the wound. The tissue within the wound is least traumatized by the use of irrigation with a physiologic solution. (Plain water irrigation is satisfactory for this if it is the only agent available.) Irrigation should be performed with copious amounts of fluid until the run off is clear.

B. **Shaving the patient.** Shaving the operation site should involve minimal area and be performed just before preparing the patient in the operating room (OR). Hair itself is cleanable, and the only purpose of shaving is to expose the skin and avoid fragments of hair getting into the wound when the incision is made. Shaving may cause small nicks that, if incurred hours before the incision, may harbor multiplying bacteria.

Use of Tourniquets

Upper extremity operations require the use of a tourniquet. There are commercially available tourniquets for fingers, but we find that a ½″ Penrose drain in an adult or a ¼″ in a small child works well when held in place by a hemostat. This must not be applied under full tension and should not be left on longer than 30 minutes.

Pneumatic tourniquets are used in the upper extremity and can be applied in most patients comfortably for 30 minutes without anesthesia, provided the extremity is exsanguinated. We therefore prefer this rather than a forearm tourniquet as favored by some surgeons for minor hand operations performed with the patient under local anesthesia.

A. **Tourniquet testing.** The safety of the tourniquet is dependent on the reliability of the valve mechanism and accuracy of the gauge. If the pressure is too low, hemostasis will not be secured and may cause a more significant complication in IV (Bier) block anesthesia. If the pressure is too high, direct injury to the underlying skin, muscle, nerves, and blood vessels may occur. Tourniquets can get rough care in the course of a day in the OR; bumping or dropping them can cause either or both of these important parts to be damaged. Tourniquets should therefore be checked daily to ensure that the valve will hold during the operation and that the gauge is recording accurate pressures. There are commercially available *aneroid testing devices.* We prefer to maintain a *mercury blood pressure manometer* in line with the tubing going from the tourniquet gauge to the cuff. This provides continuous monitoring of the pressure delivered.

B. Optimal use of tourniquet

- Direct pressure problems from a tourniquet occur at the areas of the edges. The cuff should therefore be the widest that comfortably fits the patient. This will allow a more diffuse area of pressure application.
- A protective covering should be wrapped around the arm before cuff application. This should be snug but not tight and should be applied neatly to prevent skin irritation. We routinely use cast padding. During the preparation, this must be kept dry to avoid pressure over a wet pad, which would irritate the skin. This can be done by careful preparation technique. We do not favor the use of a plastic adherent drape distal to the tourniquet. These fit snugly, and if the tourniquet is released during the operation to allow revascularization, a venous compression effect may occur at the site of this drape.
- The tourniquet pressure should be preset before inflation so that it is reached rapidly. Slow inflation may result in venous congestion.
- In patients with infections or suspected malignant tumors, extremity exsanguination with a Martin's bandage before inflation is *not* used. The arm is elevated, and then inflation is performed to prevent intravascular seeding.
- The tourniquet should not be inflated for more than 2 hours without deflating it for 15 minutes to relieve pressure and clear distally collected metabolites. In some circumstances, this can be stretched to 3 hours. The patient's age, general condition, type

of operation, and tourniquet pressure play a role in this decision.

Anesthesia

Most operations on the upper extremity can be performed with local or regional anesthesia. The need to keep the patient comfortable while wearing the tourniquet for an adequate length of time can alter the possibility of using local or IV block anesthesia. Brachial plexus blocks may be considered. Some patients are too anxious to tolerate brachial plexus block (transaxillary or superclavicular). In these patients and in patients requiring grafts from other sites (skin, nerve, tendon, bone), general anesthesia is necessary.

In performing *digital blocks,* the soft tissue should not be overdistended. Too much pressure on digital arteries for prolonged intervals can cause finger damage. Epinephrine should not be used in local anesthetics for digital blocks because vasospasm resulting from its use can be harmful.

Incisions

The surgeon should plan incisions carefully. Incisions result in scars that can alter the function of adjacent structures and thereby alter the use of the hand. Midaxial, Brunner, or Littler incisions can be used individually or in combination. The surgeon needs to have a good understanding of the use of these incisions in order to be able to satisfactorily plan the operative procedure. The margin between a skin graft and adjacent healthy skin behaves as an incision line therefore the graft pattern needs careful design.

Dressings

Dressings are used to cover and protect the wound, support repairs such as tendons and nerves, and absorb drainage. The first layer applied should be nonadherent and may contain antibiotics. Next is a layer of bulky gauze either comfortable wrapped or placed in longitudinal strips. This is held in place and made to conform by a more firm gauze wrapping. The dressing should exert less and less pressure going from distal to proximal. Compression is acceptable; constriction is not.

Splints

A. **Material for splints.** Immobilizing splints can be made of plaster, plastics, fiberglass, or metal.

B. **Degree of restriction.** Splints should restrict only the part required. The remainder of the hand should have as much freedom as possible in order to prevent stiffness. For example, volar wrist splints should not extend beyond the proximal transverse palmar skin crease. If they do, metacarpalphalangeal (MP) joint flexion will be prevented. In the extended position, MP joint collateral ligaments are in their shortest diameter. Protein containing edema fluid surrounding these ligaments will result in scar formation with permanent contracture of the ligaments and limited motion.

C. **Positioning of joints.** Large joints will tolerate immobilization better than smaller ones. To protect tendon and nerve repairs, wrists and MP joints should be properly positioned.

- ▼ The interphalangeal joint should be allowed to remain in a neutral position.
- ▼ For flexor tendons, wrists should be placed in one-half full flexion and the MP joints in 50° flexion.
- ▼ For extensor repairs, the wrists should be in 50° extension and the MP joints in a neutral position.

D. **Time period for immobilization**

- ▼ If tendons are to be kept immobilized during their healing, flexor tendons require 3 weeks and extensor tendons require 4 weeks to heal.
- ▼ Nerve repairs should be protected until axonal regrowth has progressed to approximately 1 cm into the distal stump. We favor immobilization of nerve repairs for 4 weeks.
- ▼ Mallet fingers are splinted in a neutral position for 6 weeks.
- ▼ Boutonniere proximal interphalangeal joint deformities are statically splinted for approximately 3 weeks in a neutral position while the distal interphalangeal joint is allowed freedom of motion.

When the swelling subsides a dynamic extension splint is applied for approximately 4 weeks.

- After carpal tunnel surgery, we keep the wrist immobilized for 2 weeks.
- Phalangeal fractures are usually immobilized for 3 to 4 weeks and metacarpal fractures for 6 weeks.

POSTOPERATIVE CARE

After surgery, the operated hand should be observed every hour for 4 hours, then every 4 hours until it can be determined that hemostasis is satisfactory and significant edema is not going to develop. Continued follow up should include observation for the development of further edema, temperature change, discoloration, and pain.

Edema

A. **Causes of edema.** Edema can occur after surgery, trauma, or infection. It may also be associated with a tight dressing, dependent position of the hand, and limited exercise. Its end result can be a stiff hand therefore each of its causes must be looked for and an appropriate corrective effort started immediately in order to treat the problem.

B. **Management of edema.** Atraumatic surgery, well-fitting compression dressing, elevation of the hand, and exercise can limit edema. Elevation should be above heart level in order for gravity to be beneficial. Muscle contracture works as a venous pump, and therefore suspending the limb in a static position, such as from an IV pole, should be avoided. Placing the hand at the patient's side on a folded blanket or a pillow provides a comfortable, elevated position and allows the patient to frequently exercise the hand and arm. This exercise should be performed hourly during waking hours. If the patient cannot actively move the extremity, it may be passively put through a range of motion with similar benefits. When the patient is out of bed, the hand and arm should be in a sling with the hand at heart level. The patient should remove the extremity from the sling hourly for exercise.

Temperature Changes

Operated parts frequently demonstrate temperature changes.

A. **Warmth of hand.** Regional anesthesia resulting in a sympathetic block can make the hand warm. Infection can do the same but usually does not manifest until 72 hours after the injury and is associated with pain.

B. **Coldness of hand.** A cold extremity may indicate poor circulation. Removal of a constrictive dressing or splint is often the simplest means of correction and should be considered first. Obviously, removal of a dressing or splint following a nerve or tendon repair can unnecessarily jeopardize the repair and should not be done unless sufficient indications are present to make it warranted. If a cast or dressing requires a release they should be either completely changed or cut open down to skin and then the edges spread apart.

Discoloration of Hand

Although some discoloration may be expected after trauma (accident, surgery) the presence of dead white skin indicates the intolerable situation of absent arterial blood flow. Purple discoloration indicates diminished arterial flow, poor venous outflow or both resulting in stagnated blood. Purple discoloration can also be indicative of a tight dressing, vascular injury, and dependent positioning.

A. **Testing nailbed capillary blanching and filling.** This is helpful in evaluating circulation. If filling occurs briskly in spite of some nailbed discoloration, viability of the part is presumed likely. If the refill is poor, vascular compromise is present, and an appropriate investigation is critical.

B. **Doppler pulse examination.** This may be helpful in evaluating compromised blood circulation.

C. **Arteriography.** This is the most definitive adjuvant test for evaluating the presence or disruption of circulation through a vessel.

Pain of Hand

Most hand surgery patients have minimal pain if the surgery was atraumatic, the dressing and splint properly applied, the part kept elevated, and the hand and arm regularly exercised. The presence of severe continuous pain can be indicative of a compartment compression problem. This may be present with palpable pulses. Exacerbation of pain by passively stretching the involved muscles may be a confirmatory finding. Edema and color and temperature change are also valuable signs in evaluating pain and should be assessed carefully in patients. Merely prescribing a pain medication without first looking may allow a warning signal to go unheeded, and the result can be disastrous.

PSYCHOLOGIC CARE

There is a strong emotional bond between humans and their hands. They are the only anatomic part seen continuously, and because of this, one is keenly aware of the hands and changes in them. Hands provide means of self care, earning a living, communicating (e.g., sign-language), expressing emotion (e.g., holding hands), and protection (e.g., groping in darkness). A disability to this important part may threaten any one or all of these activities, making the patient anxious and emotionally labile.

Outside pressures can cause emotional overtones affecting the results of treatment. A child with a congenital hand deformity will function well until reaching the age when peer criticism makes the child aware of the difference. The deformed hand that served the child may now be hidden. The laborer who dislikes the particular job and does not want to return it to it may become poorly motivated and not respond well to treatment. The potential for monetary gain in a liability or workers' compensation claim may prohibit improvement until the issue is cleared.

Sometimes patients demonstrate these attitudes openly, and other times they are subtle. The treating surgeon must be aware of the possibility of these psychologic problems and be prepared to work through them so that they do become stumbling blocks in achieving the goal of good posttreatment hand function.

CHAPTER 34

Burns

Donald H. Parks and Craig B. Bass

Annually, more than 500,000 persons in the United States require medical care for burns, and of these, more than 100,000 require hospitalization. There are 150 burn units in the United States treating more than 20,000 patients annually, particularly the more seriously injured. Plastic surgeons are called upon regularly to treat burn patients, and the goal of this chapter is to describe the basic principles and practice of contemporary burn care.

A first-degree burn may require first aid only, whereas a massive burn can take months of intensive hospital care, followed by 2 to 3 years of rehabilitation that may include multiple-stages reconstructive surgical procedures. Physicians should understand the initial burn assessment, inpatient hospital care, and outpatient wound management.

INITIAL CARE OF BURN PATIENTS

Evacuation

Patients should be carefully evacuated from the source of the burn.

Emergency Care at Scene

- ▼ Provide immediate cardiopulmonary resuscitation (CPR) if indicated. Check for heart beat and pulses, respiratory effort, level of consciousness and other obvious injuries. (Cardiac arrest is most commonly associated with electrical injury, and with immediate resuscitation, prognosis is excellent in these patients. Physicians should encourage the public to learn CPR.)
- ▼ Stop further injury by the following actions:

- Extinguish and remove burning clothing.
- Reduce temperature of injured tissues with cold water lavages or soaks for 10 to 20 minutes if available, avoiding hypothermia by limiting cooling to 25% of the body surface.
- Care for chemical burns by doing the following:
  - Remove immediately all contaminated clothing.
  - Use copious water lavage.
  - Initiate prolonged irrigation of eyes with saline solution or tap water eye wash.

▼ Obtain and maintain airway and ventilate, if indicated by doing the following:

- Provide humidified oxygen by mask, if available.
- Provide endotracheal intubation and ventilation when required.
- Check for the following conditions:
  - Associated trauma to neck or chest wall
  - Emergent potential for obstruction of the airway by acute upper airway edema associated with inhalation of heat

Hospital Care: Emergency Room

▼ Obtain medical history as follows:

- Determine time and circumstances of injury. Particularly note history of closed-space fire, associated fall, or type of chemical and characteristics producing injury, if applicable.
- Assess previous treatment before arrival at emergency room.
- Determine preexisting illnesses.
- Determine type and amount of medications.
- Determine allergies.

▼ Perform physical examination. (Should conform to Advanced Burn Life Support [ABLS] guidelines.)

- Primary survey (from ABLS guidelines) includes the following items:

- Airway
- Breathing
- Circulation
- Cervical spine immobilization

▼ Secondary survey (from ABLS guidelines) includes a head-to-toe physical examination to characterize other injuries.

▼ Administer fluid resuscitation, as follows: Institute intravenous (IV) fluid therapy with lactated Ringer's solution for burns of more than 15% of body surface in adults or more than 10% in children, or in special circumstances, such as preexisting dehydration in infants and small children up to 2 years, or patients with other injuries. Secure one No. 16 or No. 18 plastic cannula in an adequate vein. I do not think multiple large-bore IV catheters are necessary in most cases, and they may result in overhydration. The formula for fluid resuscitation is as follows:

■ Adults. First 24-hour fluid requirement: 4 ml × weight in kg × percent of total body burned

- Fluid: lactated Ringer's solution
- Volume: half in first 8 hours from time of injury, half in subsequent 16 hours
- Rate: infusion rate adjusted to obtain 30 to 50 ml/hr urine output and stable vital signs

■ Children (age 1 to 15). Calculate body surface area in square meters from pediatric nomogram: First 24-hour fluid requirement: 2000 ml/m^2 of total body surface area (TBSA) + 5000 ml/m^2 of total body surface area burned ($TBSA_b$)

- Fluid: lactated Ringer's + 12.5 albumin/L
- Volume: Half in first 8 hours, half in subsequent 16 hours
- In infants aged less than 1 year, a composite solution of fluid should be used: half normal saline + 20 mEq bicarbonate/L + 12.5 albumin/L
- Rate: adjust infusion rate to obtain approximately 20 ml urine output per meter of body surface area per hour and stable vital signs

- Insert indwelling urinary catheter and nasal gastric tube.
- Calculate extent and depth of burn using the "rule of nines" and rule of nines modified for children (Fig. 34-1).
- Maintain peripheral circulation as follows:
  - Remove all rings and bracelets.
  - Observe extremity burns for the following clinical signs of impaired circulation:
    - Cyanosis
    - Delayed capillary refilling
    - Progressive neurologic signs such as paresthesia and deep tissue pain

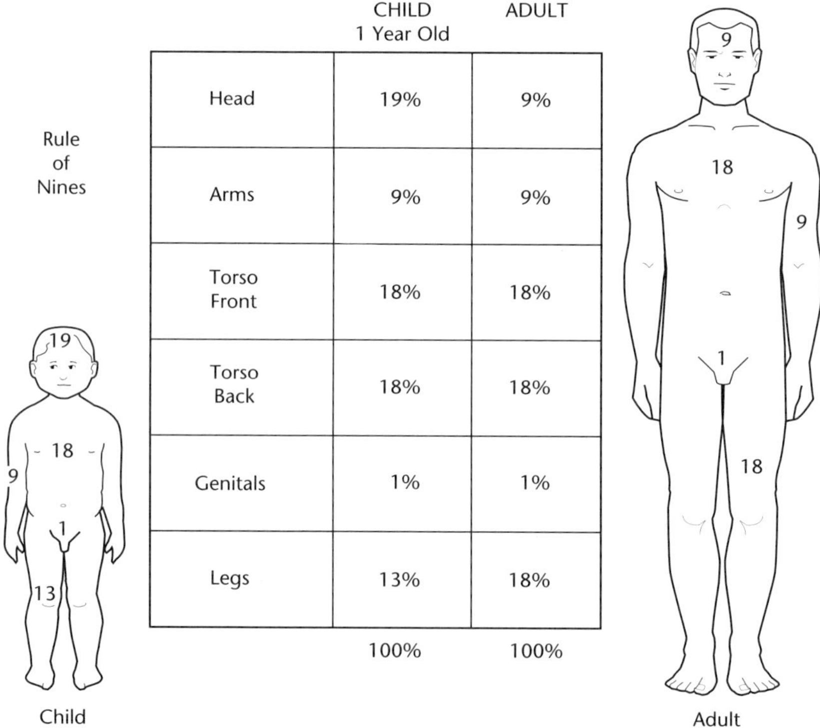

Rule of Nines	CHILD 1 Year Old	ADULT
Head	19%	9%
Arms	9%	9%
Torso Front	18%	18%
Torso Back	18%	18%
Genitals	1%	1%
Legs	13%	18%
	100%	100%

Fig. 34-1 *Rule of nines is helpful for initial estimation of extent of burned body area.*

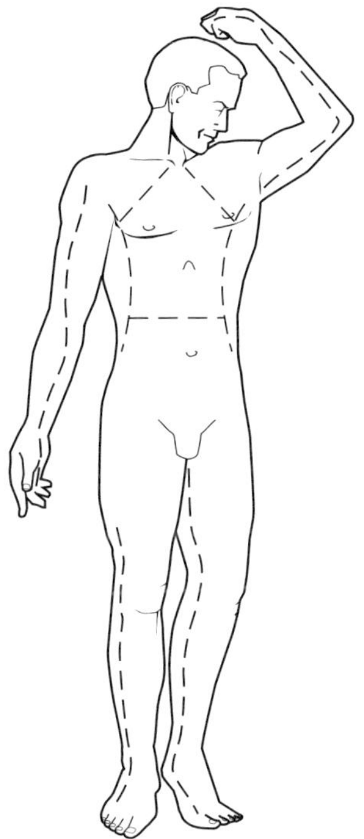

FIG. 34-2 *Frequently used escharotomy and fasciotomy incision sites.*

- Perform escharotomy if circulation is impaired (Fig. 34-2), using the following procedures:
  - Short-acting general anesthesia is recommended. Propofol has been a useful short-acting agent in my experience.
  - Use cutting current on a carefully grounded electrosurgical unit to make incisions.
  - Make incision in midlateral or midmedial line of limb.
  - Make incision to cross the involved joints if circumferentially burned.
  - Incise only to depth that allows cut edges of eschar to separate.

- Perform fasciotomy only when injury involves subfascial tissues or perfusion abnormalities persist. Fasciotomy is commonly indicated in contact (entry-exit) type of electrical injury or deep thermal burns to the forearm.
- Give analgesic medications in appropriate doses IV as needed (morphine 3 to 5 mg every 2 to 3 hours as needed for adults). Requirements may vary dramatically for individual patients.
- Administer tetanus prophylaxis according to immunization status; tetanus toxoid, 0.5 ml, and tetanus immune globulin, human, 250 units, should be given for unimmunized patients. American College of Surgeons (ACS) guidelines should be followed (Table 34-1).
- Start initial burn wound care as follows:
  - Cover burns with dry sterile dressing or cover with a clean sheet.
  - Cleanse with chlorhexidine gluconate (Hibiclens) soap solution and débride (leave blisters intact).
  - If patient is to be admitted, begin topical therapy of choice (silver sulfadiazine or others).
- Admit patient to hospital (American Burn Association Guidelines). Burn center referral criteria: burn

Table 34-1 *American College of Surgeons' Guidelines to Prophylaxis Against Tetanus in Wound Management.*

History of Tetanus Immunization (Doses)	Tetanus-Prone Wounds		Non–Tetanus-Prone Wounds	
	TD	TIG	TD	TIG
Uncertain	Yes	Yes	Yes	No
0 or 1	Yes	Yes	Yes	No
2	Yes	No	Yes	No
3 or more	No	No	No	No

TD, Tetanus and diphtheria toxoids adsorbed (for adult use); *TIG,* tetanus immune globulin (human).
From Committee on Trauma, American College of Surgeons, 1987.

injuries usually requiring referral to a burn center include the following:

- Second- and third-degree burns more than 10% of TBSA in patients less than 10 or more than 50 years of age
- Second- and third-degree burns more than 20% of TBSA in other age groups
- Second- and third-degree burns that involve the face, hands, feet, genitalia, perineum, and major joints
- Third-degree burns more than 5% of TBSA in any age group
- Electrical burns, including lightning injury
- Chemical burns
- Burn injury with inhalation injury
- Burn injury in patients with preexisting medical disorders that could complicate management, prolong recovery, or affect mortality
- Any patients with burns and concomitant trauma (e.g., fractures) in which the burn injury poses the greatest risk of morbidity or mortality (in such patients, if the trauma poses the greater immediate risk, the patient may be treated initially in a trauma center until stable before being transferred to a burn center. Physician judgment will be necessary in such situations and should be in concert with the regional medical control plan and triage protocols.)
- Burn injury in patients who will require special social or emotional or long-term rehabilitative support, including cases involving suspected child abuse and substance abuse
- Hospitals without qualified personnel or equipment for the care of children should transfer children with burns to a burn center with these capabilities.

Questions concerning specific patients can be resolved by consultation with the burn center physician. Guidelines should be modified according to the judgment and experience of the attending physician and be within the limitations of the available burn care facilities.

OUTPATIENT MANAGEMENT OF MINOR BURNS

"Minor Burns" Defined

Minor burns may be defined in the following manner:

- Superficial second-degree involving less than 10% of TBSA
- Deep second- and third-degree involving less than 2% of TBSA

My technique

- Cleanse burn wound in emergency room with chlorhexidine gluconate (Hibiclens) solution.
- Rinse with saline and pat dry with sterile gauze.
- Aspirate large blisters with a No. 18-needle under sterile conditions.
- Dress extremity and trunk burns with Xeroform gauze, apply Kerlix for absorption, and wrap with Ace bandage or elastic netting to retain dressings.
- Change dressing(s) in office at 3 to 5 days, débride blister material, and reapply Xeroform, a thin layer of gauze, and netting.
- Continue office follow-up until healed and amenable to exposure and application of moisturizer.
- Treat face and neck burns with antibiotic ointment (Polysporin) and shower daily. Apply ointment 3 to 4 times daily as long as the wound is healing.

MANAGEMENT OF HOSPITALIZED BURN PATIENT

Airway Management

Confirm airway control and ventilation.

Fluid Resuscitation and Therapy

A. **Formula for fluid resuscitation.** First 24 hours: Administer as described previously under Hospital Care: Emergency Room.

B. Directions for fluid therapy. Next 24 to 48 hours:

- Approximately half of the fluids given the first day are needed, but monitor rate according to things such as vital signs and urine output.
- Colloid: Plasmanate or 5% solution of human serum albumin is administered during the second 24-hour period as part of the total fluid requirement. An infusion of 0.5 ml/kg per percent burned is recommended.

C. Goals of fluid resuscitation

- Urine volume approximately 50 ml/hr
- Sensorium clear and lucid
- Pulse rate less than 120 a minute
- Blood pressure normal to high-normal
- Central venous pressure less than 5 cm water
- Lack of nausea and ileus

D. Considerations in fluid replacement therapy. The Parkland formula for adults, presented in this chapter, is preferred because it is simple and effective. Other fluid replacement formulas are also effective, provided that close attention is paid to individual patient responses and modifications are made according to these responses. All formulas are guidelines only and may require individual modification. There has been no consensus as to the ideal or universal fluid composition or rate and volume of fluid administration.

- Mechanisms of fluid loss are as follows:
    - Evaporation from the burn surface. It is estimated that for every 1 square meter of body surface area (BSA) burned, a patient loses 4 L of water to the environment every 24 hours.
    - Increased vascular permeability as a result of the following:
        - Direct endothelial cell injury
        - Mediator-induced endothelial injury (mediators include prostaglandins, histamine, and O_2 radicals)

- Altered microcirculatory hemodynamic parameters and particularly increased microvascular hydrostatic pressure producing fluid leakage
- Increased burn tissue osmotic pressure augmenting local fluid loss
- Decreased osmotic pressure because of hypoproteinemia

▼ Edema mobilization. At 72 hours to 5 days, mobilization of the burn wound edema occurs. During this period, laboratory values and clinical signs may be deceptive, and massive fluid diuresis may occur. There is usually a high cardiac output, and tachycardia is present secondary to the expanding blood volume produced by the fluid movement.

▼ More fluid is often required by patients with severe mechanical or electrical trauma and with large burns with delays in initiation of fluid therapy. Monitoring by invasive methods such as Swan-Ganz catheterization may be necessary in these difficult situations.

E. Subsequent fluid and nutritional support

▼ Full liquids by mouth on second day advancing to a high-protein, high-calorie diet or tube feeding by third day if tolerated

▼ Packed red blood cells (RBCs) to maintain hematocrit level above 30%

▼ Colloid as needed, provided as 25% human serum albumin to maintain blood serum albumin level at more than 2 g/dl

Nutrition

Providing adequate nutrition is one of the more important tasks that the clinician can accomplish in the care of the seriously burned patients. After a major thermal injury, a multifactorial accelerated rate of tissue breakdown occurs and by 10 days the metabolic rate dramatically increases to 2 to 2.5 times basal levels. When adequate nutrition is provided, these adverse metabolic responses can be altered and body weight can be maintained in spite of ongoing hypermetabolism. Nutritional support consists of carbohydrate, protein, fat and essential fatty acids, trace elements, and vitamin replacement.

A. **Diet.** Patients with extensive burns are prohibited food and liquid by mouth for control of gastric dilatation, ileus, and prevention of emesis for the first 12 to 24 hours. On the second day, oral feeding is instituted by mouth or more commonly in large burns via a Dobhoff tube with placement always confirmed by x-ray examination. Initially small volumes of dilute elemental feedings are instilled such as 50 ml of ½ strength Travasorb MCT. The volume is increased incrementally on the basis of patient tolerance during the subsequent 24 hours to a maximum of 120 ml/hr in most adult patients. It is also our practice to increase concentration to full strength during a 3-day interval.

B. **Nutritional goals.** Daily caloric goals in adults may be calculated according to the Curreri formula: 25 kcal/kg + (40 kcal × percent of TBSA burned.

 - ▼ It is recommended that 20% to 23% of the total caloric requirement be provided from protein sources.
 - ▼ Carbohydrate accounts for approximately 50% to 60% of caloric needs, and fat, with appropriate essential fatty acids accounting for the remainder.
 - ▼ Vitamins and trace elements are supplied according to recommended dietary allowance (RDA) recommendations.

C. **Monitoring nutrition**

 - ▼ Daily body weights are essential.
 - ▼ Nutritional assessments may include transferrin and albumin determinations, immune parameters, and other tests.
 - ▼ Use of a metabolic cart, if available. Some centers have more sophisticated methods of determining energy expenditure and thus have more accurate requirement calculations.

Systemic Antibiotics

Antibiotic coverage should be limited to specific bacterial infections, as determined by culture and sensitivity. Infection is unlikely the first 3 days after a burn, except as caused by beta-hemolytic streptococci. Some physicians in certain geographic locations such as the Midwest (U.S.) administer prophylactic penicillin to most patients and particularly children as a routine. Antibiotics should be stopped by the fifth day or given only when there is evidence of infection, based upon culture and sensitivity results. Use of broad-spectrum antibiotics should be avoided unless specific infections are to be treated.

BURN WOUND MANAGEMENT

The skin plays an essential role in thermoregulation and control of water and electrolyte balance and is an effective barrier against bacterial invasion. Burning destroys the skin and interferes with these vital functions to varying degrees, depending on the extent of the burn injury. The guiding principle of burn wound management involves restoration of these functions by resurfacing the burned areas with autogenous skin as promptly as possible. There is strong evidence that in most patient groups, early surgical excision and grafting improves mortality and morbidity statistics, although older patients may represent an exception.

Initial Treatment

- All burn wounds should be fully exposed and urgently examined after appropriate resuscitative measures have been undertaken (Table 34-2).
- The surface area burned is then assessed and documented, and an initial plan of wound care is developed (See Fig. 34-1.).
- The surface should be cleansed with a mild antiseptic solution. I prefer to use chlorhexidine gluconate and then apply the appropriate dressings.

Topical Antimicrobial Agents

Topical antimicrobials are used for the control of burn would flora. Topical antimicrobials have been most dramatically

Table 34-2 *Guide for Evaluating Degree of Burn Injury*

Criteria	First-degree Burn	Second-degree Burn (Superficial)	Second-degree Burn (Deep)	Third-degree Burn (Deep Full Thickness)
Cause	Sunburn	Spill scalds, flash, or flame	Immersion scalds, flame	Immersion scalds; flame, electricity, chemicals
Color	Pink or red	Pink or skin colored	Bright red, weeping, white	Pearly white, brown or charred
Surface	Uniform, no vesicles	Bullae or weeping	Moist	Dry
Pinprick/ touch	Present	Present	Variable	Absent
Time	Heals 5 days	Heals in 10-14 days	2-6 weeks usually grafted	Produces granulating wounds; requires grafting
Sequellae	None	Permanent pigment and textural alteration	Severe hypertrophic scar and contractures	Variable scarring and contractures

effective in the management of patients with burns involving 20 to 60% of TBSA. The ideal agent is broad-spectrum, non-toxic, easy to apply, and cost-effective among other traits.

A. **Silver sulfadiazine.** This approaches the ideal; it does not penetrate eschar well but is the most common topical antimicrobial used. I prefer to apply a 1-mm thick coating of silver sulfadiazine on the burn wound and overlay the cream with a single layer of a plain fine-mesh gauze. The mesh is then retained by elastic netting (Bandnet) allowing for ease of patient mobility and a "semiclosed" dressing. The cream is applied every 12 or 24 hours in conjunction with hydrotherapy, either tank immersion or showering. Silver sulfadiazine may be contraindicated in infants less than 1 year old.

B. **Other agents**

- Mafenide acetate (Sulfamylon) is one of the earliest and most successful broad-spectrum agents. It penetrates eschar but may be painful and is a carbonic anhydrase inhibitor that produces metabolic acidosis. Some physicians alternate mafenide with silver sulfadiazine daily for maximum antimicrobial effect.
- Silver nitrate 0.5% is a broad-spectrum but messy liquid that may produce hyponatremia and leaching of minerals. It also distorts or obscures wound appearance.

Hydrotherapy

Hydrotherapy may begin once the patient is stable. Tank immersion in water containing chlorhexidine gluconate (Hibiclens) or showering in a bench shower is used. No aggressive débridement is performed. Hydrotherapy allows the following:

- Cleansing and débridement of easily removable necrotic material before the reapplication of the topical agent
- Adequate daily inspection of the wound
- Removal of the topical agent
- Therapists to conduct range-of-motion exercises

Hydrotherapy is often prescribed daily or twice daily until second-degree partial thickness injuries heal or until full-thickness injuries are ready for grafting. Care must be taken to avoid patient hypothermia, and adequate pain control must be provided.

Surgical Management

The availability of specially trained personnel used with an efficient surgical team along with reliable anesthetic techniques and facilities conducive to major burn excision and grafting has heralded a new era of burn care from the surgical standpoint. In 1968, Janzekovic described early excision and immediate skin grafting of burns, and subsequently, many authors reported on early excision and autografting as a method to dramatically improve survival and reduce the complication rate, particularly in patients with extensive burns. Other advantages of early excision and grafting include improved functional results and cosmetic outcome particularly, with tangential excision and shortened hospital stay, thus reducing costs for hospitalization.

A. **Timing.** Surgical excision is indicated for patients with deep second-degree burns and to some extent third-degree burns and ideally is performed within the first 5 days after injury. Some physicians have reported on surgical excision and grafting performed the day of injury, but my approach is to begin the surgical management at approximately 3 to 5 days postinjury and after the emergent phase of fluid resuscitation.

B. **Prequisites.** The patient should be stable with a corrected hematocrit more than 30%, serum albumin level greater than 2/dl and with satisfactory fluid, electrolyte, and acid-base parameters. Inhalation injury, particularly if severe, may be a contraindication to early surgical incision. Informed consent must be obtained from the appropriate source whether it be the patient, parents, or guardian.

Techniques of Surgical Excision

A. Tangential excision.

- ▼ Indications and timing. Tangential excision implies the sequential removal of shavings of necrotic burned tissue, particularly with deep second-degree burns, and the immediate grafting with thin sheets of autograft. The technique is usually performed between 2 and 5 days postinjury, and theoretically its success is based on the preservation of the zone of capillary stasis that surrounds a necrotic burn wound, thereby allowing nourishment of the autograft and reversal of the capillary stasis. Failure to graft immediately may result in irreversible necrosis of the deep dermis or the zone of stasis thus providing a full-thickness or third-degree injury. Additionally, early intervention will provide removal of necrotic tissue before bacterial colonization and result in much earlier permanent wound closure and initiation of physical and occupational therapy, thereby enhancing functional recovery.

- ▼ Technique
  - ■ Tangential excision on extremities may be performed using pneumatic tourniquets to control blood loss, which otherwise might be profuse, and is accomplished using Goulian dermatomes. Sequential thin shavings of necrotic skin are removed, enhanced by traction and countertraction on the site causing tensing of the eschar. The ideal graftable surface is characterized by pinpoint bleeding, but if tourniquets are used, then surgeons must depend upon their experience in recognizing the viable tissue plane.
  - ■ Grafts are harvested while awaiting hemostasis at the excision site and are applied either as sheets or as meshed. No sutures or staples are used to retain skin grafts under any circumstance.
  - ■ My usual dressing consists of a layer of Nterface over thin grafts approximately 0.008 inches thick, moistened gauze (Kerlix), and elastic wraps. The donor site is dressed with a single layer of scarlet red gauze after obtaining hemostasis by local pressure.
  - ■ The Nterface is exposed 3 days after grafting and at 5 days is removed. Subsequently, skin moisturizers are applied to restore moisture and improve graft durability. Exercises are deferred for the first 5 days after grafting in most circumstances to avoid graft loss, but subsequently more aggressive occupational and physical therapy can be introduced.

B. Tangential débridement.

- ▼ Indications. Tangential débridement is a technique of removing sequential slices of necrotic tissue in well-defined third-degree injury or in burns in which excision has been delayed, such as with severe inhalation injury. This technique generally exposes subcutaneous fat that may have equivocal viability, and immediate grafting may or may not be indicated. If not indicated, then topical antimicrobial dressings are usually applied to the freshly excised surface after obtaining hemostasis, and the patient resumes hydrotherapy and topical antimicrobials until either further débridement is performed or granulation tissue develops that will be amenable to grafting.

- ▼ Technique
  - ■ Pneumatic tourniquets on the extremities are advised, and a Cobbett or Braithwaite knife or Goulian dermatomes may be used to excise eschar. If immediate grafting is performed, then meshed graft is generally most successful, allowing for fluid seepage through the mesh without dislodging the grafts.
  - ■ Alternatively, biologic membranes such as fresh frozen Xenograft, amnion, or other materials have been used after tangential débridement to prepare the wound for autografting.
- ▼ Aesthetic results. Aesthetic results, and to some degree the functional results, with tangential débridement may be inferior to that of tangential excision. The initial indications also vary because usually one is treating a more extensive or deeper colonized wound. The risk of sepsis is slightly greater after tangential débridement, particularly if the wound is left open for a prolonged time.

C. Excision to fascia

- ▼ Indications. Excision of a burn wound to fascia in specific anatomic areas of the body is indicated when small, local, deep third-degree burns are present, such as electrical arc injuries in which patients demonstrate burn wound sepsis and in situations where massive burns are present. This procedure occasionally produces severe cosmetic deformity and functional compromise, but the indications are specific and demand aggressive local treatment.

- Small, local third-degree burns. Well-demarcated deep third-degree burn wounds such as from hot presses, catalytic converters, and electrical arcs, and wounds such as are seen in patients pinned beneath vehicles are typical circumstances where the patient is brought to a hospital initially with deep injuries. There may be little to be gained by deferring definitive management of these deep injuries or sequentially débriding. Consequently, many such injuries are amenable to excision to the fascial layer, which is a relatively vascular, well-defined plane that readily accepts split-thickness skin graft. In virtually all circumstances, immediate closure by skin graft should be performed, and on rare occasions, local transposition flaps may be used for definitive closure.
- Burn wound sepsis. Burn wound sepsis is a common cause of death in hospitalized burn patients, although infection in burn wounds has decreased as a cause of death in recent years, being superseded by pulmonary infection. However, if overwhelming burn wound sepsis develops, then excision of the involved tissues to fascia may be a life-saving measure, as has been demonstrated in a series of 22 nonpaired burned children reported in 1979.
- Massive burns. Early and extensive excision and grafting either with autograft, biologic membranes, or synthetic skin substitutes along with subsequent sequential wound coverage have resulted in dramatic survival rates, particularly in massively burned children. Many surgeons treating massively burned patients, particularly children, adolescents, and young adults, have used early surgical excision in conjunction with synthetic skin substitutes, biologic dressings, and more recently, cultured epidermal autograft and have employed a variety of techniques and dermal substitutes. These massively burned patients often subsequently require complex plastic sur-

gical reconstruction to obtain maximum functional and aesthetic outcome.

Enzymatic Débridement of Burn Wounds

Some physicians continue to débride limited areas of deep burn with enzymatic agents. In certain selected cases, enzyme agents may be used in lieu of escharotomy, because rapid eschar softening and thus release of constricting burn may be attained.

A. **Indications.** Older adults or high-risk patients in whom surgery may pose major risks may be candidates for enzymatic débridement of burn wounds.
B. **Technique.** It is generally recommended that only small areas of burn should be treated enzymatically at a time (i.e., less than 15% of TBSA should be treated at a time and the enzyme must be activated by a moist environment). Silver sulfadiazine cream will activate or enhance enzyme activity but must be changed every 8 to 12 hours.
C. **Complications.** Enzyme débridement has been associated with wound infection, bleeding from the treated surface, and pain. The role of enzyme débriding agents varies among physicians and has never gained widespread popularity.

Skin Substitutes

A number of skin substitutes have been developed for burn management. Temporary skin substitutes should be readily available; adhere to the wound; be conducive to wound healing; reduce fluid, electrolyte, and protein loss; relieve pain; and decrease or control bacterial proliferation in the wound. Such materials must be cost-effective and nontoxic.

A. **Indications.** Indication for such materials are numerous with some of the more common indications as follows:
   - ▼ On fresh superficial second-degree burns with denuded blisters (Some materials useful in such patients include Biobrane, Nterface, and processed amnion, and xenograft among others. I prefer Biobrane, which is readily available, adheres, and is translucent.)

- In patients with large burns and limited donor sites (Temporary skin substitutes are useful in providing wound coverage and protection while preparing for autografting. Allograft provided in accordance with current tissue bank procedures has been valuable as a temporary skin substitute. Other materials include xenograft [porcine] and Biobrane.)
- As a test and preparation material for subsequent autografting in wounds that may be questionable recipient sites (Xenograft has been useful in such circumstances.)

B. **Types of skin substitutes and products.** The spectrum of available skin substitutes and adjuncts include the following:

- Natural biologic dressings
  - Allograft
  - Amnion
  - Xenograft
  - Allograft with cyclosporine
- Collagen synthetic composite membranes
  - Biobrane
  - Burke-Yannas skin
- Synthetic membranes
  - Nterface
- Medicated gauze
  - Xeroform
  - Petroleum jelly

Many other products are available with beneficial properties.

Cultured Epidermal Autografts

Since the early 1980s there has been intense activity in the culturing of autogenous epidermal cell lines in the laboratory for transplantation, particularly in patients with massive burn wounds and thus with extreme limitations in donor site availability. Processing is available commercially, as well as in some institutions, but can be expensive and requires skilled professional care during the grafting process.

There is good evidence now that a dermal equivalent is important, whether it be autogenous or allogeneous, to obtain a more stable, durable, and generally satisfactory integument. Currently, such technology however, may provide the only hope for massive surface area burns, and investigation into improving both technical and qualitative results should be pursued.

CHEMICAL BURNS

Burns caused by chemicals account for approximately 3% of all burn unit admissions. Tissue injury from chemicals varies with the following contact characteristics:

- ▼ Mechanism of action
- ▼ Concentration
- ▼ Quantity of agent
- ▼ Duration and manner of skin contact
- ▼ Immediate care rendered

General Management

A. Irrigation

- ▼ Immediate and copious irrigation with running water after removal of all jewelry and contaminated clothing is essential for treating most chemical burns. Neutralization is not popular, because exothermic reactions during neutralization may cause thermal burns.
- ▼ Alkali burns. These tend to be more severe than acid burns, and irrigation should be prolonged for 1 hour or longer.
- ▼ Acid burns. These tend to neutralize quicker on skin, and irrigation for 30 to 45 minutes at the scene may suffice in most cases.

B. Initial hospital management. Chemical burns generally require hospital admission for observation, because the initial clinical impression may be misleading. The wounds are treated with hydrotherapy and topical antibiotic ointments or creams until a clear care plan is defined.

Treatment of Special Chemical Injuries

Some chemical burns require special treatment such as the following:

- White phosphorous burns: Irrigate with 1% copper sulfate.
- Hydrofluoric acid burns: Irrigate immediately with water and apply calcium gluconate gel. With severe local burns, regional infiltration with calcium gluconate solution must be administered and serum calcium monitored.
- Muriatic acid burns: Neutralize with soap; water may enhance burn.

Every attempt should be made to identify the chemical involved; treatment should be based on such identification and reference to material available from the scene, in the emergency facility, or through regional poison control centers.

Chemical Burns of Eyes

Irrigate the eyes immediately with water, and subsequently as soon as available, is the advice in most cases. Saline irrigation may be facilitated with Morgan lenses or other emergency irrigation devices, and ophthalmology consultation should be obtained immediately.

Electrical Burns

Burn injuries resulting from electricity account for 3 to 10% of all burn center admissions and can be particularly devastating. Following are descriptions of types of electrical burns.

A. **Contact or entry-exit burns.** These burns may result from high voltage (>500 V) or low voltage. Cardiac arrest may be somewhat more frequent with lower voltages, and burns may be more severe with higher voltages. Current flows through the body and dissipates as heat when a resistance such as bone is met. There are usually multiple contact sites on the body, and such burns tend to be extremely deep. Deep periosseous muscle necrosis is often the rule to be followed with a relatively small cutaneous or surface injury.

   - If contact burns occur on the extremity, emergency fasciotomies for prevention of compartment syndromes is required. Contact burns on hands or wrists may require emergent carpal tunnel decompression as well.

- ▼ Fluid resuscitation often demands larger volumes of fluid than with thermal cutaneous burns because of deep tissue injury and the necessity to enhance urine flow and clear pigmenturia from muscle destruction, which may lead to acute renal failure.
- ▼ Ophthalmology consultation should be obtained early in the patient's course, particularly with head and neck burns, to obtain a baseline, because "electrical cataracts" are reported up to 3 years after injury. Their pathogenesis is unknown.
- ▼ Serial débridement and early reconstruction with skin grafts, local or distant, and free flaps are often indicated. Amputation rates are also significant in such patients.

B. **Arc burns.** Arcing currents travel external to the body but may reach temperatures of up to 2500° C. These burns may be extensive and are often deep as well. Early excision and reconstruction with grafts or flaps may be indicated, but generally resuscitation and wound care is similar to that for cutaneous thermal burns. The "kissing-injury" seen in flexion creases indicates the arc-type of burn, and electric cord burns to the lips in children are also produced by arc currents.

C. **Thermal flame burns.** These burns may accompany contact and arc burns and result from the ignition of the person's clothing or objects on or near the body. Electrical burns particularly of the entry-exit type may be associated with fractures from falling or from tetanic contractions at the time of current flow. Late complications are relatively common and in addition to scar and scar contractures may include neurologic abnormalities, ophthalmic changes, and posttraumatic stress disorder among others.

D. **Lightning injury.** Lightning injury is a serious type of electric burn. Prolonged periods of apnea are a unique feature of severe lightning injuries. CPR should be instituted immediately and continued as long as needed. The usual tests for death should not be accepted initially because fixed dilated pupils and apnea do not necessarily mean a fatal lightning accident. Refractory asystolic cardiac arrest and a rapid fall in body temperature unresponsive to rewarming are reasonable criteria for declaring death after lightning injury.

COMPLICATIONS OF BURNS

Pulmonary Complications of Smoke Inhalation

The inhalation of toxic products of combustion and asphyxia account for most burn deaths and most deaths that occur at the scene. Shirani et al. have shown that inhalation injury and pneumonia increased mortality in patients with cutaneous burns by 60% more than that expected because of the burn alone. Smoke inhalation thus is a most critical clinical factor in burn survival and morbidity.

A. Types of smoke inhalation injury

- ▼ Carbon monoxide poisoning
- ▼ Smoke toxicity
  - ■ Direct injury caused by the following agents:
    - Hot gases
    - Super-heated particulate matter
    - Conversion of gases to acid and alkalis
  - ■ Smoke poisoning caused by thermodegradation of the following:
    - Natural substances
    - Synthetics (e.g., polyurethane)

B. Diagnosis of smoke inhalation. History of injury in a closed space and the presence of facial burns; soot in the mouth, pharynx, and nose; hoarseness; singed nasal hair; and altered consciousness are important signs of significant inhalation injury.

- ▼ Carbon monoxide poisoning. Carbon monoxide has an affinity for hemoglobin 250 times that of oxygen, shifting the O_2 dissociation curve to the left and leading to severe tissue hypoxia. Blood gases, particularly the Po_2, may be seriously misleading, and a carboxyhemoglobin level in arterial blood must be obtained immediately. Treatment consists of the administration of 100% O_2 , preferably by endotracheal tube in symptomatic poisonings or in a hyperbaric environment, if readily available.

- ▼ Smoke Toxicity. Strong clinical judgment must be used in determining whether intubation of the patient is indicated and determining the type and parameters of artificial ventilation required. The diagnosis of smoke inhalation may be assisted by fiberoptic bronchoscopy, xenon lung scanning, and rarely by pulmonary function testing. The initial chest x-ray examination is typically not helpful.

C. **Endotracheal intubation.** Indications for intubation include symptomatic CO poisoning, potential upper airway edema or edema of the head and neck, and strong suspicion of smoke toxicity. It is critical to identify potential airway problems immediately and intubate early even if the indications are not clearly manifest. Tracheostomy is rarely if ever indicated in burn patients and in many circumstances may be contraindicated acutely.

Infection

The burn patient is prone to infection because of local and systemic breakdown of defense mechanisms. notably the immune system, the presence of necrotic or devitalized tissues, and destruction of the physical skin barrier.

A. **Pneumonia.** The most common cause of death in hospitalized burn patients is infection, and the most common infection is pneumonia. The incidence is higher in older adults and in those patients who have sustained inhalation injuries.

- ▼ Attention to pulmonary factors, including pulmonary toilet, frequent turning, chest pulmonary therapy, sitting out of bed, or ambulating early, is critical to preventing the development of pneumonias in burn patients. Skilled ventilator management may be critical in preventing such complications.

- Direct culture by bronchoscope is often helpful in determining organisms present and sensitivities with consolidation. Specific antibiotics must be administered on the basis of sensitivity patterns and kinetics.

B. **Burn wound infection.** Early wound excision, broad-spectrum antibiotics, nutritional support, and other factors have led to a decrease in the wound as a septic source, although by no means has wound infection been eliminated. Penicillin is often administered prophylactically in the first 5 days postburn to prevent beta-streptococci wound infection, insidious in certain geographic areas. However, the random infusion of broad-spectrum antibiotics is probably not indicated. Antibiotic therapy should be tailored according to cultures, kinetics, and clinical examination of the wound. Patients on systemic antibiotics are also given mycostatin orally daily to prevent yeast or fungal overgrowth.

C. **Chondritis of ear.** Burns of the external ear may result in infection and death of the cartilage, a particularly painful and ultimately disfiguring complication. Prevention of the condition by avoiding pillows on the bed and maintaining the ears against the mastoid is critical. Topical antibiotic ointment, a light gauze dressing, and elastic netting around the head that prevents folding of the ears forward have been effective. Once established, meticulous surgical débridement of involved cartilage is urgently indicated together with local and systemic antibiotics.

Late Problems in Burn Patients

Sequelae of burn injuries can range from mild alteration in skin pigment and texture to massive hypertrophic scar and scar contractures. Rehabilitation by occupational and physical therapists, psychologists, and the physician can lead to successful outcomes even from massive injury. Modalities including splints, special elastic garments, and reconstructive surgery are often required. In the final result, the outcome depends on the patient's motivation, compliance, determination, and will.

FURTHER READINGS

Baxter CR: Early resuscitation of burns. In Welch C, editor: *Advances in Surgery,* Chicago, 1970, Mosby.

Curreri PW: Nutritional replacement modalities, *J Trauma,* 19 (11):906, 1979.

Demling RH, LaLonde C, editors: *Restoration and maintenance of hemodynamic stability in burn trauma,* New York, 1989, Thieme Medical.

Guidelines for the operation of burn centers, *J Burn Care Rehabil* 16(1):20A, 1995.

Nebraska Burn Institute: *Advanced burn life support manual,* Lincoln, NE, 1990, Nebraska Burn Institute.

Parks DH, Carvajal H, Larson DL: Management of burns, *Surg Clin North Am* 57:8750894, 1977.

Parks DH, Thomson PD, Linares H: Surgical management of burn wound sepsis, *Surg Gynecol Obstetr* 153:374, 1981.

Shirani KZ, Pruitt BA, Mason AD Jr: The influence of inhalation injury and pneumonia on burn mortality. *Ann Surg* 205(1): 82, 1987.

Trunkey DD: Inhalation injury, *Surg Clin North Am* 58:1133, 1978.

CHAPTER 35

Skin Grafts and Skin Flaps

John G. Penn

The specialty of plastic and reconstructive surgery is based on the transplantation and reorganization of tissue. In many instances, this involves the replacement or coverage of tissue defects. Therefore complete proficiency in the use of skin grafts and flaps is essential in the armamentarium of the plastic surgeon.

In this specialty, possibly more than any other branch of surgery, there can be great variation in the approach to a problem. The cardinal rule, and this applies especially when planning a graft or flap, should be simplicity. The simplest approach more often than not will be the best.

CLASSIFICATIONS

Skin tissue transplantation is of two types; these involve (1) free grafts in which the tissue is detached completely from the donor site and transferred to a recipient area and (2) flaps that consist of skin and subcutaneous tissue that are removed from one part of the body to another while a vascular pedicle or attachment is maintained between it and the body for nourishment. In recent years, proficiency in microsurgery has facilitated transfer of relatively large blocks of tissue to distant sites by isolating the vascular pedicle, detaching it, and then reanastamosing it to a second vascular pedicle at a distant recipient site.

FREE GRAFTS

Free grafts may be divided into three types: (1) split-thickness skin grafts, (2) full-thickness skin grafts, and (3) composite grafts.

The transplanted tissue must be nourished in the initial stages by diffusion from the recipient site until revascularization of the graft has occurred. Thus, the thinner the graft, the more readily it will be accepted. The thinner the graft skin, however, the more it will tend to contract and cause distortion.

Split-Thickness Skin Grafts

Split-thickness skin grafts comprise the epidermis and a varying portion of the underlying dermis. They may be cut at varying levels of thickness, depending on their requirements. Thin split-thickness skin grafts, often *Thiersch grafts,* would involve only a small portion of dermis (1⁄10,000 inch), whereas thicker grafts would include larger proportions (1⁄25,000 inch).

A. Indications for use. Split-thickness skin grafts are preferred to cover raw areas rapidly. They may be applied in sheets, strips, or stamps, or may be meshed in order to enable a sheet of skin to cover a larger area. Each treatment has its own indications. Sheets are usually applied when the defect is small and the chances for contamination are few. Strips or stamps are used for larger defects or when infection is suspected in the recipient site (so that drainage can occur around the grafts). Skin grafts are most useful in covering large granulating areas, such as those occurring after full-thickness or deep partial-thickness burns. If the granulations are "beefy-red" in color and clean and a bluish epithelializing edge is evident, good acceptance of the skin graft should be anticipated. If the granulations are pale and soggy however and no epithelializing edge is apparent, the recipient site is probably not yet ready for grafting.

B. General principles of split-thickness grafting

- ▼ Contracture. Although the split-thickness skin graft has the advantages of being rapidly performed and providing easy cover, for large areas, it has the disadvantages of tending to contract and differentiating in color and texture than the adjacent skin (when applied to the face). Because of this, when using skin grafts, the surgeon should insert enough skin to allow for contracture. This applies particularly in the eyelid regions, where undermining to allow for implantation of extra skin should be performed. After time, it is a minor procedure to trim off any excess skin. For the same reason, incisions near the eyelids in the treatment of ectropion or burns should be extended beyond the canthi before one inserts the graft. This principle also applies when split-thickness skin grafts are applied to relieve contractures extending across joints, in which case the incision must be made from axis to axis, although the skin loss may not extend that far.

- ▼ Expression lines. The borders of a split-thickness skin graft applied to the face should be within the geographic expression lines as much as possible. If it is necessary to apply grafts away from these borders, the lines should be broken up by a zig-zag insertion, which not only reduces contracture deformity of the border scar but also blends the color of the graft with that of normal skin.
- ▼ Areas of shadow and highlighting. Cognizance should be taken that certain areas of the face are permanently in shadow, while others are normally highlighted. For example, a split-thickness skin graft from the body would be less obvious on the upper eyelid than on the lower eyelid and would be unacceptable on the malar eminence, where a local flap or a full-thickness retroauricular skin graft would be preferable.

C. Donor site

- ▼ Selection of donor site. Donor sites should be selected for size, texture, color match, and minimal deformity of the donor site according to individual requirements. Factors to consider in the selection of a donor site include the following:
  - ■ Quality of skin required (grafts from medial aspect of thigh or volar forearm are hairless, soft, and pliable)
  - ■ Ease of obtaining graft
  - ■ Desire to hide donor site (e.g., within "bikini line" of buttock)

    - Thickness of graft required (thicker graft can be taken from lower abdomen or back than from medial aspect of thigh)

- Preparation of donor site and taking of skin graft. There are numerous methods of taking skin grafts and applying them. Each surgeon has a favorite system, depending on the site for grafting and on the training received. The donor site should be lubricated with mineral oil and immobilized with either tongue blades or a metallic skin plate. Either a skin knife, dermatome, or power-driven grafting device may be used to cut the free-skin graft. The surgeon must ensure that the proper thickness has been met before cutting the graft. Careful observation of the cut skin and the donor site is essential to monitor the appropriate thickness. If fat is showing in the donor site, the blade is cutting too deep and must be adjusted. Skin that is too thin to function however will be obvious because it is observed on the cutting blade. Again, one should readjust the blade before completing the graft.
- Care of donor site. The donor site may be dressed with an occlusive, sterile plastic drape or may be left exposed after applying an antiseptic to the area. The type of dressing depends upon the area of the donor site, the mobility or immobility of the area, and whether the patient is being treated as an outpatient or an inpatient.

D. Graft recipient site

- Preparation
    - In the operating room (OR), with the patient under adequate anesthesia or sedation, the graft recipient site is scrubbed thoroughly with surgical soap (e.g., Betadine, pHisoHex), irrigated with copious amounts of normal saline, and draped in a sterile fashion separate from the donor site. Hair adjacent to the recipient site that could interfere with suturing or healing is shaved before beginning the surgical preparation. In order for the skin graft to successfully

grow in the recipient site, fewer than 10.5 bacteria of tissue should be present.

- The graft is applied and fixed in position with sutures or staples. It is essential that no bleeding or fluid collection occur under the skin whichever way the graft is applied to the recipient site. This may be assisted by suturing the graft to the base or by applying an adequate pressure dressing for immobilization, either by overtying the dressing or by using a plaster splint. Other methods involve leaving the graft exposed and expressing any underlying fluid accumulation several times daily. As long as there is no movement of the graft, no hematoma under the graft, and no infection, successful acceptance of the graft can be anticipated.

E. General postoperative care

▼ Pain control. With successful acceptance of a skin graft, pain in the recipient site should decrease daily and should be controlled after several days with oral analgesics such as acetaminophen with codeine or Darvocet N-100. Persistent pain in the operative site several days postoperatively often indicates the development of a wound infection, which requires localized wound care and resection of any nonviable tissues. Intramuscular (IM) injections of agents such as morphine or meperidine hydrochoride frequently are required after surgery to relieve pain in the slint-thickness donor site during the early days of reepithelialization.

▼ Nutrition. Adequate preoperative and postoperative nutrition with positive nitrogen balance is essential for any type of wound healing. When oral caloric intake is impossible, intravenous (IV) hyperalimentation as described by Dudrick may be indicated for the seriously ill patient requiring skin grafts. Multiple vitamins and minerals (vitamins B, C, E and zinc) have been shown to promote wound healing.

- Mobilization. Adequate adherence between the skin graft and its recipient site is necessary for survival of the graft through vascularization. It is believed that true blood circulation takes place in the graft on the fourth to seventh postoperative day and that lymphatic circulation occurs by the fourth or fifth day after grafting. Unwanted movement between a graft and its recipient bed damages this circulation. Although some surgeons have reported success with early ambulation, most patients with lower-extremity skin grafts are confined to bed for 1 week or more. When a skin graft is placed over a joint, it should be immobilized for several weeks by splinting.
- Discharge from hospital. Depending on the size and location of the skin graft and its rapidity of acceptance, patients may be discharged several days postoperatively when a tie-over dressing is stented on the face or 2 to 3 weeks after surgery requiring major lower-extremity grafts.

Full-Thickness Skin Grafts

Full-thickness skin grafts involve the epidermis and the whole underlying dermis. They have the advantages over split-thickness grafts of minimal contracture, usually better color match, and fuller texture. However, only limited quantities of skin are available for this purpose, and acceptance is more precarious because an excellent underlying blood supply is necessary for the survival of a full-thickness skin graft.

A. **Indications for use.** Because full-thickness skin grafts appear more similar to adjacent normal skin than do split grafts, they often are chosen over split grafts to cover defects of the face. Texture, color, and growth of hair follicles come closer to normal with full-thickness skin graft than with split-thickness skin grafts. An additional advantage of a whole graft is its lesser amount of contraction, which is especially important in decreasing facial distortion.

B. **General principles of full-thickness grafting.** Meticulous technique is required both in the removal of the graft from the donor site and in its application. It is often advisable to use low-power magnification in order to allow accurate skin apposition at the edges. As the graft is prepared for application, it should be traumatized as little as possible. Redundant fat on the deep surface should be carefully trimmed away. However, overenthusiastic trimming of subcutaneous fat may do more harm than good. Firm immobilization is achieved by anchoring the graft to its bed by means of multiple basting sutures and tie-over cotton bolus dressings.

C. Donor sites

- Selection of donor site. Favored donor sites for full-thickness skin grafts are the postauricular skin, supraclavicular skin, preauricular skin, upper eyelid skin, antecubital and inguinal region skin, prepuce, labia majora, and the areola of the nipple. Skin grafts to the face should be taken from above the clavicles to achieve a more natural color match.
- Preparation of donor site and taking of graft. Full-thickness donor sites, usually smaller in area than most split-thickness sites, are scrubbed with surgical soap and draped in a sterile fashion as in other operative procedures. While the assistant or the surgical nurse holds tension on the adjacent skin, the surgeon uses a sharp scalpel or Joseph scissors to excise the full-thickness skin graft, which was measured from an exact pattern of the recipient site. The donor site is usually sutured primarily after undermining of the adjacent skin edges to allow closure without tension. A large full-thickness donor site can be resurfaced with a split-thickness skin graft.
- Care of donor site. Usually the donor site for a full-thickness skin graft such as the postauricular sulcus or the inguinal crease can be closed primarily. An area sutured primarily is dressed with antibiotic ointment, nonadherent gauze, and paper tape like any other surgical incision. When the donor margins cannot be approximated primarily, a split-thickness skin graft can be used to cover the donor site, which now becomes a recipient site and is cared for as explained earlier.

D. **Graft recipient site.** Like a split-thickness skin graft, a full-thickness skin graft must have uninterrupted contact with a clean, vascularized recipient bed with less than 10.5 bacteria of tissue present in order for it to survive. Because of its decreased nutritional needs during the plasmatic absorption phase lasting 48 hours a thin-split skin graft is more likely to take successfully than a full-thickness skin graft. However, the thicker the skin graft, the less it will contract postoperatively.
E. **General postoperative care.** Postoperative care for the patient with full-thickness skin grafts uses the same basic principles as described earlier for patients with split-thickness skin grafts.

Composite Grafts

These involve not only the skin but also underlying tissue such as subcutaneous fat, muscle, and cartilage.

A. **Indications for use.** Examples of composite grafts include sections with underlying cartilage taken from an ear and inserted into the opposite ear; the alae, tip, or columella of the nose; or into an eyelid defect. Grafts containing significant amounts of subcutaneous fat may be used to correct defects around the nasal tip or alar rim, although this fat is known later to be absorbed. An infrequent indication for use is a triangular full-thickness section taken from the center of the lower lip, including skin, muscle, and mucous membrane, that is inserted into the upper lip for reconstruction. However, relatively large lip defects can be reconstructed with vascularized local flaps, which have a greater chance for survival than composite lip grafts.
B. **General principles of composite grafts.** Only small portions of tissue can be grafted in this way because revasularization of the graft must occur before it infarcts and dies. In order to have a chance to survive through the bridging phenomenon, a composite graft should have no point more than 1 cm from its border (0.5 cm is safer). Collateral vessels from the vascularized areas to the avascular areas provide needed circulation. Again, meticulous technique with minimal handling of the

composite graft and accurate apposition when suturing it into place is essential.

C. **Postoperative care.** The use of iced compresses is advisable for the first 48 hours after grafting because cold reduces the metabolic rate of the grafted tissue while revascularization occurs. Because composite grafts are small, the donor area is usually sutured primarily.

SKIN FLAPS

A skin flap contains both skin and subcutaneous tissue transferred from one area of the body to another while its vascular attachment is maintained intact for nourishment.

Indications for Use

A skin graft should be used if it will satisfy the requirements of the reconstruction. Among the many indications for using a skin flap are closure of wounds with a poor vascular surface, transporting padding to cover a bony projection, and reconstruction of facial features such as the lip or nose. A later operation on a deep structure can be performed through a flap whereas this usually cannot be done through a graft.

General Principles of Flaps

Skin flaps are either local or distant in origin. When a local flap is used, tissue lying adjacent to a defect is used to fill it. Therefore the same color, texture, hair distribution, and thickness that the original skin of the lost area had is usually retained. Local flaps may also provide sensation in the reconstructed region. A distant flap can be used where a local flap or free graft is not available or advisable. The distant flap carries with it body and texture not available in a free graft, but the ultimate color and texture of the flap are determined by the properties of its donor site.

Donor sites

A. **Selection of donor site.** Generally, the nearer the donor site is to the recipient, the better the color match. For example, the use of forehead skin in nasal reconstructions gives a better texture and color match than does a flap from the arm. Likewise, the use of arm or chest skin would be better than skin from the abdominal wall. It should be remembered that hair-bearing skin, when transferred by local or distant flap, will continue to grow hair. The distribution and insertion of this hair on the face and neck must be carefully considered.

- Local flaps. Many types of local flaps are used in plastic surgery. These include the following:
  - Rotation flaps. These are semicircular in design and rotate around a central pivot into the defect.
  - Transpositon flaps. These are square or rectangular in shape and are used to cover an immediately adjacent defect.
  - Interpolated flaps. These may be the same shape as transposition flaps; they cover a defect near, but not immediately adjacent to, the flap. Variation of the interpolated flaps include the *island flap,* in which an island of skin with its neurovascular or vascular pedicle is transferred through a tunnel beneath the skin to fill a distant defect.
  - Advancement flaps. These do not rotate around a pivot but move directly forward or laterally into a defect. Modifications for this principle include *V-Y advancement flaps* in which a V-shaped incision is made, and the skin on each side of the V is advanced with the incision closed as a Y and *Y-V advancement flaps,* which are just the opposite. Another modification of the advancement principle is the *bipedicle flap,* in which the blood supply is retained through both ends of the flap, and the tissue in the center is moved laterally to cover a defect nearby.
- Distant flaps
  - Distant flaps may be constructed in an area away from the defect and then transferred to it directly, as in the raising of a flap on the chest and the transfer of it to a defect of the face.

- Alternatively, distant flaps can be transferred indirectly through the use of an intermediate carrier. An example of this is the raising of a flap on the abdominal wall and using the wrist as a carrier to transfer it to cover a defect of the face or the leg. Indirect flaps are often tubed. *Tubing* is achieved by making parallel incisions, undermining the skin and subcutaneous tissues between them, and suturing these two edges together in the form of a tube. The skin of such a flap is elastic; the scar of the border is not. Because contracture of this scar is a natural phenomenon, the mobility of the flap is dependent on the length of the scar and on the skin itself. An attempt therefore should be made to establish a flap with borders that are as long as necessary, avoiding curved incisions. This may be achieved with creating the flap by making the parallel incisions in a zig-zag fashion rather than straight or curved lines.

Flap Recipient Site

A. **Preparation.** Few procedures are as satisfying functionally and aesthetically or give such rapid results as the skin flap; however, few procedures require as much common sense, technical skill, and sound patient care to effect the optimum results. Meticulous suturing without tension and careful postoperative wound care that avoids pressure and maintains cleanliness are essential in achieving the reconstructive goal. Any tight sutures compromising blood supply in the flap recipient site should be removed immediately so that the flap will survive.

   The *Z-plasty,* a technique used frequently in plastic surgery, is a type of double-transposition flap in which two triangular flaps are interchanged. It is used to increase the length of skin in the flap recipient site by a desired amount or to change the direction of a scar so that it will lie in a more favorable skin line.

B. **Timing of flap transfer.** When adequate blood supply is present, immediate transfer to the recipient site can be achieved. Other flaps may have to be treated with caution and delayed 10 days to several weeks before transfer. Numerous tests of the blood supply have been described, including temporarily clamping the tube or injections with IV fluorescein dye. Sometimes clinical evaluation and experience are the most convenient and reliable means of assessing when a tubed pedicle is ready for transfer. The wise surgeon when in doubt will follow Gillies and Millard's principle (i.e., Never do today what can honorably be put off until tomorrow.) before dividing a distant flap's essential blood supply.

C. Postoperative care

- ▼ General care. When local flaps are used, surgery and hospitalization are reduced to a minimum. By using the natural elasticity of the skin, local flaps often can be adjusted into position and the donor site closed primarily. Sometimes however to obtain full benefit of the local flap, it may be necessary to cover the donor site with a free graft, a second local flap, or even a distant flap; this requires longer hospitalization and postoperative care similar to that for patients with extensive skin grafts.

- ▼ Flap care. For a flap to survive in its recipient site, pressure, kinking, tension, infection, and hematoma must be avoided. Excessive external pressure can be relieved by repositioning the patient or removing a dressing that is too tight. Kinking can be rectified in a tube pedicle by realigning its position so that sharp angulation is avoided. Tension is relieved by removing tight sutures, incising the flap with a scalpel blade in the blanched region, or returning the flap to its original position. Infection is treated with antibiotics and frequent saline dressing changes. Hematoma under a flap should be evacuated in the OR; bleeding points must be controlled for flap survival.

CHAPTER 36

Myocutaneous Flaps

John B. McCraw and John H. Moore, Jr.

The introduction of axial cutaneous, muscular, and musculocutaneous flaps—muscle and the attached overlying skin—into the mainstream of plastic surgery has been rapid and accompanied by the impression that these procedures are so reliable and simple that complications and patient dissatisfaction are unlikely. Further experience has taught the protagonist of these procedures that this is far from the case. In fact, these procedures, although surgically straightforward, are fraught with complicated medical, social, and psychologic effects that had previously not been expected. For these reasons, it is important that we survey the entire subject of the general approach to major reconstructions with myocutaneous flaps.

Some of the more common flaps include the pectoralis major, latissimus dorsi, rectus abdominis, gluteus maximus, rectus femoris, tensor fasciae latae, gastrocnemius, and soleus muscles. Fascial flaps (superficial temporal, scapular, radial forearm, and dorsalis pedis) are also common. In addition, many of these flaps can also be used for microvascular free-tissue transfer and can include segments of bone for composite transfers.

Because all major reconstructive procedures are landmark events in the patient's life, it is requisite that all patients be carefully instructed about the medico-psycho-social ramifications of the proposed procedure. It is inherent that the surgeon correctly understand the patient's perception of the proposed procedure so that goals are realistic for both. It is common for the surgeon to overestimate or underestimate the effect of the surgical procedure on the patient's life.

We must first clarify the role of the plastic surgeon as a consultant in wound healing and tissue transfer. Many patients' conception of the plastic surgeon is simply that of a surgeon who is technically meticulous and deals mostly in surgery that relates to appearance. It is not unusual for the patient to be surprised that the internist or other surgeon is not thoroughly versed in all aspects of complicated problems of wound healing. Once patients understand that our specialty is based on tissue transfer (e.g., flaps and grafts), rearrangement (e.g., rhytidectomy), and tissue repair (e.g., lacerations), it is easier for them to realize that the specialty of plastic surgery was established long before the development of plastic materials and that the term *plastic,* in the context of reconstructive surgery, implies *moulding* or *shaping.*

In addition to patients, we must educate our referring physicians. This will improve continuity of care and enable primary care physicians to feel as a part of the team. As a secondary gain, subsequent referrals will be better prepared for the plastic surgical consultation.

CONSULTATION AND PATIENT SELECTION

Patient Education

A primary goal of the consultation should be to educate the patient. The surgeon can either maximize or minimize the extent of the surgery and the potential complications of a particular procedure. Because many procedures are somewhat elective, patients should be allowed to be active participants in their reconstructive options. In most cases, we find it helpful to explain the reconstructive options to patients and then tell them what we think is best and the reasons for that choice. Frequently, it is helpful to enlist the aid of former patients who have gone through a similar procedure. Former patients placed in this role should understand that that they are not "cheerleaders," but are "educators." Thus, the prospective patient will have enough information to arrive at a decision. (In cases of trauma or nonelective surgery, this information obviously must be modified.)

The essential points of patient education are as follows:

- Patients should be told the reasons for the choices among myocutaneous flaps, grafts, and healing by epithelialization. This helps patients to understand that the purpose of treatment is to reduce the time for healing to the minimum and to cover the wound as completely and simply as possible.
- The risks and benefits of various forms of treatment should be explained to the patient in a complete manner. The patient should understand that scarring is always concomitant with any surgery; that a donor site will result whether it is closed primarily or skin grafted; and that these sophisticated forms of treatment can fail completely and result in a worse deformity than was initially encountered. As with any surgery, patients should understand that no form of restorative surgery will necessarily return them to complete normality and that problems of contour, asymmetry, and the occasional obligatory need to revise any reconstructive operation will continue to exist. Conversely, the distinct benefits of the current methods of reconstruction with myocutaneous flaps—the blood supply through many musculocutaneous arteries augments the skin's blood supply, providing a safer flap—were not available a generation ago and must be emphasized. This fact should not be taken for granted either by the patient or the surgeon. The benefits of these capabilities clearly outweigh the risks.
- Patients must understand that all reconstructive procedures are of significant magnitude and are associated with the occasionally formidable risks of local, regional, or general anesthesia; bleeding; infection; or thickened scar formation. A skin graft can be associated with significant pain, temporary loss of mobility, prolonged healing, and significant scarring, even though it is one of the simpler forms of reconstruction. Most patients understand the risks of anesthesia, but it is only fair to iterate these risks as they apply to each patient. Surgeons are loath to have surgery on themselves, and they can better empathize with patients undergoing these major procedures by imagining themselves in their place.

Informed Consent

The most important factor in patient selection probably is the understanding by the surgeon of the patient's perceptions of the anticipated surgery after the patient has been carefully informed and instructed. It is known that informed consent is practically impossible to obtain because patients may remember or understand little of what they have been told. We feel that a better term for this is *intelligent concurrence,* which implies that the patient has a reasonable understanding of the proposed undertaking and completely concurs in every foreseeable aspect with the physician. This may be difficult to do because it requires surgeons to blend a technical education with a humanistic approach, but it is worthwhile. If the patient is not able "to concur intelligently," the patient should not be considered as a candidate for surgery. This is particularly important in elective reconstructions in which the patient actually has a choice and is not required to have a reconstructive procedure. As an example, in our consultations for breast reconstruction, at least 1 hour is allotted for this discussion, with the spouse in attendance, followed by another hour immediately before surgery. A handout can be used as a means of patient education and can serve as a focal point for discussion between the surgeon and patient after the patient has had a chance to study the material.

Confirmation of Diagnosis and Explanation of Treatment Plan

As in all major reconstructions, consultation must confirm the exact diagnosis and the appropriateness of the planned treatment. The patient should understand the length of hospital stay, the need for prolonged follow-up, and the reasonable possibility of the need for secondary revision procedures. Family support must be considered as an integral part of the recovery process, both in the hospital and after discharge to home.

Consideration of Insurance

Because insurance problems are common, they always should be considered before surgery, so that patients can determine whether they are starting on a program that is financially feasible. If any of the nonsurgical details are left unresolved before surgery, it may be more difficult for the patient to accept the traumatic experience of a difficult reconstructive procedure with myocutaneous flap. A better understanding often means better recovery.

Alternatives of Treatment

The alternatives of treatment and the consideration of no treatment must be carefully explained by the surgeon. Neither patients nor surgeons should ever enter into a procedure that any of them feels is particularly inappropriate: an unsatisfactory outcome will cause surgeons to blame patients because the surgeons were "forced" to do an operation against their will. Patients justifiably will blame surgeons because the surgeons neglected to explain the consequences of the treatment. Similarly, patients must understand that they will not reach a state of complete normality, no matter what type of reconstruction is performed.

Deferring or Declining Care of a Patient

Whether to defer or decline participation in the care of a patient is a question for the physician to consider as carefully in a reconstructive procedure as in an aesthetic procedure. The surgeon may have been taught to presume patient acceptance of all goals, plans, and proposed reconstructive surgery, but this is unrealistic in the day of the well-educated patient. When the negative factors of psychologic instability, striving toward unrealistic goals, disagreement with treatment modalities, or future noncompliance with physician's instructions are suspected, the surgeon should strongly consider not undertaking surgical reconstruction. In this situation, it is right to explain to the patient that one cannot achieve the goals that the patient expects. Another simple method of evaluation that we find helpful is the degree of rapport established at 3 minutes in the interview and again at 30 minutes after initiation of the interview. If one is quickly comfortable with the patient, and a mutual understanding remains established after 30 minutes, this has proved to be an extremely valuable prognosticator of future understanding and cooperation. Recognition of an unhappy patient is most important to physicians. Because of their disease or deformity, a patient may be justifiably sad, depressed, or neurotic. We have found that unhappy people get unhappy results, irrespective of the actual quality of the reconstruction.

Unfortunately, a few unhappy or unsettled patients can be missed in the preoperative consultation. This will become readily apparent in the first few weeks postoperatively. Frequent telephone calls, depression, concern over the results, pain, and a general ill-felling are all common indicators of patient dissatisfaction. We have found the best approach is to be available, to be precise in our comments, reinforcing what was said preoperatively, and to be honest. Patients appreciate straightforward comments, and having experience with a particular procedure will allow surgeons to reiterate the postoperative course with some reasonable sense of authority. In a few patients, an early revision of the surgical plan may be indicated to reduce potential patient dissatisfaction. At this time, the surgeon should attempt to precisely define what the patient desires, and a second opinion may be helpful. The astute surgeon knows when to listen and acts accordingly.

PREOPERATIVE EVALUATION

As is explained in Chapter 2, the general health of the patient must be clearly determined and any special health problems must be resolved or carefully monitored by an internist or family physician before and during hospitalization. It is good policy to include general or specialty internists on the medical team to ensure that all serious medical matters will be cared for adequately during reconstruction.

CHOICE OF ANESTHESIA

The choice of an anesthetic is a subject related to overall medical care, because one must carefully protect certain individuals. Regional anesthesia may be a good anesthesia for some patients but in certain other cases it may not be as advisable as controlled ventilatory anesthesia. These choices are best made by the competent anesthesiologist after the plastic surgeon has described the specific operative requirements (See Chapter 5.). The surgeon must remember that in the high-risk patient, local anesthesia may be as dangerous as general anesthesia.

The structural deformities related to major resections and reconstructions of the chest and abdominal walls must be outlined carefully to anesthesiologists, so that they will know what kind of intraoperative requirements and complications to expect. For instance, the chest or abdominal wall resection can cause significant ventilatory difficulties to the unprepared anesthesiologist, but a properly informed anesthesiologist should be capable of managing the patient for any major myocutaneous reconstruction.

WOUND PREPARATION

Before one begins any major reconstruction, it is ideal to have the wound as well prepared as possible. Obtaining a quantitative bacteriologic count of 10^3 bacteria or less/g of tissue is preferable. We routinely use *quantitative cultures* in monitoring wounds because they are better than any clinical judgement. Extensive wound-healing studies by Krizek and Robson in clinical and experimental settings have confirmed that counts of less than 10^5 bacteria/g of tissue are necessary to successful skin grafting. Important considerations in wound preparation follow.

Standard Care

A. Surgical débridement. Before initiating any local wound care, necrotic tissue is best treated by surgical débridement either in the operating room (OR) or at bedside. Catgut sutures and a disposable thermal cautery are helpful if beside débridement is planned.

B. Dressings

- Surface wounds should be protected with a *saline-moistened dressing* to prevent drying. Drying is always harmful, and almost any kind of moisture, whether water or saline, is usually helpful. This is particularly true in the inherently dry wound.
- If the wound is infected or weeping on the surface, *wet-to-dry dressings* can be used, and they still are the

standard of treatment. It is often difficult for nurses to carry out an order for wet-to-dry dressing, because nurses are not well versed in wound care, unless they have a special experience or a particular interest. The wet-to-dry dressing frequently fails because it is intended to dry out in its deepest portion and remain moist on its surface so that capillary attraction will withdraw some of the fluids, surface bacteria, and debris into the dressing. This requires frequent changes and intermittent surface wetting of the dressing so that the entire dressing does not dry out completely. If the dressing does dry out, it serves little more purpose than a simple dry dressing.

C. **Enzyme compounds.** Enzymes have been used for many years, but they are not necessarily any more effective than is careful attention to wet-to-dry dressings. All of the existing compounds, with the exception of sutilains ointment (Travase), have been singularly disappointing.

- ▼ If properly applied, *sutilains* can be helpful in removing the final adherent slough if it is less than 1 mm thick. The ointment must be applied in a thick coat and covered with a moist dressing that is neither wet nor dry, and it must be changed 4 times a day. If it has not had a significant effect in 3 or 4 days, it probably will not contribute significantly to wound preparation.
- ▼ Dextranomer (Debrisan) is another agent that has been helpful in reducing the bacterial count in weeping wounds. It is not significantly helpful for venous, arterial, or dry ulcers, but it can have a rapid effect in weeping ulcers. Dextranomer is simple to use, and this constitutes one of its major advantages from the standpoint of nursing care. A thick coat of Dextranomer is used 3 times daily and covered with a dry dressing. Glycerin solution was originally suggested as a mixture with dextranomer, but we have not found this to be efficacious. It is of utmost importance that all of the dextranomer be removed

before reapplication. If it is not, the remaining sludge of moist, sugary dextranomer is, in fact, an agent that can promote bacterial growth. We have found that the Water Pik is the best method to remove this material, and it usually does not cause significant discomfort. The combination of dextranomer and Water Pik has been helpful, and one may question whether it is the Water Pik itself that is the significant débriding agent.

D. **Showering.** If the patient is ambulatory, showers can be helpful in wound débridement. Pain may be restrictive; however, if able, most patients are amenable to showering 2 to 3 times a day.

E. **Antibiotics.** Systemic antibiotics have not been particulary helpful unless the wounds are infected. Antibiotics do not achieve any significant tissue concentration in the usual surface wound, and consequently, we seldom use systemic antibiotics in routine wound care. If used chronically, antibiotics may actually select for resistant bacteria. Open, draining wounds rarely result in systemic sepsis. Surgeons should monitor all of these infected and weeping wounds with wound biopsies, which are cultured in a quantitative manner to assess progress before reconstruction.

Management of Infected Deep Wounds

Infected deep wounds involving the major body cavities or extremities, which are not accessible to direct applications of surface-active agents or are subject to frequent dressing changes, are difficult to manage. Dextranomer and sutilains are apparently not effective in cavities and can be harmful.

A. **Wound packing.** Packing these wounds with Kling wrap can be done, but it usually acts more as a dam to the exudates than as a topical débriding agent. Proper packing is placed loosely in a wound, preventing loculations and aiding in drainage. A tightly packed wound can create an abscess. In addition, a Kling-type of bandage is recommended over 4 by 4-type of bandages, because packing with the latter may result in this material inadvertently being left in the wound, creating a new nidus of infection.

B. Irrigation

- The usefulness of in-and-out saline irrigation solutions is impressive. There are numerous methods of getting the saline in and out of the wound, but the constant irrigation must be associated with some reduction of surface bacteria by volume dilution alone.
- *Providone-iodine* (Betadine) can be used in similar fashion as an irrigation solution. We have not been impressed with reports that povidone iodine is significantly more effective than saline, but no major harmful effects of Betadine have been noted. Betadine and iodoform are toxic to fat cells and should be used with caution where a large amount of subcutaneous tissue is exposed.
- In contaminated wounds, we favor ¼ strength *Dakin's solution* (sodium hypocholorite). This decreases the bacterial count and aroma of a wound and apparently does not interfere with healing and subsequent formation of granulation tissue.

The deep infected wound remains a significant patient care problem and one for which there is no answer short of operative débridement and immediate coverage with muscle.

Timing of Coverage

It is often wise to perform separate planned sessions of débridement before coverage when the wound is severely infected (more than 10^5 bacteria/g of tissue). Most situations do not require immediate coverage, and the time spent in wound preparation is well worthwhile. If the wound can be made clean enough to accept allograft (homograft) or xenograft adherence, it is generally clean enough to primarily close with a flap. At the time of final reconstruction, it is wise to remove any foreign body or devitalized bone because it may become a residual source of infection. It is not necessary to perform a separate operation for this removal because this is usually combined with the definitive reconstruction.

Exposed Structures

A. **Exposed dried bone.** This is usually not infected or a contributor to wound infection. Its surface can be débrided easily at the time of the definitive closure without harm.

B. **Dried vessels.** These constitute a perilous situation in which the vessel can rupture at any time. Such a vessel requires coverage at the earliest possible time to prevent such a catastrophe. Vascular surgical consultation may be indicated if large, named vessels are involved.

C. **Dried nerves.** These are similar to dried vessels, in that the epineural blood supply can be destroyed by drying and can lead to a significant nerve deficit. Drying should be avoided whenever possible, but if it cannot, nerves should be revascularized with muscle flap coverage and without significant epineural débridement.

D. **Dried tendon.** This is somewhat different from vessels and nerves in that it can be covered with a vascularized flap and can completely reconstitute its substance, even though the tendon is dead and tanned. Full function can be restored in the dried tendon. However, the "soupy" tendon is autolyzed and must be excised.

E. **Metallic prostheses.** These are usually removed at the time of the coverage of exposed bone, but removal is not necessarily imperative. When it is critical to leave the metallic prosthesis in place, like in knee joints, ankle joints, and spinal fusions, successful coverage has been obtained with vascularized myocutaneous flaps when the wound has been meticulously cleansed with in-and-out saline irrigation. Leaving a prosthesis in place is not always successful, but when a total joint prosthesis is worth saving, it is certainly a worthwhile attempt, because its removal usually leads to disastrous bony malfusion. We have found irrigation with povidone- iodine and hydrogen peroxide followed-up by pulsed jet saline lavage helpful in these problematic wounds. When one is covering long bone fractures with myocutaneous flaps, it is preferable to remove a metallic prosthesis whenever possible, because the underlying bone may be infected around the penetrating screws and not accessible to the vascularized flap coverage owing to the position of the prosthesis. It is essential that the reconstructive surgeon develop a treatment plan with the orthopedic surgeon. In exposed, long bone fractures, we prefer the external fixation appliance to the internal fixation type. This minimizes orthopedic hardware and diminishes the likelihood of devitalized bone from periosteal stripping.

F. **Exposed vascular protheses.** These must be viewed more critically, because they constitute an urgent coverage problem, owing to the possibility of "blow out." The infected and exposed vascular prosthesis will not necessarily rupture in a matter of hours, but it should be treated in conjunction with the vascular surgeon with due haste. The wound may be so severely infected that it requires prior débridement, but this is most unusual. In general, vascular prostheses should be covered with an adjacent muscle after immediate débridement. The infected pseudosheath around the vascular prosthesis must be entirely excised, and all of the infected material in the area must be removed and covered in coordination with a vascular surgical reconstruction. If the prosthetic graft appears to be infected, it is best removed, and an extraanatomic bypass performed (by the vascular surgeon) away from the infected wound.

FLAP SELECTION

Types of flaps

One should be able to use any type of flap to reconstruct a defect. This sounds simple, but one must have an alternative plan for every eventuality. Whatever the case, the objective is to get the job done in the simplest manner, with the least donor defect. The alternative plan involves a choice from among similar flaps, such as the gracilis and rectus femoris in the groin and the latissimus and pectoralis in the chest. If a chosen flap is incapable of doing the job for one reason or another (e.g., vascular compromise), the surgeon must be ready to use the flap of second choice. A primary consideration is whether to use a *local flap* that is composed of skin or muscle alone or one of muscle and skin combined; or whether to use a *free flap*. Local flaps always should be used in preference to free flaps unless the special considerations of the location or problems related to local flaps weigh the balance in favor of a better-quality free flap, which might be done more reliably in a single stage.

A. **Muscle flaps.** These are used primarily to provide a vascularized surface for the defect. They may be used to eradicate infection or to revascularize bone, and when required they are vastly superior to cutaneous flaps for these purposes.

B. **Fasciocutaneous flaps.** These carry fat on the underlying fascia. They are less effective than muscle flaps in eradicating infection. Most flaps are thinner and more pliable than muscle flaps. They have a better blood supply than cutaneous flaps.

C. **Cutaneous flaps.** These carry fat on their undersurface and are less effective in satisfying the requirements. Conversely, cutaneous flaps may provide a thinner flap, which can be used for situations such as filling facial defects and covering less severe wounds.

D. **Musculocutaneous flaps.** These are used in preference to muscle flaps alone whenever a skin component is necessary for combined replacement of the deficient tissues. They are used most effectively in breast reconstruction and in treating radiated wounds. In general, a muscle flap with a skin graft in the lower extremity is a better aesthetic result than a musculocutaneous flap.

E. **Free microvascular flaps.** These are commonly used today. They yield superior results in difficult reconstructions (e.g., head and neck cancer extirpations, distal extremity wounds). They may be the best reconstructive choice for a variety of wounds with the microsurgeon's expertise being the deciding factor.

Location of Defect

The location of the defect is a particularly important factor in the surgeon's choice of the type of flap.

A. **Low pretibial area or dorsum of foot.** Many times these areas are better served by the use of a free flap than by use of local muscle flaps or cross-leg flaps. When one compares the results of the reverse soleus flap to a free latissimus dorsi flap, the inherent disadvantages of the free flap may become relatively insignificant.

B. **Perineum.** In the perineum, the gracilis flap or the inferiorly based rectus abdominis flap is the preferred standard flap, but a broader area of coverage may be required in the groin or the anterior perineum and may make the tensor fascia lata the flap of choice.

C. **Chest.** In the chest, one can repair virtually any defect with either the local island pectoralis paddle or the latissimus dorsi flap. The location of the defect and the nature of the injury allows the surgeon to choose preferentially (See Chapter 27.).

Special Requirements for Defect

Special requirements for correction of a defect dictate a special choice of flaps. For instance, when fascia is needed for structural support, the preferred flap in the abdomen is the tensor fascia lata or rectus femoris musculofascial flap. It provides structural support without the necessity for skin and adequately completes the reconstruction. Muscle itself is preferred over a cutaneous flap whenever infection is present, when a prosthesis must be covered, or when bone must be ravascularized. Myocutaneous flaps are used in preference to muscle flaps alone, particularly when sensation must be provided to the recipient area. Examples are the gastrocnemius myocutaneous flap for prepatellar coverage and the tensor fascia lata flap for reconstruction of the areas of the buttocks. In general, a muscle flap with a skin graft yields a superior aesthetic result when compared to a musculocutaneous flap.

Donor Sites

The donor site is always a significant consideration. Fortunately, most donor sites can be primarily closed. However, this consideration is particularly important in a young woman, and it may lead the surgeon to choose the groin, as opposed to the chest, as the source of a free flap. Similarly, consideration of donor site defects may encourage the surgeon to use a small latissimus free flap rather than a cross-leg flap, which disfigures both lower extremities. The functional deficit of the donor flap must always be considered. For example, a latissimus dorsi free muscle flap may pose considerable restrictions on a cross-country skier.

INTRAOPERATIVE CONSIDERATIONS

Anatomy of Muscle and Supporting Vasculature

The anatomy of the muscle and supplying vasculature is the essential consideration. The surgeon should be able to predict reliably what flaps will be useful for reconstruction of various defects. One should learn this anatomy through cadaver dissection, supervision by an experienced surgeon, or attendance at the various flap workshops dealing with these reconstructive problems. No textbook describes the anatomy as well as does a simple cadaver dissection.

One must be able to predict the smallest number of primary muscle vessels that will support any given muscle or myocutaneous flap. This may result in an *island flap,* one in which the flap is dangling by the vessels. There is nothing wrong with using an island flap; however, there is always a significant cutaneous vessel in the base of the skin portion of the flap that should not be divided unless it is absolutely necessary.

A. **Complication of vascular spasm.** A danger in using an island flap that was not initially recognized is the problem with the ill-defined entity of "*vascular spasm.*" We feel that spasm is related to undue torsion on the vessel that causes the arterial portion of the vascular tree functionally to close. The usual worst-case scenario for vascular spasm is loss of the cutaneous portion of the flap, with problematic viability of the muscle. This situation primarily affects long, thin muscles and, for whatever reason, is not a significant factor in broad, flat muscles.
B. **Management of vascular spasms.** Once vascular spasm begins, there is essentially no procedure that predictably will relieve the spasm. We have tried numerous topical and intraarterial drugs such as lidocaine without effect. The only significant relief that we have found (experimentally) is excision of the involved portion of the vessel and either reapproximation or vein grafting. Warm compresses and time are the best predictors for the relief of spasm. If dermal bleeding then ensues, the surgeon can be reasonably certain that the

flap has a good chance for survival. In the usual case of spasm, the cutaneous portion of the flap bleeds freely from the subdermal margin of the skin before the existence of spasm, but when spasm ensues, the cutaneous portion of the flap does not bleed or show fluorescence at all. This complication certainly teaches one to be less cavalier in the treatment of the primary muscular vessels and to know well the involved anatomy.

Flap Viability

A. **Clincial signs** The assessment of flap viability is important, and certain factors, such as visual inspection of color and capillary refill of the flap, have not been helpful. The only anatomic test that has been helpful is the presence of a brisk, bright red flow of blood from the superior base of the dermis. Essentially this is as good an assessment as that of proper fluorescence. When one evaluates fluorescence and obtains an area of good fluorescence, the bleeding at this subdermal margin is brisk and bright red.

B. **Fluorescein angiography.** IV fluorescein is the surgeon's mainstay in assessment of flap viability, because it is the only functional study of the intraoperative circulation. Circulating fluorescein is deposited in the interstitium at the limits of functional capillary circulation and is a highly reliable indicator. Good fluorescence shows as bright chartreuse coloration in the skin portion of the flap when observed with a Wood's light after other lights have been turned off. Spotty fluorescence, which can be equated with viability, is seen as a near confluence of the spots of chartreuse fluorescence. A blue area of nonfluorescence is ironclad evidence of nonviability.

C. **Excision of nonviable portion of flap.** It is our policy to excise the portion of the flap shown to be nonviable by its nonfluorescence unless there are supervening factors of cold or spasm. Biopsy of the questionable flap margin may be helpful in that the surgeon will visualize the dilated Sucquet-Hoyer canals at the margin of the capillary and reticular dermis. This dilatation is not understood, but it may be related to a sluggish flow through these larger vessels that bypass the capillaries; it indicates nonviability. This assessment can be done intraoperatively as a frozen section, if other modalities are inconclusive.

Intraoperative Medications

Drugs to salvage dying flaps have been used experimentally with reported good effect but have been disappointing clinically. It seems that the reconstructive flap either has an adequate blood supply or it does not, and its viability amounts to a "yes" or "no" at the time it is elevated. It is hoped that some breakthrough in pharmacologic management of the microcirculation will be found, but no pharmacologic agent to date has consistently enabled salvation of a nonviable flap. Most clinical reports on this subject are anecdotal.

We have used *isoxsuprine* and *corticosteroids* systemically and *heparin* intradermally, with variable results. *Thorazine* (25 mg orally or rectally 3 times a day) is also a useful adjunct to relieve established spasm. The patient needs to be well hydrated before beginning pharmacologic manipulation.

Operating Room Environment

A cool ambient temperature in the OR can cause problems that are not anticipated. Cold air will cause nonfluorescence or death of flaps that are exposed to cold for a prolonged time. Worse, it can cause the death of a patient who is not monitored by rectal or esophageal temperature probes and is not maintained on a heating blanket. Paper surgical gowns and caps have been a great detriment to reconstructive surgery in this respect, because the surgeon becomes so hot wearing them that an OR temperature of approximately 68° F (20° C) is necessary for comfort in a long operation. The surgeon must be exceedingly concerned about myocutaneous flap viability when the temperature of the patient falls below 95° F (35° C).

Drainage

A. **Choice of drain.** Drains are used when a large area of potential dead space is open; the Jackson-Pratt, Blake, or TLS siliconized drains are preferred.

B. **Number of drains.** We prefer to use at least two drains for a large area, as opposed to the traditional one drain. These drains are placed on wall suction for several days and their outputs are individually recorded.

C. **Positioning of drains.** The Jackson-Pratt drain is not comfortable to the patient at its exit point from the skin. Consequently, the exit point should be situated in an area of relatively denervated skin. The Blake and TLS drains have an advantage in that they are apparently less painful to the patient when removed. Adequate drainage obviates the need for any pressure dressing. In fact, pressure dressings are harmful and are not recommended in the area of a newly positioned flap.

D. **Positioning of patient.** Pressure is further averted after surgery by positioning patients in bed so that they are not lying on the myocutaneous flap. For flaps overlying a pressure area, an *air-fluidized bed* (Clinitron) has been helpful. In this bed, patients can lie directly on the flap without jeopardizing the flap viability.

E. **Removal of drains.** Drains are removed when their output is less than 15 ml in a 24- hour period per drain. If one removes a drain before this time, the likelihood of seroma accumulation is significant. We usually find it better to leave drains in place a little longer rather than remove them too soon.

POSTOPERATIVE CARE

Pain Management

One of the most important aspects of postoperative care is patient comfort. Freedom from pain is a primary consideration and, to achieve it, one may have to give large doses of a narcotic agent such as meperidine, 75 to 100 mg, with or without hydroxyzine hydrochloride, 25 to 50 mg IM every 3 to 4 hours as an antiemetic and narcotic potentiator. The patient-controlled anesthesia (PCA) pump has been helpful in reducing postoperative pain. With this pump, the patient has the ability to self-administer a narcotic (usually morphine) IV, resulting in a relatively steady state of available drug. Anesthesiologists also have been helpful in postoperative pain management. No major reconstructive surgical patient has become addicted to narcotics in our experience. Pain relievers should be given in adequate doses as long as the general condition of the patient allows. The relatively massive dose of methylprednisolone (e.g., 500 to 1,000 mg), which is commonly given on completion of surgery, has the beneficial effect not only of reducing edema formation with minimal risk related to steroid use but also of providing a sensation of euphoria for the patient in the first or second postoperative days. During this period, patients require less pain medication, because of the euphoria. Methylprednisolone has had a significant salutary effect in patient comfort.

Nutrition

Postoperative nutritional support is usually not remarkable unless the patient has an existing nutritional problem. The intention should be to correct negative nitrogen balance as much as possible during the postoperative period so that healing can progress in a normal fashion. IV hyperalimentation is seldom used because less complicated traditional alimentation is possible through small silicone intranasal gastric catheters. We find that an adequate preoperative nutritional status is essential to ensure normal healing. In major reconstructive procedures, we prefer to have the albumin level above 3 g/dl.

Most myocutaneous flap procedures involve significant blood loss, but blood replacement can usually be minimal. Patients are carried with hematocrits of approximately 25% without transfusion, unless there is a factor of hemodynamic instability (See Chapter 7.). In elective reconstructive procedures, autologous or donor-directed blood may help ease the patient's concern over the possibility of a transfusion. Plasma substitutes are used to the utmost in all cases, together with prolonged oral iron therapy to avoid unnecessary transfusion. The old rule requiring a hematocrit of 30% is now considered invalid.

Mobilization

Another aspect of patient comfort is mobility; all patients should be mobilized immediately. With the exception of distal lower-extremity flaps, there are few myocutaneous flaps that cannot be subjected to dependency during mobilization the day after surgery. We also feel that patients should shower after the second postoperative day, even with drains in place. Showering has not been a source of wound infections. Postoperative patients tend to have an improved sense of well- being following a shower. It reinforces the fact that they are definitely healing and recovering. A physician's denial of this comfort is grounded only in old teachings.

Prevention and Management of Hematoma

Surgeons should protect a myocutaneous flap from extremes of heat or cold. Hematoma formation beneath the flap is a particulary unwanted complication. The hematoma has special deleterious effects of its own that are poorly understood. If a hematoma does accumulate, it should be drained atraumatically. Sutures must be released to relieve any pressure, and a drain is usually placed to facilitate removal of this remaining fluid. Drains can be left in place for a prolonged time (weeks if necessary) without worry of infection, which is contrary to previous concepts.

Discharge from Hospital

Patients should be released from the hospital as soon as their condition allows them to return to the activities of daily living that arise in the home situation. This may be days or weeks after an extensive myocutaneous flap reconstruction. Patients should be active participants in the timing of discharge from the hospital. We routinely tell patients to let us know when they are ready to go home. All patients are different with regard to recovery time, and we must understand this. In general, the more we can do to make patients feel normal, the faster will be their recovery. It is often beneficial for patients to complete their postoperative care in an office setting after discharge, because this requires more complete mobilization than is usually undertaken in a hospital milieu. At times it may be difficult for patients and their families to do this, but it apparently promotes an earlier return to normal activity.

Removal of Sutures

Depending on their location, degree of healing, and wound tension, nonabsorbable sutures are removed 1 to 2 weeks (or sometimes longer) after surgery.

Financial and Legal Aspects

Many reconstructions have related financial problems. Patients may require social service support or disability insurance ratings. Physicians must be familiar with the insurance problems that patients may have and must be cognizant of a possible loss of income resulting from the procedure. When reconstructive procedures are performed for injuries subject to litigation, the time of settlement must be judged in part by the surgeon, so that the patient will not be penalized by the prolonged nature of multistage reconstructions.

A patient's financial problems can embroil the surgeon; there is a relatively high incidence of malpractice claims in successful reconstructive procedures. As examples, two vascular patients sued for the loss of a foot after coverage was successfully obtained for the lower third of the tibia but could not be provided for the foot. Because of the reconstructive procedure, the difference to the patient was a below-knee versus an above-knee amputation. To the plastic surgeon this represented surgical success, but to the patient it was a failure.

Lawsuits do not usually result from use of new and unusual procedures in properly informed patients but rather from patient misunderstanding of the goals of reconstruction. It should be clear to the patient and included in the informed consent form that the possibilities of abject failure are always present in attempts at reconstruction. Certainly the greatest cause of medical litigation is the loss of rapport between the surgeon and the patient. We should all remain cognizant of this situation (See Chapter 11.).

FUTURE CHANGE

Surgeons today must be wary of the rare grandiose reconstruction that salvages a "million dollar" finger. An example of this is a replanted finger that never worked and was finally amputated with a loss of 2 years to the patient and a total medical cost that was astronomic. This sort of problem seldom occurs with the myocutaneous flap reconstructive procedures, but it is always possible. One should reasonably expect that today's reconstructive procedures will save society the expense of prolonged hospital and surgical costs related to older methods and save patients from the horrors of nonhealing wounds.

CHAPTER 37

Microsurgery

SALEH M. SHENAQ AND MALCOLM A. LESAVOY

The art and practice of microsurgery essentially is the ability to anastomose vessels that are 1 mm or less in diameter by using suture material that is as small as 18 μm in diameter (with a needle of 50 μm in diameter) and the repair of 1-mm nerves (or 0.2 or 0.3-mm fascicles of nerves) with similar suture material. Students of surgery must avail themselves of the numerous laboratory manuals and books recently published in the actual technique of microsurgery. When one understands the mechanics of this technique, one must then set aside time to practice in a laboratory environment. A clinical operating room (OR) obviously is not the place to learn microsurgery. Thus, microsurgery is not a surgical discipline for the "weekend warrior." It is a surgical discipline that must be continually updated, practiced, and used. It is unlike any other type of plastic surgical construction or reconstruction; it is a pure and somewhat complex technical exercise. Little is left to imagination, with the exception of the actual applications of microsurgery.

REPLANTATION

History of Replantation

Historically, amputation has been the treatment of choice for severely injured limbs. Carrel and Guthrie performed some of the earliest experimental replantation work. They achieved limited success in the canine hind limb replantation technique, which they gained from their pioneering work in vascular repair. In 1962 Malt performed the first successful attachment of a completely amputated arm in a young boy injured in a train accident, and a functional limb was obtained. In 1968, Komatsu and Tamai reported the first successful replantation of a completely amputated digit.

Subsequently, a plethora of reports appeared describing success rate of replantation of digits, indications, and technical refinements. Replantation was extended to other types of tissues in the 1970s such as to the lower extremity and scalp. Today, replantation capabilities are widely available because of the organization of replantation teams in most major trauma centers.

Finger Anatomy

The digital arteries of the metacarpophalangeal joint level measure approximately 1 mm in outer diameter. Digital veins at this level are somewhat larger, (i.e., between 1.2 and 1.5 mm in outer diameter). A digital nerve at this same metacarpophalangeal joint level is approximately 0.8 to 0.9 mm in diameter and contains within its epineurium two or three main fascicles. Amputations proximal to the metacarpophalangeal joint level obviously have larger structures to repair. The brachial artery at the antecubital fossa usually measures 5 to 8 mm in diameter, whereas a digital artery at the middle phalangeal level measures approximately 0.6 to 0.7 mm in diameter.

Principles of Finger Replantation

Principles of reconstructive or traumatic hand surgery apply to all replantation surgery. We agree with Kleinert that all structures should be repaired. In the replantation of a finger, this means that the bone should be appropriately fixed, both flexor tendons and extensor apparatus should be repaired, at least one arterial repair should be accomplished accompanied by one or two dorsal venous anastomoses, and both ulnar and radial digital nerves should be repaired. Only in rare circumstances, such as in crush or severe avulsion, will any of these basic principles be abandoned.

Patient Selection

A. Indications

- ▼ General considerations. The basic philosophy of replantation of fingers or extremities is the restoration of function. A replantation purely for cosmetic reasons is rarely indicated. The overall function of the hand must always be considered, and many factors associated with this function must be queried before acceptance of a patient for replantation. Occupation, hand dominance, number of fingers injured, age, and the presence of systemic or psychiatric disease are important factors for the surgeon to evaluate in making the appropriate decision.

- Multiple- versus singe-digit amputations. A major indication for replantation is multiple-digit amputations proximal to the distal interphalangeal joint. Single-finger amputations usually are not indications for replantation. Single-digit amputation distal to the proximal interphalangeal (PIP) joint on the other hand warrants the replantation. Because total function of the hand is sought, a single finger (with exception of the essential thumb) that is replanted will usually downgrade the function of the entire hand and not be a positive contribution to that hand's function. When multiple digits are amputated however replantation should be attempted for all digits. Exceptions to this rule may be a single-digit amputation in a child or a special circumstance of occupation (e.g., a musician or baseball pitcher). All thumb amputations at the level of the base of the nail and proximal should be replanted. A hand without a thumb is essentially useless, as is the blacksmith's hammer without an anvil. Single-or multiple-digit amputations in children should be replanted because the functional adaptation is more favorable in this group of patients.
- Type of injury. The type of injury as ascertained by taking a complete medical history of the mechanism of amputation, and close examination of the amputated part and the proximal stump may provide positive indications for performing replantation. Clean, guillotine-type amputations are best suited to replantation; severe crush or avulsion injuries are least suited. It should be mentioned however that with the advent of interpositional vein grafts, the limiting factor for replantation today is that of the distal vascular abed. If the distal vascular bed is injured or destroyed, and replantation will be

fruitless. Many hours can be saved by carefully examining the amputated stump. If one finds longitudinal injury of the vascular bundles (as is sometimes evidenced by presence of a red line), this type of finger injury is unsuitable for replantation. If however proximal vessels are destroyed for some distance and the distal vessels are suitable for repair, interpositional vein grafts should be used. Frequently, simultaneous sural nerve grafts also are required to span the gap of damaged or absent nerve tissue.

B. **Contraindications.** Some contraindications to replantation would obviously include the following:

- Arteriosclerotic disease
- Relatively severe diabetes mellitus
- Possible neoplastic disease
- Peptic ulceration, cardiac disease, and pulmonary limitations: These illnesses may preclude the use of anticoagulants, prolonged anesthesia, or both and frequently needed secondary reconstructive procedures.
- Concomitant systemic injuries: Obviously, life-threatening injuries in addition to the amputation must be cared for immediately and replantation must be relegated to a secondary role. It has been our experience in a number of cases in which massive facial and intracranial injuries or intraabdominal penetration and bowel eviscerations were present that replantation was successfully accomplished secondarily.

C. **Patients with psychiatric disease.** Psychiatric disease can be a difficult problem with which to deal. However, it is usually best to attempt to determine as much of the medical history as possible and to try to consult with a psychiatrist before making a decision for replantation. Self-inflicted amputations are done at times of severe mental disturbance; the psychodynamics often are unknown. It is possible that such patients have never been treated on a psychiatric basis before their amputation.

Replantation should be accomplished if possible, and thorough psychiatric evaluation and intensive treatment should be carried out postoperatively. (We once treated a case of penis amputation with replantation; the patient previously had undergone no psychiatric treatment and was extremely grateful for the replantation. A similar case was that of self-inflicted hand amputation in a severely disturbed patient who subsequently underwent replantation and intensive psychiatric therapy. He was extremely grateful for the replantation.)

Preoperative Care

A. **Care at referring hospital.** The following initial preparations must be done before the patient's arrival at the replantation center:

- ▼ Once the call to the emergency room (ER) is received, instructions are given to the referring ER or paramedic team to wrap the severed part in a saline-soaked gauze sponge, enclose the part in a plastic wrapping or place it within a rubber surgical glove, and then immerse the glove in an ice bucket filled with ice and saline or water. Amputated parts must be cared for as described. If this is not carried out, it is possible for amputated parts to be damaged en route. We have had fingers packed in dry ice arrive at the replantation center frostbitten, completely destroyed, and unsuitable for replantation. It is inadvisable for amputated fingers to be immersed in an ice bucket without protective covering because they will become macerated and unacceptable for replantation.
- ▼ After this preparation, the patient, any appropriate radiographic films, and the amputated parts are sent by the fastest means to the replantation center.
- ▼ If the patient being referred for replantation has other major injuries, it is sometimes expedient to have the amputated parts and appropriate radiographic films sent by courier to the replantation center where work can immediately begin on the amputated parts. Meanwhile the patient can be

cared for at the referring hospital and any indicated emergency therapy instituted at that time. When this type of delay is foreseen, hours can be saved by having the replantation team dissect recipient vessels and other appropriate structures on the amputated parts before the patient actually arrives in the replantation center.

B. **Care at replantation center.** The following should occur when the patient arrives at the replantation center:

- ▼ A complete medical history and physical examination must performed.
- ▼ Appropriate laboratory tests should be performed. A complete blood count, prothrombin time, partial thromboplastic time, urinalysis, and other indicated blood studies should be drawn, together with a type and cross-match of four units of blood.
- ▼ If radiographic films have not come with the patient, appropriate views of the amputated parts and the proximal stump should be taken without delay.
- ▼ Broad-spectrum intravenous (IV) antibiotics should be instituted in the ER with tetanus toxoid. Two aspirin suppositories should be given rectally in the ER for their anticoagulant effect (aspirin decreases platelet cohesiveness).
- ▼ Once the decision is made for replantation, the amputated parts can be taken separately to the OR where a special team can start working under magnification and sterile conditions.

C. **Advising patient and family.** Consultation with the patient and patient's family is important in the preoperative preparation. If the patient is asked to decide whether or not to replant, the patient almost always will opt for replantation. This is normal and is to be expected. However, the replantation team should first advise the patient and family as to the possibility of successful replantation and restoration of the overall function of the hand. It is at this point that the surgeon's most difficult decision arises: To replant or not to replant? If a single finger (except the thumb) is amputated, the surgeon should not recommend replantation, although the patient almost always will ask to have the finger replanted. It is the experience of many surgeons that single-finger replantations are detrimental to the overall function of the hand and are not in the best interest of the patient. In many cases, the patient who has undergone traumatic amputation of a single finger is the employed head of a household. If replantation of a single finger is carried out, many months of rehabilitation and possibly further surgery will be needed to obtain good function. If simple closure of the amputation site is accomplished, this patient will be able to return to work after several weeks of absence and be able to provide for the family in the usual fashion. Obviously there are philosophic differences of opinion, and there are exceptions to every rule. However, surgeons in most replantation centers throughout the world have found that single-finger replantations do not serve the best interest of the patient. Simple closure usually provides the best care for the injured individual when the overall function of the hand is the prime consideration.

Intraoperative Care

A. **Anesthesia.** We prefer to use general anesthesia on the patient during replantation surgery and free flap reconstruction for many reasons. The disadvantages of axillary or brachial blocks are their relatively short duration of action and the subsequent increasing restlessness of the patient. Often, 4 to 12 hours (and sometimes longer) is needed for replantation microsurgery or free flaps. Heavy sedation and axillary blocks will not suffice. Even if an indwelling catheter is placed around the brachial plexus and the long-acting local anesthetic bupivacaine (Marcaine) is used, adequate anesthesia often may not be available. Although the positive effects of a sympathetic blockade by a regional block are accomplished, the surgeon still has difficulty in harvesting small vein grafts and sural nerve grafts from the lower extremities without a general anesthetic. For all these reasons, general anesthesia is preferred so that good control of the patient is possible and other indicated procedures can be performed without difficulty.

B. **Wound preparation.** While the patient is undergoing induction of general anesthesia, preparation of the distal amputated fingers or parts is carried out with a surgical scrub. Once the proximal limb is prepared and draped, identification of all tendons, bony structures, digital arteries, dorsal veins, and digital nerves is made both in the proximal stump and in the distal amputated parts. Tagging the tendons with micromosquito clamps and identifying each prospective artery, vein, and nerve with an 8-0 nylon suture saves much time after bone fixation has been accomplished.

C. **Sequence of repair.** It is important for the surgeon to follow this sequence of repair for the anatomic parts of the finger:

- ▼ Bony stabilization must be maintained and secured first. Kirschner wires are inserted for stabilization after the ragged ends of the bone have been débrided.
- ▼ The flexor and extensor tendons are then repaired as in other surgical procedures. It is not within the scope of this chapter to discuss the pros and cons of tenorrhaphy or of profundus and superficialis flexor tendons being repaired together. However, with few exceptions, we repair all tendons. Once the tendon repairs have been completed, stabilization of the digit is accomplished.
- ▼ Attention can now be paid to the vascular repairs:
  - ■ It is generally advisable to perform the venous repairs before the arterial repairs so that blood loss is less. If this is done, an advantage is that the proximal arm tourniquet can be inflated, and microvascular clamps will not be required on the fragile veins. Six to eight interrupted sutures usually are required to anastomose a dorsal finger vein adequately. As a rule, the anastomosis of two veins is better than one for each finger replantation. Once this has been accomplished, a 4-0 or 5-0 nylon suture should be placed approximating the skin overlying the venous anastomoses so that further movement

of the hand and fingers will not disrupt these repairs.

- The hand is then turned with the volar-side up, and the digital arterial anastomosis is accomplished. It is advisable to do this anastomosis with proximal tourniquet control so that the microvascular clamps need not be applied to the 1-mm arteries. Occasionally, these microvascular clamps will be needed to assist the surgeon in orienting and facilitating the actual anastomoses. A 1-mm artery requires 10 to 12 sutures circumferentially for a proper anastomosis. After the anastomosis, the artery is usually in a relatively severe amount of spasm. Constant irrigation with 1% xylocaine (without epinephrine) usually provides relief. Once the anastomoses have been accomplished and the spasm relieved, the proximal arm tourniquet is released, and blood flow to the amputated finger is reconstituted. It usually takes 2 to 4 minutes for good flow to be evident within the amputated part. This time is directly proportional to the duration amount of ischemia.

▼ After vascular reconstruction of the finger, the neural elements are repaired in similar microsurgical fashion. The advent of the operating microscope has added greatly to the functional return of neural repairs and to the patency rate of vascular anastomoses. Because of this, the microscope should be used for all replantations and free flaps.

The sequence of repair of bone, tendon, vein, artery, and nerve should be followed virtually with each replantation. It obviously makes no sense to perform an arterial and nerve repair first and then take the chance, at worst, of disrupting these fragile repairs or, at least, placing the vessels in severe spasm while bony stabilization and tendon repairs are completed.

D. **Maintaining length.** In earlier replantations, relatively significant bony shortening was carried out to relieve tension on arterial and nerve repairs. It now has become commonplace to try to maintain length as much as possible, limited by the amount of skin coverage that is available. Maintenance of length has been made possible by the advent of vein interpositional grafts. If there is a gap of arterial injury, vein injury, or absent segments of nerve, bony stabilization should be maintained along with bone length, and vein grafts should be taken from the dorsum of the foot or the contralateral hand to span the vascular gap. Sural nerve grafts can be harvested to span the nerve gaps.

Postoperative Management

A. **Dressing and splinting.** After the operation is completed, a bulky hand dressing is applied together with either volar or dorsal plaster splints for stabilization.

B. **Elevation.** Elevation is maintained at approximately 45° to allow for adequate venous drainage and for arterial inflow.

C. **Medications.** Postoperatively the patient should receive broad-spectrum IV antibiotics and adequate pain and sleep medication. There is much controversy about the use of postoperative anticoagulation. There are, at this point, no scientific data to support either use or nonuse. Success or failure of replantation depends on the diligence used in operative technique. We believe however that some anticoagulation should be maintained. For this reason, 500 ml of low molecular-weight dextran is given IV every 12 hours for 5 days, and two aspirin (10 grains) are taken orally daily for 2 weeks.

D. **Monitoring.** Constant monitoring of the viability of the replanted finger or the free flap is maintained by the surgeons and the nursing staff by evaluating subjective temperature, capillary fill of the nail beds, and Doppler pulses. It has been demonstrated that if there is decreased arterial flow within the first 12 hours after microvascular replantation, reexploration may salvage a failed replant. After 12 hours, exploration is often useless.

E. **Discharge.** The patient is usually hospitalized for 5 to 6 days after microsurgery and then discharged with broad-spectrum antibiotics and aspirin.

F. **Follow-up therapy.** Follow-up therapy is maintained on an outpatient basis. The usual mobilization, with guarded, passive range of motion, is begun at 4 weeks; active mobilization is begun at 6 weeks. Replanted fingers are treated no differently than other hand cases. Kirschner wires usually are removed at 6 weeks. Subsequent intensive therapy for range of motion and sensory reeducation is mandatory. The patient with replanted digits should be handled by a therapist experienced in hand therapy and rehabilitation. The overall care should be supervised by the treating hand surgeon. Frequently, these patients would require secondary procedures such as tenolysis, capsulotomies, and neurolysis. Such procedures should be carefully undertaken and properly timed when therapy is no longer helpful.

FREE FLAPS

Microvascular surgery has enabled the reconstruction of once unreconstructable cases with the advent of free-tissue transfer using microvascular anastomoses. The principles of dissection and technique are similar to those of replantation and the postoperative management is the same.

Most Common Flaps

The most commonly used free-microvascular flaps include the following:

- Latissimus dorsi musculocutaneous
- Rectus abdominis musculocutaneous
- Scapular flap
- Lateral arm flap
- Radial forearm flap
- Temporalis fascia flap
- Fibula flap
- Bowel flap
- Omental flap

Indications

The clinical applications of free flaps have expanded tremendously in the past decade. Most of the surgical disciplines as in plastic surgery, orthopedics, cardiovascular and thoracic surgery, obstetrics, gynecology, urology, and head and neck have advanced as a result of reconstruction using microsurgical free-flap transfer. Defect whether traumatic, congenital, surgical, or secondary to irradiation or infections could be salvaged with the technique of free-flap transfer regardless of age of patient or location of defect. Specific indications are primarily dictated by the composite nature of the defect and goal of reconstruction. Form and functional restoration must be achieved. The mere survival of a free flap is not a true index for the success of reconstruction.

CHAPTER 38

Free Tissue Transfer

Saleh M. Shenaq and Tue Anh Dinh

Free tissue transfer is a relatively new field in the specialty of reconstructive surgery. The advances in free tissue transfer have arrived with the advances in microsurgery, which is the specialty involving the manipulation of tissue under high optical magnification offered by the microscope or high powered loupes. Microsurgery includes microvascular surgery and microneural surgery. The history of microsurgery started with Carrel and Guthrie, the fathers of vascular surgery, who first described earlier this century the triangulation method for anastomosis of small vessels. In 1921 Nylen was the first to use the microscope to aid in surgery. However, the microscope and surgical instruments at that time were not conducive to surgery performed under the microscope. In 1960 Jacobson and Suarez were first to report patency of small vessels after microsurgical repairs. In 1962 Malt and McKhann galvanized the entire medical world with the report of a successful replantation of an amputated arm in a young boy. This is the impetus that encouraged many of the investigators to push forward and expand new frontiers of microsurgery and free flap reconstruction. Komatsu and Tamai in 1965 were first to replant a traumatically amputated thumb successfully. In the following decade Buncke, Daniel, and Taylor, and Harri and Ohmori along with many others described many flaps that could be transferred for reconstruction. Advances in microsurgery, such as improved microsurgical techniques and instruments combined with increased understanding of the flap anatomy and vascular supply, have made free flap transfer a safe and effective method for reconstruction of difficult defects. Currently, free flap transfer is an accepted method to reconstruct physical defects and has an expected success rate of more than 95%.

CONSIDERATION FOR FREE FLAP RECONSTRUCTION

Before choosing a free flap, one must consider the objective of the reconstruction. The return of function after reconstruction should be the primary objective. Whether the objective is the restoration of movement, protective coverage of exposed vital structure, or bridging a nerve gap to restore neural continuity, simple options should first be considered. The ladder of reconstruction should be followed. If equally acceptable results are achieved by a more simple method, then that method is preferred. One should consider other reconstructive options including direct closure, skin graft, local or regional flap, and tissue expansion before deciding on the use of free flap or prefabricated free flap.

Factors in Flap Selection

Once free flap reconstruction is deemed necessary, then flap selection should be based on the following factors:

- Type of tissue required for reconstruction (should resemble native tissue)
- Similarities between size and shape of flap and defect
- Anatomic consideration: length of vascular pedicle that is required to provide a tension free anastomosis with recipient vessel; vein graft should be avoided if possible
- Extent of donor site morbidity (concealed versus visible scar), need for skin graft to cover donor site, loss of function at donor site, potential complication (i.e., hernia)
- Patient factors: age (especially in children because size of their vessels are smaller and there is need for growth; arthrosclerosis should be considered in older patients)
- Ease of procedure, depending on flap's anatomy and surgeon's experience and comfort with flap

Risk Factors for Flap Failure

Before any free flap transfer, the patient should be examined carefully for factors that may increase the risk of flap failure. The following factors should be eliminated or controlled before surgery whenever possible:

- ▼ Smoking should be stopped 2 weeks before surgery, and no smoking should be allowed for 4 weeks after flap transfer.
- ▼ The use of anticoagulants and aspirin may be required after flap transfer; however, these medications are stopped before surgery.
- ▼ Other risk factors include systemic disease, such as cancer or hypercoagulable state that could increase the risk of thrombosis. Systemic diseases that decrease peripheral perfusion such as congestive heart failure or peripheral vascular disease may also compromise the flap.

SURGICAL PROCEDURE

Free Flap Transfer

After a flap has been chosen according to the previously listed factors and after optimum conditions for success have been obtained, one can proceed with free flap transfer. The surgery begins with exploration and preparation of the defect. Any débridement that is required is done at this time, and the recipient vessels and nerves are dissected and isolated. The quality of the vessels (i.e., size and blood flow) and the quality of the nerve are assessed at this time before starting the flap elevation. Then a template is usually made of the defect by tracing the defect and the location of the recipient vessel and nerve over a piece of sterile paper. The donor flap is then designed, using this template. The flap is then elevated until it is free with the exception of the supplying artery and veins. At this time, one can examine the perfusion of the flap especially at its distal edges to ensure that the flap can survive on the planned donor vessels. After this proves satisfactory, the donor vessels can be divided and transferred to the recipient site.

Anastomosis

After transfer, the arterial anastomosis is performed before the venous anastomosis. The neural anastomosis can be performed next or at the end of the case before the final setting of the flap.

A. **Type of anastomosis.** The type of anastomosis depends on the size discrepancy between the recipient and donor vessels and also the possible morbidity in diverting blood flow from the end organ. The most common anastomosis is end-to-end. This requires that the two vessels be of similar size. For size discrepancy of less than 50%, mechanical dilatation of the smaller vessel is usually sufficient for end-to-end reanastomosis. End-to-side anastomosis is usually reserved for size discrepancy of more than 100% and when the elimination of distal donor vessel blood flow is detrimental.

B. **Continuous versus interrupted suture.** The use of continuous versus interrupted suture for reanastomosis is dependent on the surgeon's preference. Continuous suture has a higher chance of vessel constricture but can be performed faster. The patency rate between continuous versus interrupted suture is similar.

C. **Assessment of patency.** The "milk test" is usually performed to assess the patency of the anastomosis. Using two microforceps, a distal segment of the vessel is emptied of blood and then the microforceps are sequentially released to assess vessel refill. During this time, one must be observant of spasm and thrombus formation inside the reanastomosed vessel. Thrombus can be of the *white clot type,* which consists mostly of fibrin, or the *red clot type,* which consists mostly of platelets. The risk of thrombus formation is decreased with gentle handling of the tissue, complete resection of the damaged vessel wall before anastomosis, and by accurate opposition of the edges. The use of heparinized solution (50 units/ml) for irrigation and avoidance of tension during the anastomosis will also help in this respect.

D. **Spasm and its management.** Spasm is a physiologic response resulting in vasoconstriction and usually leads to thrombus formation. The treatment for spasm includes the application or irrigation with 2% lidocaine solution during the entire procedure, application of external verapamil, intraarterial papaverine or Phentolamine. Mechanical dilation with jeweler's forceps, hydrodistension of the lumen of the vessels with heparinized saline, and stripping of the adventitia will also decrease the risk. Side branches of the vessel should be ligated with sutures to decrease the propagation of spasm. Despite all these precautions, one still may encounter a no-reflow phenomenon that is manifested by the failure to reperfuse the flap despite successful anastomosis. This could be as a result of intravascular aggregation of debris, swelling of the cell in the vessel wall, or a high level of vasoconstricting prostaglandin. This risk increases with increasing ischemia time. One can attempt to chemically dilate the vessel; however, most cases require resectioning of the no-flow segment and reanastomosis.

Securing of Flap and Drains

After successful anastomoses, the flap is usually inset and secured in place with absorbable sutures. Usually one or two drains are placed underneath the flap to evacuate any possible hematoma.

POSTOPERATIVE CARE

The healing of the vessel reanastomosis usually starts by 3 days and is complete within 1 month. Healing starts by formation of pseudointima and differentiation of myoendothelial cells from the reanastomosed ends to regenerate the endothelial layer.

Postoperative Monitoring

Postoperative monitoring, in our experience, is best done by clinical examination. The flap is checked for color, warmth, and capillary refill every hour for the first 24 hours, then every 2 hours for the next 24 hours, and then every 4 hours. Trained nursing staff familiar with free flap procedures and their postoperative care should be available during this critical period. A surface Doppler may be used to assess arterial patency; however, venous patency is not assessed by this method.

Environmental Control

A well-controlled postoperative environment is essential for the success of the free-flap transfer. Generally, we recommend keeping the room warm (above 35° C). Tobacco is prohibited near the patient to avoid second-hand smoke effects, and the patient is not allowed any caffeine which is found especially in tea, coffee, and chocolate.

Medications

Many postoperative medications have been used to increase the success of the transferred flap. The most common is dextran, which is a polysaccharide with a 40,000 Dalton molecular weight. Dextran affects platelet adhesion and also coagulation factor VIII (antihemophilic factor). It also increases colloid oncotic pressure that increases blood flow to the flap. However, this can cause fluid overload in a cardiovascularly compromised patient. Aspirin inhibits cyclooxygenase and platelet function and is effective at low doses (5 mg/kg/day). Streptokinase can be used to convert plasminogen to plasma, which promotes clot dissolution. Heparin acts to prevent clot formation.

A. **Dextran.** Our current recommendation for postoperative free flap care includes the routine use of dextran solution at the rate of 10 to 25 ml/hr. Dextran is usually started at the conclusion of the arterial anastomosis.
B. **Heparin and lidocaine.** Heparin and lidocaine solutions are used as a local irrigant. The use of systemic heparin is indicated if there is questionable anastomosis or the extensive use of vein graft. Usually, heparin is given in a bolus dose of 5,000 units at the beginning and 100 to 200 units/hr for prophylaxis afterwards.
C. **Streptokinase.** We occasionally use streptokinase if an established thrombus is persistent at the site of the anastomosis.

Use of Leeches

During the postoperative course if venous congestion is persistent, the use of leeches could be beneficial. The leeches are changed every 4 hours, and each leech can remove approximately 30 ml of congested blood.

COMMONLY USED FLAPS

Muscle and Musculocutaneous Flaps

A. **Latissimus dorsi flap.** The latissimus dorsi flap is a popular flap that provides a large amount of free tissue;

is easy to transfer by relatively inexperienced surgeons; and has a reliable, long, and large vascular pedicle. The latissimus dorsi muscle can be transferred in its entirety or in part and can also include the overlying skin. The muscle is supplied by the thoracodorsal artery that arises from the subscapular artery that is from the axillary artery. Venous drainage occurs from the venae comitantes that drain to the thoracodorsal and axillary veins. The muscle is also supplied by a nerve that divides into an anterior and posterior branch. This flap provides a large amount of tissue, and a large skin area measuring approximately 40 by 20 cm can be included. The length of the pedicle can be as long as 10 cm. The donor scar can be oriented transversely or obliquely across the back. Functionally, the loss of the latissimus muscle results in little morbidity. This flap is commonly the first choice in many reconstructions requiring large tissue coverage.

B. **Rectus abdominis flap.** The rectus abdominis can be transferred as a muscle and also as a musculocutaneous flap. This muscle also provides a large amount of tissue, and it gives the surgeon a choice in design variation of the flap in terms of shape and size. The muscle is supplied by the superior and inferior epigastric vessel. The main pedicle is the inferior epigastric that arises from the external iliac artery and enters the muscle from its underside. There are perforators that supply the skin that radiates from around the umbilicus. Venous drainage is along venae comitantes. The vascular supply of this muscle is reliable, and the design of the flap and its overlying skin area can be oriented transversely or obliquely. This flap is commonly used for reconstruction of the breast however removal of this muscle may result in weakness of the anterior abdominal wall. In women of child-bearing age and in an athletic individual, this may be a contraindication.

Sensate Skin Flaps

A. **Lateral arm flap.** The lateral arm flap is based on the posterior radial collateral artery, which is a branch of the profunda brachii. The posterior radial collateral artery anastomoses with the interosseous recurrent artery in the region of the lateral epicondyle. It gives out perforating branches through the lateral intermuscular septum to the skin area on the posterior lateral aspect of the upper arm. It also provides blood supply to the underlying humerus. The venous drainage is through venae comitantes. The skin is innervated by branches of the posterior cutaneous nerve of the arm, which is a branch of the radial nerve. This flap is preferable because of the thin and sensate skin that it provides along with a 6- to 10-cm vascular pedicle. There is little donor site morbidity. The skin of this flap is thin, supple, and hairless. This flap can also include vascularized bone (i.e., part of humerus). This flap is the usual first choice for coverage of any defect requiring sensate skin.

B. **Dorsalis pedis flap.** The dorsalis pedis sensate flap is based on the dorsalis artery, which is the terminal branch of the anterior tibial artery. It covers almost the entire dorsum of the foot. Venous drainage is largely through the long saphenous vein. Most of this flap is supplied by terminal branches of the superficial peroneal nerve, but the first interdigital web space is supplied by the deep peroneal nerve. This flap is useful, because it provides thin, good sensate skin. This is especially applicable for reconstruction of hand defects. However, this flap is difficult to raise, and the donor defect is difficult to close. Usually, a skin graft is required to cover the exposed extensor tendons.

Osteo and Osteomusculocutaneous Flaps

A. **Fibula vascularized osseous flap.** The fibula is an excellent donor site for vascularized bone. Almost the entire fibula except the distal 6 cm and proximal 4 cm can be transferred. The fibula receives blood supply from a nutrient artery from the peroneal artery. This artery enters the periosteum of the fibula approximately at its midpoint. The length of the pedicle can be as long as 8 to 10 cm. Venous drainage is also through venae comitantes. A segment of skin above the fibula on the lateral leg can be included in the flap; this requires that the deep fascia be included to protect the fasciocutaneous perforator. The donor defect can be closed primarily, and the resultant donor morbidity is minimal. The fibula is a strong cortical bone that is often used to reconstruct the opposite leg's defect or in mandibular reconstruction.

B. **Deep circumflex iliac osteocutaneous flap.** The deep circumflex iliac flap includes a portion of the bone from the iliac crest and the overlying skin. The flap is based on the deep circumflex iliac artery (DCIA) that is a branch of the external iliac artery arising just above the inguinal ligament. The DCIA supplies a nutrient branch to the iliac bones and also has perforators that supply the overlying skin. Venous drainage is through venae comitantes that untie to form a large single vein and drain into the external iliac vein. The flap is raised as a single block taking a portion of the iliac bone at the anterior curvature and the overlying muscle and ellipse of skin. The curvature of the iliac crest renders it suitable for replacement of bone defects in the head and neck area, especially for reconstruction of the mandible. This flap can be difficult to raise, and the vascular pedicle is short, but the donor site can be closed primarily with little morbidity.

Miscellaneous Flaps

A. **Free jejunal transfer.** The jejunum is usually used to reconstruct defects of the upper gastrointestinal tract. Usually the second loop of the jejunum is taken. The jejunum is supplied by branches from the superior mesenteric artery. Venous drainage accompanies the artery. The vascular pedicle of this flap is as long as 20 cm. The flap is reliable, however, there is additional morbidity with laparotomy.

B. **Temporoparietal fascial flap.** The temporoparietal fascial flap is based on the superficial temporal artery and vein. The procedure involves elevation of scalp flaps to expose the underlying fascia, which then can be removed. The amount of fascia available is rather small and fan-shaped, and the supplying vessel pedicle is short. However, this is an excellent vascularized fascia that can later be skin grafted, and the donor site is inconspicuous.

C. **Second toe free flap.** The second toe free flap is used to reconstruct the thumb. This flap is based on the first dorsal metatarsal artery that is a terminal branch of the dorsalis pedis vessel. The second toe with the surrounding skin, along with the second metatarsal bone and tendon, can be removed. The skin around the second toe is supplied by branches from both the superficial peroneal nerve and the deep peroneal nerve. The dissection and elevation of this flap are difficult, however, it is an excellent substitute for the thumb.

CHAPTER 39

Cutaneous Laser Surgery

Joseph Agris

Laser surgery is a fast-developing new medical field in which the range of applicability is only now becoming evident. Patient care in laser surgery is becoming more advanced and uniform as use of lasers increases. All lasers emit light in the visible portion of the electromagnetic spectrum. Common factors to all lasers are frequency, wavelength, and energy source of photons. Lasers vary in wavelength and power range. Some are used directly and others with fiberoptic cables, which can be directly coupled through microscopes on articulated arms.

Types of Lasers

There are many types of lasers: helium, neon, ruby, argon, and carbon dioxide. In the electromagnetic spectrum, the ruby laser is located in the red portion, the argon laser in the green, and the carbon dioxide laser in the infrared (Fig. 39-1). Each type of laser has its own specific characteristics; they are not interchangeable in their applications.

The argon laser emits visible light of low energy. The light is nonionizing and unlike x-radiation. As the wavelength becomes longer, there is a decrease in the ionizing effect. No dysplasia results from its use.

Properties of Laser Light

A laser beam is nothing more than an oscillating form of light created in a tube. It has a high degree of uniformity and a low degree of efficiency. In the argon laser, argon is placed into a long, resinating tube with a totally reflecting mirror at one end and a partially reflecting mirror at the other end. A high-voltage electric current is then added. The system is activated by the electric current, which raises ions of argon

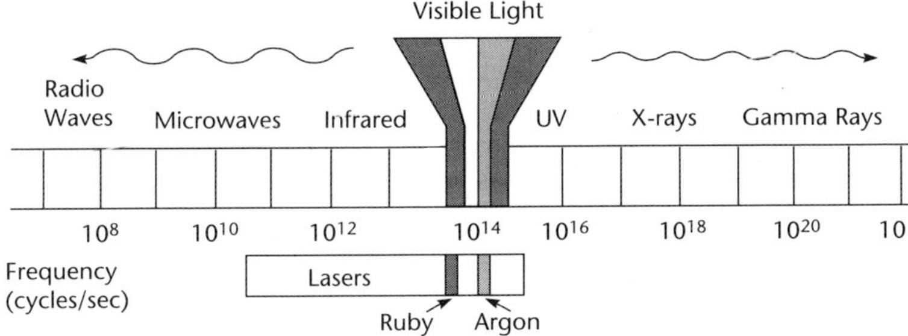

FIG. 39-1 *Argon laser photocoagulator functions within green spectrum of electric magnetic field.*

to a higher energy level, causing them to emit quanta of radiant energy (photons); the photons strike the mirrors setting up an oscillation. As the photons oscillate between the two mirrors in the tube, they begin to move up and back in parallel without divergence, stimulating emission of more photons and producing a narrow, intense, and uniform beam of light (Fig. 39-2).

A. **Wavelengths.** As the wavelength is increased, the transmittance is decreased. Therefore the short wave (green spectrum) of the argon laser has no effect in the superficial layer of the skin. Within the first 30μm of tissue depth there is no effect when the argon laser is used because of the high preferential absorption; the argon laser concentrates its effect in the dermis (Fig. 39-3). Red blood cells in the dermal layer will absorb almost 100% of the energy emitted; while blood cells absorb nothing. The light energy is converted to heat energy when it is absorbed by the vascular lesion of the dermal layer. The heat released results in protein coagulation and obliteration of vascular dermal structures. There is no effect on skin appendages such as hair follicles, sweat glands, or sebaceous glands.
B. **Argon versus carbon dioxide.** It is important to understand the difference between the action of the argon laser and the CO_2 laser. The argon laser transmits in the blue-green visible spectrum a light whose selective absorption results in the conversion of light energy to heat energy and ultimately coagulation in the dermal layer. The CO_2 laser in comparison has a long wavelength and

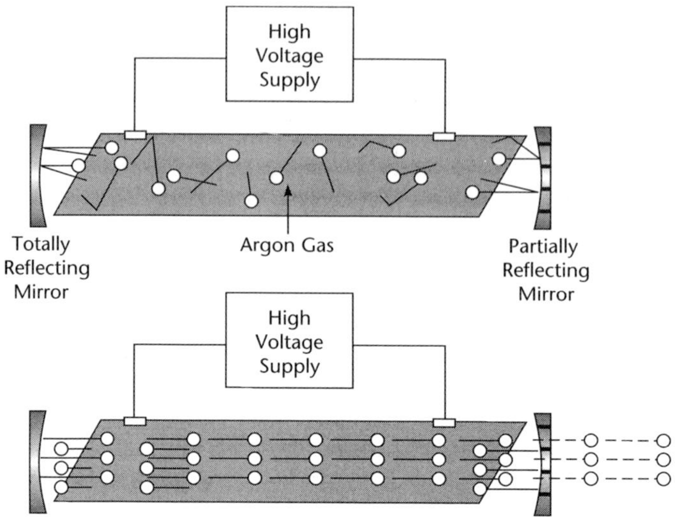

Fig. 39-2 *Argon gas molecules move randomly within laser tube. When high-voltage electric supply is added, molecules move in parallel rows. This is enhanced by reflecting mirror at each end of tube. Pure light source is produced that is released through openings in partially reflecting mirror.*

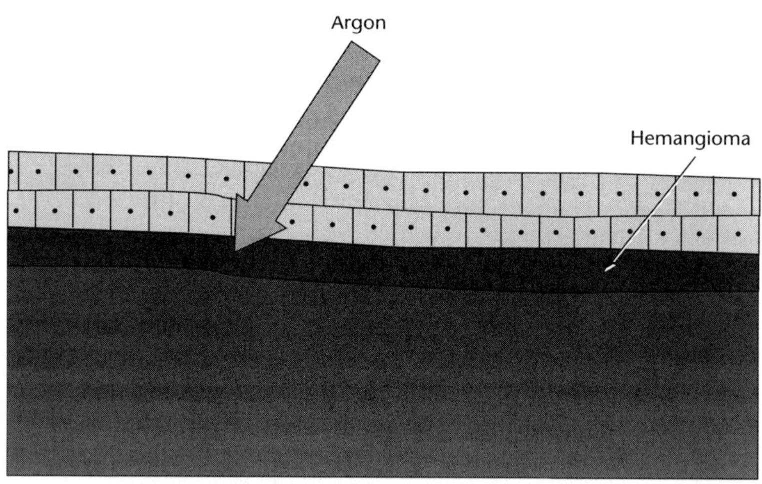

Fig. 39-3 *Argon laser does not effect first 30 μm of tissue depth and focuses on lesions below skin surface.*

operates in the infrared portion of electromagnetic spectrum (i.e. 90% of the CO_2 laser's emission is absorbed within the first 30 µm of tissue, so the CO_2 laser acts as an electrosurgical knife, vaporizing tissue with minimal bleeding, cell by cell, beginning at the skin surface). The argon laser is effective as a coagulating laser (not a cutting laser); its action is in the dermis and not on the skin surface. The CO_2 laser will destroy skin and its appendages (Fig. 39-4).

The specific characteristics of the CO_2 and argon lasers determine their interactions with biologic tissue that in turn determine their specific medical applications. They are not interchangeable in their uses.

MEDICAL USES OF ARGON LASER

The argon has been used for many years in ophthalmology for retinal photocoagulation. It also has been used for the treatment of cutaneous skin lesions such as hemangiomas (port-wine birthmarks), telangiectasia, cherry angiomata, and superficial spider varicosities. It recently has proved useful for the removal of decorative tattoos. With appropriate adjunctive equipment, the argon laser also can be used for endoscopic hemostasis throughout the gastrointestinal tract.

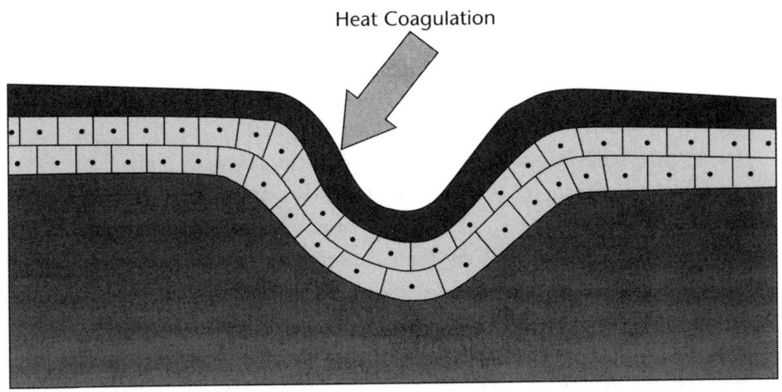

FIG. 39-4 *Carbon dioxide laser acts as "optical scalpel" that begins cutting at skin surface, removing all layers of tissue.*

In comparison, the CO_2 laser is used as an electrosurgical knife of optical scalpel. The CO_2 laser was used first to minimize bleeding, and later for debridement of pressure ulcers and burns. Its use was extended to cutaneous lesions such as veruccae, condylomata, nevi, melanomas, and other carcinomas. It has recently been adapted for treatment of lesions of the cervix and also has been modified for use by the otolaryngologist for the treatment of inner ear problems, removal of vascular nasal lesions, and in turbinectomy and tonsillectomy. The most recent application of the CO_2 laser has been its introduction into operative dentistry for the removal of intraoral lesions and the treatment of gingival disease. It must be remembered that the CO_2 dioxide laser is an electrosurgical knife (best thought of as an "optical scalpel").

TREATMENT OF PORT-WINE HEMANGIOMAS

Until the argon laser was applied to the treatment of port-wine hemangiomas, various modalities were used, none produced a satisfactory result and many left detrimental residuals.

Comparison of Modalities

A. **Radiation therapy.** Initially, radiation therapy was used with promising results; however, atrophy of the developing underlying structures, including bone and subcutaneous tissue, resulted. After many years, chronic radiation changes appeared in the skin with hyperpigmentation and hypopigmentation, telangiectasia, ulceration, and, in some cases, carcinogenic changes.

B. **Local and sclerosing agents.** Local agents such as liquid nitrogen formerly were placed on the lesion. This resulted in second- and third-degree burns with subsequent scarring. The decrease in color, if any occurred, was the result of oblation of the vessels, with deposition of scar. Sclerosing agents were injected into these lesions at repeated intervals, but they too resulted in minimal oblation and secondary scarring.

C. **Excision.** Surgical excision has always been effective, especially for smaller lesions, when the scar can be hidden in the natural cutaneous lines and shadow areas. Serial excisions of larger lesions have been attempted, but the resultant scar has always been a problem. En bloc excision and reconstruction with a flap or a skin graft can lead to injury of the underlying nerves, especially in the facial area. It is difficult because of the amount of blood in the operative field as well as the extensive blood loss that can occur. Therefore excision has not been felt to be satisfactory for large lesions.

D. **Tattooing.** Surgical overtattooing of the lesion provides some temporary benefits; however, the tattooing must be periodically "touched up" as the pigment is absorbed and removed by the action of the sunlight. With repeated tattoo procedures, hypertrophic scarring results.

E. **Argon laser.** The argon laser, with its high preferential absorption by vascular lesions in the dermal layer, has proved to be the most useful modality available today for the treatment of these lesions. At present, the argon laser's selective coagulation at 0.5 mm below the skin surface while sparing skin appendage and producing minimal histopathologic changes without ionization currently makes it the modality of choice. The original investigative work was carried out by Goldman and later by Maser, Apfelberg, and Lash. Port-wine hemangiomas are common congenital vascular lesions that can occur anywhere on the body but are seen most frequently in the head and neck area. They are noninherited, congenital, disfiguring, and functionally disabling lesions. Port-wine hemangiomas persist into adult life, often becoming more pronounced (elevated or corrugated) as the individual advances in age and loses the supporting elastic fiber of the skin and around the vessels. It is common for these lesions to attain a deeper color as the patient gets older.

Facial Quadrants

If the face is divided into four quadrants by drawing a line transversely through the pupils of the eyes and a second line vertically down the midline, some interesting relationships are developed (Fig. 39-5). Lesions that involve three or more quadrants of the face have a 10% association of unilateral glaucoma. The involved eye, as would be expected, is on the side of the face that is most involved with the hemangioma. In addition, patients with three or more quadrants of the face involved have a 5% incidence of seizure. This is a result of involvement of the choroid and the pia mater with hemangioma. Seizures may appear shortly after birth and any time until puberty. They are easily controlled with the standard antiepileptic medications such as phenytoin (Dilantin); in addition, when lesions involve two quadrants of

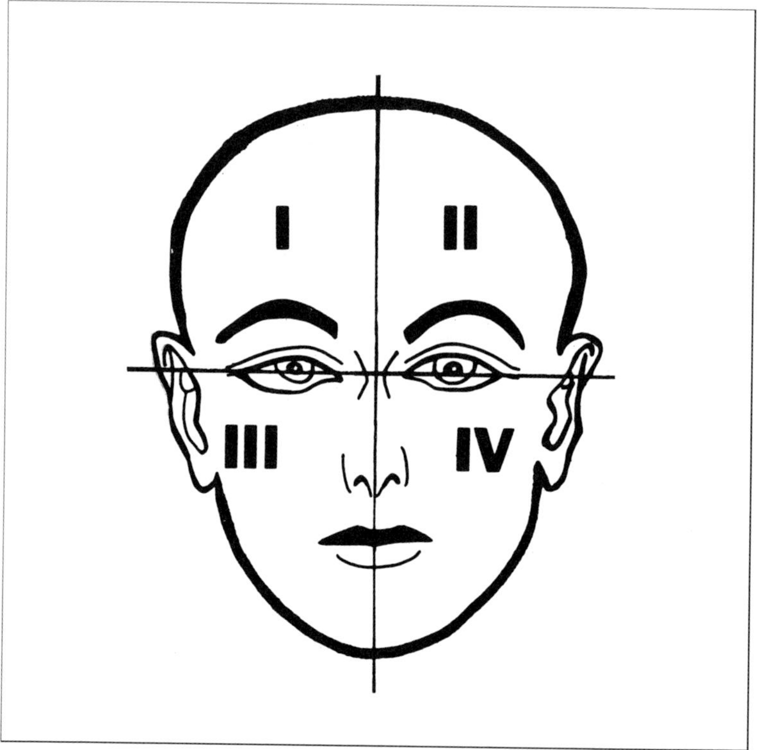

Fig. 39-5 *Face has been divided into four quadrants. When nevus flammeus involves any three quadrants, there is 10% incidence of glaucoma in eye on most affected side and 5% incidence of seizures. When both occur together, it is called Sturge-Weber syndrome.*

the face, to the right and left of the midline, as well as a third area at some other location on the body, secondary anomalies such as glaucoma and seizure also may occur. Parents and responsible parties should be made aware of the possibility of these problems when a child is found to have three or more quadrants of the face involved. When both glaucoma and seizure are present, the condition is known as *Sturge-Weber syndrome.*

Patient Treatment Procedures

A. **Test patch.** After a complete medical history and examination, all patients receive a "test patch." The purpose of the test patch is to determine the response of the lesion to the argon laser. An area of approximately 2 cm^2 is selected. The Cooper model 770-05 Photocoagulator is maintained in an outpatient surgical suite, which provides safety and an operating room atmosphere, with the option of both local and general anesthesia.

The majority of the patients (more than 90%) are treated as outpatients under local anesthesia (lidocaine, 1%, without epinephrine). The laser delivers a maximum power of 5 watt through a fiberoptic cable to a pencil-tipped hand piece that emits a 5-mm laser beam. The 2-cm^2 test patch takes approximately 10 to 15 minutes using a 5-mm probe at 1.6 to 1.8 watt with a pulsation of 0.5 seconds. Photographs are taken before and after using color-control patches to insure uniformity. Meticulous records are kept that include date, time, area treated, watt seconds, and pulsation. When the test patch is completed, the immediate effect of the laser treatment is noted. The area is much lighter in color than the surrounding tissue because the blood vessels in the treated area have become coagulated. Within 3 to 5 days, a scab or small crust may form. This usually persists for 10 to 15 days. The patient is given a topical antibiotic and is directed to apply it to the test patch area tid. In addition, the patient is instructed to keep the area as clean as possible. The patient is warned not to pick at the scab but to allow it to separate spontaneously. The only restriction it to minimize strenuous physical activities that would cause excessive perspiration. Other than this, the patient can conduct any normal daily activities unhindered.

After the crusting has separated spontaneously, the test patch will remain lighter than the surrounding tissue for 2 to 3 weeks. It gradually attains a pink hue. This does not indicate that the hemangioma is recurring. This pink hue is the usual reaction of the skin to the laser treatment. It will fade gradually over the next 12 to 18 months. However, the majority of the fading occurs within 3 to 4 months after treatment. At this time, the patient returns for reevaluation of the test patch. If fading is substantial and there is minimal depression with little or no surrounding scarring, a treatment program is established with 6-week to 3-month intervals between each treatment.

B. **Dividing treatments.** A treatment plan is established, dividing the facial area into temporal, orbital, facial, submandibular, and postauricular quadrants. Depending on the size of the lesion, from one to six outpatient visits are required to complete treatment. The Cooper model 770-05 Photocoagualtor is used with a 5-mm probe. From 1.6 to 2.2 watt is administered depending on the response of the lesion and the results of the test patch. The laser is used in a present mode to fire every 0.5 seconds.

   Lesions smaller than 4 cm^2 are treated en bloc. Larger lesions are treated by using a striping technique (i.e., 4-mm bands of treated tissue are alternated with 2-mm bands of untreated tissue). The striping follows the direction of the lines of the facial contour. The cheek and temporal area is treated by directing the laser beam in transverse direction, whereas the lip is treated in a vertical direction.

   With completion of the laser surgery, a topical antibiotic is applied. The patient is instructed to keep the area clean with a mild soap-and-water solution and to reapply the antibiotic ointment 3 times a day until any scabs that have developed separate spontaneously. The patient is instructed to avoid exposure to the sun. Vigorous exercise is forbidden. When treating the eyelids and periorbital area, moderate edema beginning shortly after treatment and lasting 3 to 5 days can be expected. This is explained to the patient before treating this area. Edema in the brow and facial area is minimal and presents no problem.

The striping technique alternates 4-mm stripes of treated with nontreated tissue. However, when the patient returns in 6 weeks to 3 months for continued therapy, it is noted that the untreated areas are usually 1 to 2 mm in width. It is thought that the action of the laser extends beyond the treated area. Vessels are being coagulated that feed the adjacent untreated 4-mm bands. Therefore fading of the lesion occurs beyond the treated area. This has several definite advantages.

A smaller area (25% to 50%) or less will require laser surgery on subsequent visits. This in turn reduces the operating time, minimizes the anesthetic need, reduces the chances of scarring, decreases the total watt seconds of exposure, and adds to the patient's comfort. Economically the cost and time factor is appreciably reduced.

The patient returns at 6-week to 3-month intervals until the entire area has been treated. A touch-up is undertaken in any of the previously healed quadrants as needed, and a new quadrant is then treated by the striping technique.

LIMITATIONS OF ARGON LASER TREATMENT

Incomplete Obliteration

It is important to realize that the argon laser photocoagulator will not completely eliminate all hemangiomas. At best, the laser will produce a noticeable lightening of the birthmark. The degree of lightening that occurs depends on:

- ▼ Color of the birthmark (pink, pink-red, red, red-purple, purple, and purple-black)
- ▼ Patient's natural skin tone (lighter the complexion of individual, better the result)
- ▼ Consistency of the skin

For example, deep-purple birthmarks may exhibit remnants with a light-violet hue, while birthmarks that are red in color often exhibit pale-pink remants. Currently, we are just beginning to touch up these areas; however, neither enough time has elapsed nor have enough patients been completely treated to permit accurate assessment of the secondary treatment to these areas. Patients are usually able to eliminate the use of makeup or switch from tedious, time-consuming applications of thick makeup (e.g., Cover Mark) to standard over-the-counter makeup. In no case has 100% obliteration of the birthmark resulted after laser treatment.

In older lesions that are elevated, corrugated, and spongy in appearance, not only is the coloration altered, but a striking improvement is noted in the surface texture. The corrugations become flat, and the sponginess shrinks, resulting in a much smoother surface. This effect on older lesions with the reduction in pigmentation allows the patient who was previously unable to apply makeup the opportunity to use it.

Scarring

Another potential limitation of laser treatment is that a number of patients (approximately 15%) develop some scarring.

A. **Site of lesion.** When scarring does occur, it seems more frequent in the nasolabial fold area, along the upper lip, and at the base of the nose and columella. Rarely does scarring occur in the periorbital area, brow, or face.

B. **Age of patient.** Scarring is more likely to occur in younger individuals and remain raised, red, and indurated for longer periods. This is particularly true in infants and young children. Because of the prolonged period of induration and erythema and the necessity for general anesthesia in infants, we prefer to wait until the child is older. However, this does not preclude the conducting of a test patch area at any age using local anesthesia on an outpatient basis. This still can be used as one of the criteria for treating or not treating a lesion at that time.

NEW LASER DEVELOPMENT

Application of the laser and its effect are the deciding factors in which type of laser to use and where to apply it. In the treatment of port-wine lesions, the argon laser made a significant improvement and was the recognized treatment modality for these lesions. However, there are some inherent problems with the use of the argon laser, especially in children. Specifically, unwanted scarring occurred. This is not scarring as we usually think of it but usually hypopigmentation or depigmentation of the area treated. In addition, specific areas such as upper lip, the commissure, and the angle of the mandible seemed more prone to this type of scarring, especially in younger individuals. Also, the use of the argon laser requires experience and skill to determine the endpoints, and when adhered to, good results can be obtained.

With the desire to treat children sooner in order to avoid some of the psychologic and sustained physical handicaps of the port-wine lesions, other lasers were developed. Damage to the skin could be controlled at least in part by the choice of the wavelength. With this in mind, research was directed at the absorption spectrum of oxyhemoglobin. Oxyhemoglobin demonstrates three peaks on the chromophore. The third peak (577 nm) was selected because of the advantages of better depth of penetration and less competitive absorption from other pigments such as melanin, which is also present in the skin. This type of wavelength control confined the absorbed laser energy. This reduces scarring and pigmentation changes.

Pulsed Tunable Dye Laser

The pulsed tunable dye laser at 577 nm can selectively target oxyhemoglobin, lessening peripheral damage. There is less risk of change in pigmentation and scarring, especially in children. The pulsed tunable dye laser uses a pulsed width of 450 μsec, which causes minimal epidermal damage while vascular destruction is achieved with a transient local temperature rise destroying the blood vessels. Yet minimal extravascular damage is incurred. No studies have shown that this laser's wavelength affects endothelial cells or peripheral fibroblasts except for the thermal damage to blood vessels.

Copper Vapor Lasers

The copper laser uses a yellow light. The reason for using a yellow light is because it would be less sparing of nontarget tissue. In addition, the yellow light has a better absorption by oxyhemoglobin. There is also more filtering of skin melanin. Therefore the laser penetrates deeper with greater energy to the selected target. As such, there is less tissue damage to nontarget areas with the yellow copper vapor laser than with other modalities. Copper also has an intrinsic high gain. This results in low cooling requirements and is more efficient than other visible light sources. The light of the copper vapor laser is delivered in short pulses at high repetition rates appearing continuous to the naked eye. The copper vapor laser also gives one the choice of precise wavelengths. A yellow wavelength (578.2 nm) or a green wavelength (510.5 nm) is available.

TREATMENT OF LESIONS

Red, Almost Purple Lesions

These lesions, especially if they are cobblestone or corrugated, can most effectively be removed with an argon laser. The thick elevated lesions are usually seen in adults. With increasing age the lesions become thicker, elevated above the skin and often bleed with minimal trauma. The first stage in treating these lesions is to reduce their bulk and prevent further occurrences of bleeding. The argon laser seems to do this most effectively and with minimal scarring.

Telangiectatic and Light Colored Lesions

These lesions do better with the pulsed tunable dye laser and the copper vapor laser. Patient's selection, age of patient, and the type of lesion will determine which of these lasers will be most effective. In some cases the lesion may exhibit several different components, and it is advisible to stage the treatment using different lasers for different areas of the lesion.

Laser technology is advancing rapidly and continued improvement modalities are becoming quickly available. A krypton laser has made its appearance, but there are no comparative studies or extensive experiences yet. In addition, a new laser for the treatment of *brown lesions* such as giant nevi has also been made available. Large series have not yet been published supporting its efficacy.

SKIN RESURFACING

Fine wrinkles (rhytids), scars, postacne changes (pitting), and other skin irregularities are often treated with dermabrasion or chemical peel. They are now also treated with a new laser, the Ultra Pulsed 5000 and other similar lasers. These lasers produce an exfoliation of the upper layers of skin. Most cells consist of water. The laser's heat causes the water in the cell to expand rapidly. The cell ruptures, and a superficial exfoliation occurs. One can increase the depth by going over the same area two or three times if the wrinkles are deep. Similar to a dermabrasion, the area is kept moist with a topical antibiotic or moisturizer for approximately 5 days. Depending on the depth of the treatment, it takes 5 to 6 weeks for the erythematous hue to dissipate. Makeup can be used to cover the area after 4 to 5 days. Laser resurfacing is faster, more comfortable, and has less of a chance of scarring than chemical peel for fine and intermediate rhytids. For deep rhytids and scars, a phenol peel is still superior.

CHAPTER 40

Genital Surgery

Charles E. Horton, Charles E. Horton, Jr.,
and John A. Dean

Reconstructive surgery has played a major role in genital surgery since Mettauer performed the first hypospadias repair in 1836. Male and female genitalia have been reconstructed for a variety of congenital, traumatic, neoplastic, endocrine, and psychologic reasons. Such conditions, unless corrected, interfere with normal urinary function and the ability to perform sexually. There can also be serious secondary psychologic problems in many patients if the physical problem is allowed to persist. A team approach, involving surgeons familiar with reconstructive and urologic techniques, leads to a better understanding of the pathology and to improved results.

The majority of genital surgery is performed on infants and children and can be technically challenging. Because of the small size of the structures, their delicate blood supply, and the potential for wound contamination, the risks of hematoma formation and infection are increased when compared with other reconstructive surgeries.

Patient care extends from the initial consultation to the postoperative visits after discharge from the hospital. Many patients, including children, have had multiple previous procedures and are therefore familiar with hospital protocol. Each previous surgery increases the amount of scarring within the genitalia and makes subsequent surgery more difficult. Careful and comprehensive surgical correction, followed by meticulous care, is the best guarantee of success in these patients.

CONGENITAL AND PEDIATRIC PROBLEMS

Hypospadias

Hypospadias is a congenital condition in which the urethral meatus is proximal and ventral to the tip of the glans. With the meatus located more ventrally, the likelihood of an associated ventral curvature of the penis, or chordee, is greatly increased. Three percent of hypospadias patients have a primary intersex condition. Hypospadias is preferably corrected in a single-stage surgical procedure performed before the age of memory recall (i.e., by the age of 2). Patients have reached adequate size by this age, making reconstruction safe and predictable.

A. Preoperative care

- ▼ If hypospadias is associated with impalpable testes, appropriate tests to exclude an intersex condition should be performed at birth. These tests include a complete endocrine screen, chromosome analysis, intravenous pyelogram (IVP), cystourethrogram or sinogram, and endoscopy.
- ▼ Rarely do hypospadias patients have an associated abnormality of the upper urinary tract; therefore routine screening of the kidneys is not necessary. If however the degree of hypospadias is severe, and especially if there is an abnormality of a second organ system (e.g., hypospadias and spina bifida), then a renal ultrasound should be obtained to rule out problems of the upper urinary system.
- ▼ Analysis of urine, including microscopy, cultures, and testing for sensitivities is always done to ensure urine sterility before any operative intervention. We use perioperative broad-spectrum cephalosporin antibiotics IV.
- ▼ Occasionally a boy will have a small penis with a paucity of skin available to use in the repair. In these patients, administration of testosterone enanthate, 3 mg/kg, intramuscularly (IM), 5 and 2 weeks preoperatively has been shown to increase penile size, amount of prepuce, and perhaps the

vascularity of the penile tissues, all of which help to make hypospadias repair technically easier and more successful.

B. Intraoperative care

- A large variety of reconstructive options exist. A procedure suitable for each patient's problems must be chosen. No surgeon can be an expert with all hypospadias repairs; however, all surgeons performing these repairs must be competent with the procedure applicable to each type of hypospadias deformity. Similarly, a variety of methods of dressing, urinary diversion, and drainage are currently used. Optical magnification with loupes is beneficial.
- Surgical procedures
  - Distal hypospadias. Distal cases, not associated with chordee, can be corrected with meatal advancement glansplasty incisions (MAGPI), urethral advancement procedures, or flip-flap urethroplasty. Each of these procedures is relatively less invasive and requires less penile dissection than those required for the proximal condition.
  - Proximal hypospadias. More proximal hypospadias require extensive dissection of the penis, correction of chordee, and the reconstruction of long lengths of urethra with either pedicled or free preputial skin. Hairless full-thickness groin skin grafts, bladder mucosal, or buccal mucosal grafts can be used if the patient has already been circumcised.
- Methods of urinary diversion. The following methods of urinary diversion are commonly used:
  - Distal hypospadias. In distal cases urinary diversion is not necessary. We commonly stent the meatus with a small Silastic catheter that resides only in the distal penis. Patients can urinate through the stent, which is usually removed after 3 to 5 days.
  - Midshaft and proximal hypospadias. Suprapubic cystostomy is recommended for midshaft and

more proximal cases. Kits that enable a percutaneous suprapubic tube to be placed are commercially available. These kits are used in addition to a Silastic tube placed in the distal penis, across the urethroplasty, but not into the bladder. Transurethral bladder drainage is avoided because of the tendency of this type of drainage to transmit shear forces to the urethroplasty. Urinary diversion is usually maintained for 7 to 10 days or longer with more complex cases.

- ▼ Hemostasis. Hemostasis is achieved with the preoperative use of 1:200,000 epinephrine solution in 0.5% lidocaine injected into the operative field, together with the careful ligation of large vessels and the use of a fine-point electrocautery. Intraoperatively, we rarely find it necessary to use a tourniquet, because gentle pressure by an assistant can control most bleeding. Meticulous technique must be used in this hematoma-prone area.
- ▼ Fluorescein angiography. Fluorescein given intraoperatively can be used to confirm vascularity of flaps. Ten minutes after the fluorescein is injected, the flap is viewed under ultraviolet light, and if it fluoresces, adequate circulation is demonstrated.
- ▼ Drainage. A small closed-suction drain is used to avert possible hematoma. Tubing of the size of a 16 or 19 butterfly needle is fenestrated and placed under the dissected flaps through a separate stab incision. The needle is attached to a small vacutainer to achieve constant suction. These vacutainers (Minivacs) are changed every 2 to 4 hours, and the blood collection is measured. We have a strong preference toward the use of drains. We have never encountered problems resulting from their use, but problems have resulted when we failed to use drains.
- ▼ Dressings. Suture lines are covered with antibiotic ointment (e.g., bacitracin) to seal them and to avoid adherence of the clear, semipermeable, elastic dressing (e.g., Opsite) that is used to wrap around the

phallus. This dressing applies gentle pressure to help minimize hematomas and allows for the visualization of skin flaps and suture lines. All catheters and stents must be sutured and taped into position so that they cannot exert pressure on the neourethra.

C. Postoperative care

- Bedrest. Bedrest is required for all patients with proximal and midshaft hypospadias reconstruction. This minimizes the detrimental effects of venous engorgement and edema formation associated with dependency of the genital area. The bedrest period usually lasts throughout the period of maximum edema formation (i.e., approximately 4 days postopertively). A bed cradle device is used to keep the bed covers from the penis during this bedrest period.
- Pain management. Most pediatric anesthesiologists can administer a caudal block, which provides complete pain relief for 8 to 12 hours postoperatively. Beyond that time, appropriate narcotic analgesia is used to both treat postoperative pain and minimize the hypertensive response to this pain, thereby decreasing the chance of hematoma formation. This analgesia should be changed from a parenteral to an enteral route once the patient can tolerate a diet.
- Dressings. The transparent dressing is inspected frequently for evidence of flap ischemia or hematoma. The dressing is removed on the third postoperative day, and the penis is not redressed.
- Suture line care. Suture lines are gently cleansed with peroxide-soaked swabs, followed by coating with an antibiotic ointment (e.g., Bacitracin) every 8 hours. In particular, the new urethral meatus must be kept clean and moist to avoid crusting of old blood that could partially obstruct the urethra once voiding has resumed.
- Bladder care. Bladder spasms can be distressing and can result from the mere presence of a catheter. These spasms may produce leakage of urine around the catheter and therefore must be controlled:

  - Adequate control can usually be obtained by using belladonna and opium suppositories in appropriate dosage. Anticholinergic drugs such as propantheline bromide (Pro-Banthine) or oxybutynin chloride (Ditropan) may also help.
  - Occasionally, bladder spasms will be severe and refractory; in these patients we have had good response to intravesical instillations of oxybutynin or lidocaine solutions. One must be sure that the suprapubic catheter or the Silastic stent is not blocked. A blocked catheter can be cleared by gentle saline irrigation. If this is not successful, the catheter should be changed. Extreme caution is necessary for dealing with a blocked catheter that passes through a newly constructed urethra.

- Removal of urethral stents and suprapubic drainage. Urethral stents are normally removed after 3 to 5 days. Suprapubic drainage is used 7 to 8 days after a complex repair using flaps, bladder mucosa, or skin grafts. The suprapubic tube is first clamped and a voiding test is performed. If initial problems arise, such as fistula formation, the clamp can be removed to extend the time of urinary diversion. Oral cephalosporins are continued until the urinary drainage catheter is removed.

Fistulas and Sequelae of Hypospadias Repair

Complications of hypospadias repair may pose difficult surgical problems. A urethral fistula is rare with distal repairs: it occurs in less than 10 to 15 % of proximal hypospadias repairs. However, there is an unfortunate group of patients in whom numerous surgical repairs have failed on a larger scale. These patients are called *hypospadias cripples.* They may be older children, teenagers, or older men who have had multiple operative procedures for ongoing problems, such as chordee, urethral fistulas, urethral stenosis, urethral diverticula, or the presence of hair-bearing skin in the neourethra. The last situation occurs if scrotal skin is used in the reconstruction of the urethra, so that after puberty, hair develops and may become the focus of a persistent urinary tract infection or even calculus formation. Emotional problems associated with genital deformities and surgical failures are common in this group.

A. Preoperative care

- In all hypospadias cripples, urine culture and renal function testing (blood urea nitrogen (BUN), serum creatinine, urea, and electrolytes) are routinely performed.
- Renal ultrasonography may be necessary to assess the upper urinary tracts if long-standing obstruction is suspected.
- Urethrography, both voiding and retrograde studies, is of benefit in the older patient or when the anatomy is thought to be complex.

B. Intraoperative care

- At surgery, urethroscopy is performed to confirm the urethral anatomy and determine the pathologic disorder. A urethral sound is passed to calibrate the diameter of the lumen and to assess areas of stenosis in particular.
- Urethral fistulas sometimes are small and difficult to find. A useful technique is injection of dilute methylene blue solution into the urethra through the external meatus while occluding the proximal urethra; using moderate pressure, a fine stream will identify all openings. Spraying of the urinary stream can be demonstrated intraoperatively by creating an artificial stream with an injection of saline through a perineal urethral puncture site. Chordee can be demonstrated using artificial erection testing. This is done by injecting saline into the corporal bodies through a butterfly needle. while occluding their base, until an erection occurs.
- A simple fistula is repaired by excision and closure in layers of the urethral wall, subcutaneous tissue, and skin. Closure of a larger fistula may require advancement or rotation of additional penile skin flaps into the urethral defect so that the urethral lumen is not narrowed. These repairs cannot suc-

ceed in the presence of distal obstruction, and a recurrent fistula is an indicator that other pathologic disorders are within the urethra.

- When the urethra is not satisfactory owing to a combination of stenosis, multiple fistulas, or diverticulum formation, excision of the unhealthy tissue entirely and formation of a new urethra with flaps or a tube graft of full-thickness hairless skin or bladder mucosa is preferable. This surgery is fraught with difficulties because of scarring, tenuous blood supply, and dwindling supplies of good local donor tissues.

C. **Postoperative care.** After a simple fistula repair, no stent or catheter is used. In more complicated cases, the stent is left in for 3 to 5 days and bedrest is prolonged, according to the hypospadias regimen. The care of drains and the use of antibiotics and other drugs is similar to those in the routine hypospadias patient.

Exstrophy-Epispadias Complex

The exstrophy-epispadias complex is a rare group of defects that range from isolated epispadias to classic bladder exstrophy associated with epispadias, to the most severe form, cloacal exstrophy.

A. **Preoperative care.** In newborns with exstrophy-epispadias, the delicate bladder surface is protected from desiccation from the time of birth by implementing the following procedures:

- The child is placed in an incubator without a diaper, and petroleum jelly is applied to the exposed bladder epithelium, which is covered with a sheet of plastic wrap.
- A full physical examination is performed, and tests of renal function are done.
- Renal ultrasnography is performed to assess the upper urinary tract, but these newborns are usually robust babies without other organ system abnormalities.

B. **Intraoperative care.** A staged, functional approach is advocated in repair of this grievous anomaly. In this scheme, immediate bladder closure is followed by a continence procedure at age 2 to 3 years, with subsequent epispadias repair at 4 to 5 years. A multispecialist team composed of surgeons, neonatal pediatricians, and anesthesiologists is necessary for optimal management of these problems.

- ▼ Bladder closure. Bladder closure, when possible, is performed in the first 24 hours of life. When the bladder patch is small and thick, with no elasticity or contractility, excision and urinary diversion has been classically advocated. Smaller initial bladders are now being reconstructed than would have been considered before, with plans for eventual bladder augmentation at a later stage. All attempts to avoid permanent loss of bladder function are now being made. Practically speaking however if the bladder patch has an estimated capacity of less than 5 ml or cannot be inverted by the tip of the examining finger, then such a bladder is not suitable for closure. If the bladder is not closed early, mucosal thickening with edema and fibrosis occurs. Neonatal closure has the potential for preserving vesicle function and averting mucosal metaplasia and possible later neoplastic changes. If bladder closure is performed in the first 24 to 48 hours of life, the bony pelvis and the abdominal wall tissues are malleable and usually can be approximated in the midline anteriorly, thus eliminating the diastasis associated with exstrophy. If bladder closure is performed after the first 24 to 48 hours of life, iliac osteotomy is required and greatly enhances the success of bladder closure. The bladder is usually closed around a Malecot suprapubic catheter, which is left in place for 4 weeks. The ureters are catheterized with No. 5 French feeding tubes, which are left in for 5 to 7 days, while edema from the bladder closure subsides. If iliac osteotomy has been performed, the patient is placed in Bryant's traction or external pelvic fixation for 3 to 4 weeks to allow firm, fibrous healing of the pelvic ring.

C. **Follow-up.** After bladder closure, epispadias and incontinence persist. The bladder outlet is calibrated with a sound, 4 to 6 weeks after closure, to ensure that an adequate outlet exists. Ultrasonography and cystography studies, and BUN, serum creatinine, and creatinine clearance tests are performed to assess renal status, bladder capacity, and degree of vesicoureteral reflux, which is always present. Urine cultures are obtained at frequent intervals, and patients are maintained on a suppressive dose of antibiotics.

- Bladder neck and urethra reconstruction. When the patient is aged 3 to 5 years, the bladder is assessed as follows with the possibility of a possible continence procedure:
  - If the bladder capacity is 50 ml or more, then bladder neck reconstruction may be done as the next step. This entails concomitant bilateral ureteral reimplantation for the treatment of reflux. Ureteral and suprapubic catheters are again used. Perioperative medication including antibiotics and antispasmodics are used as previously described.
  - If bladder capacity is less than 50 ml, the epispadias repair should be undertaken before bladder neck reconstruction. The moderate increase in bladder outlet resistance provided by an intact urethra can stimulate a previously small bladder to grow to a size acceptable for repair.
- Epispadias repair. In men, epispadias repair may require multiple procedures. These include mobilizing the crura to lengthen the penis, releasing the chordee, and using dermal grafts to lengthen the shortened dorsum of the corpora cavernosa to create a straight dangling penis of sufficient length. A neourethra must be constructed and brought to the tip of the glans. Additionally, soft tissue must be brought into the suprapubic area to allow the penis to dangle and to provide adequate coverage for the area. This can be achieved using local cutaneous flaps or pedicled rectus abdominis myocutaneous flaps. When the bladder is excised, urinary diversion is necessary and can be accomplished in various ways, such as colon or ileal loop urinary conduit.

Intersex Conditions

The most common type of intersex state that requires surgical correction is *female pseudohermaphroditism.* This is the result of the adrenogenital syndrome, also known as congenital adrenal hyperplasia, in which an enzymatic defect in the metabolic pathways of cortisone leads to an excess of androgenic steroids, thereby causing virilization of the female embryo. The degree of phallic enlargement and of urogenital sinus fusion is variable and depends on the extent and timing of the androgenic stimulus. The spectrum varies from clitoral enlargement only to labioscrotal fusion with a single external orifice and urogenital sinus. It is imperative that these infants with 46xx chromosomes be diagnosed accurately, because with appropriate reconstruction, they have the potential to live as completely normal, fertile women.

A. Diagnosis

- ▼ At birth, an endocrine screen that includes urinary 17-ketosteroids, urinary pregnanetriol, and serum electrolytes is performed.
- ▼ Other studies include a buccal smear, chromosome analysis, (IVP), cystourethrography sinography and endoscopy.
- ▼ If appropriate sex assignment is difficult, a *diagnostic laparoscopy* may be indicated.

B. Management

- ▼ Some intersex cases have severe metabolic abnormalities because of their inability to handle salt and water appropriately. These patients need careful adjustment of electrolytes and blood volume status and administration of corticosteroids (prednisone) and mineralocorticoids (fludrocortisone acetate) before any surgical interventions.
- ▼ For female pseudohermaphroditism, reconstructive surgery is performed as early as possible and involves clitoral reduction surgery and vaginoplasty.

PEYRONIE'S DISEASE

Peyronie's disease is a condition of unknown cause that occurs in middle-aged men. A thick fibrous plaque, which may even become calcified, develops along the penile shaft in the tunica albuginea of the corpora cavernosa, causing a bend in the erect penis and thereby making sexual intercourse difficult or impossible. Not all men with Peyronie's disease are appropriate for surgery. Before surgery is undertaken, the condition should have been present for at least 1 year and should have progressed to the point where sexual function is not possible.

Preoperative Care

Some patients with Peyronie's disease may have the associated problem of impotence that must be evaluated before any surgery. Excision of the plaque, and dermal grafting will straighten the penis in a man who is capable of having erections, but these measures will not cure impotence caused by lack of erectability of the penis. For this reason, a nocturnal penile tumescence study is performed. If this study documents the occurrence of erections, we can proceed to surgical removal of the Peyronie's plaque, supported by sex therapy.

Intraoperative Care

Surgery offers correction of the bend in the penis. Surgical straightening of the penis involves excision of the plaque and the placement of a dermal graft in the tunica albuginea of the corpora to fill the defect.

The technique of artificial erection is used several times intraoperatively. A No. 21 butterfly needle is inserted into either of the corpora and a minimum of 50 ml of saline is injected, while pressure is manually applied around the base of the penis, thereby creating an erection. This test is used initially to document the site and degree of angulation of the penis. After excision of the plaque and placement of the dermal graft, this test will confirm that the bend in the penis has been completely corrected.

A urethral catheter may be inserted and left in position for 24 hours in patients in whom there has been extensive dissection. A Minivac drain made from a butterfly needle connected to a vacuum blood-collecting tube is used beneath the flaps. The penis is wrapped with a clear, semipermeable dressing (e.g., Opsite) to apply gentle pressure while allowing visualization of the penis.

Postoperative care

A. **Medications.** Diazepam and amyl nitrite spansules at bedside as needed are used for 2 to 3 days to prevent erections, which would be painful and could cause bleeding. Antibiotics are used in the perioperative period.

B. **Drains.** The Minivac drains are removed 1 to 2 days postoperatively, and the patient is allowed to ambulate after removal of the drains.

C. **Discharge and follow-up care.** The patient leaves the hospital 3 to 4 days after the surgery; he should avoid sexual activity for a least 6 weeks. Vitamin E, 200 IU 3 times a day, is given for 1 year postoperatively, because it may prevent the recurrence of fibrosis.

PENILE RECONSTRUCTION

Reconstruction of the penis may be indicated when there has been traumatic loss or resection is required for malignancy. Another group requiring penile construction is the female-to-male transsexual.

Free Flap Penile Formation

Penile formation using innervated free tissue transfer has allowed the phallus to be constructed in a single stage, to have sensation, to carry a urethra to the tip of the flap, and to be more aesthetically acceptable than previous techniques. The results of this type of reconstruction are steadily improving as further experience is being gained. Besides the usual genital management, a free flap requires careful observation and care, particularly in the early postoperative period. The flap must be inspected frequently, observed for color, consistency, and capillary refill, and tested for Doppler impulses in the pedicle. Careful monitoring will lead to an early diagnosis of flap failure and enhance the chance of flap salvage by early reexploration. The reexploration rate is approximately 10% with a 50% salvage rate in this group.

Replantation of Amputated Penis

The amputated penis can be successfully replanted by using microvascular techniques. The preoperative and postoperative care in this instance does not vary from the usual free flap technique, with the exception that the amputated penis should be secured promptly, wrapped in a sterile gauze, placed in a plastic bag, and brought to the replantation center. This plastic bag should be placed in a larger plastic bag containing ice water. The amputated part should never be frozen.

IMPOTENCE

The truly impotent patient can now be offered a variety of options for the treatment of this problem. Rigid and inflatable prostheses and intracorporal self-injection therapy for pharmacologic erections are available. Vacuum erectile devices can also be used.

Preoperative Procedures

If surgical treatment is chosen, the following preoperative procedures are implemented:

- ▼ Nocturnal penile tumescence (NPT) studies are performed to ensure that the patient is in fact impotent. Nocturnal erections occur at the time of rapid eye movement (REM) sleep, and therefore NPT studies are often done in conjunction with electroencephalography.
- ▼ Sexual counseling is given, because psychologic factors are important.
- ▼ If impotence is demonstrated on NPT, vascular studies, such as penile Doppler ultrasound with pharmacologic erection, are done to determine whether a correctable vascular problem can be identified.

Perioperative and Intraoperative Procedures

Cephalosporin antibiotics are used in the perioperative period. The prosthesis itself is soaked in cephalsoporin solution before implantation. Liberal irrigation of the penile wound with antibiotic solution is also performed throughout the procedure. A catheter may be left in the urethra for 24 hours but is not essential.

Postoperative Care

Postoperatively the patient remains in the hospital for 1 to 2 days. If the inflatable device is used, it is left in a partially inflated state at the time of discharge from the hospital. With either type of device, no sexual activity should be undertaken for at least 6 weeks.

VASOVASOSTOMY AND VASOEPIDIDYMOSTOMY

These procedures are routinely used for obstructive causes of infertility in men. The most common indication is the reversal of the vasectomy operation. A vasovasostomy can be performed with ordinary macroscopic techniques, but the use of microsurgical methods gives better results. Patency rates of 75 to 85% can be expected, with pregnancy resulting in 40 to 50% of cases. In general, the more time that elapses after the vasectomy, the less is the chance that vasovasostomy will result in pregnancy.

Vasovasostomy is an outpatient surgical procedure. A scrotal athletic support may aid in the patient's comfort. The patient is advised against sexual intercourse and heavy lifting for 2 weeks.

Sperm counts are obtained 3 months and 1 year after the procedure. Sometimes sperm do not return to the semen for a period of 3 to 6 months but are present in maximum numbers within 1 year.

VAGINAL RECONSTRUCTION

Vaginal reconstruction is performed in patients after ablative surgery for carcinoma and also in patients with inadequate or absent vagina (atresia, intersex, and transsexuals). Preoperative counseling and evaluation is a team effort, involving the gynecologist, oncologist, psychiatrist, urologist, endocrinologist, and plastic surgeon.

Patients with Carcinoma

Postablative reconstruction preferably should be performed under the same anesthetic as the extirpative surgery. Tumor patients are usually of an older age group, and careful preoperative cardiovascular and pulmonary evaluation is essential before undertaking such a lengthy procedure. By providing immediate coverage of the "perineal burn" produced by the resection, morbidity and mortality rates are decreased with immediate reconstruction.

All tumor patients have a preoperative IVP and cystoscopy. Sigmoidoscopy may also be of value after a thorough mechanical preoperative bowel preparation. Perioperative broad-spectrum antibiotics are administered. These patients are at risk of thromboembolic complications because of their age, current neoplastic disease, and nature and length of the procedure. Antiembolism measures such as pneumatic compression stockings and "mini dose" heparin, 5,000 U every 12 hours subcutaneously (SC) should be considered and instituted preoperatively. Central venous pressure monitoring and arterial line measurements may prove valuable.

Postablative vaginal reconstruction uses either bilateral gracilis myocutaneous flaps or a rectus abdominis myocutaneous flap brought through the peritoneal cavity to the pelvis.

Jackson-Pratt drains are used in the donor sites to decrease hematoma or seroma formation. They can be removed when the output is less than 30 ml/day, usually on approximately the fifth postoperative day.

Patients with Atresia or Intersex

Atresia and intersex patients are reconstructed using skin grafts placed within a pocket created by dissecting between the bladder and the rectum. We prefer to use full-thickness grafts harvested from the groin areas rather than McIndoe's traditional split-thickness grafts, because of the improved donor sites and the tendency toward less contracture of these grafts. A preoperative bowel preparation and antibiotics are also administered in these patients. The skin graft is secured around a condom-shaped stent and sutured to the labial outlet. The stent remains for 7 to 10 days. After removal, the split-thickness skin-grafted patients must be instructed in performing routine dilatations of the neovagina using a commercially available dilator. In patients with full-thickness skin grafts, minimal dilatation is necessary. Sexual activity is permitted 4 to 6 weeks after surgery.

Some centers are now performing vaginal reconstruction using isolated loops of colon. Postoperative problems include those associated with all laparotomies in addition to the possibility of excess neovaginal mucus production and neovaginal prolapse.

Transsexuals

In the male-to-female transsexual patient, a multitude of described procedures are available, generally involving local flaps and grafts for vaginal construction. Stents and drains are used as desired by the surgeon, but the same protocol applies as with atresia patients.

CHAPTER 41

Pressure Ulcers

JOSEPH AGRIS

Pressure sores, also called *bed sores* and *decubitus ulcers,* are a serious and frustrating problem for the spinal cord-injured patient, the stroke patient, and the debilitated or comatose patient. When the patient is hospitalized for the treatment of a pressure sore, it is estimated that the total direct and indirect cost, including a 6-to-8 week hospitalization, surgery, and loss of individual productivity, approaches $30,000. Pressure ulcers are an age-old problem that still remain with us today. Patients with pressure ulcers are encountered in all medical and surgical practices. Although physicians in some subspecialties will see more cases than others, all physicians at some time will be required to provide immediate treatment for pressure ulcers and to prescribe long-term management and prevention measures. Until the 1930s, the only form of treatment was the application of topical medication to encourage healing. Since 1938 surgical treatment for pressure ulcers, combined with antibiotic therapy, has proved successful.

In recent years the increased incidence of spinal cord injuries owing to automobile accidents (75% of all spinal injuries in the United States) and the increased number of geriatric patients have stimulated interest in the problem of pressure ulcer prevention and treatment.

GENERAL PATHOPHYSIOLOGY

The major cause of all decubitus ulcer cases is *pressure.* Other factors predisposing to the formation of such ulcers include *paralysis, paresis, shearing forces, malnutrition, infection,* and advanced age. However, the patient who lacks protective sensation, regardless of the cause, or who cannot change body position because of debilitation or fixation devices is prone to the development of a pressure ulcer.

Prolonged periods of minimal pressure are just as injurious as intense pressure of short duration. When pressure exceeds the normal capillary blood pressure of 32 mm Hg, tissue anoxia and cell death result. At first, vasodilation appears as a reactive hyperemia in the surrounding skin. If pressure is removed as soon as the skin reddens (reactive hyperemia), perfusion of the tissue will occur together with removal of toxic byproducts. The damage at this stage is reversible; however, if continued pressure is applied, the damage becomes irreversible. Depending on the overall health of the patient, the blood supply to the area, the condition of the skin, and the amount of pressure applied, irreversible damage can be produced in 1 to 6 hours. It is possible that fat necrosis and muscle damage may have occurred beneath the skin by the time the hyperemia is recognized.

CLASSIFICATION AND TREATMENT STAGES

Stage I

A. **Pathophysiology and clinical signs.** The initial changes consist of erythema, edema, and punctate hemorrhages. The overlying skin acquires a pink-to-red color and feels warmer than the adjacent tissue. If shear stresses or friction caused by spasms also are involved, the overlying skin will blister. Small blebs will form like those seen in a second-degree burn. The dermis is intact, as are the skin appendages. At this point, damage is still reversible if immediate care is provided.

B. **Treatment**

- ▼ First and foremost, treatment consists of removing the pressure and eliminating the shearing forces on the area.
- ▼ Next, the area is cleansed every 6 to 8 hours with a mild soap-and-water solution.
- ▼ The wound is then covered with a topical antibiotic and a fine-mesh gauze dressing. This will permit drainage, minimize the bacterial count, and allow epithelialization to occur undisturbed. A dry sterile dressing is placed over this and changed every 8 hours. Benzoin is applied to the adjacent skin to

toughen and protect it. Porous paper tape is used to hold the dressing in place, and with each dressing change, the tape is applied to a different area so that irritation does not occur.

- ▼ Epithelialization will occur in 14 to 21 days with conservative management.

Stage II

A. **Pathophysiology and clinical signs.** If pressure persists, the hyperemia and edema increases, blisters rupture, and the overlying skin sloughs. A full-thickness skin loss develops. An erythematous halo of 1 to 2 cm usually surrounds the area and represents a localized cellulitis. Bacterial contamination leads to secondary localized cellulitis and to secondary infection of the wound. If the defect is larger than 1 cm, healing by secondary intention is unlikely. In fact, considering the difficulty these patients have in bowel, bladder, and personal hygiene, even small full-thickness lesions, if not treated immediately, are likely to result in major surgical intervention.

B. **Treatment.** In stage II defects (full-thickness skin losses larger than 1 cm), conservative management consists of immediate treatment. In lesions 1 to 3 cm with sufficient surrounded unscarred tissue and adequate underlying adipose tissue, immediate excision and primary closure should be undertaken as follows:

- ▼ Many of these patients lack sensation in the area and do not require the use of an anesthetic. With a minimal number of instruments, the wound is excised in the clinic or office, the margins are cauterized, and primary 3-0 monofilament suturing is undertaken. The wound is then dressed.
- ▼ The patient is instructed in care of the wound and then can go home in the care of a family member or attendant. Before being discharged the patient is instructed in home care as follows:
  - ■ After 48 hours, the patient is allowed to bathe and wash directly over the area.
  - ■ With the help of family or attendant, the wound is dressed twice each day.

- The patient is advised to remain in bed the first week to minimize any tension on the suture area. After 1 week, the patient is allowed to sit up for 1 hour in the morning and the evening. This time is used for personal hygiene, bath, and toilet regimen. During the third week, the patient may add 15 minutes to the sitting time each day.

C. **Follow-up.** The patient is followed-up on an outpatient basis. As long as no erythema is present around the sutures, they are left in place. If erythema develops around a suture, that particular suture is removed, and the rest is left in place. Final suture removal is in 3 to 5 weeks, depending on the activities of the patient. If small defects are closed immediately, operation and hospitalization may not be necessary, and loss of work and its associated socioeconomic difficulties will not result. The best physical and psychologic result is thus obtained.

Stage III

A. **Pathophysiology and clinical signs.** In the stage III defect, usually a full-thickness skin loss greater than 3 cm is present, with no laxity of the surrounding tissues. Maceration beyond the area of the ulcerative defect and scarring from previous ulcers or surgical procedures may be observed.

B. **Treatment.** In the stage III patient, primary closure using adjacent tissue is not possible. However, because only full-thickness skin is lost and adequate muscle and subcutaneous tissue remain, a skin graft is appropriate. This is applied when an adequate granulating bed is present.

- ▼ Wound preparation for stage III is as follows:
  - Initial treatment consists of eliminating pressure from the area, reducing the shearing stresses, and preventing spasms.
  - Devitalized tissue is débrided to encourage formation of granulation tissue and to minimize bacterial contamination.

- Wet-to-dry dressings are applied every 6 hours. Gauze pads (4 by 4 inches) that do not contain cotton are dampened with sterile saline solution and squeezed until almost dry. These are then applied to the open wound only. Wet dressing should *not* extend beyond the wound margins, because the continuous moisture results in the maceration of uninvolved skin.
- After applying the wet dressings to the wound area only, several dry gauze sponges are applied over the wet dressings and benzoin and porous paper tape are applied to the adjacent skin.
- The dressing is removed every 6 to 8 hours. The wound is cleansed with a mild soap-and-water solution, and a new wet-to-dry dressing is applied.
- If soilage occurs as a result of bladder or bowel contamination, the dressing is immediately removed, the wound is washed, and the wet-to-dry dressing is reapplied.

The patient, attendant, and family are instructed in wound management and dressing changes. In many cities, a visiting nurse service is available, and the patient can be seen daily. The visiting nurse will help with dressing changes and aid in general hygiene and care of the patient.

▼ Skin grafting

- The patient is seen biweekly in the office. When the wound is ready for grafting, hospital admission is scheduled. The patient is usually admitted 2 or 3 days before surgery at which time Hubbard tank (whirlpool) therapy is instituted.
- Wet-to-dry dressing is continued, with the addition of 0.5% acetic acid solution. This further reduces the bacterial count before grafting.
- The graft is undertaken in the operating room under sterile conditions, using skin from the posterior aspect of the calf in a nonsensory area. Anesthesia is not required, and the procedure can be undertaken quickly and easily because both the donor and recipient sites usually lack sensation.

- When the graft is secure, usually in 7 to 10 days, the patient can be discharged for continued care at home. This consists of staying off the graft site for an additional week and maintaining good hygiene. Lanolin is gently massaged onto the graft and into the donor area twice a day for 2 months or more.

By using family, attendants, the visiting nurse service, and ancillary personnel, hospitalization can be minimized and the patient's recovery maximized.

Stage IV

A. **Pathophysiology and clinical signs.** Once the overlying skin sloughs, subcutaneous tissue is exposed and bacterial contamination occurs. When contamination exceeds 10^5 bacteria/g of tissue, the body defenses are unable to meet the bacterial invasion. At this point, contamination becomes infection. In 3 to 5 days, a well-circumscribed focus of necrosis results. Initially, this appears as a reddish-gray area surrounded by an erythematous halo; a yellowish-gray eschar then forms with a waxy, shiny surface. An exudate develops (pus), which is discharged from the periphery of the eschar. The surrounding erythematous halo becomes brighter and larger, and bleeding may occur at the margins of the halo. Centrally, a gray-to-black area of necrosis develops; putrefaction becomes evident. Bacterial infection results in continued fat necrosis, edema, thrombosis, and enlargement of the wound.

   There is no such thing as a small pressure ulcer. The visible skin defect is merely "the tip of the iceberg." At this point, the ulcer becomes a cone-type of defect. The point of the cone is at the skin surface. The larger, underlying defect forms at the base. Beginning at the skin extensive lateral destruction of each subsequent layer is evident as one progresses from skin to subcutaneous tissue, to deep fascia, muscle, and bone. This would be analogous to passing through a small cave entrance only to enter a high-vaulted cavern.

B. **Treatment.** Preparing this type of ulcer for surgical closure usually takes 2 to 3 weeks. If the patient is cooperative and there is good family support or an attendant available, much of the work can be done at home. This can be supported with such ancillary personnel as the visiting nurse service or community volunteers. The following basic principle of wound care should not be forgotten or replaced by the application of topical medication to improve or cure pressure ulcers: no topical medication promotes healing faster than the technique of *sharp débridement* and *wet-to-dry dressing changes.* The rate of healing may even be hindered by the application of many of these topical medications, not to mention the added risk of allergic reaction and superinfection. Depending solely on a surface application of such medication is unwise, and much time is wasted waiting for the promised magical result.

- ▼ Débridement. All necrotic tissue must be sharply débrided. The use of topical medications is a waste of time, money, and effort. No topical medication will remove necrotic tissue, sterilize the wound, and cause epithelialization to occur. Sharp débridement is the only effective method of removing devitalized tissue, decreasing the bacterial count, and preparing the wound for surgical closure. Because the majority of these patients lack sensation in the area of the defect, surgical débridement can be undertaken in most well-equipped office facilities with a minimal number of instruments. All that is required is a scalpel, sharp scissors, toothed forceps, a good light, and a cautery unit. If a cautery unit is not available, silver nitrate sticks will provide cauterization in most cases. The surrounding tissue and wound are washed with surgical soap solution and gently rinsed. Devitalized tissue is sharply excised until punctate bleeding occurs. Further excision is not necessary because it only produces extensive hemorrhage, which is difficult to control. Sharp débridement should not produce bleeding that cannot be controlled by pressure alone.
- ▼ Control of bleeding. Once all the devitalized tissue is excised, the minimal bleeding that occurs is controlled by direct pressure with a moistened

gauze sponge held in place for five to ten minutes. Any bleeding that remains is controlled with a portable cautery unit or silver nitrate sticks.

- Dressings. After bleeding is controlled, the wound is packed. Any of the commercially available roll gauze dressings are used during the following procedure:
  - The portion of the gauze to be packed into the wound is first dampened with sterile saline solution. Some may prefer to use one of the commercially available iodine-containing solutions if the patient is not allergic to iodine. However, the most important step in this procedure is that once the gauze packing has been dampened, it should be wrung out so that no excess fluid is present that will cause maceration of the surrounding uninjured tissue. Packing can be performed with forceps or with the use of a cotton-tipped applicator (Q-tip) to direct the gauze into the depths of the wound; otherwise it is ineffective. Packing should continue from the deepest portion of the wound surface.
  - At the skin surface, the packing should be dry. Having a wet dressing on the skin surface serves no purpose except to macerate the surrounding skin and enlarge the defect. The packing should be cut flush with the skin surface.
  - Dry gauze sponges are placed over the packing, and benzoin and porous paper tape are applied to the surrounding skin.
  - The procedure is repeated every 8 hours. With each dressing change, the position of the paper tape is changed so that irritation of the skin does not occur.
- Treatment of wound contamination. If contamination occurs from an incontinent bladder or bowel, the dressing is removed. The wound is washed with a mild soap-and-water solution and repacked. Additional mechanical débridement (as with a high-pressure water system, a pulsating showerhead, or

Water Pik-type of devices) and syringe irrigation have been helpful in deeper wounds. These devices are inexpensive, readily available, and easily adapted for home use.

- Hospitalization for surgical closure. If the home environment is suitable and community ancillary personnel are available, the patient can be treated at home and followed-up in the office biweekly for dressing changes. When the wound is clean and ready for surgical closure, the patient is admitted to the hospital 2 or 3 days before the planned surgery. (See p. 647, Hospital Admission.). This permits a more extended examination and workup required for those patients who have multiple problems, and any continued necessary débridement and Hubbard tank (whirlpool) therapy to further reduce bacterial contamination.

Stage V

A. **Pathophysiology and clinical signs.** In special circumstances, the pressure ulcer appears to be a typical cone-type of defect. The skin opening is relatively small compared to the extensive undermining and cavern formation. In these circumstances, débridement is difficult if not impossible, and packing is inadequate unless the skin defect is enlarged.

B. **Treatment**

- Extention of wound. Because the majority of stage IV ulcers lack sensation, the wound can be extended appropriately to allow for adequate débridement and packing in an office or outpatient facility. The most important consideration is the direction of the incision to the extent of the wound. The wound should be extended in a direction that will enhance future operative reconstruction. Preplanning of the operative procedure (type of flap to be used) should be noted in the records before one extends the wound. In this way, the blood supply to a needed flap will not be endangered. One then incises the skin to allow adequate drainage, débridement, and ease of packing.

- Control of bleeding, drainage of wound, and packing. In most patients, a minimal amount of bleeding occurs, usually along the skin margin only, which can usually be controlled with direct pressure; However, clamping of vessels, and ligation, or use of a cautery may occasionally be required. Any remaining subcutaneous tissue that is incised is usually avascular and does not present a problem. The remaining deep fascia is already undermined, owing to the typical cone-type of deformity produced by the pressure ulcer. Therefore no deep incisions are required. If the patient is febrile, the wound is adequately opened, drained, and packed; no antibiotic coverage is needed. If the wound meets all the above criteria and the patient is febrile, one must look for a secondary source of infection (e.g., abscess, osteomyelitis, urinary tract infection, respiratory tract infection). Urinary tract infection is the most common cause of death. Pressure ulcers are the second most common.

Stage VI: Chronic Ulcerative Defects

A. **Pathophysiology and clinical signs.** In stage VI patients, the acute processes have long since abated. A large cavity defect with skin undermining is present. The base of the ulcer is a bony prominence. The cavity is lined by a fibropseudosheath known as a *bursa*. Drainage is usually a clear or yellow nonviscous discharge. Gross pus is not encountered. The surrounding skin margins are usually indurated, show active epithelialization, and may even be hypertrophic. The tissue beyond the skin margins is usually soft, supple, and uninvolved. The bacterial flora present within the bursa cavity and within the chronic granulations are synergistic with the patient. The bone itself usually is not involved, and x-ray examination will show the typical decalcification seen in the lower extremity and pelvis of spinal cord-injured patients. This decalcification should not be confused with osteomyelitis.

   If these patients develop a sudden onset of fever with a well-drained bursal-lined pressure defect, secondary sources of infection must be considered. It is rare under these circumstances that the pressure ulcer will be the cause of the fever. More likely, the urinary tract or respiratory tract will be the site of the sepsis.

Pressure ulcers are chronically contaminated wounds, and all contain a mixed bacterial flora. The basic characteristic of a chronically contaminated wound is the formation of granulation tissue, which in itself, will not occur in the absence of bacterial contamination.

B. Treatment

- ▼ Antibiotics. Topical antibiotics do not penetrate the depth of granulation tissue and therefore are ineffective. Systemically administered antibiotics do not lead to adequate tissue levels in granulating wounds. Therefore systemic antibiotics have little or no effect on the bacterial level of chronic pressure ulcers. As with any potent therapeutic agent, the antibacterial should be introduced at the time when it will be most effective, therefore systemic antibiotics should be introduced in the immediate preoperative, intraoperative, and postoperative periods surrounding surgical excision and closure of the pressure ulcer. At this time, new tissue planes are opened, and an adequate antibiotic level will inhibit the establishment of new foci infection. Therefore in the management of pressure ulcers, *systemic antibiotics are used only as an adjunct to surgical management.*
- ▼ Hospital admission. Patients with stage VI defects can be admitted directly to the hospital for surgical closure of the ulcer 2 to 3 days before the procedure. When plans are made for hospital admission of a patient with type VI pressure ulcers, special equipment and a special treatment plan are required, to prevent other areas of tissue breakdown and to provide for the patient's general comfort. A hospital-type bed with electric controls should be provided. This will enable the patient to change position and will provide ease of nursing care. The bed should have a water mattress, an egg-crate mattress, or a foam mattress. Additional pillows

should be available to support the patient appropriately. A trapeze, or overhead bar, is often helpful.

- Positioning. The most common site of pressure sores is directly over a bony prominence. Of all pressure defects, 80% to 90%, occur below the waist. Two thirds of these occur around the hips and buttocks, in the ischial, sacral, and trochanteric areas. Knee and heel defects are the next most common occurrences. If the patient is placed in the prone position, (i.e., on the abdomen), 90% of these bony prominences (pressure points) are alleviated. (Fig. 41-1). Any standard hospital bed appropriately prepared with an egg-crate mattress on which five or six pillows are placed will more than adequately remove pressure from 90% of the areas that are prone to ulcerative defects. Pillows should be placed so that the knees and the feet are not in contact with the mattress or the back of the bed. Additional pillows are placed under the thighs so that the knees are elevated from the bed. Sheepskin knee pads can be applied for additional protection. Several pillows are placed under the abdomen and chest, with the anterior iliac crest suspended between them. Additional pillows are used as needed to support the

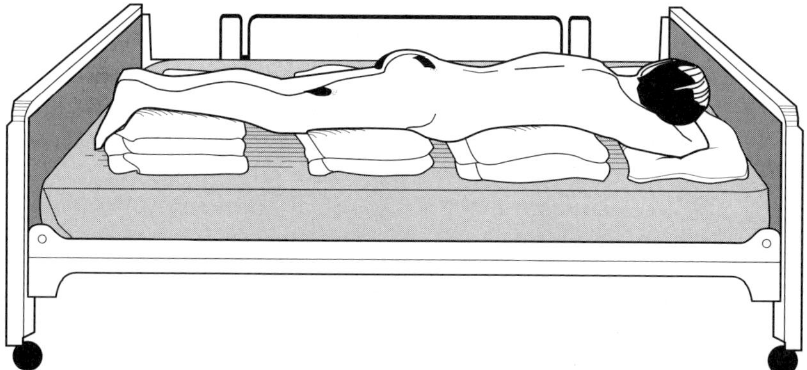

Fig. 41-1 *Of all pressure ulcers, 80% occur posteriorly. If patient has no respiratory tract problems, majority of pressure ulcers can be prevented if patient is maintained in prone position as shown. Not only is position helpful for patient care in hospital but it should also be used during sleep for rest of patient's life.*

head and arms. With the patient elevated in this manner, contamination from the bladder and bowel is also minimized. With this type of positioning, the patient can easily be rotated every 2 hours to the left or right lateral decubitus position by angulating the position of the pillows under the chest and abdomen. This ability to be rotated allows the patient to be fed while in a comfortable position and provides for maintenance of bladder and bowel. The patient will henceforth sleep in the prone position. For patients not used to being in this position for a prolonged period, they must be started 3 to 5 days before the surgical procedure is done, so that the patient will be prepared to maintain this position for 2 or 3 weeks after surgery. Once this pattern has been established, the patient will use the prone position at home while sleeping and for rest periods during the day.

- ▼ Nutrition. Bedridden and debilitated patients tend to have generalized muscle atrophy and nutritional imbalance, even if they have the best of home and hospital care. Because most of these patients exhibit a negative nitrogen balance, restoration of their nutritional status, with emphasis on maintenance of a serum protein level higher than 6 mg/dl, is of immediate importance. Ideally, surgery should not be performed unless the patient's serum proteins exceed 6 mg/dl. The choice of measures to correct nutritional deficiencies will depend on the general status of the patient and the severity of the lesions present. Treatment of these problems can usually be categorized as follows:
  - ■ If the patient is able to take food orally, this is the best and most convenient method of correcting any nutritional deficiencies. A high-protein high-caloric diet with supplemental feeding between meals is used, augmented by vitamin supplements, including trace minerals. Dietary intakes of 3,800 to 4,600 calories per day are required. The calorie count is recorded on a daily basis, and the patient is weighed two times a week to monitor progress.

- If oral feeding is inadequate to produce desired caloric intake, supplemental nasogastric feedings with commercially prepared products are instituted. We use a slow-drip technique, flowing 24 hours per day, and calorie intake approaching 4,800 calories per day can be achieved. In addition, the patient is encouraged to eat as much as is desired. With combined oral and nasogastric feeding, intakes exceeding 5600 calories per day have been obtained.
- If the patient is unable to tolerate oral or nasogastric feedings, intravenous (IV) hyperalimentation is required.

▼ Spasms. Spasms are short, sudden, involuntary, and uncontrollable muscle contractions that occur as a result of a spinal cord injury. Spasms may be mild and infrequent and therefore will not present a problem. However, moderate or severe spasms, particularly spasms that produce long spastic states bordering on rigidity, will only become worse with the attempts of patients to position themselves comfortably after surgery and must be controlled before any elective procedure. Patients with spasms tend to abrade their skin against clothing, bedding, and supportive appliances, resulting in abrasion, secondary infection, and ulcer formation. In addition, spasms are usually increased as a result of surgical manipulation, and if severe, will result in dehiscence in the suture line and separation flap. Every effort must be made to reduce or eliminate spasms, or the surgery will inevitably be unsuccessful.

- Drug therapy. The introduction in recent years of pharmacologic agents for the control of spasticity in spinal cord-injured patients has simplified treatment. Currently the two most effective medications are diazepam (Valium) and sodium dantrolene (Dantrium). These medications are administered orally and may be used together in severe cases. The amount given is gradually increased for several weeks until spasms are brought under control. The use of these agents is the easiest way to control spasms.

- Auterior rhizotomy or alcohol injection. When oral medications are ineffective, a neurosurgeon should be consulted about the advisability of anterior rhizotomy or alcohol injection. These treatments are effective; however, the side effects (such as loss of any remaining bladder control or sexual function) must be seriously considered and discussed with the patient before the treatment. If the patient is severely incapacitated and bedridden as a result of pressure ulcers secondary to spasms, the decision to control spasm, even with the loss of bladder or sexual function, may have to be made.

▼ Contractures. In 20% to 30% of paraplegic patients, varying degrees of contractures are present. These create difficulty in maintenance of certain positions, in mobility, and in daily hygiene. The contractures force the patient to favor and maintain one position over another for long periods, resulting in pressure ulcer formation. To correct an existing ulcerative defect and prevent further ulceration from occurring, measures to also correct the contractures must be undertaken.

▼ Treatment for these contractures is as follows:

- Mild to moderate flexion contractures, particularly of the hips and knees, often can be prevented by keeping the patient in the prone position and prescribing both active and passive exercise to be done at least twice daily. As indicated, orthopedic appliances, splints, and braces ban can be used.
- For moderate to severe contractures of the hip and knee area, surgical release is often necessary to prevent new pressure ulcers from forming and to ensure adequate treatment for existing ones. Without release of contractures, it may be impossible to change the patient's position to provide adequate surgery and postsurgical nursing care.

▼ Bladder and bowel care. The majority of spinal cord injury patients have incontinence of both bladder and bowel. Most of these patients have a bladder and bowel regimen. The patient's present problem should be discussed in detail, and, if difficulty with repeated soilage from bladder or bowel has been encountered, appropriate changes should be made as follows:

- A rigid bowel program, including the use of digital stimulation, rectal suppositories, and enemas, if needed, should be established, and a particular time of each day or every other day should be set aside for bowel care.
- A bladder program should also be established, which will depend on the level of lesion, the age and intelligence of the individual, and the ability to manipulate a catheter and adjunctive aids. The regimen can range from intermittent catheterization to periodic changes of an indwelling catheter. While the patient is in bed, gravity drainage to a bedside receptacle is all that is necessary. When the patient is again mobilized, the use of a leg bag is begun.

▼ Laboratory studies. Because of the many facets of problems associated with most spinal cord-injured patients, laboratory studies should include the following tests:

- Complete blood count (CBC), electrolyte, blood uria nitrogen (BUN), creatinine, and protein levels.
- Urinalysis (mandatory for all of these patients), including a culture and sensitivity testing. A fresh catheter sample is preferable.
- Chest radiograph and a radiograph of the bony area underlying the ulcerative defect. The latter is especially important in chronic defects in which osteomyelitis or joint involvement is believed to have occurred.
- Blood typing and crossmatching, because many of these patients are anemic and a significant blood loss is anticipated in surgery.
- In addition, most hospitals require a rapid plasma reagin test (RPR) for syphilis.

- Anesthesia considerations. Before surgery, the patient's level of sensation is determined by pricking with a sharp-pointed instrument. Most patients with spinal cord injuries have an area of normal sensation followed by a transition zone and then an area below which no sensation is present. When the ulcerative defect is well within the area of sensory loss, surgery may be performed without general anesthesia. When the ulcer borders on the transition zone, local anesthesia will usually suffice, and again the procedure can be undertaken without a general anesthetic. In fact, 80% to 90% of paraplegics and quadriplegics can be managed with minimal sedation, adequate monitoring, and no general anesthesia. Surgical procedures can be performed safely under these circumstances. When sensation is present at the surgical site, general anesthesia is required. Even when general anesthesia is not required, an anesthesiologist should be present throughout the procedure to monitor blood pressure and pulse rate.
- Preoperative orders
  - Bowel preparation. Because most ulcers occur in areas that are easily contaminated by both bladder and bowel excretion, a preoperative bowel preparation is given. Most spinal cord-injured patients have decreased bowel mobility, and the mechanical preparation therefore is begun 2 to 3 days before surgery. Preparation consists of a mild laxative given 2 days before surgery followed by a soapsuds enema each morning and evening for 2 days until clear.
  - Diet and fluids. During this time, the patient is on a clear liquid diet. On the day before surgery, an IV 16- or 18-gauge peripheral catheter is placed, and supplemental IV fluid is started.
  - Antibiotics. On the night before surgery, IV antibiotics are started. The antibiotics administered should cover gram-positive and gram-negative organisms, because 80% of these lesions are contaminated with *Pseudomonas, Escherichia coli,*

and *Aerobacter.* Appropriate antibiotics are chosen. These are correlated with the results obtained from the culture and sensitivities taken on the day of admission.

- Other measures. Operative sedation is ordered by the anesthesia service. In addition, whirlpool cleansing (Hubbard tank) is suggested before surgery to help reduce the bacterial flora in the wound and provide adequate hygiene needed for these patients.

▼ Planning of the operative procedure. Planning of the operation begins at the bedside with both digital and manual examination of the ulcerative defect and surrounding tissue. The defect, the extent of undermining, and any fistulas are outlined. The surrounding skin is observed, and the amounts of skin loss, maceration, previous scars, and old surgical incisions are noted. A sketch is made in the patient's chart. The type of flap is designed at bedside and a pattern is constructed to ensure that the flap will cover the anticipated defect. In addition, the position in which the patient is to be placed in the OR is determined. This planning will allow for adequate exposure and prior preparation of donor and recipient areas.

▼ Intraoperative procedure

- Electrocardiographic leads are attached and automatically monitored.
- Preoperative medication is administered and additional sedation provided during surgery by the anesthesiologist as needed.
- A 16- or 18-gauge catheter is inserted in a vein, and IV fluid is administered. Should blood be needed, this will be a more than adequate site for transfusion.
- Special care is taken in the OR to protect bony prominences from extensive pressure during surgery. The OR table is first covered with a foam or eggcrate mattress. Additional foam pads or

sheepskin covers are applied to vulnerable areas, such as knees, heels, and elbows. After the pads are in place, the patient is positioned and reexamined to ensure that there are no pressure sites. The proper positioning of the patient during and after surgery is one of the most important factors in obtaining a successful result.

- Intraoperative IV antibiotics are started before the incision is made.
- Once the skin incision is made, blood loss will be minimized by using the electrosurgical knife. All attempts are made to remove the ulcer en bloc without violating the ulcer cavity. Normal skin must not be sacrificed. The surrounding cicatrix, bursa, and granulation tissue must be totally removed. The incision is extended to allow for adequate exposure and removal of all devitalized tissue, but extension is performed in such a manner that blood supply to the planned closure is not jeopardized. The bony prominence is removed.
- Direct pressure and the electrocautery will control most bleeding.
- Copious saline irrigation is used before closure.
- All wounds are drained adequately by using two or more drains placed into the depths of the wound and brought externally to the most inferior and dependent portion of the wound to allow for adequate drainage. In addition, some form of suction is advisable.

▼ Postoperative care

- Beginning on the second postoperative day, the wound is dressed and examined each morning and evening.
- Drains are left in place for 3 to 10 days, depending on the extent of the surgery and the degree of drainage. Drainage is recorded every 8 hours and totaled every 24 hours. When the drainage total is less than 10 ml, all drains can safely be removed. As drainage decreases, it is often advisable

to remove the drains in stages, removing one and then the others at 1- to 2-day intervals.

- The patient is kept on IV fluid and receives IV antibiotics for ten to fifteen days after surgery.
- The patient is maintained on a clear-liquid diet for the first 5 postsurgical days. This is changed to a low-fiber diet for the next 3 to 5 days, and then to a high-protein, high-calorie diet of 3,600 to 4,500 calories per day. Snacks are provided between meals, and supplemental feeding is given as needed.
- After the first week, the bowel program is reinstituted, with digital stimulation, rectal suppositories, or enemas as needed. Stool softeners will also help.
- The patient is kept in the prone position on pillows, as was previously described, for 3 to 6 weeks and is rotated gently for meals, changing bed linen, bowel program, and general hygiene to the nonaffected side. The lateral decubitus positions are used after 2 weeks, and should not exceed 2 hours at any one time. The patient will always sleep in the prone position.
- If primary closure has been accomplished, the patient may begin to sit during the second week. If a muscle flap was used and followed by primary closure, sitting is not allowed until the third week. If a rotation or advancement flap was used to close the defect, the patient may sit in bed during the third week and begin sitting in a wheelchair in the fourth week. When a musculocutaneous flap is used, the patient may be rotated during the first week and begin sitting toward the end of the second week or the beginning of the third week. Sitting begins with two 45-minute periods per day. It is suggested that these periods be during mealtimes to make eating more enjoyable and to make it easier for both the patient and the nursing staff. Moreover, this allows time for the bed linen to be changed. When

the patient is returned to the bed, the wound and surrounding tissue is inspected, and, if no erythema is present, 15 minutes is added to the sitting time every second day. This is continued until a sitting time of 2 hours has been achieved.

- Sutures remain for 3 to 6 weeks. The wound is inspected daily, and as soon as erythema is noted around a particular suture, that stitch is removed. As long as there is no induration or erythema, the sutures are left in place until the patient is sitting.

▼ Prevention

- Evaluation of wheelchair and cushions. Once the wound is healed and the patient is again sitting, the patient's cushion and wheelchair are evaluated. Most patients will do well with a 3- to 4-inch Tempra Foam Cushion and cushion cover. Most cushions last less than 6 months. The patient should be informed that the cushion should be replaced twice a year. Today there are many centers around the United States (similar to the Texas Institute of Rehabilitation and Research in Houston) that provide pressure pad evaluation for spinal cord-injured patients. If such a facility is accessible, it is advisable to have the patient evaluated so that the best cushion available can be provided for the individual patient's size, weight, contour, and shape. Because more than 40 different types of cushions are now available—air, foam, water, gels—a pressure pad evaluation can determine which type would be most effective for the individual patient.
- Evaluation of patient's position in wheelchair. The patient's position in the wheelchair is evaluated by a biomedical engineer to determine the best chair for the patient's needs, comfort, and prevention of further recurrences. This evaluation includes the proper adjustment and alignment of the seat, back, arm rest, and foot rest of the wheelchair.

- Skin care. The skin must be kept clean and dry at all times. Areas of the body where sweating occurs and fluids collect, (inguinal, scrotal, perineal) must be cleansed several times a day with a mild soap-and-water solution. These areas should then be rinsed and gently patted dry. After washing and drying is completed, a lotion, preferably containing lanolin, is applied and gently massaged into the skin without leaving any moist areas that may lead to maceration or irritation. Coarse soaps or solutions containing alcohol remove oil from the skin, causing drying, cracking, and resultant breakdown. A fine talcum powder may be applied to areas where moisture tends to develop and should be lightly dusted over a dry skin surface, leaving a fine, even application. If the powder is applied to moist skin, the powder will form small granules. These will abrade the skin during position changes or when muscle spasms occur, and the patient will be in a worse condition than if the powder had not been applied at all. Overvigorous rubbing and excessive application of lotions and powders can result in maceration, abrasion, and ulceration. The combination of moisture, heat, friction, and pressure must be avoided. Some benefit may be derived from gentle massage of vulnerable skin areas with a sparing amount of lotion.

  With incontinent patients, more frequent examination is required. Particular care must be directed to keeping the skin clean and free of moisture. The urethral catheter must be checked regularly and replaced every 2 weeks or as needed. If leakage occurs from the catheter or a leg receptacle, skin should be cleansed immediately, rinsed, and patted dry. The same skin care is required in the presence of bowel incontinence to eliminate skin soilage and prevent embarrassment to the patient.

  Ultimately, skin inspection is the basis of ulcer prevention. A rigid inspection schedule must become a part of the patient's daily routine. The skin is examined on a regular basis each morning and evening. In addition, each time the patient is turned or receives specific treatment, the skin should be examined. Particular attention is directed to skin area over bony prominences. Long-handled, flexible mirrors are available to allow paraplegics to view all areas of the body without difficulty. These are inexpensive, are easily obtained, and are a simple and adequate means of inspecting all areas of the body. At the first sign of redness, abrasion, or irritation, pressure must be removed immediately so that an ulcerative defect does not result. Prevention is the key to the well-being and comfort of the long-term, bed-ridden patient.

Index

A

Page numbers in italics indicate illustrations; *t* indicates tables.

B

D

E

F

G

H

I

J

K

L

M

Q

R

S

Z